The Female Athlete

The Female Athlete

Edited by

RACHEL M. FRANK, MD
Associate Professor
Director, Joint Preservation Program
Department of Orthopaedic Surgery
University of Colorado School of Medicine
Denver, CO, United States

ASSOCIATE EDITORS

ELIZABETH G. MATZKIN, MD
Department of Orthopaedic Surgery
Brigham and Women's Hospital
Boston, MA
United States

Harvard Medical School
Boston, MA
United States

MARY K. MULCAHEY, MD
Associate Professor
Department of Orthopaedic Surgery
Tulane University School of Medicine
New Orleans, LA, United States

ELSEVIER

The Female Athlete

ISBN: 978-0-323-75985-4

Copyright © 2022 Elsevier Inc. All rights reserved.

Publisher: Dolores Meloni
Acquisitions Editor: Lauren Boyle
Editorial Project Manager: Susan Ikeda
Project Manager: Kiruthika Govindaraju
Cover Designer: Alan Studholme

3251 Riverport Lane
St. Louis, Missouri 63043

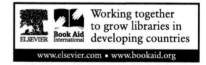

Working together to grow libraries in developing countries

www.elsevier.com • www.bookaid.org

Table of Contents

Dedication

Rachel M. Frank, MD

This book is dedicated to Laura Redmond Ramirez (1984–2017), a person unlike any other, who was taken from this world much too soon. She embodied the definition of female athlete, but more important, was an outstanding human being, sister, daughter, wife, and to me, the best of friends. I'd also like to take this opportunity to thank several people, although there are countless other individuals who deserve to be recognized. First, thank you coeditors Mary and Liz—their expertise, experience, passion, and talent are unmatched, and I am so incredibly humbled and honored to have worked on this book with you. They define what it means for women to support women, and I am so grateful to have had this opportunity to work together with them. Next, to my family, both at home in Chicago and in Colorado—thank you for your support and understanding of my long nights and sometimes very brief FaceTime calls. Next, I'd like to thank Janet Rayfield, my University of Illinois soccer coach, turned mentor, turned friend—no words can describe how grateful I am for your support, guidance, mentorship, and friendship. To Lindsay Tarpley, the most unusual of circumstances allowed us to meet (but maybe not so unusual if you think about it), and I'm so thankful for your friendship and for your willingness to be part of this project. To my college soccer teammates—you are all powerful, strong, and incredible women—thank you all for helping me become the best version of myself (and may each of you forever pass the beep test). To my Chair, Dr. Evalina Burger—I'm not sure where to start, but suffice to say, thank you for absolutely everything, including always, and I mean always, being available for me and for being a mentor for myself and female orthopods all over the world. Lastly, I'd like to acknowledge and thank several of the male mentors/colleagues/friends in my life, who have always supported me and never treated me different simply because I am a woman—Drs. Charles A. Bush-Joseph, Bernard R. Bach Jr., Anthony A. Romeo, Brian J. Cole, Aaron G. Rosenberg, Armando F. Vidal, and Eric C. McCarty (and many others)—thank you for supporting me for who I am and not simply to check a box.

Mary K. Mulcahey, MD

I am honored to have had the opportunity to serve as a coeditor of this phenomenal book. Working with Rachel and Liz, two of my closest friends and colleagues in sports medicine, has been amazing. I believe in the importance and power of this book, not only in its content but also in the authorship and leadership that came together to make this happen.

Understanding gender-related differences in the incidence and outcomes of sports medicine injuries is critical for us as orthopedic sports medicine surgeons and for all members of the sports medicine team. This will help us take better care of our patients. My passion for women's sports medicine is grounded in my experience as a sprinter and long jumper at Dartmouth and has grown in my role as Director of our Women's Sports Medicine Program at Tulane. This book details what is currently known about how patient gender impacts injuries, outcomes, and return to play. The passion and drive of many orthopedic researchers and the support of our sports medicine societies and journals will continue to further our progress. I am excited and honored to be part of this journey!

Elizabeth G. Matzkin, MD

I would like to dedicate this book to all the female athletes who have inspired me in so many ways and have trusted me to help them in their journey to return to play after injury. More specifically, I want to dedicate this book to my three athletic daughters. Abby—your perseverance and "never give up" attitude is infectious and reminds me to always give 100% in everything I do. Sami—your heart and passion for the game, your teammates, and your coaches remind me how important it is to love what you do in life. Emily—your intensity mixed with your sense of humor allow you to always play hard and have fun and remind me that this is a great way to succeed in all facets of life. My husband, Eric, who may be the biggest and most genuine supporter of female athletes and female orthopedic surgeons, thank you. My coeditors, Rachel Frank and Mary Mulcahey, continue to raise the bar and pave the way for many to follow. Your energy and dedication to make orthopedics better for women and treatments better for female athletes is never ending. Lastly, my support system that allows these collaborations to be successful—my family, work team, my many mentors, the Panda 6, and my amazing female colleagues in sports medicine.

List of Contributors

Sheila M. Algan, MD
Clinical Associate Professor of Orthopaedic Surgery
University of Oklahoma
Oklahoma City, OK, United States

Kelsey Andrews, BS
Medical Student
PGY-3
University of Colorado School of Medicine
Aurora, CO, United States

Sherrie Ballantine-Talmadge, DO, FACSM
CU Sports Medicine & Performance Center
Assistant Professor
Department of Orthopedics
University of Colorado
Boulder, CO, USA

Jennifer J. Beck, MD, FAAOS
Associate Professor of Orthopaedic
    Surgery-DGSOM
Director of Outreach and Research-OIC
Department of Orthopaedic Surgery
Orthopaedic Institute for Children/UCLA
Los Angeles, CA, United States

Jamie R. Birkelo, PA-C
Department of Orthopedics
Rush University Medical Center
Midwest Orthopaedics at Rush
Chicago, IL, United States

Ljiljana Bogunovic, MD
Orthopedic Associates of Wisconsin
Pewaukee, WI, United States

Hannah L. Bradsell, BS
Department of Orthopaedic Surgery
University of Colorado School of Medicine
Aurora, CO, United States

Jacqueline M. Brady, MD
Department of Orthopaedics and Rehabilitation
Oregon Health & Science University
Portland, United States

Katherine C. Branche, MD
Department of Orthopaedic Surgery
University of Missouri-Kansas City
Kansas City, MO, United States

Scott Buzin, DO
Department of Orthopaedic Surgery
Robert Wood Johnson Barnabas Health
Jersey City Medical Center
Jersey City, New Jersey, United States

Ellen K. Casey, MD
Associate Professor
Weill Cornell Medicine
Associate Attending
Department of Physiatry
Hospital for Special Surgery
New York, NY, United States

Caitlin C. Chambers, MD
Department of Orthopedic Surgery
University of Minnesota
Minneapolis, MN, United States
TRIA Orthopedic Center
Woodbury, MN, United States

Sarah M. Cheney, BS
Georgetown University School of Medicine
Washington, DC, United States

Stephanie Chu, DO
Associate Professor
University of Colorado School of Medicine
Aurora, CO, United States

Heather R. Cichanowski, MD, CAQ
Medical Director of Women's Sports Medicine
Department of Sports Medicine
TRIA Orthopedic Center
Woodbury, MN, United States

Kelly E. Cline, MD
Sports Medicine and Pediatric Orthopedic Surgery
Texas Orthopedics
Austin, TX, United States

Sara Edwards, MD
Associate Professor
UCSF Department of Orthopaedic Surgery
San Francisco, CA, United States

Claire D. Eliasberg, MD
Department of Orthopaedic Surgery
Hospital for Special Surgery
New York, NY, United States

Elizabeth A. Fierro, DO
Resident Physician
Department of Physical Medicine & Rehabilitation
NYU Grossman School of Medicine
New York, NY, United States

Alison Dittmer Flemig, MD
Department of Orthopedic Surgery
University of Colorado
Aurora, CO, United States

Rachel M. Frank, MD
Associate Professor
Director, Joint Preservation Program
Department of Orthopaedic Surgery
University of Colorado School of Medicine
Denver, CO, United States

Nicole A. Friel, MD, MS
Co-Director of Sports Medicine
Shriners Hospitals for Children Northern California
Assistant Clinical Professor
Department of Orthopedic Surgery
University of California at Davis
Sacramento, CA, United States

Kirsten D. Garvey, MS
Department of Orthopaedic Surgery
Brigham and Women's Hospital
Boston, MA, Unites States

Harvard Medical School
Boston, MA, Unites States

Arianna L. Gianakos, DO
Harvard - Massachusetts General Hospital
Department of Orthopedic Surgery
Boston, MA, United States

Elan Golan, MD
Northside Orthopedic Specialists
Northside Orthopedic Institute
Snellville, GA, United States

Mia S. Hagen, MD
Surgical Director
Sports Medicine Center at Husky Stadium

Assistant Professor
Department of Orthopedics & Sports Medicine
University of Washington
Seattle, WA, United States

Megan Lisset Jimenez, DO
Emory University
LaGrange, GA, United States

Pamela J. Lang, MD
Department of Orthopedics and Rehabilitation
University of Wisconsin School of
    Medicine and Public Health
Madison, WI, United States

Jody Law, BA
Department of Orthopedic Surgery
Washington University School of
    Medicine in St. Louis
St. Louis, MO, United States

Tiffany Liu, MD
Resident, UCSF
San Francisco, CA
United States

Matthew T. Lopez, PT, DPT
Senior Sports Specialist Physical Therapy
Northside Hospital Orthopedic Institute − Sports
    Medicine
Atlanta, GA, United States

Natalie A. Lowenstein, BS
Department of Orthopaedic Surgery
Brigham and Women's Hospital
Boston, MA, Unites States

Harvard Medical School
Boston, MA, Unites States

Elizabeth G. Matzkin, MD
Department of Orthopaedic Surgery
Brigham and Women's Hospital
Boston, MA, Unites States

Harvard Medical School
Boston, MA, Unites States

Stephanie W. Mayer, MD
Associate Professor of Orthopedic Surgery
University of Colorado
Denver, CO, United States

Laura Moore, MD
Chief Resident, UCSF
San Francisco, CA, United States

Mary K. Mulcahey, MD
Associate Professor
Department of Orthopaedic Surgery
Tulane University School of Medicine
New Orleans, LA, United States

Warren Nielsen, MD
Department of Orthopaedics and Rehabilitation
University of Vermont
Burlington, VT, United States

Kate M. Parker, BS
Department of Orthopedics & Sports Medicine
University of Washington
Seattle, WA, United States

Stephanie S. Pearce, MD
Department of Orthopaedic Surgery and
    Sports Medicine
Children's Hospital of the King's Daughters
Norfolk, Virginia, United States

Elise B.E. Raney, MD
University of Wisconsin Department of Orthopedics
    and Rehabilitation
Madison, WI, United States

Beth E. Shubin Stein, MD
Department of Orthopedic Surgery
Hospital for Special Surgery
New York, NY, United States

Luis J. Soliz, MD
Assistant Professor
Loyola University Medical Center
Department of Orthopaedic Surgery and
    Rehabilitation
Chicago, IL, United States

Andrea M. Spiker, MD
University of Wisconsin Department of
    Orthopedics and Rehabilitation
Madison, WI, United States

Katherine Sprouse, MD
Resident Physician Surgery
Birminham, AL, United States

Sabrina M. Strickland, MD
Department of Orthopaedic Surgery
Hospital for Special Surgery
New York, NY, United States

Karen M. Sutton, MD
Associate Professor
Weill Cornell Medicine
Associate Attending
Department of Orthopaedic Surgery
Hospital for Special Surgery
New York, NY, United States

Erika L. Valentine, MD
Resident Physician
Department of Orthopedic Surgery
University of California at Davis
Sacramento, CA, United States

Leslie B. Vidal, MD
Sports Medicine Surgeon
The Steadman Clinic
Vail, CO, United States

Kathleen Weber, MD, MS
Assistant Professor
Director of Primary Care Sports Medicine
Department of Orthopedics
Rush University Medical Center
Midwest Orthopaedics at Rush
Chicago, IL, United States

Sarah Weinstein, DO
Sports Medicine Fellow
University of Colorado School of Medicine
Aurora, CO, United States

Vonda Wright, MD, MS
Chief- Northside Hospital Orthopedic
    Institute Sports Medicine
Atlanta, GA, United States

John W. Yurek, DO
Jersey City Medical Center, Department of
    Orthopaedic Surgery
Jersey City, NJ, United States

About the Editors

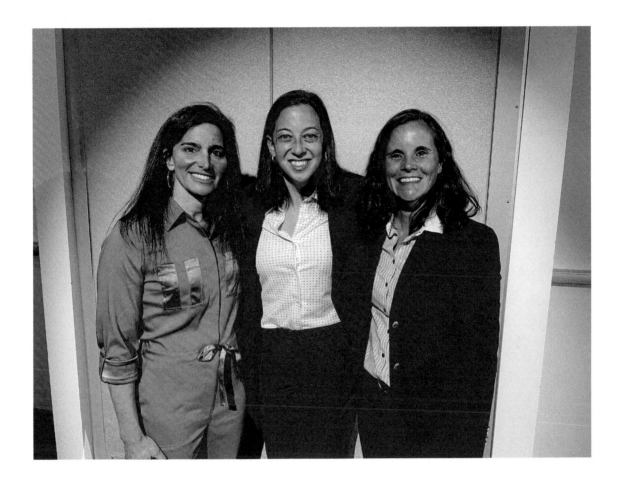

Rachel M. Frank, MD. Dr. Frank is a board-certified orthopedic surgeon and sports medicine specialist. She is an associate professor and director of the Joint Preservation Program in the Department of Orthopaedic Surgery at the University of Colorado School of Medicine. After playing 4 years of Big Ten Soccer at the University of Illinois, she completed medical school at the Northwestern University Feinberg School of Medicine, orthopaedic surgery residency at the Rush University Medical Center, a research fellowship at the Rush University Medical Center, and sports medicine fellowship at the Rush University Medical Center. Dr. Frank has authored or coauthored over 300 peer-reviewed publications and her research focuses on joint preservation and posttraumatic osteoarthritis. Dr. Frank is the head team orthopedic surgeon for the Colorado Rapids, team physician for the University of Colorado, and a U.S. Soccer Network Team Physician. Dr. Frank enjoys cycling, hiking, and long-distance triathlon, and she is especially passionate about her French bulldog, Murphy.

Mary K. Mulcahey, MD. Dr. Mulcahey is a board-certified orthopedic surgeon specializing in shoulder and knee surgery and sports medicine. She is a New Hampshire native, who received her Bachelor of Arts in Biochemistry from the Dartmouth College and her

Doctor of Medicine from the University of Rochester School of Medicine. She completed her orthopedic residency at the Brown University, followed by a fellowship in Orthopaedic Trauma at the same institution. Dr. Mulcahey then went on to do a fellowship in sports medicine at the San Diego Arthroscopy and Sports Medicine. She is an associate professor in the Department of Orthopaedic Surgery at the Tulane University School of Medicine, and she serves as the director of the Women's Sports Medicine at Tulane. Dr. Mulcahey was a sprinter and long jumper while in college at Dartmouth, and she has a passion for taking care of female athletes.

Elizabeth G. Matzkin, MD. Dr. Matzkin is a board-certified orthopedic surgeon and sports medicine specialist at the Brigham and Women's Hospital. She serves as the chief of Women's Sports Medicine, and her clinical interests are focused on preventing and providing care for sports injuries. Dr. Matzkin completed medical school at the Tulane University, residency at the University of Hawaii, and fellowship at the Duke University. Dr. Matzkin's goals are to return her patients to the activities they love. Dr. Matzkin's research has focused on the female athlete and gender differences in musculoskeletal medicine.

Foreword

As a young girl, I loved to climb, run, jump, throw, race, and compete. Thankfully, my parents not only kept from stifling those impulses but also encouraged them. I am so grateful that my father recognized that his daughter loved and could benefit from the lessons of sport as much as his son. Decades later, many of those years spent coaching, I celebrate the impact of the female athlete. Female athletes are running companies. Female athletes are engineering solutions to world problems. Female athletes are impacting governments and cultures around the world, and female athletes are competing on the highest stages of professional sports. Equality is still a future aspiration but young girls dream proudly of being athletes.

Dr. Rachel Frank was one of those young girls. She played as a goalkeeper for the University of Illinois where I was and still am the head women's soccer coach. "Frankie", long before Dr. Frank was a title on the horizon, embraced her competitiveness and drive to be great. She welcomed the opportunity to push her body to its limits and tested herself to be better every day. Her unquenchable thirst for knowledge was in the classroom and on the field. As she pushed to and sometimes past her physical limits, she sought knowledge and understanding about every injury she sustained and dealt with. Fueled by that exploration, "Frankie" pursued and accomplished her dream of becoming an orthopedic surgeon, and now Dr. Frank has leveraged the intersection of her athletic and academic worlds. The entire female athletic community will reap the benefit of that juncture.

My experience through the years in women's sports has also taught me that in the journey toward equality, we must close the gap of knowledge, data, and information about the female athlete. A gap has been created by the male dominance of this arena not only on the field, track, and courts but also in the research studies, the medical labs, and the performance data collection across all sports. I am not a doctor but as a female athlete and coach of female athletes, this book is groundbreaking and validating. The culmination of medical expertise targeting the female athlete written by female practitioners and surgeons fills a void that has existed for far too long. Injuries, issues, and struggles that are unique to the female athlete have been acknowledged and addressed. Thank you, Dr. Frank, for recognizing the need, gathering the expertise, and sharing it with the medical community. Also thank you to every contributing author for helping close the knowledge gap for female athletes. Your collective work will impact the next female athlete who can use her experience to impact the world in the way you have with this book.

To the readers—read and learn from the pages that follow. Remember as you do to keep pushing the limits, keep fighting for equality in your own way, and keep challenging the world to grow.

We are our best selves when we ask the best of ourselves.

Janet Rayfield

My name is Lindsay Tarpley and I am a two-time Olympic Gold Medalist in soccer who suffered a career-ending knee injury during the prime of my career. I played for the Women's National Soccer Team over 120 times and loved being able to compete at the highest level.

Unfortunately, in a send-off game to the World Cup in 2011, I suffered a huge knee injury. My injury was very complex and I was never able to recover from it, but I certainly learned a lot throughout the difficult process to my new normal.

One of the most important lessons I learned from this journey is to use your athletic mindset and take the process as a challenge to overcome. I set goals physically and mentally, worked hard before and after surgery, and stayed in communication to meet expectations. There are good days and tough days, but after going through this process, I came out with a different perspective and a new outlook on my life.

Anterior cruciate ligament injuries in women happen at a much higher rate and I experienced firsthand how difficult the process can be; however, it is important to surround yourself with a positive support system. I highly recommend keeping a journal to keep track of your progress and thus you can look back on how far you have progressed.

I was fortunate to have wonderful doctors, Dr. Frank being one of them, who guided me through my surgeries and my recoveries and helped me reevaluate my expectations. I had trust in my doctors that they had my best interest in mind and aligned my vision and invested in my recovery.

This injury changed my life, and although it wasn't the outcome I wanted, I appreciate being surrounded by doctors, physical therapists, family, and teammates who had my best interest in mind. Having a healthcare team that understands me, my injuries, my goals, and my needed recovery was critical in this process. Now, I am using a similar mindset in this next chapter of my life diving into being an entrepreneur, a mother, and a businesswoman. My experiences as an athlete and as a patient have influenced me, and I'm sure they have a lasting impact on so many athletes every single day.

The concept of this textbook is exciting, as it focuses exclusively on the female athlete and is written by female authors. This is really a "first" on so many levels. Female athletes-turned-patients, such as myself, benefit from the content and knowledge contained within the book, and this book also provides opportunities for women in orthopedic surgery to take center stage. In a society where women often get passed over for leadership opportunities, career opportunities, etc., this book stands out.

Lindsay Tarpley

Introduction

RACHEL M. FRANK, MD • MARY K. MULCAHEY, MD • ELIZABETH G. MATZKIN, MD

In the field of sports medicine, patients, physicians, and the public have all come to expect good to excellent outcomes for the vast majority of athletes, regardless of the injury. In the high-level athlete, treatment that does not result in the ability to return to preinjury level of play can have detrimental implications. Not only can the athlete's physical, mental, and/or emotional health suffer, but also injuries may impact the athlete's career longevity as well as future financial productivity. Thus efforts must be made to optimize care for athletes on an individual, patient-specific level.

Of all the important factors that must be considered when assessing and treating an athlete, the impact of patient gender is perhaps the most critical, yet, historically, has often been neglected. Certainly, the "same injury" in a male patient may present differently in a female patient and may also require a different treatment approach. As these differences may be subtle, a better understanding of the ways in which seemingly common sports medicine injuries present in female patients versus male patients is needed. This book will describe recent literature analyzing gender-related differences in injury patterns and treatment options relevant to several "hot topics" in sports medicine. The book provides a comprehensive overview of the more common sports medicine injuries of the lower and upper extremities, with specific focus on these injuries in the female patient population. The final section of the book focuses on more general sports medicine issues that either are more common (or exclusively) in the female athlete than in the male athlete (i.e., female athlete triad/RED-S [relative energy deficiency in sports], exercise considerations in pregnancy, etc.) or impact the female athlete differently than the male athlete (i.e., concussions, overuse injuries, etc.). The information in the chapters in this section is critical for all sports medicine physicians and allied professionals to understand in order to provide appropriate care for female patients presenting with both acute and chronic injuries and/or sports medicine-related conditions. We will discuss not only the incidence, presentation, and treatment of such injuries and conditions but also their prevention strategies, with the ultimate goal of helping our athletes avoid preventable injuries and/or conditions.

In addition to providing content critical for the sports medicine clinician, including orthopedic surgeons, non-operative sports medicine physicians, primary care and family medicine physicians, physician assistants, nurse practitioners, nurses, athletic trainers, medical assistants, physical therapists, occupational therapists, exercise physiologists, and sports medicine specialists of all disciplines, this book serves another purpose. When planning for the creation of this book, certainly, one main goal was to discuss all things related to the female athlete. Another goal, however, was to provide a platform for female sports medicine specialists to share their knowledge and expertise. To that end, the primary and/or senior author of *all chapters* in this book is female. We did not intend for this to be exclusionary of males, and each of us are so grateful for our supportive male colleagues, mentors, and trainees. We did this to give females an opportunity to be included, when so often, particularly in orthopedic surgery, females are either looked over or, in some cases, blatantly excluded. To be clear, each author was invited based on their qualifications and expertise as a sports medicine clinician and not to increase diversity or "check a box." So often, the same experts get asked to write chapters, speak at symposiums, etc., and they get invited back year after year. In sports medicine, those individuals tend to be mostly, if not entirely, males, and the cycle repeats itself. We hope this book helps break that cycle and give females, who are equally able and affable, an opportunity to shine. We are so grateful to our authors for contributing to this book and sharing their expertise and experience with the readers.

Finally, we encourage everyone to really take some time to read each Foreword, with powerful statements provided by two internationally recognized female athlete superstars, including the University of Illinois Head Soccer Coach (and former All-American and Nike Player of the Year), Janet Rayfield, and two-time Olympic Gold Medalist, Lindsay Tarpley. These two incredible women have had experiences as athletes, patients, and professionals in the sports medicine world, and they offer a unique perspective on what it means to be a female athlete and a female professional.

We hope you find the educational content of this book helpful for your clinical practice and thank you for taking this journey with us.

CHAPTER 1

Knee Anatomy and Biomechanics

KATE M. PARKER, BS • MIA S. HAGEN, MD

INTRODUCTION

Important morphologic differences have been found between the female and male knee. In addition to these anatomic differences, there are also significant neuromuscular differences between genders. This chapter outlines these differences, as they specifically pertain to the female athlete and risk for injury. The important characteristics of female knee bones, alignment, and soft tissues (ligament, meniscus) are covered first, followed by neuromechanical differences. The majority of research in this topic is directed at anterior cruciate ligament (ACL) tears and patellar instability, and as such, this chapter focuses on these injuries in particular.

OSSEOUS DIFFERENCES

When comparing male to female knee osseous anatomy, comparative studies in sports medicine focus on femoral notch morphology, tibial slope, femoral condyle geometry, and patellofemoral articulation.

Femoral Notch Width

Gender differences in femoral notch anatomy has been a topic of research because of the proposition that notch morphology relates to ACL injury risk, yet its significance remains unclear. It is possible that a small notch indicates a small ACL making it more susceptible to injury[1-3] or that a narrower notch impinges the ACL resulting in shear force leading to tears.[4] It is also possible a smaller ratio of notch width to bicondylar width (notch width index, or NWI) leads to ACL injury,[5-7] yet some studies have found this risk to be nonexistent.[8,9]

In a study using axial plane magnetic resonance imaging (MRI) and three-dimensional analysis to measure femoral notch anatomy, Charlton et al.[10] collected measurements of femoral notch volume and femoral bicondylar width, considering patient gender, height, and weight. Compared with males, females had a statistically smaller femoral notch volume, but this difference was primarily related to weight and height. Comparing male and female femoral bicondylar width, they found a statistically significant difference between males and females, with males having a larger bicondylar width (difference, 4.4 mm; $P = .001$). This study excluded subjects with a history of previous knee injury or surgery, which may have introduced a selection bias, creating a cohort of subjects possessing certain anatomic or physiologic differences from those prone to injury. Additionally, they found that notch width did not directly increase with height, as did femoral bicondylar width, which led the authors to question the use of the NWI as a standardizing tool.

Shelbourne et al.[1] measured the intercondylar notch width intraoperatively and performed radiographic measurements on 714 ACL-deficient patients. In agreement with prior studies,[11] they found that females, on average, had smaller notches than males. They also found that the NWI changed with height because the femoral condylar width increased more than the notch width in taller subjects. They critiqued the use of NWI, as it was assumed that both the notch width and the femoral bicondylar width increase similarly with increasing height. Consequently, they recommended comparison of different subjects with absolute notch width measurements rather than NWI. In a later study by Anderson et al.[12] utilizing MRI measurements in high-school students, notch width was found to increase with height for male subjects, but not for females. The NWI was stable with increasing height in male players, but it reduced with increasing height in female players. This study suggested that, in contrast to males, as females grow taller, the size of the femoral notch does not increase with the absolute width

The Female Athlete. https://doi.org/10.1016/B978-0-323-75985-4.00006-4

of the femoral condyles. This discrepancy may cause intercondylar notch stenosis and lead to an increased risk of ACL tear (Fig. 1.1).

In summary, differences in femoral notch volume and bicondylar width between males and females may mostly be due to height and weight rather than gender specifically. However, the aforementioned disproportionate growth between femoral notch width and bicondylar width in growing females, resulting in a lower NWI with increased height, may be a significant contributor to ACL injury risk from notch stenosis. This phenomenon has not been seen in males, who have a much more proportionate growth of both notch and bicondylar widths. Further research between genders considering age, race and body type is needed to support this theory.

Tibial Plateau Slope

Several studies suggest that females have a steeper angle to the anterior to posterior slope of the tibial plateau than males.[13,14] This increased slope is thought to increase the risk of ACL rupture because of the relationship

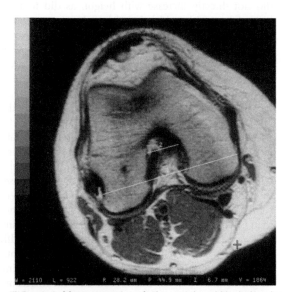

FIG. 1.1 Measurements of the notch width index by Anderson et al.,[12] performed at the level of the popliteal recess. The larger line measures the total condylar width. Line 2 measures the notch width at 2/3 of the notch height. (Reprinted with permission from Anderson AF, Dome DC, Gautam S, Awh MH, Rennirt GW. Correlation of anthropometric measurements, strength, anterior cruciate ligament size, and intercondylar notch characteristics to sex differences in anterior cruciate ligament tear rates. *Am J Sports Med.* 2001;29(1):58–66, Copyright (2001) SAGE Publications.)

between the slope of the tibial plateau and the anterior tibial translation of the knee. With steeper tibial slopes, the application of large compressive joint loads exposes greater magnitudes of anteriorly directed force on the proximal part of the tibia, and this may lead to an increased risk of ACL injury as the ACL attempts to provide restraint to this anteriorly directed force.[15–19] Several studies have suggested that higher tibial slope increases the risk for ACL tears, especially in females.[20–23]

Hohmann et al.[25] compared males and females who suffered ACL injuries and found that females had a significantly greater posterior tibial slope, which was thought to place the female knee at an increased risk for a pivot shift injury. Utilizing MRI, Hashemi et al.[24] measured the medial, lateral and coronal slopes of the tibial plateau in 33 female and 22 male patients. This study found the mean medial and lateral tibial slopes for the female subjects were significantly greater than those for the male subjects (medial: 5.9 degrees compared with 3.7 degrees; $P = .01$; lateral: 7.0 degrees compared with 5.4 degrees; $P = .02$) (Fig. 1.2). Weinberg et al.[26] utilized 545 bilateral cadaver specimens to establish normative values of medial and lateral posterior tibial slope and to determine differences in genders, age and race. Tibial slope measurements were taken with radiographic measurement and digital laser-derived three-dimensional analysis. The mean medial and lateral tibial slopes were greater in females than those in males, and regression analysis confirmed gender to be an independent predictor for increased slope.

In opposition, Karimi et al.[27] used MRI to measure posterior tibial slope in an Iranian population and found no significant correlation between genders. Given contradictory evidence, there may be factors other than gender that contribute to tibial slope, such as age, body mass index (BMI), or ethnicity and these should be considered in future research.

Femoral Trochlear Groove

It has been theorized that compared to males, females may have lower medial and lateral femoral condyles anteriorly, resulting in a shallower trochlear groove. Yet when correcting for size of the distal femur, these differences may not be significant. In a detailed radiographic study of 400 knees in 1964, Brattstrom[28] found females had, on average, 1.5 mm lower lateral and 1.1 mm lower medial condyles anteriorly. However, when adjusted for size, males and females had similar anterior condylar measurements. Similarly, Poilvache et al.[29] reported an average 1.4 mm lower lateral condyle and a 1.6 mm lower medial condyle for females compared with males. However, these data points were direct, absolute measurements, uncorrected for the

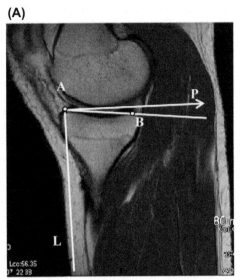 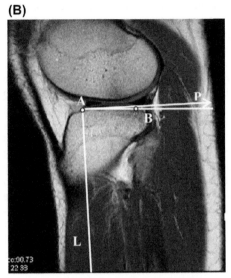

FIG. 1.2 Magnetic resonance imaging by Hashemi et al.[24] illustrates the utilized method for the measurement of the medial and lateral tibial slopes. Line L indicates the longitudinal axis, line P is perpendicular to line L, and line AB represents the tibial slope. **(A)** Medial tibial slope. **(B)** Lateral tibial slope. (Reprinted with permission from Hashemi J, Chandrashekar N, Gill B, et al. The geometry of the tibial plateau and its influence on the biomechanics of the tibiofemoral joint. *J Bone Joint Surg Am.* 2008;90(12):2724–2734, Copyright 2008, Wolters Kluwer Health, Inc.)

size of the distal femur or the patient and thus may have been secondary to smaller overall femora for females compared to males. Varadarajan et al.[30] studied the gender differences in trochlear groove orientation. The proximal portion of the trochlear groove was found to be oriented significantly more medially in females than in males, which was hypothesized to contribute to differences in patellar tracking.

Gender Differences in Coronal and Rotational Alignment and Clinical Implications

The quadriceps angle, or the "Q-angle", was first described by Brattstrom in 1964.[31] The Q-angle is the angle between the line of pull of the quadriceps (anterior superior iliac spine to mid-patella) and the line connecting the center of the patella with tibial tuberosity. An increased Q-angle is thought to create excessive lateral forces on the patella through a bowstring effect. The literature describing "normal" values of the Q-angle is variable. In general, the average normal Q-angle should fall between 12 and 20 degrees.[32–37] Some studies have illustrated that values between 8 and 10 degrees for males and up to 15 degrees for females are deemed normal, with higher values indicating potential pathoanatomy.[38,39]

Greater femoral anteversion and/or tibiofemoral angles result in greater Q-angles. Changes in the

tibiofemoral angle have a substantially greater impact on the magnitude of the Q-angle compared with femoral anteversion. As such, the Q-angle seems to largely represent a frontal plane alignment measure. As many knee injuries appear to result from a combination of both frontal and transverse plane motions and forces, this may in part explain why the Q-angle has been found to be a poor independent predictor of lower extremity injury risk.[32]

Historically the literature seems in agreement that females have wider Q-angles than males, with mean differences from 3 to 5.8 degrees depending on the resource.[28,32–36,40] This difference may be because on average, females have shorter femora and more widely spaced hips than males.[41,42] Theoretically, the combination of wider hips and shorter femora would increase the valgus of the lower limbs, thus increasing the Q-angle.

However, when data are corrected for the difference in height between males and females the difference in Q-angle may disappear. After measuring the Q-angle in 69 subjects, Grelsamer et al.[43] found that males and females had similar Q-angles and that despite the gender, shorter individuals had slightly greater Q-angles than those who were taller. This study suggested that the historically proposed slight difference in Q-angles between males and females may simply be explained by the fact that males tend to be taller. In a systematic review of Q-angle measurements, Livingston[44] concluded that "the common belief that females have wider hips than males is not supported by scientific data, nor is the assumption that Q angles are bilaterally symmetric. These outdated assumptions must be replaced by a new approach to the study of the Q angle."

In a clinical study on lower extremity alignment, Nguyen et al.[45] found significant gender differences in hip anteversion between males and females, along with pelvic angle, genu recurvatum and Q-angle. They concluded that although the reasons contributing to these gender differences are not entirely known, there is evidence to suggest that many of these gender differences are developmental in nature and emerge after puberty. Their finding that females showed greater femoral anteversion than males agreed with that of other studies[46,47]; however, these studies did not conclude this difference to be statistically significant. Thus further research is required to definitively show significant gender differences in lower extremity alignment.

The Q-angle is of importance, as elevated Q-angles may increase the risk for anterior knee pain or patellar dislocation. The larger the angle, the greater the lateralization force on the patella, increasing retropatellar pressure between the lateral facet of the patella and the lateral femoral condyle.[48] A 10% increase in the Q-angle has been shown to increase the stress on the patellofemoral joint by 45%.[49] Continuous compressive forces may give rise to patellofemoral pain syndrome and cause degeneration of the joint.[50,51] If the lateral force becomes large enough the patella may potentially sublux or dislocate over the femoral sulcus, with quadriceps activation and knee extension.[48] However, some case-control studies have not supported the hypothesis that larger Q-angle is a risk factor for patellofemoral pain syndrome, as this condition is likely multifactorial[52–54] (Fig. 1.3).

The Q-angle's direct relationship with the risk of ACL injury is somewhat controversial because of the multitude of factors that constitute lower limb alignment. For example, if the patella sits laterally, or if the subject stands in an internally rotated position, the value of the Q-angle may be affected. Studies on female athletes have thus found no significant association between Q-angle and ACL injury when comparing injured and noninjured groups.[56,57] However, if the Q-angle were interpreted simply as increased valgus alignment it could represent the relation between valgus force and ACL tear. Studies have produced significant ACL strain with pure valgus torque.[58,59] Additionally, the knee joint responds to increased lateral axial pressure by increasing the internal and anterior rotation, which increases ACL strain dramatically.[60] In support of this, training programs that reduce knee abduction moments have been shown to reduce risk of injury to the ACL.[61]

Anatomic alignment differences are one of the many factors believed to contribute to the higher incidence of ACL injury in females. An increase in femoral anteversion has been considered a risk for ACL injury because excessive internal rotation at the hip may lead to knee valgus alignment.[57] Femoral rotation also affects the patellofemoral joint. Forces of the femoral trochlea and the peripatellar retinaculum combine to act on the central portion of the patella. With the femur rotated internally, the lateral articular surface of the trochlea encroaches upon the patella's lateral articular surface and presses it medially. With the femur rotated externally, the medial articular surface of the trochlea impinges upon the patella's medial articular facet and pushes it laterally. The degree of femoral rotation is important in its potential to alter the biomechanics of the patellofemoral joint. Lee et al.[62] concluded that femoral rotations greater than 20 degrees, often caused by trauma, congenital abnormality or infection of the bone result in severe alterations to the natural biomechanics of the patellofemoral joint.

External tibial rotation has also been associated with possible increased risk of ACL and patellar injury. A gender-specific in vivo study of knee laxity and stiffness suggested that external tibial rotation and abduction were associated with the impingement of the ACL.[63] In this position the ACL would be compressed against the lateral wall of the intercondylar notch, making it more prone to injury. In addition to ACL injury, external tibial rotation has been associated with a variety of patellofemoral dysfunctions, including instability[64,65] and patellofemoral pain syndrome.[66] Biomechanical studies have shown that fixing the tibia in 15 degrees of external tibial rotation will significantly increase lateral facet patellofemoral joint contact pressure at all knee flexion angles.[67] To date, no gender differences have been established in tibial torsion[45,68–70]

SOFT TISSUE DIFFERENCES
Anterior Cruciate Ligament Anatomy

It has been well documented that females are more susceptible to ACL tears than males. There are 350,000 ACL injuries in the United States each year,[71] with a disproportionate number of these injuries occurring in female athletes.[72,73] Numerous studies have been done to analyze gender differences in ACL characteristics such

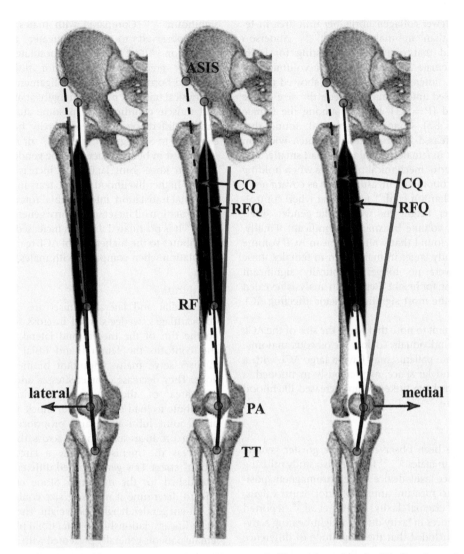

FIG. 1.3 Effect of patellar displacement on quadriceps angle (Q-angle), as described by Freedman et al.[55] Center image: Method for measuring Q-angle utilizes anterior superior iliac spine (ASIS), patella (PA), and tibial tuberosity (TT). RFQ represents the rectus femoris myotendinous junction, and the true directional pull of the quadriceps muscles. The outside images represent shifts in the Q-angle (CQ) with movement of the PA laterally (left image) and medially (right image). Lateral PA movement causes the CQ to decrease to zero and the RFQ to become negative, and medial PA movement causes the CQ and RFQ to become larger. (Reprinted with permission from Freedman B, Brindle T, Sheehan F. Re-evaluating the functional implications of the Q-angle and its relationship to in-vivo patellofemoral kinematics. *Clin Biomech*. December 2014; 29(10):1139–1145. Published online 2014 Oct 7. https://doi.org/10.1016/j.clinbiomech.2014.09.012, Copyright (2014) Elsevier.)

as cross-sectional area, volume, tensile strength and mechanical properties. While studies have found significant differences in these categories between genders, many conclude that these may more closely be related to differences in weight and height.

Studies have shown the female ACL has inferior mechanical properties than the male ACL, including a lower tensile modulus of elasticity and ultimate failure load.[74] This apparent weakness has been thought to be due to smaller ACL cross-sectional area, smaller ACL volume and fewer collagen fibrils per unit area in female ACLs than in male ACLs.[12,74,75] Anderson et al.[12] found that even when adjusting for body weight, the female ACL has a smaller volume than the male ACL. Interestingly, their data showed that as height increased among male subjects the size of the ACL increased ($P = .03$), but not among the female subjects ($P = .82$). Chandrashekar et al. found that ACL size increased in proportion to notch width in males but not in females: female ACLs had smaller volumes and inferior mechanical properties when holding age and anthropometric measurements as covariates.[74] In contrast, Charlton et al.[10] found that when controlling for gender, height and weight, the gender differences in ACL volume became nonsignificant. Finally, Fayad et al.[76] found that while the mean ACL volume was significantly larger in males than in females these differences were no longer statistically significant when adjusting for height. Regression analysis revealed height to be the most significant factor affecting ACL volume.

It is important to note that while the size of the ACL varies among individuals, so does the osseous anatomy. However, some patients may have a large ACL with a small intercondylar space; as previously mentioned, a small NWI has been linked to an increased likelihood of ACL rupture.[76,77]

Joint Laxity

Females have been observed to have greater general joint laxity than males.[78–81] In an in vivo study utilizing a Vermont knee laxity device and electromagnetic position sensors to measure anteroposterior, varus-valgus, internal and external laxity, Shultz et al.[78] reported gender differences in laxity during weight-bearing activities. They concluded that the magnitude of difference was fairly consistent across all non-weight-bearing measures, with females having 25%–30% greater motion than males for anterior, varus-valgus and internal-external rotations (posterior laxity measures were not statistically significant in difference). When an axial compressive load of 40% body weight was applied to the knee joint, the total motion decreased in all knees but the magnitude of the difference between genders increased, with females having 50%–60% greater motion during weight bearing than males.

Other studies looking at gender-based differences in tibial external and internal rotations consistently report greater rotational laxity in females than in males, with differences ranging from 3 to 8 degrees.[81–83] Notably, when considering varus-valgus laxity the differences between genders seemed smaller and, in some cases, not

significant.[83,84] Compared with males, females have been observed to exhibit greater anterior tibial translation.[78,85–90] Liu et al.[91] speculated the explanation for greater female anterior tibial translation involved hormonal differences, ligament size, the state of physical training, muscle strength, anatomic structure and muscle coordination. In some studies, however, gender differences in anterior laxity have only been exhibited in 50 degrees of flexion,[83] or not at all.[92,93]

Interest in better understanding gender-based differences in knee joint laxity has increased due to the known higher likelihood of ACL tears in females. Anterior tibial translation, internal tibial rotation and valgus tibial rotation all increase the force generated within the ACL.[60] It is postulated that this increased internal laxity contributes to the higher rate of ACL tears in the female population when compared with males.

Meniscus

The medial and lateral menisci are crescent-shaped fibrocartilages, wedge-shaped in cross section, that sit on the rim of the medial and lateral tibial plateaus and conform the femoral and tibial contours. The menisci serve many important biomechanical functions. They decrease contact stresses and increase contact area of the tibiofemoral joint. They also contribute to load transmission, shock absorption, stability, joint lubrication and proprioception. Weight bearing produces axial forces across the knee, which compress the menisci causing a circumferential or "hoop" stress. Few gender-based differences have been established for the meniscus. Stone et al.[94] utilized MRI to determine if meniscal size could be predicted by patient gender, height and weight. They found height had a linear relationship to total tibial plateau and that female patients generally presented with smaller dimensions than males. Additionally, groups with higher BMI presented with significantly larger meniscal dimensions than groups with lower BMI at any given height, thus making BMI a better predictor for meniscal size than height or gender.

NEUROMUSCULAR DIFFERENCES

Studies have shown that the contraction of the quadriceps muscle group applies an anterior shear force to the tibia through the patella tendon. This shear force may increase the load on the ACL when the knee flexion angle is less than 30 degrees. In this position, if the hamstring muscles do not apply sufficient posterior shear force as counter the ACL is at risk of tear.[84,95] Wojtys and Huston found that with maximum contraction of the knee musculature females reduced anterior tibial translation by 217%, whereas males reduced translation by 473%. In terms of injury to the knee, they proposed that these gender differences in strength and the hamstring-to-quadriceps (H/Q) ratio suggest that the ACL in females may be subjected to higher strain than the ACL in males during sports activities.[95] In a review on female and male peak torque H/Q ratios, Hewett et al.[96] found that gender differences in isokinetic H/Q ratios were not observed at slower angular velocities. They did find, however, that at high knee flexion/extension angular velocities (seen during sports activities) there were significant gender differences in the H/Q ratios. Unlike males, females did not show an increased H/Q torque ratio at velocities approaching those of functional activities. They also found with isokinetic dynamometer measurements that male athletes demonstrated significantly greater hamstring peak torque with increasing maturity, while females' peak hamstring torque remained stable with increasing maturity. Hewett proposed that the decreased H/Q ratio of female athletes relative to males could possibly be related to imbalances in neuromusculature with the onset of puberty and hypothesized that this may be a contributing factor in the increased risk of ACL injury in postpubertal female athletes.

Many studies on neuromuscular control agree that females tend to be more "quadriceps dominant" compared to males.[11,95] The lateral pull of a dominant quadriceps muscle, in addition to an increased Q-angle, may contribute to the higher risk of patellar dislocation seen in females over males. Analyzing the epidemiology and natural history of acute patellar dislocation, Fithian et al.[97] reported that between the ages of 10 and 17 years, the risk of primary dislocation is about 33% higher in girls than boys.

In addition to this, ACL tears in young athletes are associated with poor neuromuscular control leading to altered lower limb biomechanics including increased knee valgus and foot pronation angles, decreased hip and knee flexion, and hip abduction during cutting and landing.[98,99] Female athletes commonly demonstrate imbalances in strength, timing of activation and recruitment patterns of the lower extremity muscles. These gender differences in neuromuscular control of the knee appear to become prominent with the onset of puberty, as studies on younger adolescents have detected no significant difference in neuromuscular control with various athletic tasks until the age of 14 years.[100] In a study including postpubertal females,

Myer et al.[101] found that risk factors for ACL tears in females (increased knee valgus and foot pronation angles, decreased hip and knee flexion, and hip abduction during cutting and landing) were exacerbated as they matured and peaked following the postpubertal stage of development.

It has been shown that implementation of neuromuscular training (NMT) programs that alter knee biomechanics and reduce abduction knee motion during the landing phase of a jump appear to reduce ACL injury risk in youth athletes.[102] These findings have been paramount in designing effective NMT in female athletes. There may be a potential window of opportunity to decrease ACL injury risk in young female athletes if NMT is implemented prior to the onset of puberty.[103] After a 6-week NMT intervention inclusive of strength training, plyometric training and balance training, teenage female basketball, volleyball and soccer athletes have been found to significantly increase their knee flexion angle and decrease internal knee valgus in response to a drop vertical jump task.[104] The effects of NMT in preventing the incidence of ACL injury have been extensively studied in adolescent basketball, soccer and volleyball athletes.[62,104,105] NMT programs have been shown to be effective in improving lower limb alignment on a drop-jump test,[106] increasing hamstring strength, increasing knee flexion angles on landing and reducing deleterious moments and ground reaction forces.[107−109] The reduction of injurious forces on the knee after NMT suggests that risk factors such as lower H/Q ratios and uncoordinated muscle recruitment are modifiable.

CONCLUSION

The male and female knee anatomy and biomechanics are generally quite similar. However, there are subtle differences that may account for a slightly higher risk of specific injuries in females compared with males, such as ACL tears and/or patellar dislocations. Neuromuscular patterns may also play a role in injury risk and could potentially represent modifiable risk factors. It should be noted that many studies on gender differences have concluded that other factors such as patient height, weight and even ethnicity may have substantial impacts on knee anatomy and neuromuscular patterns. Future research on female and male knee anatomy and biomechanics should attempt to control for these factors when searching for gender-specific differences.

REFERENCES

1. Shelbourne KD, Davis TJ, Klootwyk TE. The relationship between inter- condylar notch width of the femur and the incidence of anterior cruciate ligament tears: a prospective study. *Am J Sports Med.* 1998;26:402–408.
2. Davis TJ, Shelbourne KD, Klootwyk TE. Correlation of the intercondylar notch width of the femur to the width of the anterior and posterior cruciate ligaments. *Knee Surg Sports Traumatol Arthrosc.* 1999;7(4):209–214.
3. Dienst M, Schneider G, Altmeyer K, et al. Correlation of intercondylar notch cross sections to the ACL size: a high resolution MR tomographic in vivo analysis. *Arch Orthop Trauma Surg.* 2007;127(4):253–260.
4. Simon RA, Everhart JS, Nagaraja HN, Chaudhari AM. A case-control study of anterior cruciate ligament volume, tibial plateau slopes and intercondylar notch dimensions in ACL-injured knees. *J Biomech.* 2010;43(9):1702–1707.
5. Fung DT, Zhang LQ. Modeling of ACL impingement against the intercondylar notch. *Clin Biomech.* 2003;18:933–941.
6. Herzog RJ, Silliman JF, Hutton K, Rodkey WG, Steadman JR. Measurements of intercondylar notch by plain film radiography and magnetic resonance imaging. *Am J Sports Med.* 1994;22:204–210.
7. Ireland ML, Ballantyne BT, Little K, McClay IS. A radiographic analysis of relationship between the size and shape of ICN and ACL injury. *Knee Surg Sports Traumatol Arthrosc.* 2001;9:200–205.
8. Lombardo S, Sethi PM, Starkey C. Intercondylar notch stenosis is not a risk factor for anterior cruciate ligament tears in professional male basketball players: an 11 year prospective study. *Am J Sports Med.* 2005;33:29–34.
9. Alizadeh A, Kiavash V. Mean intercondylar notch width index in cases with and without anterior cruciate ligament tears. *Iran J Radiol.* 2008;5:205–208.
10. Charlton W, St. John TA, Ciccotti M, Harrison N, Schweitzer M. Differences in femoral notch anatomy between males and female, a magnetic resonance imaging study. *Am J Sports Med.* 2002;30(3) (American Orthopaedic Society for Sports Medicine).
11. Anderson AF, Lipscomb AB, Liudahl KJ, et al. Analysis of the intercondylar notch by computed tomography. *Am J Sports Med.* 1987;15:547–552.
12. Anderson AF, Dome DC, Gautam S, Awh MH, Rennirt GW. Correlation of anthropometric measurements, strength, anterior cruciate ligament size, and intercondylar notch characteristics to sex differences in anterior cruciate ligament tear rates. *Am J Sports Med.* 2001;29(1):58–66.
13. Beynnon BD, Hall JS, Sturnick DR, et al. Increased slope of the lateral tibial plateau subchondral bone is associated with greater risk of non- contact ACL injury in females but not in males: a prospective cohort study with a nested, matched case-control analysis. *Am J Sports Med.* 2014;42(5):1039–1048.
14. Brandon ML, Haynes PT, Bonamo JR, Flynn MI, Barrett GR, Sherman MF. The association between posterior-inferior tibial slope and anterior cruciate ligament insufficiency. *Arthroscopy.* 2006;22(8):894–899.
15. Wang D, Kent III R, Amirtharaj M, et al. Tibiofemoral kinematics during compressive loading of the ACL-intact and ACL-sectioned knee roles of tibial slope, medial eminence volume, and anterior laxity. *J Bone Joint Surg Am.* 2019;101:1085–1092.
16. Dejour H, Bonnin M. Tibial translation after anterior cruciate ligament rupture. Two radiological tests compared. *J Bone Joint Surg Br.* 1994;76:745–749.
17. Slocum B, Devine T. Cranial tibial wedge osteotomy: a technique for eliminating cranial tibial thrust in cranial cruciate ligament repair. *J Am Vet Med Assoc.* 1984;184:564–569.
18. Torzilli PA, Deng X, Warren RF. The effect of joint-compressive load and quadriceps muscle force on knee motion in the intact and anterior cruciate ligament-sectioned knee. *Am J Sports Med.* 1994;22:105–112.
19. Beynnon BD, Fleming BC, Labovitch R, Parsons B. Chronic anterior cruciate ligament deficiency is associated with increased anterior translation of the tibia during the transition from non-weightbearing to weightbearing. *J Orthop Res.* 2002;20:332–337.
20. Terauchi M, Hatayama K, Yanagisawa S, Saito K, Takagishi K. Sagittal alignment of the knee and its relationship to noncontact anterior cruciate ligament injuries. *Am J Sports Med.* 2011;39:1090–1094.
21. Todd MS, Lalliss S, Garcia E, DeBerardino TM, Cameron KL. The relationship between posterior tibial slope and anterior cruciate ligament injuries. *Am J Sports Med.* 2010;38:63–67.
22. Hudek R, Fuchs B, Regenfelder F, Koch P. Is noncontact ACL injury associated with the posterior tibial and meniscal slope? *Clin Orthop Relat Res.* 2011;469(8):2377–2384.
23. Dare DM, Fabricant PD, McCarthy MM, et al. Increased lateral tibial slope is a risk factor for pediatric anterior cruciate ligament injury: an MRI-based case-control study of 152 patients. *Am J Sports Med.* 2015;43(7):1632–1639.
24. Hashemi J, Chandrashekar N, Gill B, et al. The geometry of the tibial plateau and its influence on the biomechanics of the tibiofemoral joint. *J Bone Joint Surg Am.* 2008;90(12):2724–2734.
25. Hohmann E, Bryant A, Reaburn P, Tetsworth K. Is there a correlation between posterior tibial slope and noncontact anterior cruciate ligament injuries? *Knee Surg Sports Traumatol Arthrosc.* 2011;19(suppl 1):S109–S114.
26. Weinberg D, Williamson D, Gebhart J, Knapik D, Voos J. Differences in medial and lateral posterior tibial slope. An osteological review of 1090 tibiae comparing age, sex, and race. *Am J Sports Med.* 2016;45(No. 1).
27. Karimi E, Norouzian M, Birjandinejad A, Zandi R, Makhmalbaf H. Measurement of posterior tibial slope using magnetic resonance imaging. *Arch Bone Jt Surg.* November 2017;5(6):435–439.

28. Brattstrom H. Shape of the intercondylar groove normally and in recurrent dislocation of the patella; a clinical and x-ray anatomical investigation. *Acta Orthop Scand Suppl*. 1964;68:1–148.

29. Poilvache PL, Insall JN, Scuderi GR, Font-Rodriguez DE. Rotational landmarks and sizing of the distal femur in total knee arthroplasty. *Clin Orthop Relat Res*. 1996;331: 35–44.

30. Varadarajan K, Gill TJ, Freiberg AA, Rubash HE, Li G. Sex differences in trochlear groove orientation and rotational kinematics of human knees. *J Orthop Res*. July 2009; 27(7):871–878. https://doi.org/10.1002/jor.20844.

31. Brattström H. Shape of the intercondylar groove normally and in recurrent dislocation of patella: a clinical and X-ray anatomical investigation. *Acta Orthop Scand*. 1964;35:1–148. https://doi.org/10.3109/ort.1964.35.-suppl-68.01.

32. Nguyen A-D, Boling MC, Levine B, Shultz SJ. Relationships between lower extremity alignment and the quadriceps angle. *Clin J Sport Med Off J Can Acad Sport Med*. May 2009;19(3):201–206.

33. Jaiyesimi A, Jegede O. Influence of sex and leg dominance on Q-angle among young adult Nigerians. *Afr J Physiother Rehabil Sci*. 2009;1:18–23.

34. Omololu BB, Ogunlade OS, Gopaldasani VK. Normal Q-angle in an adult Nigerian population. *Clin Orthop*. 2009; 467:2073–2076.

35. Raveendranath R, Nachiket S, Sujatha N, Priya R, Rema D. Bilateral variability of the quadriceps angle (Q angle) in an adult Indian population. *Iran J Basic Med Sci*. 2011;14:465–471.

36. Tella B, Ulogo UU, Odebiyi D, Omololu A. Sex variation of bilateral Q-angle in young adult Nigerians. *Nig Q J Hosp Med*. 2010;20:114–116.

37. Davies G, Larson R. Examining the knee. *J Am Phys Ther Assoc Sports Med*. 1978;6:49–67.

38. Loudon JK. Biomechanics and pathomechanics of the patellofemoral joint. *Int J Sports Phys Ther*. 2016;11: 820–830.

39. Tanifuji O, Blaha JD, Kai S. The vector of quadriceps pull is directed from the patella to the femoral neck. *Clin Orthop*. 2013;471:1014–1020. https://doi.org/10.1007/s11999-012-2741-5.

40. Horton MG, Hall TL. Quadriceps femoris muscle angle: normal values and relationships with sex and selected skeletal measures. *Phys Ther*. 1989;69:897–901.

41. Outerbridge RE. Further studies on the etiology of chondromalacia patellae. *J Bone Join Surg [Br]*. 1964;46: 179–190.

42. Simmons K. The Bush Foundation study of child growth and development. *Monogr Soc Res Child Dev*. 1944;9(1): 1–87.

43. Grelsamer RP, Dubey A, Weinstein CH. Males and female have similar Q angles. *J Bone Joint Surg Br*. 2005;87: 1498–1501.

44. Livingston LA. The quadriceps angle: a review of the literature. *J Orthop Sports Phys Ther*. 1998;28:105–109.

45. Nguyen AD, Shultz S, Schmitz R. Landing biomechanics in participants with different static lower extremity alignment profiles. *J Athl Train*. 2015;50(5):498–507.

46. Braten M, Terjesen T, Rossvoll I. Femoral anteversion in normal adults. Ultrasound measurements in 50 males and 50 female. *Acta Orthop Scand*. 1992;63:29–32.

47. Prasad R, Vettivel S, Isaac B, Jeyaseelan L, Chandi G. Angle of torsion of the femur and its correlates. *Clin Anat*. 1996;9:109–117.

48. Brechter H, Powers CM. Patellofemoral stress during walking in persons with and without patellofemoral pain. *Med Sci Sports Exerc*. 2002;34(10):1582–1593.

49. Huberti HH, Hayes WC. Patellofemoral contact pressures. The influence of q-angle and tendofemoral contact. *J Bone Joint Surg Am*. 1984;66(5):715–724.

50. Emami MJ, Ghahramani MH, Abdinejad F, Namazi H. Q-angle: an invaluable parameter for evaluation of anterior knee pain. *Arch Iran Med*. January 2007;10(1):24–26.

51. Tállay A, Kynsburg A, Tóth S, et al. Prevalence of patellofemoral pain syndrome. Evaluation of the role of biomechanical malalignments and the role of sport activity. *Orv Hetil*. October 10, 2004;145(41):2093–2101.

52. Boling MC, Padua DA, Marshall SW, Guskiewicz K, Pyne S, Beutler A. A prospective investigation of biomechanical risk factors for patellofemoral pain syndrome: the Joint Undertaking to Monitor and Prevent ACL Injury (JUMP-ACL) cohort. *Am J Sports Med*. 2009;37(11): 2108–2116.

53. Thijs Y, Pattyn E, Van Tiggelen D, Rombaut L, Witvrouw E. Is hip muscle weakness a predisposing factor for patellofemoral pain in female novice runners? A prospective study. *Am J Sports Med*. 2011;39(9):1877–1882.

54. Ramskov D, Jensen ML, Obling K, Nielsen RO, Parner ET, Rasmussen S. No association between q-angle and foot posture with running-related injuries: a 10 week prospective follow-up study. *Int J Sports Phys Ther*. 2013;8(4): 407–415.

55. Freedman B, Brindle T, Sheehan F. Re-evaluating the functional implications of the Q-angle and its relationship to in-vivo patellofemoral kinematics. *Clin Biomech*. December 2014;29(10):1139–1145. https://doi.org/10.1016/j.clinbiomech.2014.09.012. Published online 2014 Oct 7.

56. Mohamed EE, Useh U, Mtshali BF. Q-angle, Pelvic width, and Intercondylar notch width as predictors of knee injuries in female soccer players in South Africa. *Afr Health Sci*. June 2012;12(2):174–180.

57. Loudon JK, Jenins W, Loudon KL. The relationship between static posture and ACL injury in female athletes. *J Orhtop Sports Phys Ther*. August 1996;24(2):91–97.

58. Withrow TJ, Huston LJ, Wojtys EM, Ashton-Miller JA. The effect of an impulsive knee valgus moment on in vitro relative ACL strain during a simulated jump landing. *Clin Biomech*. 2006;21(9):977–983.

59. McLean SG, Huang X, Su A, Van Den Bogert AJ. Sagittal plane biomechanics cannot injure the ACL during side-step cutting. *Clin Biomech*. 2004;19(8):828–838.

60. Markolf KL, Burchfield DM, Shapiro MM, Shepard MF, Finerman GA, Slauterbeck JL. Combined knee loading states that generate high anterior cruciate ligament forces. *J Orthop Res.* 1995;13(6):930−935.

61. Hewett TE, Lindenfeld TN, Riccobene JV, Noyes FR. The effect of neuromuscular training on the incidence of knee injury in female athletes. *Am J Sports Med.* 1999; 27:699−706. https://doi.org/10.1177/03635465990270 060301.

62. Lee T, Morris G, Csintalan R. The influence of tibial and femoral rotation on patellofemoral contact area and pressure. *J Orthop Sports Phys Ther.* November 2003;33(11).

63. Park HS, Ahn C, Zhang LQ. A knee-specific finite element analysis of the human anterior cruciate ligament impingement against the femoral intercondylar notch. *J Biomech.* July 20, 2010;43(10):2039−2042.

64. Fox TA. Dysplasia of the quadriceps mechanism: hypoplasia of the vastus medialis muscle as related to the hypermobile patella syndrome. *Surg Clin North Am.* 1975;55:199−226.

65. Turner MS. The association between tibial torsion and knee joint pathology. *Clin Orthop.* 1994:47−51.

66. Andriacchi TP, Andersson GB, Fermier RW, Stern D, Galante JO. A study of lower-limb mechanics during stair-climbing. *J Bone Joint Surg Am.* 1980;62:749−757.

67. Lee TQ, Yang BY, Sandusky MD, McMahon PJ. The effects of tibial rotation on the patellofemoral joint: assessment of the changes in in situ strain in the peripatellar retinaculum and the patellofemoral contact pressures and areas. *J Rehabil Res Dev.* 2001;38:463−469.

68. Kristiansen LP, Gunderson RB, Steen H, Reikeras O. The normal development of tibial torsion. *Skeletal Radiol.* 2001;30:519−522.

69. Shultz SJ, Nguyen AD, Windley TC, Kulas AS, Botic TL, Beynnon BD. Intratester and intertester reliability of clinical measures of lower extremity anatomic characteristics: implications for multicenter studies. *Clin J Sport Med.* 2006;16:155−161.

70. Staheli LT, Corbett M, Wyss C, King H. Lower-extremity rotational problems in children. Normal values to guide management. *J Bone Joint Surg Am.* 1985;67:39−47.

71. Griffin LY, Albohm MJ, Arendt EA, et al. Understanding and preventing noncontact anterior cruciate ligament injuries: a review of the Hunt Valley II meeting, January 2005. *Am J Sports Med.* 2006;34(9):1512−1532.

72. Agel J, Arendt EA, Bershadsky B. Anterior cruciate ligament injury in national collegiate athletic association basketball and soccer: a 13-year review. *Am J Sports Med.* 2005;33(4):524−530.

73. Arendt E, Dick R. Knee injury patterns among males and female in collegiate basketball and soccer. NCAA data and review of literature. *Am J Sports Med.* 1995;23(6): 694−701.

74. Chandrashekar N, Mansouri H, Slauterbeck J, Hashemi J. Sex-based differences in the tensile properties of the human anterior cruciate ligament. *J Biomech.* 2006;39(16): 2943−2950.

75. Chaudhari AM, Zelman EA, Flanigan DC, Kaeding CC, Nagaraja HN. Anterior cruciate ligament-injured subjects have smaller anterior cruciate ligaments than matched controls: a magnetic resonance imaging study. *Am J Sports Med.* 2009;37(7):1282−1287.

76. Fayad L, Rosenthal E, Morrison W, Carrino J. Anterior cruciate ligament volume: analysis of sex differences. *J Magn Reson Imag.* 2008;27:218−223.

77. Shelbourne KD, Facibene WA, Hunt JJ. Radiographic and intraoperative intercondylar notch width measurements in males and female with unilateral and bilateral anterior cruciate ligament tears. *Knee Surg Sports Traumatol Arthrosc.* 1997;5:229−233.

78. Shultz SJ, Shimokochi Y, Nguyen AD, Schmitz RJ, Beynnon BD, Perrin DH. Measurement of varus-valgus and internal-external rotational knee laxities in vivo—part II: relationship with anterior-posterior and general joint laxity in males and females. *J Orthop Res.* 2007; 25(8):989−996.

79. Scerpella TA, Stayer TJ, Makhuli BZ. Ligamentous 988. laxity and non-contact anterior cruciate ligament tears: a sex based comparison. *Orthopaedics.* 2005;28:656−660.

80. Larsson LG, Baum J, Mudholkar GS. Hypermobility: features and differential incidence between the sexes. *Arthritis Rheum.* 1987;30:1426−1430.

81. Chung JH, Ryu KJ, Lee DH, et al. An analysis of normative data on the knee rotatory profile and the usefulness of the Rotatometer, a new instrument for measuring tibiofemoral rotation: the reliability of the knee Rotatometer. *Knee Surg Sports Traumatol Arthrosc.* 2015;23(9): 2727−2733.

82. Hsu W, Fisk JA, Yamamoto Y, et al. Differences in torsional joint stiffness of the knee between sexes: a human cadaveric study. *Am J Sports Med.* 2006;34:765−770.

83. Boguszewski D, Cheung E, Joshi N, Markolf K, McAllister D. Male-female differences in knee laxity and stiffness a cadaveric study. *Am J Sports Med.* October 13, 2015;43(12):2982−2987.

84. Chappell JD, Yu B, Kirkendall DT, Garrett WE. A comparison of knee kinetics between male and female recreational athletes in stop-jump tasks. *Am J Sports Med.* 2002;30:261−267.

85. Hutchinson MR, Ireland ML. Knee injuries in female athletes. *Sports Med.* 1995;19:288−302.

86. Rozzi SL, Lephart SM, Gear WS, et al. Knee joint laxity and neuromuscular characteristics of male and female soccer and basketball players. *Am J Sports Med.* 1999;27: 312−319.

87. Rosene JM, Fogarty TD. Anterior tibial translation in collegiate athletes with normal anterior cruciate ligament integrity. *J Athl Train.* 1999;34:93−98.

88. Shultz SJ, Kirk SE, Sander TC, et al. Sex differences in knee laxity change across the female menstrual cycle. *J Sports Med Phys Fitness.* 2005;45:594−603.

89. Beynnon BD, Bernstein I, Belisle A, et al. The effect of estradiol and progesterone on knee and ankle joint laxity. *Am J Sports Med.* 2005;33(9):1298−1304.

90. Uhorchak JM, Scoville CR, Williams GN, et al. Risk factors associated with non-contact injury of the anterior cruciate ligament. *Am J Sports Med.* 2003;31:831−842.

91. Liu SH, Al-Shaikh R, Panossian V, et al. Primary immunolocalization of estrogen and progesterone target cells in the human anterior cruciate ligament. *J Orthop Res.* 1996;14:526−533.

92. Daniel DM, Malcom LL, Losse G, et al. Instrumented measurement of anterior laxity of the knee. *J Bone Joint Surg.* 1985;67A:720−726.

93. Weesner CL, Albohm MJ, Ritter MA. A comparison of anterior and posterior cruciate ligament laxity between female and male basketball players. *Physician Sportsmed.* 1986;14(5):149−154.

94. Stone K, Freyer A, Turek T, Walgenback AW, Wadhwa S, Crues J. Meniscal sizing based on sex, height and weight. *Arthroscopy.* May 2007;23(5):503−508.

95. Huston LJ, Wojtys EM. Neuromuscular performance characteristics in elite female athletes. *Am J Sports Med.* 1996;24:427−436.

96. Hewett TE, Myer GD, Zazulak BT. Hamstrings to quadriceps peak torque ratios diverge between sexes with increasing isokinetic angular velocity. *J Sci Med Sport.* September 2008;11(5):452−459. Epub 2007 Sep. 17.

97. Fithian DC, Paxton EW, Stone ML. Epidemiology and natural history of acute patellar dislocation. *Am J Sports Med.* 2004;32:1114−1121.

98. Hewett TE. Biomechanical measures of neuromuscular control and valgus loading of the knee predict anterior cruciate ligament injury risk in female athletes: a prospective study. *Am J Sports Med.* 2005;33:492−501. https://doi.org/10.1177/0363546504269591.

99. Hewett TE, Myer GD, Ford KR. Anterior cruciate ligament injuries in female athletes: part 1, mechanisms and risk factors. *Am J Sports Med.* 2006;34:299−311. https://doi.org/10.1177/0363546505284183.

100. Westin BS, Noyes F, Galloway M. Jump-land characteristics and muscle strength development in young athletes. A sex comparison of 1140 athletes 9-17 years of age. *Am J Sports Med.* 2006;34(3).

101. Myer GD, Ford KR, Divine JG, Wall EJ, Kahanov L, Hewett TE. Longitudinal assessment of noncontact anterior cruciate ligament injury risk factors during maturation in a female athlete: a case report. *J Athl Train.* 2009;44:101−109. https://doi.org/10.4085/1062-6050-44.1.101.

102. Hopper AJ, Haff EE, Joyc C, Lloyd RS, Haff GG. Neuromuscular training improves lower extremity biomechanics associated with knee injury during landing in 11−13 year old female netball athletes: a randomized control study. *Front Physiol.* 07 November 2017:883.

103. Myer GD, Sugimoto D, Thomas S, Hewett TE. The influence of age on the effectiveness of neuromuscular training to reduce anterior cruciate ligament injury in female athletes: a meta-analysis. *Am J Sports Med.* 2013;41:203−215. https://doi.org/10.1177/0363546512460637.

104. Myer GD, Ford KR, Palumbo JP, Hewett TE. Neuromuscular training improves performance and lower extremity biomechanics in female athletes. *J Strength Cond Res.* 2005;19:51−60. https://doi.org/10.1519/13643.1.

105. Pfile KR, Hart JM, Herman DC, Hertel J, Kerrigan DC, Ingersoll CD. Different exercise training interventions and drop-landing biomechanics in high school female athletes. *J Athl Train.* 2013;48:450−462. https://doi.org/10.4085/1062-6050-48.4.06.

106. Noyes FR, Barber-Westin SD, Fleckenstein C, Walsh C, West J. The drop-jump screening test: difference in lower limb control by sex and effect of neuromuscular training in female athletes. *Am J Sports Med.* 2005;33:197−207.

107. Hewett TE, Stroupe AL, Nance TA, Noyes FR. Plyometric training in female athletes: decreased impact forces and increased hamstring torques. *Am J Sports Med.* 1996;24:765−773.

108. Huston LJ, Vibert B, Ashton-Miller JA, Wojtys EM. Sex differences in knee angle when landing from a drop-jump. *Am J Knee Surg.* 2001;14:215−219.

109. Prapavessis H, McNair PJ. Effects of instruction in jumping technique and experience jumping on ground reaction forces. *J Orthop Sports Phys Ther.* 1999;29:352−356.

CHAPTER 2

Anterior Cruciate Ligament Injury in the Female Athlete

ERIKA L. VALENTINE, MD • NICOLE A. FRIEL, MD, MS

INTRODUCTION

Anterior cruciate ligament (ACL) injuries are one of the most common injuries seen by orthopedic surgeons and sports medicine specialists. Annually in the United States, there are 68.6 isolated ACL tears per 100,000 person-years.[1] Worldwide there are roughly 1.4 million noncontact ACL tears annually.[2] The ACL is subject to injury most commonly in sports that require movements such as cutting, pivoting, and jumping. These are significant injuries for both recreational and elite athletes alike, and these are associated with delayed recovery and/or inability to return to sport. In addition to the initial acute loss of function, even when the ACL is reconstructed the player then has a predisposition to early-onset osteoarthritis.[3]

The highest incidence of ACL tears overall occurs in teenage female athletes. Age-specific patterns differ between males and females, with a peak incidence in males between 19 and 25 years of age (241.0 per 100,000) and the peak incidence in females between 14 and 18 years of age (227.6 per 100,000).[1]

In the past 30 years, there has been a 10-fold increase in high-school and a 5-fold increase in collegiate sports participation by females.[4,5] As the number of females participating in high-level sports continues to increase since the passage of Title IX in 1972, the prevalence of ACL injuries is expected to increase as well. Prior to Title IX, fewer than 10,000 female athletes competed in collegiate sports. More recently, in the 2016–17 academic year, it was reported that there were a record-setting 494,992 collegiate athletes. In 2018, there were 10,586 women's teams and 9159 men's teams competing in the NCAA (National Collegiate Athletic Association) championship sports.[4]

Although there is an overall higher number of ACL tears among male athletes than females, female athletes have a higher incidence rate of ACL injury. Multiple studies have shown that the relative risk of ACL injury in female athletes, compared to male athletes, is roughly 1.40–9.74.[6,7] Females in the military have been reported to have a relative risk of ACL injury of 2.44 when compared to males.[6]

The increased incidence of ACL injuries in female athletes is most likely multivariate, stemming from mechanical, endocrinologic, and psychologic factors.

MECHANICAL FACTORS

Anatomically, the ACL is made up of two bands, the anteromedial and posterolateral, and extends from the region anterior to the tibial intercondylar eminence to the medial portion of the lateral femoral condyle. It works in conjunction with the surrounding muscles to stabilize the knee. With the knee in extension the posterolateral band is the tightest, and during knee flexion the anteromedial band is the tightest.[8] During weight bearing, the ACL prevents the tibia from translating anteriorly. During flexion and extension moments, it works with the posterior cruciate ligament to control movement of the femur on the tibia. It also provides stabilization during internal rotation moments of the tibia and during varus and valgus stresses of the knee joint.[9]

The miserable malalignment syndrome, consisting of a high quadriceps angle (Q-angle), increased pelvic width, anteverted femur, valgus knee, tibial external rotation, and pronated foot, is related to ACL injury.[10] (Fig. 2.1) Together, these individual factors create an environment that encourages extensor mechanism malalignment. This places strain on the patellofemoral joint and ultimately leads to pain. In 2003, Uhorchak et al.[11] showed that other significant risk factors for ACL injury, aside from the miserable malalignment syndrome, include a small femoral notch width, generalized joint laxity, higher than normal body mass index, and anterior to posterior knee laxity values that were one standard deviation or more above the mean. This

The Female Athlete. https://doi.org/10.1016/B978-0-323-75985-4.00022-2

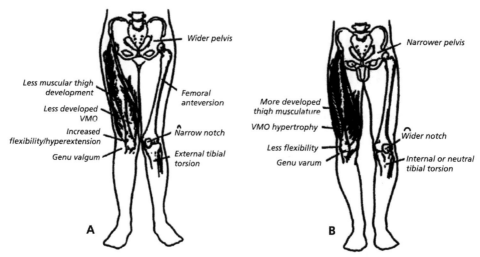

FIG. 2.1 Gender differences between **(A)** females and **(B)** males that can predispose athletes to anterior cruciate ligament injuries, as well as other lower extremity pathology. *VMO*, vastus medialis oblique. (Printed with permission from Fu F, Stone DA. 1984. Permission from publisher pending.)

was further characterized in 2018 in a retrospective study that used magnetic resonance imaging (MRI) to look at anatomic risk factors associated with ACL injury. The group of ACL-injured patients was found to have a more narrow femoral intercondylar notch width index (<0.252), a larger β-angle (>38.5 degrees), and a larger lateral tibial slope (>7.5 degrees).[12]

Femoral notch width and shape is related to the risk of ACL injury. van Eck et al. suggested that ACL injury is associated with the shape of the notch. Using arthroscopy, the authors defined three different notch shapes, which included A-shape, U-shape, and W-shape. Notches with an A-shape were found to be narrower in all width dimensions than the U-shaped variety. Patient height was correlated with notch shape, and there was a positive association with tall height and U-shaped and W-shaped notches. Females were found to have smaller notch widths at the base and in the middle.[13]

A valgus knee is often implicated in knee injuries. Three-dimensional kinematic analyses have shown that while jumping, female athletes have a higher amount of knee valgus. A prospective study assessed 291 female high-school athletes newly enrolled in basketball and handball. They analyzed dynamic knee valgus during single-leg drop jumps. The participants were then followed up for 3 years specifically looking for ACL injury. In the injured group, there was a significantly greater amount of dynamic knee valgus. They concluded that dynamic knee valgus is a risk factor for noncontact ACL injuries in female high-school athletes.[14]

A person's Q-angle is the angle that is formed from the combined vectors for the pull of the quadriceps muscle and the patellar tendon.[15] The average Q-angle in uninjured males is 12.1 degrees, and 16.7 degrees in uninjured females. This higher Q-angle in females increases the lateral pull of the quadriceps on the patella and potentiates disorders of the knee.[16] Q-angles exceeding 15 degrees in males and 20 degrees in females are considered to be abnormal.[17] An increased Q-angle may contribute to an increased risk for ACL injury by increasing the obliquity of the femur, increasing the knee valgus, and thus increasing the contact pressure applied to the patellofemoral joint. The ligament is under varying degrees of tension throughout all movements. There have been multiple studies that sought to establish an association between knee injury and Q-angle. Two of them showed that there was not a significant association.[18,19] However, there have been a couple of other studies that did note an association between Q-angle and increased risk for knee injury.[16,20] The opposing outcomes of these studies raise the question of how much a Q-angle measured in a static position correlates to dynamic motion such as in sports. When looking at collegiate basketball players, there was a significant difference in Q-angles between males and females, especially when measuring with the knee in 30 degrees in flexion.[20] This is clinically relevant, because Xerogeanes et al.[21] have shown that the greatest magnitudes of force on the ACL are incurred with the knee in 30 degrees of flexion. Thus having a larger Q-angle in this position is not favorable. This is likely multifactorial considering that Emami et al.[16] also found that 16% of the males and 20% of the females who had an abnormally high Q-angle did not present with a knee injury.

Q-angle has also been associated with a larger moment of tibial internal rotation.[22] Internal rotation of the tibia affects tibiofemoral contact forces and the force seen by the ACL during impact. In model simulations, it has been shown that ACL forces were highly correlated with contact forces on the anterior component of the tibiofemoral joint during impacts with larger knee abduction moments, internal tibial rotation, and larger contact forces.[23]

In animal models, hamstring (HS) contraction helps resist anterior tibial shear force at 30 degrees in flexion, which reduces the amount of force on the ACL.[24] This has also been shown in human subjects.[25,26] Activation of the quadriceps had the most significant effect on ACL strain.[27] The HSs are activated independently from the quadriceps, and they act as a protagonist force to the ACL. When the HSs contract, they decrease the amount of anterior tibial translation and internal tibial rotation. They also reduce tension on the ACL, with the knee between 15 and 45 degrees of flexion.[28]

When the pelvis is examined, females have a relatively wider and/or different shaped pelvis compared with males.[29] Several authors have found a significant association between pelvic width and the risk of knee injuries in females. The structural differences of the wider pelvis in females are thought to increase the risk of knee injury by creating a larger coxa vara/genu valgum alignment, with a simultaneous increase in tibiofemoral rotation forces in the transverse plane, which ultimately places a greater force onto the ACL.[26,30] With the hip being the most proximal link in the lower extremity, excessive hip adduction and internal rotation while weight bearing affects the kinematics of the entire extremity below it. Hip adduction and internal rotation can cause the mechanical axis of the knee to move medially and results in dynamic knee valgus.

In addition to laxity of the knee, females also demonstrate increased joint laxity of the foot. Excessive pronation in the subtalar joint has been found to be common in the American population. This increase in ligamentous laxity of the foot has been brought up as a potential cause for increased navicular drop in females. Patients with an increased amount of pronation have been found to have an increased amount of knee rotation when the knee is flexed to 5 degrees.[31] In the stance phase of the gait cycle, subtalar pronation and internal rotation of the tibia occur simultaneously and the ACL becomes taut as the tibia rotates.[32]

Navicular drop has been reported as a significant predictor of tibial translation by Trimble et al. They also suggested there was a relationship between increased subtalar joint pronation and increased anterior translation of the tibia. When increased navicular drop causes the tibia to move forward, this would ultimately place an increased amount of strain on the ACL.[33] A couple groups have in fact shown that there was an association between increased subtalar joint pronation and ACL injury.[19] They measured the navicular drop height from seated to standing in 22 athletes with an injured ACL and 22 control subjects with an uninjured ACL. What they found was that the subjects with an uninjured ACL dropped an average of 5.9 mm and the ACL-injured subjects dropped an average of 8.4 mm, which was statistically significant.[32]

As early as 1982, differences in the transverse plane, in the form of femoral anteversion, have been discussed as a factor in ACL injuries.[34] Greater femoral anteversion (as seen in females compared to males) as well as a smaller pelvic angle have been found to be a predictor of greater hip internal rotation and knee excursion.[35] It is these motions, as described in this chapter, that play a significant role in the higher incidence of ACL injuries in female athletes.

There are likely multiple mechanical variables that factor into the increased ACL injury risk for females, as discussed earlier. One of the functions of the ACL is to prevent internal rotation of the tibia. When the knee is at 30 degrees of flexion, there is an increase in tibial internal rotation. At this position, there is also a decrease in the HSs-to-eccentric quadriceps strength ratio. This means that during deceleration with the knee at 30 degrees of flexion the joint is taking on two simultaneous forces that compromise the ACL.[33]

Many of the forces on the knee and the ACL are easiest to describe in a static state. However, it is more realistic to think about forces during a dynamic movement. Motion perturbations (contact with another player) also likely have a role in altering the biomechanics associated with ACL injuries. During videographic and biomechanical analysis, it has been shown that motion perturbation changes an athlete's coordination and movement. When looking at a group of injured basketball players, they all sustained their injuries while handling the ball and within the first 0−3 steps.[36] During side-cutting in the presence of a nearby opponent, females were found to have greater amount of knee valgus, greater variability in knee valgus, an increase in foot pronation angles, and increased tibial internal rotation. Looking at hip biomechanics, females also had a decreased amount of hip and knee flexion as well as hip abduction during cutting.[37] These results combined suggest that the dynamic lower extremity biomechanical changes at the hips, knees, and ankles play a significant role in the higher rate of ACL injuries seen in female athletes.

Biomechanical differences between genders, as described earlier, are further exacerbated by muscular fatigue. This increases the alterations in the trunk, pelvis, and lower extremity kinematics involved in injuries to the ACL. As shown in a study, when landing from a single-leg drop after being fatigued, males had a greater amount of trunk flexion than females. Males also had a decrease in peak knee flexion and a higher amount of gluteus maximus and biceps femoris activation than their female counterparts.[38]

NEUROMUSCULAR FACTORS

There are many systems within the human body that operate automatically and subconsciously to maintain the body in its homeostatic state. One of these systems is the sensorimotor system, which incorporates all the afferent, efferent, and central integrating and processing components that are involved in providing functional joint stability during motion. A prior study showed that mechanoreceptor density in the ACL is highest at its most proximal and distal osseous attachments.[39] About 1% of the ligament's dry weight is made up of neural tissue.[40]

A neurologic link between the cerebral cortex and the ACL has been documented using electroencephalographic signals by stimulating the ACL during arthroscopy.[41] Following an injury to the ACL, multiple sensorimotor impairments may occur. These include proprioceptive deficits,[42] decreased strength of the stabilizing muscles of the knee, and alterations in muscle activation onset patterns.[43]

One proposed method to reduce ACL injuries is to implement a neuromuscular training regimen into adolescent female athlete training programs. In a large study looking at 23,554 female athletes, four variables were found to reduce ACL injury risk. The variables included a younger participant age, neuromuscular training performed for at least 20 min and at least twice per week, a greater number of exercise variations, and more usage of verbal feedback.[44]

ENDOCRINOLOGIC FACTORS

A higher magnitude of knee joint laxity has been seen in females[45] and has also been associated with a higher risk of ACL injury.[46] There is a known correlation between estrogen and ACL laxity, as well as progesterone levels and ACL laxity. As the concentration of the hormones in the serum increases, so does ACL laxity (measured using a knee arthrometer).[47] Estrogen concentrations in the blood fluctuate substantially during the menstrual cycle. Musculoskeletal function is closely related to estrogen concentrations. Estrogen works to improve muscle protein homeostasis and increases collagen content. These physiologic effects of estrogen have been shown to contribute to decrease in power and performance, which makes females more prone for injury.[48]

It has been shown that females have about 25% overall decreased stiffness of the knee, 30% greater frontal plane (varus-valgus) knee laxity, and about 35% greater transverse plane (internal and external rotation) knee laxity compared with males.[49] The previously described joint laxities that are greater in the frontal and transverse planes occur in females during low, externally applied loads and are most pronounced during initial loading of the knee joint.[50]

Shultz et al. showed that females experience larger cyclic variations in anterior knee laxity, genu recurvatum, and generalized joint laxity compared with frontal and transverse plane laxity and stiffness. In addition, females have significantly greater overall transverse and frontal plane laxity and lower stiffness when than males.[51] One study used the KT-1000 arthrometer to measure anterior-posterior knee laxity throughout the menstrual cycle and found that the fluctuations in cyclic estrogen and progesterone levels during menstruation do not have a defined relationship with anterior-posterior laxity of the knee joint.[52] In another study by the same author, a case-control study of recreational alpine skiers was performed and it was found that the likelihood of sustaining an injury to the ACL fluctuates during the menstrual cycle. The risk of sustaining a disruption of the ACL is significantly greater during the preovulatory phase than the postovulatory phase.[45]

Estrogen receptors are present in all musculoskeletal tissues, including ligament. Immunohistochemical localization was performed in 17 human specimens and showed that both estrogen and progesterone receptors were localized to fibroblasts in the ACL stroma and cells in the blood vessel walls of the ligament. These estrogen receptors have a relationship with the ACL and most likely have a periodic effect on ligament laxity.[53] Acute cyclic variations in the menstruating female athlete have been shown to cause physiologic changes in fibroblast proliferation and procollagen synthesis, which are markers of collagen synthesis. During days of high estradiol concentration (days 1 and 3 of the

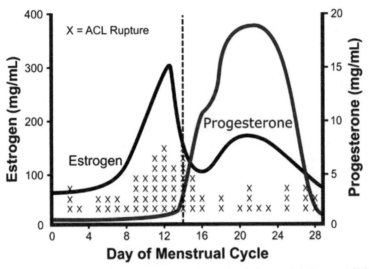

FIG. 2.2 The relationship between estrogen concentration and anterior cruciate ligament (ACL) rupture in a normal menstrual cycle. There is a correlation between the rise of the concentration of estrogen and the timing of the majority of ACL ruptures in this study. (Pending permission from Wojtys EM, Huston LJ, Boynton MD, Spindler KP, Lindenfeld TN. The effect of the menstrual cycle on anterior cruciate ligament injuries in women as determined by hormone levels. *Am J Sports Med.* April 2002;30(2):182–188.)

menstrual cycle), subjects have been found to have a decreased amount of fibroblast proliferation. During days 7, 10, and 14 of the menstrual cycle, this effect was attenuated.[54]

Multiple studies have shown a statistically significant association between noncontact ACL injury and the phases of the menstrual cycle. There is a significant increase in injuries in teenage female athletes during the ovulatory phase when compared to the other phases[55–57] (Fig. 2.2). It has even been shown that there is more laxity in the ankle joint during ovulation.[51]

There is limited evidence that suggests oral contraceptive use in females may reduce the risk of injury to the ACL. However, there has yet to be any conclusion drawn regarding differences in ACL injury risk among oral contraceptive users and nonusers throughout different points of the menstrual cycle.[2]

GENETIC FACTORS
If one could predict an individuals' risk for injury based on genomic testing, this would allow for identified predisposed athletes to undergo more specific prevention programs and perhaps guide future treatment technologies. It is known that type V collagen plays a crucial role in the regulation of size and structure of other fibrillar collagens that support many tissues in the body, which include ligaments such as the ACL. This collagen is

coded by the COL5A1 gene, which is located on chromosome 9q34.3.[58] Mutations of this gene result in a 50% reduction in the quantity of type V collagen, which leads to poorly organized fibrils, decreased tensile strength, and reduced stiffness of connective tissue.[59] Prior studies have shown variants of multiple DNA genes that have been associated with an increased propensity for ACL injury. These include COL1A1, COL3A1, COL5A1, COL12A1, ELN, FBN2, matrix metalloproteinase, and genes encoding multiple proteoglycans.[60–64]

While the aforementioned genes have been associated with ligamentous injury risk, there has not been translational work performed to figure out how to modify them. However, with the information we do have at this time, athletes and trainers theoretically are able to figure out those athletes who are most at risk for ACL injury and to work toward prevention.

PSYCHOLOGIC FACTORS
Elite athlete training requires special consideration. Performance efforts in high-intensity sports are defined by explosive strength and speed. Athletes use their mental fortitude to push past physical limits and commit to difficult goals and exceptional performance. Injury in these athletes is a stressful and adverse event. To improve the efforts of prevention and management of

sports injuries among athletes, it is important to focus on athlete health and performance outcomes as well as psychologic factors. Career longevity and performance depend on both physical and mental health. Psychology and socioculture are both involved in sports injury risk, response, and recovery.[65]

It has been shown that an individual's expectations, motivation, and satisfaction before, during, and after rehabilitation after ACL reconstruction are associated with return to preinjury sport activity at 1-year follow-up. Prior to ACL reconstruction, most patients expect to return to their preinjury activity level. One study included 65 individuals (male and female) who underwent ACL reconstruction. Those who returned to their preinjury sport level were found to have been more motivated during rehabilitation. They were also more satisfied with their activity level and knee function at 1-syear follow-up. The authors concluded that facilitating motivation may be important to support individuals in achieving their goals after ACL reconstruction.[66]

When looking at female football players with ACL injuries who underwent reconstruction, there were three core themes of psychosocial factors that characterized their resilience during rehabilitation. Those three cores were constructive communication and rich interaction with significant others, strong belief in the important and efficacy of one's own actions, and the ability to set reasonable goals.[67] These findings are the start of a conversation regarding how coaches and athletic trainers can facilitate and optimize their athletes' return to sport.

Continuing efforts in researching and protecting athletes' physical and mental health are necessary in preventing and rehabbing injuries such as ACL tears.

Other proposed mechanisms of increased ACL injury risk include the weather conditions and type of ground surface, both of which equate to the quality of interactions between the player and the ground. A study out of Australia found that low water evaporation and high rainfall significantly lowered the risk of ACL injuries in the sport of football. The proposed mechanism is that the ground softens and the shoe-surface traction is decreased as a result. They suggested that consistent extra watering and covering of grounds during periods of high water evaporation may lower ACL injury rates.[68]

PREVENTION

A recent emphasis on preventing ACL injuries has been highlighted. With the identification of specific risk factors for ACL injury, rather than intervene on an entire population, athletes who are predisposed could undergo targeted intervention.

The idea of prophylactic knee bracing and its effect is controversial. Looking retrospectively at a group of athletes, 2% of their acquired ACL injuries occurred while the affected leg was braced.[69] When assessing six different brace designs for patients with ACL deficiency and chronic instability, anterior tibial translation and neuromuscular function have been questioned. Bracing in these ACL-injured subjects was shown to decrease anterior tibial translation by 29–39% without accounting for the activation and stabilization provided by the surrounding muscles. When bracing and muscle activation were combined, anterior tibial translation was found to decrease between 70% and 85%. Notably, the study also did find that the braces caused a decrease in the HS muscle reaction times.[70]

Sports-related injuries can be minimized with comprehensive injury prevention training, which includes plyometrics, agility, and balance. Trunk control is a significant pillar of this concept. To examine the isolated effects of core muscle training on lower body neuromuscular control and biomechanics, female collegiate basketball players in Japan were split into two groups. One group underwent core muscle training, while the other group underwent standard training for 8 weeks. When three-dimensional hip, knee, and trunk mechanics were measured at the posttraining phase, there were significant differences between the two groups. During the drop-jump test and the single-leg squat, the maximum trunk-flexion angle increased and the peak knee valgus moment decreased in the core training group. These alterations in neuromuscular control and biomechanics would be favorable in the prevention of sports-related knee injuries.[71]

RECONSTRUCTION

ACL reconstruction is the typical management of ACL injuries. It has been estimated that in the United States, 90% of patients who sustain an ACL injury eventually undergo reconstruction.[72] The rate at which ACL reconstruction is successful in restoring knee stability and patient satisfaction is 90%.[73] In both adults and the pediatric population, it is common for ACL injuries to be further complicated by meniscus or cartilage damage. When left untreated, ACL deficiency can lead to recurrent instability and medial meniscal damage. This subsequently predisposes a patient to radiographic signs of osteoarthritis.[74] The likelihood that they will be symptomatic enough to eventually require a total knee replacement is quoted to be as high as five times as much when compared to non-ACL-injured patients.[75] The appropriate treatment in a timely manner is crucial to patient outcome. Depending on the patient, the treatment options are conservative or surgical in nature. Conservative treatment entails focusing on the prevention of further episodes of instability, which likely involves lifestyle changes and activity modifications.[76]

A study out of Canada looked to assess the association between the time from ACL injury to ACL reconstruction. Consistent with prior studies, the study found that increases in time to reconstruction were associated with medial meniscal tears, irreparable medial meniscal tears, medial femoral condyle damage, and early medial compartment degenerative changes at the time of reconstruction. However, increases in the time to surgery were not found to be associated with degenerative changes of the lateral or patellofemoral compartments of the knee.[77] Some studies report that patients have a higher incidence of subsequent intra-articular pathology when they are 12 months or more out from injury.[78−81]

Notably, one study has found that intra-articular pathology can be associated as early as 3 months following injury.[82]

While there are many differences in the implications of an ACL injury in males versus females, significant differences in surgical techniques have not been established. The optimal choice of graft tissue for ACL reconstruction remains a topic of ongoing debate. There is even less consensus regarding graft choice in young, female athletes. Salem et al.[83] reviewed the outcomes of two different age groups undergoing ACL reconstruction. In females aged 15−20 years undergoing ACL reconstruction, the bone-patellar tendon-bone (BPTB) autograft may lead to fewer graft ruptures than HS autograft. This difference was not observed in females aged 21−25 years. Important to note, however, is that BPTB autograft significantly increased the risk of kneeling pain as compared with HS, regardless of age. Similarly, in a smaller patient cohort, Shakked et al.[84] found that there were significantly fewer subsequent procedures and a lower rate of graft failures in the BPTB group than the HS group. On the contrary, Kautzner et al.[85] concluded that graft choice for reconstruction in female patients should be surgeon specific and individualized, as both grafts studied achieved comparable results.

OUTCOMES AFTER RECONSTRUCTION

Overall, ACL reconstruction is a reliable surgery with successful clinical outcomes. However, it has been shown that it does not restore normal knee kinematics during gait. In the transverse plane, it has been shown that there are differences in tibial rotation during the gait cycle in ACL-reconstructed knees when compared to a patient's contralateral knee. When comparing graft type, there is a reduced amount of knee varus in the HS group after reconstruction, which may relate to the graft harvest. The HS group also had a reduction in the amount of internal tibial rotation postoperatively. These alterations in the joint kinematics could be an important factor in the increased incidence of osteoarthritis of the knee after reconstruction.[86] The identification of modifiable risk factors that affect outcomes would provide future interventions to improve ACL reconstruction. Some of those that have been identified are body mass index, smoking status, allograft, and lateral meniscus pathology.[87] Lower socioeconomic status has been associated with worse patient reported outcomes after many orthopedic procedures. ACL reconstruction is one of those procedures. Given that a large proportion of the ACL reconstructions performed in the United States are of children, different factors have to be taken into account. It has been demonstrated that lower neighborhood socioeconomic status is associated with worse patient reported outcomes after ACL reconstruction and that the patient's age and education have a significant interaction in a younger population.[88]

When evaluating the success of ACL reconstruction surgery, return to sport is an important outcome. One important end-stage outcome for athletes is being able to play their sport specifically at preinjury levels of performance. This decision is made on a regular basis by surgeons, athletes, and coaches. Defining return to sport is a continuum and includes return to participation, return to sport, and return to performance.[89] Progressions in postoperative management have been made possible because of the advances in techniques and protocols. When the ACL is reconstructed without other pathologic conditions, it is currently standard to let the patient weight-bear immediately. About 67% of surgeons stated they allow patients to return to sport between 6 and 9 months, and 94% stated they allowed patients to return to sport between 6 and 12 months. About 84% of surgeons used braces postoperatively, and 48% used braces after return to sport.[90]

Overall, females are less likely to return to their preinjury sport level, or even return to any sport, after an ACL injury and reconstruction. In a meta-analysis of 69 published articles that reported return-to-sport outcomes postoperatively, there were two primary factors that favored return to sport: younger age and male gender. On average, 75% of females compared to 80% of males returned to any sport. About 52% of females returned to preinjury levels of sport, compared with 61% of males. About 68% of females returned to competitive level sport, compared with 78% of males.[91]

In a cohort of 222 patients in Australia who had ACL reconstruction and completed a 12-month postoperative assessment, along with follow-up of at least 2 years, 61% of patients reported that they had returned to their preinjury level of performance. There was not a significant difference between males and females, with 59% of males and 63% of females reporting preinjury level of performance. The investigators did find a significant association with return to sport and higher psychologic readiness, greater limb symmetry, higher subjective knee scores, and a higher activity level. However, when they looked at the multivariate model, psychologic readiness was the only variable that remained a significant predictor.[92]

After ACL injury, female athletes have a poorer functional recovery than males. Studies have shown that they also have lower activity levels than males at both 2 and 6 years after reconstruction.[87] When females do return to sport, statistics show that they are more likely than males to sustain a second ACL injury. Patients of both genders who underwent reconstruction are roughly six times more likely to sustain an ACL injury within the first 2 years after returning to sport. After reconstruction, female athletes were almost five times more likely to sustain another ACL injury than females without any history of ACL injury. About 30% of athletes who underwent reconstruction and then returned to cutting and pivoting sports sustained a second ACL injury within 2 years after reconstruction and returning to sport. Of those patients who did sustain a second ACL injury, there was no significant difference between the times to return to sport.[93]

In a randomized controlled trial out of the University of Delaware, 40 females 3–9 months after primary ACL reconstruction were randomized to 10 strength, agility, plyometrics, and secondary prevention (SAPP) exercises with or without perturbation training. They found that the perturbation training provided no added benefit. However, among young, high-level female athletes who have undergone ACL reconstruction, 10 sessions of return-to-sport training, compared with criterion-based postoperative rehab alone, yielded statistically significant and clinically meaningful higher 2-year functional outcomes.[94]

Following ACL reconstruction, it has been suggested that knee proprioception returns to normal. The amount of time it takes to get back to a normal baseline has been a recent question. Past studies had reported that it took 12 months to regain normal sensorimotor function. One of those studies compared males and females postoperatively and found that by the 12-month mark after surgery, patients had recovered their sagittal plane alignment (knee flexion angle and extension moment) equally in both genders.

Overall, the literature has been somewhat conflicting when looking at return of proprioception and the type of ACL reconstruction performed. When comparing ACL reconstruction using HSs or BPTB autograft, one study found that there is no statistically significant difference in postoperative knee proprioception at any time point up to 12 months.[42] Yet, others have suggested that the type of reconstruction may be an important factor in the impairment of sensorimotor control. It has been reported that the semitendinosus and the gracilis tendons regenerate after being harvested for ACL reconstruction. Using postoperative MRI, one group found that the semitendinosus tendon is regenerated at or below the joint line, and no gracilis tendon was observed below the joint line. Yet, the ACL-reconstructed knees, when compared to the healthy knees, had no significant difference in HS muscle activation during and after knee flexion. Their results indicated that both the semitendinosus and the gracilis muscles were highly recruited during flexion of the knee regardless of the amount of tendon regeneration.[95] A group out of Italy looked at postoperative sensorimotor control after ACL reconstruction. When they compared results between HS tendon and the BPTB groups, they found that between 6 and 12 months after surgery there was no significant difference in steadiness and onset of muscle activation. There was also no significant difference between those who underwent reconstruction and the uninjured control group.[96] When combining all these studies and data, it appears as though the selected surgical approach for ACL reconstruction does not affect the knee joint sensorimotor function to a significant degree. Further research would be necessary to further characterize this by gender.

Compared to healthy individuals, patients who have undergone ACL reconstruction have also been found to have diminished quadriceps submaximal force control, which is reflective of their medial quadriceps and HS altered muscular activity patterns and deficits in coordination.[43] In addition, the knee adduction moment has been shown to be increased following ACL reconstruction surgery. One study found that the knee adduction moment was 23% greater in females than in males, where both had undergone reconstructions. This higher knee adduction moment seen in females may suggest an increased risk of developing osteoarthritis in ACL-reconstructed females down the road.[97]

As discussed earlier in this chapter, the use of preinjury braces in athletes is controversial.

Functional bracing after ACL reconstruction surgery and its effect on graft reinjury rates is also a topic of debate. In one prospective, randomized, multicenter study, athletes were randomized into two groups postoperatively: braced and nonbraced. After reconstruction the braced group wore a functional knee brace on the affected limb for 1 year during all activities that involved jumping, pivoting, and/or cutting. The nonbraced group did not use any brace for these activities. The investigators found that there were no significant differences between the two groups in regard to stability or function of the knee, range of motion, strength of the knee, or subjective knee scores, which suggests that bracing postoperatively does not change outcomes and is not recommended.[98]

REFERENCES

1. Sanders TL, Maradit Kremers H, Bryan AJ, et al. Incidence of anterior cruciate ligament tears and reconstruction: a 21-year population-based study. *Am J Sports Med*. June 2016;44(6):1502—1507.
2. Samuelson K, Balk EM, Sevetson EL, Fleming BC. Limited evidence suggests a protective association between oral contraceptive pill use and anterior cruciate ligament injuries in females: a systematic review. *Sports Health*. December 2017;9(6):498—510.
3. Graham GP, Fairclough JA. Early osteoarthritis in young sportsmen with severe anterolateral instability of the knee. *Injury*. July 1988;19(4):247—248.
4. smeyers@ncaa.org. *Number of NCAA College Athletes Reaches All-Time High*. NCAA.org - The Official Site of the NCAA; 2018. Available from: http://www.ncaa.org/about/resources/media-center/news/number-ncaa-college-athletes-reaches-all-time-high.
5. National Federation of State High School Associations. *High School Participation Survey Archive*; 2019. Available from: https://www.nfhs.org/sports-resource-content/high-school-participation-survey-archive/.
6. Gwinn DE, Wilckens JH, McDevitt ER, Ross G, Kao TC. The relative incidence of anterior cruciate ligament injury in men and women at the United States Naval Academy. *Am J Sports Med*. February 2000;28(1):98—102.
7. Arendt EA, Agel J, Dick R. Anterior cruciate ligament injury patterns among collegiate men and women. *J Athl Train*. April 1999;34(2):86—92.
8. Moeller JL, Lamb MM. Anterior cruciate ligament injuries in female athletes: why are women more susceptible? *Phys Sportsmed*. April 1997;25(4):31—48.
9. Levangie PK, Norkin CC, eds. *Joint Structure and Function: A Comprehensive Analysis*. 5th ed. 2011, 624 p.
10. James S. Chondromalacia of the patella in the adolescent. In: Kennedy JC, ed. *The Injured Adolescent Knee*. Baltimore, MD: Williams and Wilkins; 1979:205—251.
11. Uhorchak JM, Scoville CR, Williams GN, Arciero RA, St Pierre P, Taylor DC. Risk factors associated with noncontact injury of the anterior cruciate ligament: a prospective four-year evaluation of 859 West Point cadets. *Am J Sports Med*. December 2003;31(6):831—842.
12. Shen L, Jin Z-G, Dong Q-R, Li L-B. Anatomical risk factors of anterior cruciate ligament injury. *Chin Med J (Engl)*. December 20, 2018;131(24):2960—2967.
13. van Eck CF, Martins CAQ, Vyas SM, Celentano U, van Dijk CN, Fu FH. Femoral intercondylar notch shape and dimensions in ACL-injured patients. *Knee Surg Sports Traumatol Arthrosc*. September 2010;18(9):1257—1262.
14. Numata H, Nakase J, Kitaoka K, et al. Two-dimensional motion analysis of dynamic knee valgus identifies female high school athletes at risk of non-contact anterior cruciate ligament injury. *Knee Surg Sports Traumatol Arthrosc*. February 2018;26(2):442—447.
15. Hungerford DS, Barry M. Biomechanics of the patellofemoral joint. *Clin Orthop*. October 1979;(144):9—15.
16. Emami M-J, Ghahramani M-H, Abdinejad F, Namazi H. Q-angle: an invaluable parameter for evaluation of anterior knee pain. *Arch Iran Med*. January 2007;10(1):24—26.
17. Horton MG, Hall TL. Quadriceps femoris muscle angle: normal values and relationships with gender and selected skeletal measures. *Phys Ther*. November 1989;69(11):897—901.
18. Mohamed EE, Useh U, Mtshali BF. Q-angle, Pelvic width, and Intercondylar notch width as predictors of knee injuries in women soccer players in South Africa. *Afr Health Sci*. June 2012;12(2):174—180.
19. Loudon JK, Jenkins W, Loudon KL. The relationship between static posture and ACL injury in female athletes. *J Orthop Sports Phys Ther*. August 1996;24(2):91—97.
20. Moul JL. Differences in selected predictors of anterior cruciate ligament tears between male and female NCAA division I collegiate basketball players. *J Athl Train*. April 1998;33(2):118—121.
21. Xerogeanes JW, Takeda Y, Livesay GA, et al. Effect of knee flexion on the in situ force distribution in the human anterior cruciate ligament. *Knee Surg Sports Traumatol Arthrosc*. 1995;3(1):9—13.
22. Hartley A. *Practical Joint Assessment: A Sports Medicine Manual*. St. Louis: Mosby-Year Book; 1991.
23. Navacchia A, Bates NA, Schilaty ND, Krych AJ, Hewett TE. Knee abduction and internal rotation moments increase ACL force during landing through the posterior slope of the tibia. *J Orthop Res Off Publ Orthop Res Soc*. August 2019;37(8):1730—1742.
24. Aune AK, Ekeland A, Nordsletten L. Effect of quadriceps or hamstring contraction on the anterior shear force to anterior cruciate ligament failure. An in vivo study in the rat. *Acta Orthop Scand*. June 1995;66(3):261—265.
25. Hewett TE, Myer GD, Ford KR. Decrease in neuromuscular control about the knee with maturation in female athletes. *J Bone Joint Surg Am*. August 2004;86(8):1601—1608.
26. Ireland ML. Anterior cruciate ligament injury in female athletes: epidemiology. *J Athl Train*. April 1999;34(2):150—154.

27. Dürselen L, Claes L, Kiefer H. The influence of muscle forces and external loads on cruciate ligament strain. *Am J Sports Med*. February 1995;23(1):129−136.

28. More RC, Karras BT, Neiman R, Fritschy D, Woo SL, Daniel DM. Hamstrings−an anterior cruciate ligament protagonist. An in vitro study. *Am J Sports Med*. April 1993; 21(2):231−237.

29. Haycock CE, Gillette JV. Susceptibility of women athletes to injury. Myths vs reality. *J Am Med Assoc*. July 12, 1976; 236(2):163−165.

30. Hirst S, Armeau E, Parish T. Recognizing anterior cruciate ligament tears in female athletes: what every primary care practitioner should know. *Internet J Allied Health Sci Pract*. January 1, 2007;5(1). Available from: https://nsuworks.nova.edu/ijahsp/vol5/iss1/10.

31. Coplan JA. Rotational motion of the knee: a comparison of normal and pronating subjects. *J Orthop Sports Phys Ther*. 1989;10(9):366−369.

32. Woodford-Rogers B, Cyphert L, Denegar CR. Risk factors for anterior cruciate ligament injury in high school and college athletes. *J Athl Train*. December 1994;29(4): 343−346.

33. Trimble MH, Bishop MD, Buckley BD, Fields LC, Rozea GD. The relationship between clinical measurements of lower extremity posture and tibial translation. *Clin Biomech*. May 2002;17(4):286−290.

34. Feagin JA, Cabaud HE, Curl WW. The anterior cruciate ligament: radiographic and clinical signs of successful and unsuccessful repairs. *Clin Orthop*. April 1982;(164):54−58.

35. Nguyen A-D, Shultz SJ, Schmitz RJ, Luecht RM, Perrin DH. A preliminary multifactorial approach describing the relationships among lower extremity alignment, hip muscle activation, and lower extremity joint excursion. *J Athl Train*. June 2011;46(3):246−256.

36. Olsen O-E, Myklebust G, Engebretsen L, Bahr R. Injury mechanisms for anterior cruciate ligament injuries in team handball: a systematic video analysis. *Am J Sports Med*. June 2004;32(4):1002−1012.

37. McLean SG, Lipfert SW, van den Bogert AJ. Effect of gender and defensive opponent on the biomechanics of sidestep cutting. *Med Sci Sports Exerc*. June 2004;36(6):1008−1016.

38. Lessi GC, Dos Santos AF, Batista LF, de Oliveira GC, Serrão FV. Effects of fatigue on lower limb, pelvis and trunk kinematics and muscle activation: gender differences. *J Electromyogr Kinesiol*. February 2017;32:9−14.

39. Zimny ML, Wink CS. Neuroreceptors in the tissues of the knee joint. *J Electromyogr Kinesiol*. September 1991;1(3): 148−157.

40. Schutte MJ, Dabezies EJ, Zimny ML, Happel LT. Neural anatomy of the human anterior cruciate ligament. *J Bone Joint Surg Am*. February 1987;69(2):243−247.

41. Pitman MI, Nainzadeh N, Menche D, Gasalberti R, Song EK. The intraoperative evaluation of the neurosensory function of the anterior cruciate ligament in humans using somatosensory evoked potentials. *Arthroscopy*. 1992; 8(4):442−447.

42. Angoules AG, Mavrogenis AF, Dimitriou R, et al. Knee proprioception following ACL reconstruction; a prospective

43. Telianidis S, Perraton L, Clark RA, Pua Y-H, Fortin K, Bryant AL. Diminished sub-maximal quadriceps force control in anterior cruciate ligament reconstructed patients is related to quadriceps and hamstring muscle dyskinesia. *J Electromyogr Kinesiol*. August 2014;24(4):513−519.

44. Sugimoto D, Myer GD, Barber Foss KD, Pepin MJ, Micheli LJ, Hewett TE. Critical components of neuromuscular training to reduce ACL injury risk in female athletes: meta-regression analysis. *Br J Sports Med*. October 2016; 50(20):1259−1266.

45. Beynnon BD, Johnson RJ, Braun S, et al. The relationship between menstrual cycle phase and anterior cruciate ligament injury: a case-control study of recreational alpine skiers. *Am J Sports Med*. May 2006;34(5):757−764.

46. Scerpella TA, Stayer TJ, Makhuli BZ. Ligamentous laxity and non-contact anterior cruciate ligament tears: a gender-based comparison. *Orthopedics*. July 2005;28(7): 656−660.

47. Heitz NA, Eisenman PA, Beck CL, Walker JA. Hormonal changes throughout the menstrual cycle and increased anterior cruciate ligament laxity in females. *J Athl Train*. April 1999;34(2):144−149.

48. Chidi-Ogbolu N, Baar K. Effect of estrogen on musculoskeletal performance and injury risk. *Front Physiol*. 2018; 9:1834.

49. Hsu W-H, Fisk JA, Yamamoto Y, Debski RE, Woo SL-Y. Differences in torsional joint stiffness of the knee between genders: a human cadaveric study. *Am J Sports Med*. May 2006;34(5):765−770.

50. Schmitz RJ, Ficklin TK, Shimokochi Y, et al. Varus/valgus and internal/external torsional knee joint stiffness differs between sexes. *Am J Sports Med*. July 2008;36(7): 1380−1388.

51. Shultz SJ, Pye ML, Montgomery MM, Schmitz RJ. Associations between lower extremity muscle mass and multiplanar knee laxity and stiffness: a potential explanation for sex differences in frontal and transverse plane knee laxity. *Am J Sports Med*. December 2012;40(12):2836−2844.

52. Beynnon BD, Bernstein IM, Belisle A, et al. The effect of estradiol and progesterone on knee and ankle joint laxity. *Am J Sports Med*. September 2005;33(9): 1298−1304.

53. Liu SH, al-Shaikh R, Panossian V, et al. Primary immunolocalization of estrogen and progesterone target cells in the human anterior cruciate ligament. *J Orthop Res Off Publ Orthop Res Soc*. July 1996;14(4):526−533.

54. Yu WD, Liu SH, Hatch JD, Panossian V, Finerman GA. Effect of estrogen on cellular metabolism of the human anterior cruciate ligament. *Clin Orthop*. September 1999;(366): 229−238.

55. Adachi N, Nawata K, Maeta M, Kurozawa Y. Relationship of the menstrual cycle phase to anterior cruciate ligament injuries in teenaged female athletes. *Arch Orthop Trauma Surg*. May 2008;128(5):473−478.

56. Wojtys EM, Huston LJ, Boynton MD, Spindler KP, Lindenfeld TN. The effect of the menstrual cycle on

anterior cruciate ligament injuries in women as determined by hormone levels. *Am J Sports Med*. April 2002; 30(2):182–188.

57. Wojtys EM, Huston LJ, Lindenfeld TN, Hewett TE, Greenfield ML. Association between the menstrual cycle and anterior cruciate ligament injuries in female athletes. *Am J Sports Med*. October 1998;26(5):614–619.

58. Birk DE, Fitch JM, Babiarz JP, Doane KJ, Linsenmayer TF. Collagen fibrillogenesis in vitro: interaction of types I and V collagen regulates fibril diameter. *J Cell Sci*. April 1990;95(Pt 4):649–657.

59. Wenstrup RJ, Florer JB, Davidson JM, et al. Murine model of the Ehlers-Danlos syndrome. col5a1 haploinsufficiency disrupts collagen fibril assembly at multiple stages. *J Biol Chem*. May 5, 2006;281(18):12888–12895.

60. Khoury LE, Posthumus M, Collins M, et al. ELN and FBN2 gene variants as risk factors for two sports-related musculoskeletal injuries. *Int J Sports Med*. April 2015;36(4): 333–337.

61. Khoschnau S, Melhus H, Jacobson A, et al. Type I collagen alpha1 Sp1 polymorphism and the risk of cruciate ligament ruptures or shoulder dislocations. *Am J Sports Med*. December 2008;36(12):2432–2436.

62. Mannion S, Mtintsilana A, Posthumus M, et al. Genes encoding proteoglycans are associated with the risk of anterior cruciate ligament ruptures. *Br J Sports Med*. December 2014;48(22):1640–1646.

63. Posthumus M, September AV, O'Cuinneagain D, van der Merwe W, Schwellnus MP, Collins M. The association between the COL12A1 gene and anterior cruciate ligament ruptures. *Br J Sports Med*. December 2010;44(16): 1160–1165.

64. Posthumus M, Collins M, van der Merwe L, et al. Matrix metalloproteinase genes on chromosome 11q22 and the risk of anterior cruciate ligament (ACL) rupture. *Scand J Med Sci Sports*. August 2012;22(4):523–533.

65. Wiese-Bjornstal DM. Psychology and socioculture affect injury risk, response, and recovery in high-intensity athletes: a consensus statement. *Scand J Med Sci Sports*. October 2010;20(Suppl. 2):103–111.

66. Sonesson S, Kvist J, Ardern C, Österberg A, Silbernagel KG. Psychological factors are important to return to pre-injury sport activity after anterior cruciate ligament reconstruction: expect and motivate to satisfy. *Knee Surg Sports Traumatol Arthrosc*. May 2017;25(5):1375–1384.

67. Johnson U, Ivarsson A, Karlsson J, Hägglund M, Waldén M, Börjesson M. Rehabilitation after first-time anterior cruciate ligament injury and reconstruction in female football players: a study of resilience factors. *BMC Sports Sci Med Rehabil*. 2016;8:20.

68. Orchard J, Seward H, McGivern J, Hood S. Rainfall, evaporation and the risk of non-contact anterior cruciate ligament injury in the Australian Football League. *Med J Aust*. April 5, 1999;170(7):304–306.

69. Boden BP, Dean GS, Feagin JA, Garrett WE. Mechanisms of anterior cruciate ligament injury. *Orthopedics*. June 2000; 23(6):573–578.

70. Wojtys EM, Kothari SU, Huston LJ. Anterior cruciate ligament functional brace use in sports. *Am J Sports Med*. August 1996;24(4):539–546.

71. Sasaki S, Tsuda E, Yamamoto Y, et al. Core-muscle training and neuromuscular control of the lower limb and trunk. *J Athl Train*. September 2019;54(9):959–969.

72. Linko E, Harilainen A, Malmivaara A, Seitsalo S. Surgical versus conservative interventions for anterior cruciate ligament ruptures in adults. *Cochrane Database Syst Rev*. April 18, 2005;(2):CD001356.

73. Razi M, Moradi A, Safarcherati A, et al. Allograft or autograft in skeletally immature anterior cruciate ligament reconstruction: a prospective evaluation using both partial and complete transphyseal techniques. *J Orthop Surg*. March 21, 2019;14(1):85.

74. Øiestad BE, Engebretsen L, Storheim K, Risberg MA. Knee osteoarthritis after anterior cruciate ligament injury: a systematic review. *Am J Sports Med*. July 2009;37(7): 1434–1443.

75. Simon D, Mascarenhas R, Saltzman BM, Rollins M, Bach BR, MacDonald P. The relationship between anterior cruciate ligament injury and osteoarthritis of the knee. *Adv Orthop*. 2015;2015:928301.

76. Shea KG, Carey JL, Richmond J, et al. The American Academy of Orthopaedic Surgeons evidence-based guideline on management of anterior cruciate ligament injuries. *J Bone Joint Surg Am*. April 15, 2015;97(8):672–674.

77. Sommerfeldt M, Goodine T, Raheem A, Whittaker J, Otto D. Relationship between time to ACL reconstruction and presence of adverse changes in the knee at the time of reconstruction. *Orthop J Sports Med*. December 2018;6(12), 2325967118813917.

78. Chhadia AM, Inacio MCS, Maletis GB, Csintalan RP, Davis BR, Funahashi TT. Are meniscus and cartilage injuries related to time to anterior cruciate ligament reconstruction? *Am J Sports Med*. September 2011;39(9): 1894–1899.

79. Church S, Keating JF. Reconstruction of the anterior cruciate ligament: timing of surgery and the incidence of meniscal tears and degenerative change. *J Bone Joint Surg Br*. December 2005;87(12):1639–1642.

80. Fok AWM, Yau WP. Delay in ACL reconstruction is associated with more severe and painful meniscal and chondral injuries. *Knee Surg Sports Traumatol Arthrosc*. April 2013; 21(4):928–933.

81. Granan L-P, Bahr R, Lie SA, Engebretsen L. Timing of anterior cruciate ligament reconstructive surgery and risk of cartilage lesions and meniscal tears: a cohort study based on the Norwegian National Knee Ligament Registry. *Am J Sports Med*. May 2009;37(5):955–961.

82. Papastergiou SG, Koukoulias NE, Mikalef P, Ziogas E, Voulgaropoulos H. Meniscal tears in the ACL-deficient knee: correlation between meniscal tears and the timing of ACL reconstruction. *Knee Surg Sports Traumatol Arthrosc*. December 2007;15(12):1438–1444.

83. Salem HS, Varzhapetyan V, Patel N, Dodson CC, Tjoumakaris FP, Freedman KB. Anterior cruciate ligament

reconstruction in young female athletes: patellar versus hamstring tendon autografts. *Am J Sports Med.* July 2019; 47(9):2086–2092.

84. Shakked R, Weinberg M, Capo J, Jazrawi L, Strauss E. Autograft choice in young female patients: patella tendon versus hamstring. *J Knee Surg.* March 2017;30(3): 258–263.

85. Kautzner J, Kos P, Hanus M, Trc T, Havlas V. A comparison of ACL reconstruction using patellar tendon versus hamstring autograft in female patients: a prospective randomised study. *Int Orthop.* January 2015;39(1):125–130.

86. Webster KE, Feller JA. Alterations in joint kinematics during walking following hamstring and patellar tendon anterior cruciate ligament reconstruction surgery. *Clin Biomech.* February 2011;26(2):175–180.

87. Spindler KP, Huston LJ, Wright RW, et al. The prognosis and predictors of sports function and activity at minimum 6 years after anterior cruciate ligament reconstruction: a population cohort study. *Am J Sports Med.* February 2011;39(2):348–359.

88. Jones MH, Reinke EK, Zajichek A, et al. Neighborhood socioeconomic status affects patient-reported outcome 2 years after ACL reconstruction. *Orthop J Sports Med.* June 2019;7(6), 2325967119851073.

89. Ardern CL, Glasgow P, Schneiders A, et al. 2016 consensus statement on return to sport from the first world congress in sports physical therapy, Bern. *Br J Sports Med.* July 2016; 50(14):853–864.

90. Marshall NE, Keller RA, Dines J, Bush-Joseph C, Limpisvasti O. Current practice: postoperative and return to play trends after ACL reconstruction by fellowship-trained sports surgeons. *Musculoskelet Surg.* April 2019; 103(1):55–61.

91. Ardern CL, Taylor NF, Feller JA, Webster KE. Fifty-five per cent return to competitive sport following anterior cruciate ligament reconstruction surgery: an updated systematic review and meta-analysis including aspects of physical functioning and contextual factors. *Br J Sports Med.* November 2014;48(21):1543–1552.

92. Webster KE, McPherson AL, Hewett TE, Feller JA. Factors associated with a return to preinjury level of sport performance after anterior cruciate ligament reconstruction surgery. *Am J Sports Med.* September 2019;47(11): 2557–2562.

93. Paterno MV, Rauh MJ, Schmitt LC, Ford KR, Hewett TE. Incidence of second ACL injuries 2 years after primary ACL reconstruction and return to sport. *Am J Sports Med.* July 2014;42(7):1567–1573.

94. Capin JJ, Failla M, Zarzycki R, et al. Superior 2-year functional outcomes among young female athletes after ACL reconstruction in 10 return-to-sport training sessions: comparison of ACL-SPORTS randomized controlled trial with Delaware-Oslo and MOON cohorts. *Orthop J Sports Med.* August 2019;7(8), 2325967119861311.

95. Takeda Y, Kashiwaguchi S, Matsuura T, Higashida T, Minato A. Hamstring muscle function after tendon harvest for anterior cruciate ligament reconstruction: evaluation with T2 relaxation time of magnetic resonance imaging. *Am J Sports Med.* February 2006;34(2):281–288.

96. San Martín-Mohr C, Cristi-Sánchez I, Pincheira PA, Reyes A, Berral FJ, Oyarzo C. Knee sensorimotor control following anterior cruciate ligament reconstruction: a comparison between reconstruction techniques. *PLoS One.* 2018;13(11):e0205658.

97. Webster KE, McClelland JA, Palazzolo SE, Santamaria LJ, Feller JA. Gender differences in the knee adduction moment after anterior cruciate ligament reconstruction surgery. *Br J Sports Med.* April 2012;46(5):355–359.

98. McDevitt ER, Taylor DC, Miller MD, et al. Functional bracing after anterior cruciate ligament reconstruction: a prospective, randomized, multicenter study. *Am J Sports Med.* December 2004;32(8):1887–1892.

CHAPTER 3

Anterior Cruciate Ligament Injuries: Sex-Based Differences

ELAN GOLAN, MD • MATTHEW T. LOPEZ, PT, DPT • VONDA WRIGHT, MD, MS

INTRODUCTION AND EPIDEMIOLOGY

In spite of years of research and evolving techniques, rupture of the anterior cruciate ligament (ACL) continues to represent one of the most common traumatic injuries in competitive sports.[1] Female athletes have been noted to be at particular risk for ACL tears, with injury rates as high as two to eight times as those experienced by males,[2-5] especially in sports requiring quick or repetitive lateral movement.[6] In addition to being at increased risk for primary rupture, females are more likely to sustain a contralateral injury or undergo revision surgery, experiencing rates of secondary ACL sequela as high as 34%.[7]

Interestingly, several well-designed studies have failed to identify female gender as an independent risk factor for ACL injury on multivariate regression analysis.[8-10] This has led to the suggestion that the observed increase in risk for female ACL injury is a mere reflection of increasing sports participation. However, this theory has been largely discredited by multiple surveillance studies, which failed to find an increase in ACL injury risk when expressed as a percentage of active female athletes. In one such study, performed by the National Collegiate Athletic Association, no significant change in the rate of ACL injury was noted over a 15-year period, in spite of increased female sports participation rates.[11]

Given these findings, the increased propensity for female ACL injury is likely multifactorial, attributed to factors such as variations in anatomic size and morphology, hormonal levels, and alterations in neuromuscular control. Accordingly, this chapter reviews the current understanding of the female ACL, summarizing potential contributing causes for increased risk, while also discussing strategies for injury prevention, surgical reconstruction, and rehabilitation.

ANTERIOR CRUCIATE LIGAMENT ANATOMY AND FUNCTION

The ACL is the primary contributor of anteroposterior and rotatory stability to the knee, especially in lower flexion angles.[12] It is composed of two distinct segments, the anteromedial and posterolateral bundles, which are named based on their respective insertion sites on the tibia. The native ACL is covered by synovial tissue, with the deeper areas being largely avascular, minimizing healing potential. Limited vascularity is supplied to the femoral insertion via the posterior soft tissues, with the tibial insertion site receiving a small vascular contribution from the anterior horn of lateral meniscus.[13] The ACL is also rich in mechanoreceptors, functioning to provide proprioceptive feedback while initiating protective muscular reflexes.[14-18]

The ACL's femoral insertion site is oval in shape and smaller in size than the ligament's broad tibial insertion. The isthmus of ACL exists at mid-substance, with a cross-sectional area of less than half of the tibial or femoral insertions. The intra-articular portion of the ACL is quite dynamic, demonstrating its shortest length at 90 degrees of knee flexion and increasing to its maximal size in full extension.[19]

When viewed arthroscopically, the ACL can be readily appreciated originating from the posterior aspect of the lateral femoral condyle, coursing in an anteromedial direction to insert at the interspinous area of the tibia. This intra-articular course is located within the 'femoral notch,' composed of the area between the medial and lateral condyles of the femur. Femoral notch size and the shape often play an important role in ACL injury, with several gender-specific differences noted.[20-22] Notch size can also affect intraoperative visualization, complicating the creation of anatomic tunnels, one of the most impactful metric on return-to-play outcomes.

The Female Athlete. https://doi.org/10.1016/B978-0-323-75985-4.00024-6

GENDER-BASED ANATOMIC DIFFERENCES

The size of the ACL itself has been postulated to contribute to gender-based differences in ACL injury patterns. When compared with their male counterparts, ACLs in females tend to be smaller in overall volume,[23] while also possessing less tensile resistance, demonstrating decreased elongation distances to failure.[24] Such mechanical differences have also been noted clinically, with females' knees exhibiting less resistance to rotation and anterior translation as measured on KT-1000.[3]

Females also possess a larger quadriceps angle or 'Q-angle',[25] resulting from a wider and shorter pelvis. The Q-angle is formed via the composite of two lines, originating from the anterior superior iliac spine and tibial tubercle, that course through the center of the patella. Increases in the Q-angle result in a more laterally based quadriceps force vector, placing the knee in increased valgus, thus predisposing to ACL rupture with athletic activity.[23,26]

In a 2020 systematic review, Bayer et al. examined the morphologic risk factors for ACL injury. Of all the factors considered, an A-shaped notch, sometimes referred to as 'notch stenosis,'[27] was the most commonly cited cause for increased risk of ACL injury.[21] This finding seems to correlate with increased injury risk,[27,28] as a review of patients undergoing ACL reconstruction noted a greater percentage of A-shaped notches in females than males.[22] Other authors have reported similar findings, noting a decreased notch size in females.[29]

Several morphologic factors have also been demonstrated to contribute to increased risk for ACL injury based on condylar anatomy. In one study,[30] ACL-injured females were noted to demonstrate an increased condylar offset ratio, defined as the difference between the anatomic and transcondylar axes of the femur. A second study reported a lateral femoral condylar offset of >63% to similarly correlate with increased ACL injury.[31] With regard to tibial morphology, multiple authors have reported an increased tibial slope to correlate with increased injury risk.[21,32–34] In one such study, small variations seemed predictive, with a mean lateral tibial slope of 6.3 degrees noted in individuals experiencing ACL injury, compared to just 4.1 degrees in their uninjured counterparts.

In an examination of risk factors for subsequent injury to the contralateral anterior cruciate ligament (CACL), Davey et al.[35] noted a rate of 20% for CACL injury following an index ACL tear. In this cohort of 61 female athletes, at a mean follow-up of 45 months, younger females with increased hip anteversion and increased contralateral knee laxity were noted to be at the greatest risk for CACL rupture. Interestingly, while younger patients were at higher risk of CACL pathology, increased sports participation was somewhat protective, with prior competitive play associated with decreased overall injury risk.

MENSTRUAL HORMONES AND ORAL CONTRACEPTION

The effects of menstrual hormones and oral contraceptive (OCP) use represent an oft debated risk factor for female ACL injury. Indeed, over the past decade, the amount of research dedicated to hormonal effects on ACL injury has more than doubled, allowing for an increasingly evidence-based approach to an often controversial topic.

With regard to specific menstrual hormones, estradiol has been demonstrated to result in a dose-dependent reduction of fibroblast and collagen production.[36] The resulting increase in ligamentous laxity has been correlated with increased risks for female ACL injury, especially in the preovulatory phase of the menstrual cycle.[36–38] Conversely, progestins have been found to inhibit such increases in laxity,[39,40] suggesting a decreased risk for ACL injury during the luteal phase (Fig. 3.1).

In examining several high-quality studies investigating knee laxity during phases of the menstrual cycle,[41–43] a significant increase in laxity was noted in the ovulatory phase compared with the follicular phases. Further supporting this assertion, several studies have found ligamentous laxity to be the highest with increasing levels of estradiol.[44–46] However, a similar reduction in laxity was not noted during the luteal phase, calling into question the overall importance of laxity in ACL injury and suggesting that the potential increases in risk are likely multifactorial.

The suppression of follicular development and ovulation with OCP use has been postulated to mitigate this cyclic increase in laxity, possibly resulting in a lower rate of ACL injury. However, the ability to demonstrate the protective effect of OCP use is complicated by the need to compare large numbers of female athletes of similar demographics, with readily available data regarding OCP usage. To date, two large, high-quality studies exist that have demonstrated a similar risk reduction of around 20%.[47,48]

The first study, a Danish registry-based study,[48] drew information from the country's knee ligament register as well as a prescription drug registry. Through this anonymized information, 4497 females undergoing ACL

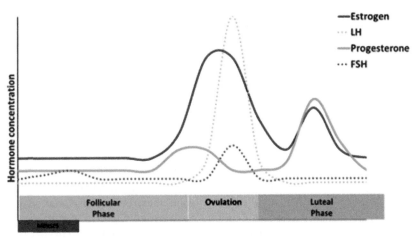

FIG. 3.1 Hormonal fluctuations during the menstrual cycle. *FSH,* follicle-stimulating hormone; *LH,* luteinizing hormone. (Modified from Senanayake and Potts, 2008.)

reconstruction surgery were compared to 8858 age-matched controls. Analysis of this data demonstrated an 18% risk reduction for ACL injury with OCP use. In a second US-based study,[47] 12,819 ACL injuries were compared to 38,457 matched controls by using a commercial insurance database. Analysis of this cohort demonstrated a near 20% risk reduction for eventual ACL reconstruction in females on regular OCP use.

Also of recent interest has been the potential effect of hormones on muscle activation and knee alignment. In this regard, several studies have investigated the role of female hormonal fluctuation on neuromuscular activity. Specifically, electromyographic studies have demonstrated differences in muscle activation in the quadriceps and hamstrings (HSs) throughout the menstrual cycle. In one study,[44] alterations to the lateral HSs were found to be most pronounced during the follicular phase. In a second similar investigation, Khowailed et al.[49] noted ovulatory phase alterations to medial quadriceps activation that placed the knee in a position of risk for increased ACL loads.

Importantly, it must be mentioned that a 2017 systematic review[50] noted overall evidence to be 'very low' utilizing the GRADE (Grading of Recommendations Assessment, Development and Evaluation) approach to analyze the effect size of the aforementioned studies (GRADEWorkingGroup.org). Thus in spite of substantial increase in the amount of recent literature, concrete ramifications of menstrual hormones on ACL injury will likely remain controversial for the foreseeable future.

GENDER DIFFERENCES IN KNEE KINEMATICS

Aside from downstream hormonal effects, it has long been postulated that one contributor to the overall increase in risk for female ACL injury stems from variations in neuromuscular control between genders. Females have been noted to be 'quadriceps dominant,' possessing a relatively larger percent of their lower extremity mass in the quadriceps muscles when compared to the HSs.[26] Such imbalances can result in athletes landing in a more upright position, with females demonstrating relatively increased knee extension, thus placing increased strain on the ACL upon impact.

Females have also been demonstrated to exhibit differences in the mechanics of athletic movements such as sidestep cutting.[51] Indeed, in an investigation of female soccer athletes with and without the presence of a defender, the defended condition resulted in increased medial ground reaction forces. The defended position was also noted to result in increases in flexion and abduction of the hip and knee, potentially predisposing for ACL injury. Similar results were noted in a subsequent study of stop-jump kinetics, with females' knees demonstrating increased anterior tibial shear force as well as valgus and extension during landing.[52]

In an attempt to mitigate such inherent risk factors, Hewett et al. prospectively analyzed two cohorts of female soccer, basketball, and volleyball athletes. The first group received neuromuscular preventative training before and throughout their seasons, while the second group was left to coach-led participation alone. When compared with females in a neuromuscular prevention program, untrained females were 3.6 times more likely to sustain a traumatic ACL event, with smaller but significant reductions in the rate of noncontact ACL injuries also noted between the groups.[53] Such imbalances are of particular concern in the setting of fatigue, which may compromise the ability to alter muscle activation patterns due to the inhibition of rapid neuromuscular feedback.[54,55]

In a biomechanical study employing three-dimensional motion analysis during vertical jumping, male and female landing kinematics was compared.[56] Female athletes were found to land with greater total knee valgus and overall lower extremity valgus angles than their male counterparts. Females were also found to demonstrate significantly greater muscle activation differences between the dominant and nondominant extremities. Based on these findings, the authors postulated that females were at increased risk for ACL injury owing to the lack of dynamic knee stability.

In an analysis of gender differences during a single-leg squat maneuver,[57] alterations to ankle, hip, and trunk mechanics demonstrated females to have tendency toward a valgus position during increasing lower extremity loads. Specifically, the authors identified females to demonstrate increased ankle dorsiflexion and pronation, increased hip adduction and external rotation, and decreased lateral trunk flexion compared to males. Taken together, these differences were found to result in a decreased ability to maintain a varus knee position, potentially increasing anterior forces on the ACL.

In a seminal paper, Hewett et al.[26] was able to identify the aforementioned alterations to knee mechanics in a clinical setting. In a study of 205 high-risk female athletes, the authors performed three-dimensional analysis of knee kinetics and kinematics during simulated jump landings. Athletes were then followed up throughout their respective competitive seasons. Compared to their uninjured colleagues, those who went on to sustain an eventual ACL injury were noted to share several distinct alterations to drop landing joint angles and forces. These included a decreased stance phase and an almost 10-degree difference increase in abduction angle. Furthermore, those with ACL injury demonstrated 2.5 times greater abduction moments and increase in ground reaction forces of 20%. The authors further identified abduction moments to be highly predictive of ACL injury, with a sensitivity of 73% and sensitivity of 78%. Dynamic valgus also demonstrated a strong correlation coefficient, with a noted r^2 of 0.88 for eventual ACL pathology.

Taken together with other factors predictive of risk, such as age, morphologic characteristics, and increased level of competition, the abovementioned biomechanical data provide a framework for ever-increasing strategies for ACL injury prevention and rehabilitation. Consideration of the many factors introduced earlier also plays an important role in the operative approach to reconstruct the female ACL.

PREVENTION

With the complexity of anatomic and knee kinematic differences in the female knee, an ACL prevention program must be multifactorial in nature. Three meta-analyses indicate that, in females, exercise-based injury prevention programs are effective in reducing the risk of all ACL injuries.[58-60] The injury prevention programs are found to be most effective when they incorporate multiple exercise components, such as trunk/core strengthening, plyometrics, strengthening, stretching, and proprioception.[61] Programs including only one exercise component did not show a significant reduction of injuries.[61] Additionally, feedback on form during tasks including drop jumps and single-leg squat maneuvers was found to be effective in reducing injury.[62-64] The feedback provided to athletes allows for addressing the changes in knee kinematics discussed earlier. Interestingly, programs without a balance training component were found effective in preventing ACL injuries in females. In fact, one study found an inverse relationship between the time spent performing balance activities and the protective effect of the program.[2]

Time to return to sport (RTS) postoperatively is a highly studied aspect of ACL rehab, but equally important can be the appropriate time to implement a prevention program. When compared with females over 18 years of age, two meta-analyses found that females under the age of 18 years have a greater reduction in ACL injuries when completing exercise-based ACL prevention programs.[58-60] A meta-regression by Sugimoto et al.[65] found a 17% lower risk of ACL injury in athletes aged 14–18 years compared with their 18+-year-aged peers when completing a prevention program.

Implementation of a prevention program has become more commonplace in the preseason, but preseason training alone was not effective in reducing ACL injuries.[60] Exercise-based prevention programs that began in the preseason, continued throughout the season, and consisted of greater than 20 min of duration multiple times per week have been shown to be most effective in reducing ACL injuries.[60,65,66] Compliance of athletes to their exercise program during that time has a potential inverse dose-response relationship, with the incidence of ACL injury in adolescent female athletes, according to Sugimoto et al.[67] With a compliance percentage of >66.6%, athletes demonstrated an 82% lower ACL injury incidence than their less compliant counterparts.[67]

A gold standard for exercise-based ACL prevention programs has not been established, but two programs have shown to be very effective in the female adolescent population. The Knakontroll program was implemented with over 4500 female soccer players aged 12–17 years.[68] The intervention group saw a 64% reduction in ACL injuries and 30% reduction in severe knee injuries.[68] The PEP (Prevent injury and Enhance Performance) program was studied by Mandelbaum et al.[69] in females aged 14–18 years and found an 89% decrease in ACL injuries in the first season of implementation and a 74% decrease in the second season. Similar nonsignificant decreases in ACL injuries were found by Gilchrist et al.[70] in college-aged females.

OPERATIVE CONSIDERATIONS

Perhaps the single largest preoperative consideration in surgical reconstruction of the female ACL is the choice of graft selection. In a large, multicenter study examining outcomes at 6 years, the Moon (Multicenter Orthopaedic Outcomes Network) Knee Group identified three independent risk factors for ACL revision and contralateral injury. These included a high-grade preoperative pivot shift, young age, and choice of autograft. While gender was not identified as a risk factor, the choice of graft did impart a significant impact, with patients receiving a HS autograft demonstrating an odds ratio of 2.1 for reinjury compared to those reconstructed with a bone-patellar tendon-bone (BTB).[8]

Salem et al.[71] noted a similar finding in an examination of outcomes in 256 athletes, with the authors limiting their investigation to females between the ages of 15 and 20 years. In this cohort, the authors noted a significantly lower rate of rerupture between the BTB (6.4%) and HS (17.5%) groups. However, BTB grafts were associated with a much higher rate of prolonged kneeling pain (12%) when compared with HS grafts (2%). Given these findings, the current literature does suggest an advantage to graft survivability when electing for a BTB-based over an HS-based reconstruction.

More recently, quadriceps tendon (QT) ACL reconstruction has gained increased attention due to the readily available access to a larger sized graft,[72,73] with the quadriceps also noted to possess a larger cross-sectional area and increased load to failure compared to a patellar tendon graft.[74] A second potential advantage to QT grafts is that similar clinical outcomes can be achieved utilizing partial- and full-thickness grafts,[75] in contrast to BTB grafts, which require harvesting of full tendon depth. In an examination of postoperative extension strength, Hunnicutt et al.[76] reported similar quadriceps function between BTB and QT groups at 8 months following ACL reconstruction. The authors also noted no difference in patient-reported outcomes between the two groups, a finding that was again verified by a subsequent prospective study, this time at 2-year follow-up.[77] In a second systematic review and meta-analysis,[78] QT ACL reconstruction demonstrated similar survivability to HS- and BTB-based procedures. Several findings were also reported favoring QT ACL reconstruction, including decreased donor-site pain and increased Lysholm scoring at final follow-up.

SURGICAL TECHNIQUE

As previously mentioned, several authors have noted females to be more likely to possess a narrowed or 'A'-shaped intercondylar notch.[79] Therefore a surgical approach that allows for consistent, anatomic ACL reconstruction in the setting of a narrowed intra-articular working space should be preferentially chosen to optimize outcomes. Notably, we would caution against routine reliance on a 'notchplasty', as it is our preference to preserve as much native anatomy as possible. Ultimately, whichever method allows for the most repeatable creation of anatomic tibial and femoral tunnels should be elected, as improper tunnel placement has been identified as the most common surgical risk factor for suboptimal patient outcomes, and highly predictive of the need for revision.[80–82]

It is our preference to perform knee arthroscopy with a standard two portal approach, modifying the medial portal to allow for both meniscal work while maintaining an appropriate trajectory for separate, anteromedial drilling. A second accessory medial portal can also be utilized; however, in our experience, this is rarely necessary if medial portal placement is appropriately planned employing outside-in localization techniques.

While we hesitate to make concrete recommendations with regard to routine graft choice, several key points warrant emphasis in the decision-making process. First, in the absence of complicating factors, allograft use in the young female athlete should be avoided to mitigate the risk of graft failure,[83,84] while avoiding the increased cost associated with allograft use.[85] Second, practitioners should be confident in their abilities to obtain an autograft of appropriate size with their preferred autograft, as sizes of less than 8 mm are associated with higher failure rates.[86–89]

Our preference is to elect for either a BPTB- or a QT-based reconstruction, noting the benefits of faster incorporation and bone to bone healing with patellar tendon,[90] with potentially easier access to a larger graft size employing a QT. Furthermore, it is our tendency to avoid HS reconstruction as a primary choice; although admittedly, the choice of autograft remains nuanced and highly controversial.[90–92] Finally, multiple studies of graft fixation methods have failed to identify any one method to exhibit clear superiority[93–96]; however, a more recent study did note larger metal screws to act as a potential risk factor for revision.[97] The most common methods of fixation include aperture-based methods in the form of screws and cross-pins versus suspensory fixation with a button-based device.

Aside from the restoration of ACL's integrity, special attention should also be paid to address secondary pathology encountered at the time of reconstruction, such as meniscal tears, compromise of collateral stabilizers, or cartilaginous lesions.[98–100] Indeed, multiple authors have demonstrated the presence of meniscal injury to negatively impact outcomes following ACL reconstruction, with tears identified later on more likely to be complex and associated with degenerative progression.[101] We do caution against the routine use of lateral tenodesis procedures, as the need for extra-articular augmentation can often be mitigated by emphasizing an anatomic reconstruction,[102] while minimizing the risk for potential overconstraint. However, benefits in such extra-articular stability procedures have been demonstrated in select at-risk groups, such as younger individuals undergoing revision surgery, a grade III pivot shift, or those exhibiting signs of advanced ligamentous laxity.[103]

RETURN TO SPORT

RTS after ACL reconstruction is a highly debated topic, with time frames ranging anywhere from 6 months to 2 years.[104] Adolescent athletes can find themselves under pressure to return quickly after ACL reconstruction, including external pressure from coaches, parents, and teammates as well as internal pressure. Hewett and Nagelli[104] postulate that after the 2-year mark in the adolescent population, the risk of repeat ACL injury is significantly decreased. This reduction is likely due to resolution of a multitude of risk factors including bone bruises, decreased proprioception, ligamentization, and decreased knee strength.[104] Delaying for

2 years in adolescents comes at a potential separate cost of decreased social/team engagement and scholarship potential, and certainly, further study is needed. Grindem[15] articulated that for each month the RTS was delayed until 9 months, the reinjury rate was significantly reduced by 51% for each month.

Perhaps even more important is the use of a criterion-based RTS battery of tests to reduce the risk of reinjury. Kyritsis et al.[105] defined a set of RTS criteria as follows:

- zero to trace effusion on stroke test,
- one-repetition maximum quadriceps limb symmetry index (LSI) >90% on knee extension,
- one-repetition maximum HSs LSI >90% on HS curl,
- good neuromotor control with no increased pain/effusion with sports-specific activities,
- functional hop testing >90% LSI for all four tests with good neuromotor control,
- running t-test <11 s.

Two studies have shown that if an athlete does not pass all the RTS criteria, they are at a four times greater risk of ACL reinjury.[105,106] In a prospective 2-year cohort study, Grindem et al.[106] reported a 38.2% ACL reinjury rate for level I sport athletes who failed the RTS criteria. In contrast, athletes who passed the RTS testing demonstrated a 5.6% reinjury rate.[106] In this same study, postoperative quadriceps strength was shown to be directly related to reinjury risk. For every 1% increase in quadriceps LSI, there was a resultant 3% decrease in reinjury risk.[106] Examining quadriceps strength as an individual RTS criterion shows a 33.3% reinjury risk for LSI <90% versus a 12.5% reinjury risk for those with LSI >90%.[106] The current gold standard of knee extension isokinetic testing is oftentimes unavailable to clinicians outside the research setting. Thus knee extension one-repetition maximum testing is more commonly used.

In 2017, Wellsandt[107] proposed that LSI was underestimating the true strength required postoperatively. Due to the bilateral resultant atrophy that occurs postoperatively, Wellsandt[107] recommended utilizing an Estimated Preinjury Capacity (EPIC) value in place of LSI. EPIC utilized an uninvolved limb quadriceps strength measurement taken preoperatively. The resultant value required a higher involved limb quadriceps strength to meet the 90% RTS criteria and did show lower reinjury rates compared to LSI testing.[107] Thus far, further study is required on EPIC, as LSI remains the commonplace testing strategy.

Neuromotor deficits are linked to a risk of reinjury, and thus it is essential to complete neuromuscular training prior to RTS. Neuromuscular training targets deficient muscles, utilizes muscle coactivation patterns associated with sports, and helps modify preexisting mechanics shown to increase injury risk.[108] It is important to include bilateral training to address mechanical faults that may exist, as well as trunk proprioception to decrease external knee abduction loads.[108] Progression should be form-dependent on the correct execution of each task and will vary greatly between athletes.[108]

REFERENCES

1. Bonazza N, Smuin DM, Sterling N, et al. Epidemiology of surgical treatment of adolescent sports injuries in the United States: analysis of the MarketScan commercial claims and encounters database. *Arthrosc Sports Med Rehabil.* 2019;1:e59–e65.
2. Al Attar WS, Soomro N, Pappas E, Sinclair PJ, Sanders RH. How effective are F-MARC injury prevention programs for soccer players? A systematic review and meta-analysis. *Sports Med.* 2016;46:205–217.
3. Renstrom P, Ljungqvist A, Arendt E, et al. Non-contact ACL injuries in female athletes: an International Olympic Committee current concepts statement. *Br J Sports Med.* 2008;42:394–412.
4. Toth AP, Cordasco FA. Anterior cruciate ligament injuries in the female athlete. *J Gend Specif Med.* 2001;4:25–34.
5. Arendt E, Dick R. Knee injury patterns among men and women in collegiate basketball and soccer. NCAA data and review of literature. *Am J Sports Med.* 1995;23: 694–701.
6. Hagglund M, Walden M. Risk factors for acute knee injury in female youth football. *Knee Surg Sports Traumatol Arthrosc.* 2016;24:737–746.
7. Allen MM, Pareek A, Krych AJ, et al. Are female soccer players at an increased risk of second anterior cruciate ligament injury compared with their athletic peers? *Am J Sports Med.* 2016;44:2492–2498.
8. Group MK, Spindler KP, Huston LJ, et al. Anterior cruciate ligament reconstruction in high school and college-aged athletes: does autograft choice influence anterior cruciate ligament revision rates? *Am J Sports Med.* 2020; 48:298–309.
9. Kaeding CC, Pedroza AD, Reinke EK, Huston LJ, Consortium M, Spindler KP. Risk factors and predictors of subsequent ACL injury in either knee after ACL reconstruction: prospective analysis of 2488 primary ACL reconstructions from the MOON cohort. *Am J Sports Med.* 2015;43:1583–1590.
10. Yabroudi MA, Bjornsson H, Lynch AD, et al. Predictors of revision surgery after primary anterior cruciate ligament reconstruction. *Orthop J Sports Med.* 2016;4, 232596 7116666039.
11. Mihata LC, Beutler AI, Boden BP. Comparing the incidence of anterior cruciate ligament injury in collegiate lacrosse, soccer, and basketball players: implications for anterior cruciate ligament mechanism and prevention. *Am J Sports Med.* 2006;34:899–904.
12. Lipke JM, Janecki CJ, Nelson CL, et al. The role of incompetence of the anterior cruciate and lateral ligaments in anterolateral and anteromedial instability. A biomechanical study of cadaver knees. *J Bone Joint Surg Am.* 1981;63:954–960.
13. Ferretti M, Levicoff EA, Macpherson TA, Moreland MS, Cohen M, Fu FH. The fetal anterior cruciate ligament: an anatomic and histologic study. *Arthroscopy.* 2007;23: 278–283.
14. Freeman MA, Wyke B. The innervation of the knee joint. An anatomical and histological study in the cat. *J Anat.* 1967;101:505–532.
15. Grindem H, Snyder-Mackler L, Moksnes H, et al. Simple decision rules can reduce reinjury risk by 84% after ACL reconstruction: the Delaware-Oslo ACL cohort study. *Br J Sports Med.* 2016;50:804–808.
16. Grigg P, Greenspan BJ. Response of primate joint afferent neurons to mechanical stimulation of knee joint. *J Neurophysiol.* 1977;40:1–8.
17. Johansson H, Sjolander P, Sojka P. A sensory role for the cruciate ligaments. *Clin Orthop Relat Res.* 1991:161–178.
18. Johansson H, Sjolander P, Sojka P. Receptors in the knee joint ligaments and their role in the biomechanics of the joint. *Crit Rev Biomed Eng.* 1991;18:341–368.
19. Fujimaki Y, Thorhauer E, Sasaki Y, Smolinski P, Tashman S, Fu FH. Quantitative in situ analysis of the anterior cruciate ligament: length, midsubstance cross-sectional area, and insertion site areas. *Am J Sports Med.* 2016;44:118–125.
20. Anderson AF, Dome DC, Gautam S, Awh MH, Rennirt GW. Correlation of anthropometric measurements, strength, anterior cruciate ligament size, and intercondylar notch characteristics to sex differences in anterior cruciate ligament tear rates. *Am J Sports Med.* 2001;29:58–66.
21. Bayer S, Meredith SJ, Wilson K, et al. Knee morphological risk factors for anterior cruciate ligament injury: a systematic review. *J Bone Joint Surg Am.* 2020;102:703–718.
22. Ireland ML, Ballantyne BT, Little K, McClay IS. A radiographic analysis of the relationship between the size and shape of the intercondylar notch and anterior cruciate ligament injury. *Knee Surg Sports Traumatol Arthrosc.* 2001;9:200–205.
23. Giugliano DN, Solomon JL. ACL tears in female athletes. *Phys Med Rehabil Clin N Am.* 2007;18:417–438 (viii).
24. Chandrashekar N, Mansouri H, Slauterbeck J, Hashemi J. Sex-based differences in the tensile properties of the human anterior cruciate ligament. *J Biomech.* 2006;39: 2943–2950.
25. Conley S, Rosenberg A, Crowninshield R. The female knee: anatomic variations. *J Am Acad Orthop Surg.* 2007; 15(Suppl. 1):S31–S36.
26. Hewett TE, Myer GD, Ford KR, et al. Biomechanical measures of neuromuscular control and valgus loading of the knee predict anterior cruciate ligament injury risk in female athletes: a prospective study. *Am J Sports Med.* 2005;33:492–501.
27. Wolf MR, Murawski CD, van Diek FM, van Eck CF, Huang Y, Fu FH. Intercondylar notch dimensions and

graft failure after single- and double-bundle anterior cruciate ligament reconstruction. *Knee Surg Sports Traumatol Arthrosc.* 2015;23:680–686.

28. van Eck CF, Kopf S, van Dijk CN, Fu FH, Tashman S. Comparison of 3-dimensional notch volume between subjects with and subjects without anterior cruciate ligament rupture. *Arthroscopy.* 2011;27:1235–1241.

29. Chandrashekar N, Slauterbeck J, Hashemi J. Sex-based differences in the anthropometric characteristics of the anterior cruciate ligament and its relation to intercondylar notch geometry: a cadaveric study. *Am J Sports Med.* 2005;33:1492–1498.

30. Hoshino Y, Wang JH, Lorenz S, Fu FH, Tashman S. Gender difference of the femoral kinematics axis location and its relation to anterior cruciate ligament injury: a 3D-CT study. *Knee Surg Sports Traumatol Arthrosc.* 2012;20: 1282–1288.

31. Pfeiffer TR, Burnham JM, Hughes JD, et al. An increased lateral femoral condyle ratio is a risk factor for anterior cruciate ligament injury. *J Bone Joint Surg Am.* 2018;100: 857–864.

32. Alentorn-Geli E, Pelfort X, Mingo F, et al. An evaluation of the association between radiographic intercondylar notch narrowing and anterior cruciate ligament injury in men: the notch angle is a better parameter than notch width. *Arthroscopy.* 2015;31:2004–2013.

33. Meister K, Talley MC, Horodyski MB, Indelicato PA, Hartzel JS, Batts J. Caudal slope of the tibia and its relationship to noncontact injuries to the ACL. *Am J Knee Surg.* 1998;11:217–219.

34. Zeng C, Yang T, Wu S, et al. Is posterior tibial slope associated with noncontact anterior cruciate ligament injury? *Knee Surg Sports Traumatol Arthrosc.* 2016;24:830–837.

35. Davey AP, Vacek PM, Caldwell RA, et al. Risk factors associated with a noncontact anterior cruciate ligament injury to the contralateral knee after unilateral anterior cruciate ligament injury in high school and college female athletes: a prospective study. *Am J Sports Med.* 2019;47: 3347–3355.

36. Agel J, Bershadsky B, Arendt EA. Hormonal therapy: ACL and ankle injury. *Med Sci Sports Exerc.* 2006;38:7–12.

37. Adachi N, Nawata K, Maeta M, Kurozawa Y. Relationship of the menstrual cycle phase to anterior cruciate ligament injuries in teenaged female athletes. *Arch Orthop Trauma Surg.* 2008;128:473–478.

38. Wojtys EM, Huston LJ, Boynton MD, Spindler KP, Lindenfeld TN. The effect of the menstrual cycle on anterior cruciate ligament injuries in women as determined by hormone levels. *Am J Sports Med.* 2002;30: 182–188.

39. Yu WD, Panossian V, Hatch JD, Liu SH, Finerman GA. Combined effects of estrogen and progesterone on the anterior cruciate ligament. *Clin Orthop Relat Res.* 2001: 268–281.

40. Yu WD, Liu SH, Hatch JD, Panossian V, Finerman GA. Effect of estrogen on cellular metabolism of the human anterior cruciate ligament. *Clin Orthop Relat Res.* 1999: 229–238.

41. Hertel J, Williams NI, Olmsted-Kramer LC, Leidy HJ, Putukian M. Neuromuscular performance and knee laxity do not change across the menstrual cycle in female athletes. *Knee Surg Sports Traumatol Arthrosc.* 2006;14: 817–822.

42. Hicks-Little CA, Thatcher JR, Hauth JM, Goldfuss AJ, Cordova ML. Menstrual cycle stage and oral contraceptive effects on anterior tibial displacement in collegiate female athletes. *J Sports Med Phys Fitness.* 2007;47: 255–260.

43. Park SK, Stefanyshyn DJ, Ramage B, Hart DA, Ronsky JL. Relationship between knee joint laxity and knee joint mechanics during the menstrual cycle. *Br J Sports Med.* 2009;43:174–179.

44. Hoffman M, Harter RA, Hayes BT, Wojtys EM, Murtaugh P. The interrelationships among sex hormone concentrations, motoneuron excitability, and anterior tibial displacement in women and men. *J Athl Train.* 2008;43:364–372.

45. Shultz SJ, Levine BJ, Nguyen AD, Kim H, Montgomery MM, Perrin DH. A comparison of cyclic variations in anterior knee laxity, genu recurvatum, and general joint laxity across the menstrual cycle. *J Orthop Res.* 2010;28:1411–1417.

46. Shultz SJ, Sander TC, Kirk SE, Perrin DH. Sex differences in knee joint laxity change across the female menstrual cycle. *J Sports Med Phys Fitness.* 2005;45:594–603.

47. Gray AM, Gugala Z, Baillargeon JG. Effects of oral contraceptive use on anterior cruciate ligament injury epidemiology. *Med Sci Sports Exerc.* 2016;48:648–654.

48. Rahr-Wagner L, Thillemann TM, Mehnert F, Pedersen AB, Lind M. Is the use of oral contraceptives associated with operatively treated anterior cruciate ligament injury? A case-control study from the Danish Knee Ligament Reconstruction Registry. *Am J Sports Med.* 2014;42: 2897–2905.

49. Khowailed IA, Petrofsky J, Lohman E, Daher N, Mohamed O. 17beta-estradiol induced effects on anterior cruciate ligament laxness and neuromuscular activation patterns in female runners. *J Womens Health (Larchmt).* 2015;24:670–680.

50. Herzberg SD, Motu'apuaka ML, Lambert W, Fu R, Brady J, Guise JM. The effect of menstrual cycle and contraceptives on ACL injuries and laxity: a systematic review and meta-analysis. *Orthop J Sports Med.* 2017;5, 2325967117718781.

51. McLean SG, Lipfert SW, van den Bogert AJ. Effect of gender and defensive opponent on the biomechanics of sidestep cutting. *Med Sci Sports Exerc.* 2004;36: 1008–1016.

52. Chappell JD, Yu B, Kirkendall DT, Garrett WE. A comparison of knee kinetics between male and female recreational athletes in stop-jump tasks. *Am J Sports Med.* 2002;30:261–267.

53. Hewett TE, Lindenfeld TN, Riccobene JV, Noyes FR. The effect of neuromuscular training on the incidence of knee injury in female athletes. A prospective study. *Am J Sports Med.* 1999;27:699–706.

54. McEldowney KM, Hopper LS, Etlin-Stein H, Redding E. Fatigue effects on quadriceps and hamstrings activation in dancers performing drop landings. *J Dance Med Sci.* 2013;17:109−114.

55. Ballantyne BT, Shields RK. Quadriceps fatigue alters human muscle performance during a novel weight bearing task. *Med Sci Sports Exerc.* 2010;42:1712−1722.

56. Ford KR, Myer GD, Hewett TE. Valgus knee motion during landing in high school female and male basketball players. *Med Sci Sports Exerc.* 2003;35:1745−1750.

57. Zeller BL, McCrory JL, Kibler WB, Uhl TL. Differences in kinematics and electromyographic activity between men and women during the single-legged squat. *Am J Sports Med.* 2003;31:449−456.

58. Myer GD, Sugimoto D, Thomas S, Hewett TE. The influence of age on the effectiveness of neuromuscular training to reduce anterior cruciate ligament injury in female athletes: a meta-analysis. *Am J Sports Med.* 2013;41:203−215.

59. Taylor JB, Waxman JP, Richter SJ, Shultz SJ. Evaluation of the effectiveness of anterior cruciate ligament injury prevention programme training components: a systematic review and meta-analysis. *Br J Sports Med.* 2015;49:79−87.

60. Yoo JH, Lim BO, Ha M, et al. A meta-analysis of the effect of neuromuscular training on the prevention of the anterior cruciate ligament injury in female athletes. *Knee Surg Sports Traumatol Arthrosc.* 2010;18:824−830.

61. Sugimoto D, Myer GD, Foss KD, Hewett TE. Specific exercise effects of preventive neuromuscular training intervention on anterior cruciate ligament injury risk reduction in young females: meta-analysis and subgroup analysis. *Br J Sports Med.* 2015;49:282−289.

62. Donnell-Fink LA, Klara K, Collins JE, et al. Effectiveness of knee injury and anterior cruciate ligament tear prevention programs: a meta-analysis. *PLoS One.* 2015;10:e0144063.

63. Gagnier JJ, Morgenstern H, Chess L. Interventions designed to prevent anterior cruciate ligament injuries in adolescents and adults: a systematic review and meta-analysis. *Am J Sports Med.* 2013;41:1952−1962.

64. Sadoghi P, von Keudell A, Vavken P. Effectiveness of anterior cruciate ligament injury prevention training programs. *J Bone Joint Surg Am.* 2012;94:769−776.

65. Sugimoto D, Myer GD, Barber Foss KD, Pepin MJ, Micheli LJ, Hewett TE. Critical components of neuromuscular training to reduce ACL injury risk in female athletes: meta-regression analysis. *Br J Sports Med.* 2016;50:1259−1266.

66. Sugimoto D, Myer GD, Foss KD, Hewett TE. Dosage effects of neuromuscular training intervention to reduce anterior cruciate ligament injuries in female athletes: meta- and sub-group analyses. *Sports Med.* 2014;44:551−562.

67. Sugimoto D, Myer GD, Bush HM, Klugman MF, Medina McKeon JM, Hewett TE. Compliance with neuromuscular training and anterior cruciate ligament injury risk reduction in female athletes: a meta-analysis. *J Athl Train.* 2012;47:714−723.

68. Walden M, Atroshi I, Magnusson H, Wagner P, Hagglund M. Prevention of acute knee injuries in adolescent female football players: cluster randomised controlled trial. *BMJ.* 2012;344:e3042.

69. Mandelbaum BR, Silvers HJ, Watanabe DS, et al. Effectiveness of a neuromuscular and proprioceptive training program in preventing anterior cruciate ligament injuries in female athletes: 2-year follow-up. *Am J Sports Med.* 2005;33:1003−1010.

70. Gilchrist J, Mandelbaum BR, Melancon H, et al. A randomized controlled trial to prevent noncontact anterior cruciate ligament injury in female collegiate soccer players. *Am J Sports Med.* 2008;36:1476−1483.

71. Salem HS, Varzhapetyan V, Patel N, Dodson CC, Tjoumakaris FP, Freedman KB. Anterior cruciate ligament reconstruction in young female athletes: patellar versus hamstring tendon autografts. *Am J Sports Med.* 2019;47:2086−2092.

72. Heffron WM, Hunnicutt JL, Xerogeanes JW, Woolf SK, Slone HS. Systematic review of publications regarding quadriceps tendon autograft use in anterior cruciate ligament reconstruction. *Arthrosc Sports Med Rehabil.* 2019;1:e93−e99.

73. Slone HS, Romine SE, Premkumar A, Xerogeanes JW. Quadriceps tendon autograft for anterior cruciate ligament reconstruction: a comprehensive review of current literature and systematic review of clinical results. *Arthroscopy.* 2015;31:541−554.

74. Shani RH, Umpierez E, Nasert M, Hiza EA, Xerogeanes J. Biomechanical comparison of quadriceps and patellar tendon grafts in anterior cruciate ligament reconstruction. *Arthroscopy.* 2016;32:71−75.

75. Kanakamedala AC, de Sa D, Obioha OA, et al. No difference between full thickness and partial thickness quadriceps tendon autografts in anterior cruciate ligament reconstruction: a systematic review. *Knee Surg Sports Traumatol Arthrosc.* 2019;27:105−116.

76. Hunnicutt JL, Gregory CM, McLeod MM, Woolf SK, Chapin RW, Slone HS. Quadriceps recovery after anterior cruciate ligament reconstruction with quadriceps tendon versus patellar tendon autografts. *Orthop J Sports Med.* 2019;7, 2325967119839786.

77. Perez JR, Emerson CP, Barrera CM, et al. Patient-reported knee outcome scores with soft tissue quadriceps tendon autograft are similar to bone-patellar tendon-bone autograft at minimum 2-year follow-up: a retrospective single-center cohort study in primary anterior cruciate ligament reconstruction surgery. *Orthop J Sports Med.* 2019;7, 2325967119890063.

78. Mouarbes D, Menetrey J, Marot V, Courtot L, Berard E, Cavaignac E. Anterior cruciate ligament reconstruction: a systematic review and meta-analysis of outcomes for quadriceps tendon autograft versus bone-patellar tendon-bone and hamstring-tendon autografts. *Am J Sports Med.* 2019;47:3531−3540.

79. van Eck CF, Martins CA, Vyas SM, Celentano U, van Dijk CN, Fu FH. Femoral intercondylar notch shape and dimensions in ACL-injured patients. *Knee Surg Sports Traumatol Arthrosc.* 2010;18:1257–1262.

80. Rothrauff BB, Jorge A, de Sa D, Kay J, Fu FH, Musahl V. Anatomic ACL reconstruction reduces risk of post-traumatic osteoarthritis: a systematic review with minimum 10-year follow-up. *Knee Surg Sports Traumatol Arthrosc.* 2020;28:1072–1084.

81. Group MK, Spindler KP, Huston LJ, et al. Ten-year outcomes and risk factors after anterior cruciate ligament reconstruction: a MOON longitudinal prospective cohort study. *Am J Sports Med.* 2018;46:815–825.

82. Borchers JR, Kaeding CC, Pedroza AD, et al. Intra-articular findings in primary and revision anterior cruciate ligament reconstruction surgery: a comparison of the MOON and MARS study groups. *Am J Sports Med.* 2011;39:1889–1893.

83. Engelman GH, Carry PM, Hitt KG, Polousky JD, Vidal AF. Comparison of allograft versus autograft anterior cruciate ligament reconstruction graft survival in an active adolescent cohort. *Am J Sports Med.* 2014;42:2311–2318.

84. Rice RS, Waterman BR, Lubowitz JH. Allograft versus autograft decision for anterior cruciate ligament reconstruction: an expected-value decision analysis evaluating hypothetical patients. *Arthroscopy.* 2012;28:539–547.

85. Mistry H, Metcalfe A, Colquitt J, et al. Autograft or allograft for reconstruction of anterior cruciate ligament: a health economics perspective. *Knee Surg Sports Traumatol Arthrosc.* 2019;27:1782–1790.

86. Magnussen RA, Lawrence JT, West RL, Toth AP, Taylor DC, Garrett WE. Graft size and patient age are predictors of early revision after anterior cruciate ligament reconstruction with hamstring autograft. *Arthroscopy.* 2012;28:526–531.

87. Mariscalco MW, Flanigan DC, Mitchell J, et al. The influence of hamstring autograft size on patient-reported outcomes and risk of revision after anterior cruciate ligament reconstruction: a Multicenter Orthopaedic Outcomes Network (MOON) cohort study. *Arthroscopy.* 2013;29:1948–1953.

88. Snaebjornsson T, Hamrin-Senorski E, Svantesson E, et al. Graft diameter and graft type as predictors of anterior cruciate ligament revision: a cohort study including 18,425 patients from the Swedish and Norwegian national knee ligament registries. *J Bone Joint Surg Am.* 2019;101:1812–1820.

89. Snaebjornsson T, Hamrin Senorski E, Ayeni OR, et al. Graft diameter as a predictor for revision anterior cruciate ligament reconstruction and KOOS and EQ-5D values: a cohort study from the Swedish national knee ligament register based on 2240 patients. *Am J Sports Med.* 2017;45:2092–2097.

90. Gabler CM, Jacobs CA, Howard JS, Mattacola CG, Johnson DL. Comparison of graft failure rate between autografts placed via an anatomic anterior cruciate ligament reconstruction technique: a systematic review, meta-

analysis, and meta-regression. *Am J Sports Med.* 2016;44:1069–1079.

91. Mohtadi N, Chan D, Barber R, Oddone Paolucci E. A randomized clinical trial comparing patellar tendon, hamstring tendon, and double-bundle ACL reconstructions: patient-reported and clinical outcomes at a minimal 2-year follow-up. *Clin J Sport Med.* 2015;25:321–331.

92. Rahr-Wagner L, Thillemann TM, Pedersen AB, Lind M. Comparison of hamstring tendon and patellar tendon grafts in anterior cruciate ligament reconstruction in a nationwide population-based cohort study: results from the Danish registry of knee ligament reconstruction. *Am J Sports Med.* 2014;42:278–284.

93. Browning 3rd WM, Kluczynski MA, Curatolo C, Marzo JM. Suspensory versus aperture fixation of a quadrupled hamstring tendon autograft in anterior cruciate ligament reconstruction: a meta-analysis. *Am J Sports Med.* 2017;45:2418–2427.

94. Lubowitz JH, Schwartzberg R, Smith P. Cortical suspensory button versus aperture interference screw fixation for knee anterior cruciate ligament soft-tissue allograft: a prospective, randomized controlled trial. *Arthroscopy.* 2015;31:1733–1739.

95. Saccomanno MF, Shin JJ, Mascarenhas R, et al. Clinical and functional outcomes after anterior cruciate ligament reconstruction using cortical button fixation versus transfemoral suspensory fixation: a systematic review of randomized controlled trials. *Arthroscopy.* 2014;30:1491–1498.

96. Hurley ET, Gianakos AL, Anil U, Strauss EJ, Gonzalez-Lomas G. No difference in outcomes between femoral fixation methods with hamstring autograft in anterior cruciate ligament reconstruction - a network meta-analysis. *Knee.* 2019;26:292–301.

97. Snaebjornsson T, Hamrin Senorski E, Svantesson E, et al. Graft fixation and timing of surgery are predictors of early anterior cruciate ligament revision: a cohort study from the Swedish and Norwegian knee ligament registries based on 18,425 patients. *JB JS Open Access.* 2019;4:e0037.

98. Musahl V, Rahnemai-Azar AA, Costello J, et al. The influence of meniscal and anterolateral capsular injury on knee laxity in patients with anterior cruciate ligament injuries. *Am J Sports Med.* 2016;44:3126–3131.

99. Dejour D, Pungitore M, Valluy J, Nover L, Saffarini M, Demey G. Preoperative laxity in ACL-deficient knees increases with posterior tibial slope and medial meniscal tears. *Knee Surg Sports Traumatol Arthrosc.* 2019;27:564–572.

100. Logan CA, Aman ZS, Kemler BR, Storaci HW, Dornan GJ, LaPrade RF. Influence of medial meniscus bucket-handle repair in setting of anterior cruciate ligament reconstruction on tibiofemoral contact mechanics: a biomechanical study. *Arthroscopy.* 2019;35:2412–2420.

101. Hagmeijer MH, Hevesi M, Desai VS, et al. Secondary meniscal tears in patients with anterior cruciate ligament

injury: relationship among operative management, osteoarthritis, and arthroplasty at 18-year mean follow-up. *Am J Sports Med.* 2019;47:1583—1590.

102. Golan EJ, Tisherman R, Byrne K, Diermeier T, Vaswani R, Musahl V. Anterior cruciate ligament injury and the anterolateral complex of the knee-importance in rotatory knee instability? *Curr Rev Musculoskelet Med.* 2019;12:472—478.

103. Getgood AMJ, Bryant DM, Litchfield R, et al. Lateral extra-articular tenodesis reduces failure of hamstring tendon autograft anterior cruciate ligament reconstruction: 2-year outcomes from the STABILITY study randomized clinical trial. *Am J Sports Med.* 2020;48:285—297.

104. Nagelli CV, Hewett TE. Should return to sport be delayed until 2 years after anterior cruciate ligament reconstruction? Biological and functional considerations. *Sports Med.* 2017;47:221—232.

105. Kyritsis P, Bahr R, Landreau P, Miladi R, Witvrouw E. Likelihood of ACL graft rupture: not meeting six clinical discharge criteria before return to sport is associated with a four times greater risk of rupture. *Br J Sports Med.* 2016;50:946—951.

106. Grindem H, Snyder-Mackler L, Moksnes H, Engebretsen L, Risberg MA. Simple decision rules can reduce reinjury risk by 84% after ACL reconstruction: the Delaware-Oslo ACL cohort study. *Br J Sports Med.* 2016;50:804—808.

107. Wellsandt EFM, Snyder-Mackler L. Neuromuscular training to target deficits associated with second anterior cruciate ligament injury. *J Orthop Sports Phys Ther.* November 2017;43(11):777—792.

108. Di Stasi S, Myer GD, Hewett TE. Neuromuscular training to target deficits associated with second anterior cruciate ligament injury. *J Orthop Sports Phys Ther.* 2013;43, 777—792, A771—711.

Anterior Cruciate Ligament Injuries in Female Soccer Players

HANNAH L. BRADSELL, BS • RACHEL M. FRANK, MD

INTRODUCTION

Since the passing of Title IX in 1972, female participation in sports at every level has increased tremendously and continues to grow.[1,2] With that, however, the prevalence of sports-related musculoskeletal injuries has also greatly increased in the female athlete. In particular, anterior cruciate ligament (ACL) injuries have become a critical issue for a variety of reasons, including the severity of the injury itself; time loss from participation in sports, recovery, and rehabilitation from surgery; and long-term consequences of injury, such as osteoarthritis. In addition to the substantial impacts an ACL injury has on an individual, the healthcare costs of reconstruction surgery and postoperative rehabilitation, as well as costs associated with nonsurgical treatment, are extremely high, surpassing $100 million per year.[3] Female soccer players especially are a high-risk population, and among all athletes in general, they are some of the most frequent to be affected by ACL injuries. Female soccer players are at a significantly greater risk of sustaining a sprain or tear to the ligament compared with other female athletes participating in a variety of other sports, and even more so when compared with male soccer players.

The ACL functions as a knee stabilizer by preventing anterior translation of the tibia and providing rotational stability. The knee support provided by the ACL is key for multidirectional cutting, landing, and pivoting sports such as soccer.[4] With a functional deficit of the ACL, performing these actions are challenging and it risks further injury, resulting in many ACL-injured athletes to be unable to return to their preinjury level of play, or even to quit playing. After reconstruction, athletes remain at high risk for reinjury of the index knee and for injury of the contralateral ACL, and female soccer players have been reported to be among athletes with the highest risk for these occurrences. Awareness of the prevalence and the severity of multiple factors related to ACL injury among female soccer players is an important step toward implementing prevention techniques to ultimately decrease the incidence of injury. Additionally, a better understanding of the mechanisms and multifaceted risk factors that cause this injury, as well as awareness of the additional risks and frequency of graft failure and second ACL injuries, are valuable information for proper treatment. Finally, knowledge of the efficacy of current prevention programs that exist and placing high importance on the need for intervention can provide athletes, coaches, trainers, and parents with methods in which they can minimize the risk of ACL injury.

EPIDEMIOLOGY

With increasing awareness of the severity of ACL injury in the athletic population, many epidemiology studies have been conducted on high-risk populations, such as female soccer players, particularly highlighting the difference in injury rates between males and females. In 2005, Agel et al.[5] reported the ACL injury rate for basketball and soccer at the collegiate level in a 13-year review. Overall, there was a total of 1268 ACL injuries with 586 sustained while playing soccer, and within soccer, there were 394 ACL injuries in females versus 194 in males. It was also observed that soccer players sustained consistently more ACL injuries than basketball players. Throughout the study, the incidence of ACL injury in males reduced, whereas the rate in females remained constant, widening the magnitude of the disparity of injury rate between males and females. In an updated review of ACL injury rates across 15 different sports at the collegiate level over a 9-year period, Agel et al.[6] observed a similar trend within soccer that female athletes sustained significantly more ACL injuries than male athletes at over double the rate. Overall, 71 females and 26 males experienced an

The Female Athlete. https://doi.org/10.1016/B978-0-323-75985-4.00021-0

ACL injury, signified by rates of 0.10 versus 0.04 per 1000 athletic exposures (AEs), respectively. Interestingly, there was a significant increase in injury rate per year over the course of this study, but these results also represented a 64% decrease in overall ACL injury rate in females and 56% decrease in males compared to the researchers' original data from their previous study.

To further emphasize the consistency of the epidemiology of ACL injuries in female soccer players, a review published in 1995[7] found a higher prevalence of knee injuries in female soccer players than in males over the course of the 5-year study period, despite the fact that there were significantly more men's teams included in the study (461 men's teams vs. 278 women's teams). The ACL injury rate was over double in the female athletes (0.31 vs. 0.13 per 1000 AEs) and 68% of females who sustained an ACL injury required surgery versus 59% of males. Notably, females also had a consistently higher rate of injury in any given year throughout the study period by at least double compared to males, in addition to a higher overall average rate.

Prodromos et al.[8] also noted that the rate of ACL injury was three times higher in female soccer players than in male soccer players (5% vs. 1.7%, respectively) participating in year-round high-level competition. Hootman et al.,[9] who studied the epidemiology of all injuries at the collegiate level over a 16-year study period, reported that soccer players sustained 579 of the 4800 ACL injuries among 15 sports. Within soccer, 411 of the ACL injuries occurred in females, whereas just 168 were suffered by males, represented by a difference in injury rate of 0.28 versus 0.09 per 1000 AEs, respectively. At the high-school level, Joseph et al.[10] also performed a multisport epidemiology study specifically comparing ACL injury patterns. The greatest prevalence of ACL injury was found in female soccer players, at a rate of 12.2 per 100,000 AEs, and among all the female athletes included in the study, 53.2% of ACL injuries occurred in soccer players. Overall, girls were twice as likely to sustain an ACL injury playing soccer compared to any other sport included in this population of high-school athletes. In a study, Larruskain et al.[11] prospectively compared injuries between male and female elite soccer players over the course of eight seasons. A total of 50 males and 35 females participated and they all belonged to the same club and had the same medical staff. At this high level of play, ACL ruptures were 5 times more common in females, which resulted in over 40% of the absences from play that

female athletes experienced. Females had a 21% greater amount of total days lost from participation, representing an injury burden twice as high compared to males, as well as a higher proportion of severe injuries overall.

When observing the incidence of ACL injuries in female soccer players compared to the risk of other injury types, ACL ruptures may always account for the majority, but they are still considered to be among the most severe type of injury with a high injury burden.[6,11,12] Faude et al.[12] prospectively analyzed injury incidences in female soccer players in the German National League over the course of a single season. A total of 165 players were included in the study, and on average, each player participated in 183 h of training and spent 31 h in matches. Overall, 241 injuries were sustained by 115 players (70% of the athletes) and 58% of the total injuries were severe injuries of the knee. Among them were 11 ACL ruptures sustained by 10 players (6% of all athletes), resulting in an incidence rate of 2.2 per 1000 match-hours. The average time lost from participation because of ACL injury was half of the year (178 days), which the authors noted that the severity of this injury and the high amount of time lost comes at a great disadvantage to the team and cost for the club. Not only is the team impacted but also the consequences for the athlete include risks of permanent disability of the injured knee, emphasizing the importance of finding effective prevention methods. Giza et al.[13] also reported injuries in professional female soccer players and found that ACL injuries consisted of 4.6% of all injuries (8 of 173) and 14.6% of all knee injuries (8 of 55), and the incidence of ACL tears was 0.09 per 1000 player-hours. Le Gall et al.[14] studied the incidence of injuries in young elite female soccer players prospectively over eight seasons, and out of the 119 players that participated in this study, 110 (92.4% of the athletes) experienced a total of 619 injuries. A majority of the injuries occurred in the youngest team (Under-15) and the least amount of injuries occurred in the oldest team (Under-19). Of the 619 injuries, a total of 12 ACL injuries were sustained by 11 players, with 7 of them occurring in the nondominant leg. Interestingly, no ACL injuries were reported in the last 3 years of the study, which the authors attributed to the introduction of a prophylactic conditioning program. Despite this, it was noted that the overall risk of ACL injury was comparable to adult elite female soccer players, which confirms the ongoing importance for intervention in the entire population of female soccer athletes and a further understanding of the many aspects associated with this specific injury.

MECHANISMS AND RISK FACTORS
Mechanisms of Injury

Understanding the most prominent mechanisms of ACL injury in female soccer players is crucial for minimizing injury risk. This necessary information can help develop targeted training programs toward avoiding the conditions that create the highest risk. Among female athletes in general, noncontact mechanisms are typically reported as the more common cause of injury compared with contact mechanisms.[6,7,12,13,15-17] Agel et al.[6] found that within 15 different collegiate-level sports, 60% of the ACL injuries sustained by female athletes were caused by noncontact mechanisms. Specifically with respect to soccer, a significantly higher incidence of noncontact ACL injuries has been reported compared with contact ACL injuries, although both mechanisms occurred more frequently in females than males (161 females vs. 66 males injured by noncontact; 115 females vs. 72 males injured by contact).[5] In a separate study, females were two times more likely to sustain an ACL injury after contact with another player and three times more likely as a result of noncontact mechanisms when compared with males. Overall, more females were injured from noncontact methods than they were from player-to-player contact incidences.[7] A 2-year retrospective study[18] reported the mechanisms of injury in high-school athletes and found that overall, noncontact ACL injuries were more common in female soccer players than contact ACL injuries at this level. Researchers further divided noncontact injuries into three categories and found that female soccer players suffered significantly more ACL injuries related to stopping and cutting than those related to landing. Within contact injuries, it was also reported that females sustained significantly more indirect ACL injuries, defined as contact with other body parts before and at the moment of injury, than direct contact injuries, which involved direct contact to the knee. Faude et al.[12] also supported these findings and reported that 7 of 11 ACL ruptures sustained by female soccer players in a season were caused by a change in direction, described as deceleration with a quick turn inducing high forces on the knee. The authors explained that their results reflected the observation that in quick stopping and cutting sports, such as soccer, increased incidence of ACL injury due to noncontact mechanisms is expected in female athletes. They also speculated that these patterns and higher rates of noncontact ACL injury could be attributed to the continuing progression in women's soccer with respect to game dynamics and the athleticism of the players.

Anatomic, Biomechanical, and Neuromuscular Risk Factors

The noteworthy occurrences of ACL injuries in female athletes, particularly soccer players, and the consequences that exist after suffering an injury have led researchers to attempt to understand the various intrinsic and extrinsic risk factors that cause such severe injuries. Various areas of study have been analyzed in an effort to explain the gender differences in ACL injury rates and mechanisms, including anatomic, biomechanical, muscle strength, and neuromuscular patterns, and to ultimately attempt to limit risk exposure to high-risk female athletes. Anatomic risk factors of ACL injury that have been mentioned, and notably reported, to occur more frequently in female athletes include smaller ligament size, decreased femoral notch width, increased posterior-inferior slope of the lateral tibia plateau, increased knee and generalized laxity, and higher body mass index.[4] In both supine and standing positions, the quadriceps angle (Q-angle) has been shown to be greater in females than males, leading the quadriceps to be pulled more laterally at the knee, causing the ACL to be placed in a position where it is at a greater risk of rupture.[19] Further related to the Q-angle, variances in pelvic structure and lower extremity alignment between males and females have also been argued as a potential explanation for the gender differences seen in ACL injury rates.[17] Additional structural factors reviewed by Sutton and Bullock[19] that potentially increase risk of ACL rupture include a narrower intercondylar notch, smaller ACL size, and an increased posterior tibial slope, although contradictory results have been reported regarding the role these factors have in injury. Hewett[17] also published a review article addressing the multifaceted risk factors associated with ACL injuries in female athletes and described that the overarching evidence for anatomic theories continues to be contradictory. Additionally, given the lack of opportunity for intervention with respect to anatomy, other theories attempting to explain the high incidence of ACL injury in female athletes have the potential to provide viable solutions for prevention and may arguably deserve more focus, such as muscle strength deficits and neuromuscular theories.

Several studies have observed mechanisms in which alterations in muscle strength are related to ACL injury risk. Ryman Augustsson and Ageberg[20] studied 225 high-school athletes and analyzed the role of lower extremity muscle strength in traumatic knee injury. The researchers categorized athletes into the weak or strong group based on the results of a one-repetition maximum barbell squat test. Within the population, a total 18 ACL injuries occurred and 14 of them were sustained by female athletes. Among these injuries, 12 were suffered by athletes categorized in the weak group compared to only 2 in the strong group. It was reported that the odds of experiencing an ACL injury was seven times greater for female athletes in the weak muscle strength group compared with the strong group ($P = .011$). Notably, the ACL injury rate was also significantly higher for female athletes in the weak group compared with male athletes in the weak group, and the injury rate was similar between weak and strong males. A correlation between lower extremity muscle strength deficits and future ACL injury was seen only in the female athletes of this youth population, indicating that screening female athletes for muscle strength at a young age could be a key factor in injury prevention training. The authors also mentioned an additional concern for the young, talented female soccer players who play extra matches with other teams, especially those who play at a higher level with more physically matured and skilled opponents, which further increases the chance of injury in this already high-risk population.

In a study by Hannon et al.[21] researchers analyzed hip and knee strength within two age groups of adolescent female soccer players to establish normative strength data for muscle groups where weakness has been previously associated with ACL injury risk. A total of 64 female soccer players aged 10−18 years were included in this study and were split up into two groups based on age. Group 1 included athletes between 10 and 14 years of age and group 2 included athletes between 15 and 18 years of age. No significant difference was found between the groups for quadriceps strength, hamstring strength, or hip external rotation strength when comparing dominant and nondominant limbs. However, a significant difference in hip abduction strength was observed between the two groups, measured by a handheld device as the subject pushed maximally into it for 3−5 s. On the dominant leg, group 1 had an average hip abduction strength, normalized to body mass, of 0.21 kg/mass compared to 0.18 kg/mass in group 2 ($P = .014$). On the nondominant leg, the same difference in strength values was seen between the two groups (group 1: 0.21 kg/mass; group 2: 0.18 kg/mass) and was found to be statistically significant ($P = .019$). Overall, the younger cohort had greater hip abduction strength and the authors mentioned that similar findings have been reported by other authors, which have observed a decrease in strength consistent with a change in pubertal status

(from prepubertal to pubertal status). Furthermore, these results can be explained by the change in fat-free mass that females experience as they progress through puberty, and when combined with the skeletal growth that occurs during this period, which causes a change in location of center of mass, these factors have been shown to increase injury risk.[22,23] As stated by the authors, the importance of publishing normative strength values for this high-risk population is to improve clinical decision-making for return to sport after an ACL injury.[21] In order to be cleared to return to sport, the strength of the injured limb should be equal to that of the healthy limb, but calculations of this symmetry can be altered by bilateral muscle strength changes that occur after ACL injury. In these circumstances, the symmetry exists, but the strength value has not been fully restored to preinjury levels, leading to athletes prematurely returning to play. Therefore the normative values taken from healthy individuals within this population can act as an accurate comparator for more appropriate clinical decision-making of when an athlete is fully ready to return to activity. Moreover, a hip strengthening program implemented during this transitional period might be advantageous for this population as they age because of the increase in ACL injury risk as hip abduction strength decreases.[21]

When muscle activity fails to stabilize the knee joint, there is an increase in the loads placed on the passive restraints of the knee leading to the eventual failure of the ACL.[19] A study by Marotta et al.[24] measured the activation time of muscles before contact with the ground in 20 professional soccer players. Surface electromyography was used to separately calculate the activation times of the rectus femoris, vastus medialis, biceps femoris, and semimembranosus muscles, while the athlete dropped from a platform and maintained a single-leg (the testing leg) landing for 5 s. They found that males had correct activation time in all the muscles examined, which related to a lower risk of ACL injury. On the contrary, females had delayed activation of the vastus medialis, which is related to an increase in anterior shear force, a known risk factor in sustaining an ACL injury. The clinical significance of these results, as noted by the authors, is that the testing protocol used in this study could be implemented in screening high-risk athletes and for developing interventions that target injury risks caused by specific muscle activation imbalances. Similarly, in his detailed review of neuromuscular factors associated with ACL injury, Hewett[17] reported gender differences in muscle usage and recruitment patterns that provide theories as to why females are at a significantly higher risk of ACL injury. Males appear to be muscle-dominant in regard to joint control strategies, while females are ligament-dominant. Additionally, males primarily use hamstring and gastrocnemius musculature, which act as a protective method to counteract landing forces, and have been shown to contract their hamstrings first in response to anterior tibial translation. On the contrary, female athletes tend to contract their quadriceps first in response to this anteriorly directed force on the back of the calf. The combination of strong quadriceps contraction during deceleration and a low flexion angle below 45 degrees leads to increased strain on the ACL.[25] Stronger contraction of the hamstrings, on the other hand, acts as an important knee stabilizer by restricting anterior tibial motion and ultimately decreasing anterior shear forces, thus significantly reducing the load placed on the ACL.[17]

Multiple studies have supported the correlation between a lower hamstring-to-quadriceps strength ratio and ACL injury, also indicated by a deficiency in hamstring strength and recruitment.[17,19,26,27] On average, females experience this muscle imbalance more frequently than males, who have a significantly higher strength ratio as well as proper coactivation patterns of these muscles. Thus the knee joint in males is naturally more protected from ACL injury risks related to unstable positions, such as knee abduction and dynamic valgus.[27] Additional risks of sustaining an ACL injury mentioned in Hewett's[17] review include off-balance, unstable landings in varus or valgus lower extremity alignment, and increased magnitude of adduction and abduction moments at the knee, which impact the hamstring and gastrocnemius functions in stabilizing the knee joint. Increased anterior knee laxity and lower knee flexor strength, also seen more commonly in females than males, have also been described as risk factors.[25] The significance of observing these neuromuscular risk patterns is that conditioning of the muscles involved in ACL stabilization and developing proper training programs to correct imbalances have the ability to correct these imbalances in high-risk female athletes and ultimately decrease the risk of ACL injury.[17]

Observing the role of improper neuromuscular control patterns in ACL injury risk provides a better understanding of the muscles involved in knee stabilization and their impact on the ACL. Developing proper training programs to condition these muscles and correct imbalances can improve strength deficits and modify activation patterns in high-risk female soccer athletes and ultimately reduce the risk of ACL injury.[17] In one study, Hewett et al.[27] used biomechanical measures of neuromuscular control and valgus loading to predict the risk of ACL injury in female athletes. Researchers prospectively screened 205 female soccer, basketball, and volleyball players prior to the start of their season during a reliable jump-landing task in which the subject dropped directly down off of a box and immediately performed a maximum vertical jump with arms raised. Neuromuscular control and joint loads were measured using three-dimensional kinematics (joint angles) and kinetics (joint moments) while the athletes performed this task, known as a drop vertical jump. By the end of their respective seasons, a total of nine ACL injuries were reported and seven of them occurred in soccer players. Notably, the nine athletes who suffered an ACL rupture had significantly different knee posture and loading compared to the 196 athletes who did not sustain an ACL rupture. More specifically, ACL-injured athletes had significantly greater dynamic lower extremity valgus and knee abduction than the uninjured athletes, indicating altered neuromuscular control characteristics. Additionally, the injured group had greater knee valgus motion and moments during ground impact of the jump-landing task compared with the uninjured athletes. This was determined to be a key component of the mechanism that led to ACL rupture and the main predictors of ACL injury risk in this study. In relation to the above-described findings, anterior tibial translation and loads on the ACL have been shown to be increased by valgus torques, and valgus loading is known to place a great amount of strain on the ACL.[28] This was further demonstrated in the study by Hewett et al. by the significantly greater values of knee abduction angles and moments observed in the ACL-injured athletes, which are factors that contribute to dynamic knee valgus and joint loading. Interestingly, statistical analysis performed by the researchers showed that knee abduction moments had a sensitivity of 78% and specificity of 73%, indicating that screening for this component has a high probability of accuracy in predicting true positive results and true negative results of the ACL injury status.[27] Based on these findings and as suggested by the authors, avoiding excessive dynamic valgus alignment and high abduction loads at landing, cutting, and/or decelerating can minimize athletes' risk of knee injury. Notably, the results from this study can facilitate the development of training programs that aim to prevent the observed ACL injury predictors through modifications of neuromuscular control patterns, ultimately guiding female athletes toward more effective, targeted interventions.[27]

In a similar study, Ford et al.[23] analyzed gender differences during landing of the drop vertical jump test and measured the maximum knee abduction angles and external moments in young athletes. Subjects participated in two testing sessions that were separated by 1 year and comparisons were made between year 1 and year 2 among pubertal females, postpubertal females, pubertal males, and postpubertal males. Researchers found that the knee abduction angle significantly increased in the pubertal female group between year 1 and year 2, during this period of rapid adolescent growth, but no change was seen in pubertal males. Postpubertal females also had a greater overall abduction angle than postpubertal males, but neither group saw a significant change between year 1 and year 2. In regard to landing with knee abduction motion and moment (torque), which are reported risk factors, both were significantly greater overall and across consecutive years in postpubertal females compared with postpubertal males following an adolescent growth spurt. The importance of these results is that they reflect an increase in ACL injury risk in female athletes during the early stages pubertal development, an important period for maturation.[23] During this time, when sex hormonal profiles are noticeably different between males and females, there is also a divergence in ACL injury rates between genders, with a disproportionate increase in females, further exemplifying the multifaceted aspects involved in ACL injuries.[19,22]

Hormonal Risk Factors

The effects of underlying hormonal influences on ACL injuries have been researched in an attempt to further understand the multifactorial nature of this significant injury. One study observed sex hormones in female athletes participating in a variety of sports[29] and found a significant difference in hormonal profiles between athletes who suffered an ACL rupture and those who did not. Overall, ACL-injured athletes had significantly lower concentration of testosterone, 17β-estradiol, and progesterone than uninjured athletes, which led the authors to believe that females with these indications are predisposed to ACL rupture. The authors acknowledged that based on the significant difference in testosterone levels between the groups, it can be said that this hormone may act in a protective manner. Likewise, various direct and indirect influences of testosterone on the ACL have been previously reported, such as greater collagen synthesis and ligament resilience, and decreased joint laxity, among many others.[22,29] With respect to 17β-estradiol, results indicated a significant difference in hormone concentrations between the ACL-injured group and the control group, specifically during the luteal phase of the menstrual cycle. Compared to the follicular phase, the luteal

phase is expected to have a 90% higher concentration of 17β-estradiol, which was seen in the control group, but only a 30% higher concentration during the luteal phase was observed in the injured group. Regarding progesterone levels, lower concentrations were also seen in the injured group during both the follicular and luteal phases, and although the magnitude of the concentration increase between phases was the same in both groups, the injured group had lower levels overall.

Based on the available data, hormone concentrations appear to be more crucial in determining ACL injury risk than the phase of the menstrual cycle, as suggested by previous studies, particularly due to the observation that differences in hormone concentrations can be misleading as to which phase of the menstrual cycle an individual is in. Furthermore, it has been reported by multiple studies that there is a greater risk of ACL injury during the preovulatory phase[30,31]; however, Stijak et al.[29] linked this generally accepted finding to the low concentrations of 17β-estradiol and progesterone seen during this phase, rather than the phase itself. Similarly, the researchers noted that individuals with even lower hormone levels than normal are at twice the risk of sustaining an ACL injury during the preovulatory phase because in general, females have naturally lower hormone concentrations during this stage.[29] Hewett et al.[31] further supported this theory in a systematic review based on the observation that a higher risk of ACL injury in females was correlated with times when hormone levels were most varied.

The mechanisms in which hormonal fluctuations appear to affect knee stability are mainly neuromuscular control and muscle strength, while the reported effects on the structure of ligaments is not well understood. For example, different levels of physical performance, neuromuscular firing patterns, motor skills, muscle function, and tendon and ligament strength have all been observed during different menstrual cycle phases.[32–35] These influences have also been tied to estrogen effects,[31] as it is a sex hormone that drastically changes throughout the duration of the menstrual cycle. Additionally, in support of the findings that fluctuating estrogen levels may increase the risk of ACL injury, Hewett[17] and Hansen[22] reported that female athletes who use oral contraceptives, which generally function to minimize surges of female sex hormones, have lower rates of ACL injury than those who do not use oral contraceptives. Researchers related the difference in injury incidence to increased overall knee stability through decreased knee laxity, increased hamstring-to-quadriceps strength ratios, and reduced valgus torques, among other stabilizing methods that were observed in oral contraceptive users.

Relaxin, a hormone with collagenolytic effects, has also been studied for its potential role in ACL tears. Interestingly, introducing relaxin to an animal model resulted in a significant weakening of the ACL, suggesting that relaxin concentration has damaging effects on the structure of collagen.[36] Similarly, it has been shown that females with higher serum relaxin concentration (SRC) have greater incidences of ACL tears.[37] In a study consisting of female athletes during the course of their college athletic career, there was a 21.9% incidence rate of complete ACL tears, and among the athletes who suffered an ACL injury, the mean SRC was 6.0 pg/mL compared to a mean SRC of 1.8 pg/mL in female athletes without a tear. Overall, it was found that individuals with SRC levels greater than 6.0 pg/mL had over 4 times the risk of sustaining an ACL tear compared with individuals with lower levels of relaxin.[37] Furthermore, researchers found relaxin receptors located on the ACL of nonpregnant females, but no receptors were found on the ACL of males. Although the mechanism of the risk of high levels of relaxin on ACL tears remains unclear, it is suggested that the integrity of the ACL in females is altered over time due to long-term exposure effects.[37] With this knowledge, it may be possible to develop medications to block relaxin receptors as an alternative to the unreasonable suggestion that individuals with predisposed risks should avoid participating in sports.

Overall, understanding the roles that various hormones may play in ACL injury risk is an additional key factor in developing all-encompassing prevention programs that better target each aspect of ACL injuries. Being aware of all areas capable of intervention can help athletes, trainers, and physicians more efficiently reduce risk, which is especially important for the vulnerable population of female soccer players.

Other Novel and Noteworthy Observations

In addition to the neuromuscular and hormonal influences on ACL injury risk in female soccer players, other modifiable risk factors, including fatigue related to playing volume, have been studied in this population. A study by Snyder et al.[38] analyzed the effects of two consecutive soccer matches on landing mechanics in Division I collegiate female athletes. The first match was played on a Friday evening and the second match was played 43 h later on a Sunday afternoon, and results were based off of physical performance and biomechanical measurements during a sidestep cutting movement. It was observed that biomechanical risk factors related to ACL injury significantly increased after playing a single soccer match and intensified further after playing in consecutive matches with less than 48 h of rest. In particular, there was a significant increase in ground reaction force leading to greater tibial compression and in lateral tibial shear joint force after the first match. After the second match, there was an even greater increase in each measurement, in addition to an increase in anterior tibial shear force, a known risk factor of ACL injury.[17,24] Significant findings of changes in physical performance parameters were also seen 12 h after the first match, including reduced knee extension strength and countermovement jump (an indication of muscle function). After the second match, countermovement jump was further reduced, and increased knee flexion and decreased knee flexion strength were also observed. Reduced knee flexion strength has been previously related to serious knee injury and observed to be more prominent in females than in males after intermittent high-intensity exercises, as commonly experienced in soccer.[39] The authors of this study also mentioned that playing in a second consecutive match with this imbalanced strength between knee flexors and extensors significantly impacts knee mechanics. Collectively, each of these risk factors, caused by excessive musculoskeletal stress and fatigue without optimal recovery time for neuromuscular and strength improvements, has the potential to greatly increase the incidence of ACL injury.[20,38] A similar finding has also been observed by Ryman Augustsson and Ageberg,[20] who reported that playing two matches in a week with a maximum of 4 days of recovery in between significantly increases injury risk in youth athletes compared to playing only one match per week. In the same sense, greater training per game hours is beneficial for reducing injury risk based on the potential for heightened performance and ideal physical conditioning.[12]

Another study[40] observed the effect of season-long participation on ACL volume in the bilateral knees of 17 female soccer players using MRI scans. Overall, there was a significant increase in average ACL volume from preseason to postseason (1426 vs. 1556 cc, respectively; $P = .006$), with a greater increase observed in the right knee than the left knee. All the athletes included in the study were right-leg dominant, and the difference in volume between limbs was attributed to the different types forces that act on each leg. The left leg is the planting leg, which causes stress at the knee during a kick, and the right leg is the kicking leg, which has additional external forces on it during contact with the ball. The authors proposed that the increase in ACL volume could be explained by repetitive trauma creating microscopic tears over the course of the season, resulting in inflammation and edema of the ligament. The results of this study reflect the process of ligament healing, which occurs in three stages: the acute inflammatory stage, followed by the proliferative repair stage (rebuilding of tissue matrix), and finally the remodeling phase.[41] The researchers did not report any ACL injuries in this population and therefore were unable to determine the effects of ACL volume on injury risk. However, these findings provide clinically relevant data on ligament healing and the functional changes that result from remodeling after injury, encouraging further research to analyze these effects on injury.

In a separate study, Kosaka et al.[42] prospectively studied a potential psychologic aspect of ACL injury with respect to competitiveness in female high-school athletes. Among the 300, 15-year-old athletes studied over the course of the 3-year study, 25 ACL injuries occurred through noncontact mechanisms. It was found that the athletes who sustained ACL injuries had significantly higher scores in competitiveness based on a Diagnostic Inventory of Psychological Competitive Ability (DIPCA.3) questionnaire that was completed at the beginning of the study. More specifically, these athletes scored higher in aggressiveness, volition for self-realization, volition for winning, judgment, and cooperation. Overall, it was observed that a higher confidence in ability was related to a higher risk of sustaining a noncontact ACL injury. The authors proposed that an explanation for this could be that the more competitive players pursued a higher level of their own performance and therefore placed themselves in higher risk situations by participating in training and competitive matches in a more aggressive manner. In addition, a noteworthy correlation between the history of concussion incidences and lower extremity injuries in collegiate athletes has been observed by multiple studies.[43-45] Each study found that athletes who reported a history of concussions were more likely to also report a history of a knee injury and were at a greater risk for knee injury than those who did not have a concussion history. Further investigation is necessary to understand the underlying mechanisms of this observation, but it is worth mentioning that a consistent relationship has been established by several studies. The importance of investigating the various mechanisms of ACL injury that have been analyzed by countless studies is to emphasize that there is no single factor that is solely responsible for this severe, unpredictable injury. It has been shown that it is not possible to visually predict which female soccer athletes may be at a greater risk of ACL injury during an activity.[46] This further indicates the need for screening these athletes to determine the specific risk factors an individual may have in order to better predict injury risk and more effectively prevent ACL injury.

POSTRECONSTRUCTION OUTCOMES AND REINJURY RISKS

Aside from the high incidence of a primary ACL injury in female soccer players, they also have an increased risk of secondary ACL injuries, such as graft failure or contralateral ACL injury. A 2020 study reported a higher risk of further ACL injury of ACL-reconstructed soccer players in a 10-year follow-up.[47] Among the 684 respondents of a questionnaire that was used to obtain results about return to play and additional knee injuries at 10 years after subjects' primary ACL injury, 51% reported that they had returned to soccer while 49% did not return. Within the players who did not return, 65.4% reported that it was due to causes related to knee. Among the players who did return to playing soccer, it was found that they had a significantly higher risk of graft failure and rerupture, contralateral ACL injury, and new injury to the affected knee. In this population, 28.7% sustained a new injury overall, where 9.7% had a rerupture and 20.6% suffered a contralateral ACL tear. Notably, further ACL injury was more prominent in females of this study, but this was not found to be statistically significant, and no significant difference in risk of rerupture was found between the types of graft used (bone-patellar tendon-bone vs. hamstring). In a similar study of a 5-year follow-up post-ACL injury,[48] 5.0% of patients underwent a contralateral ACL reconstruction surgery and 4.1% had a revision surgery of the affected knee overall. Particularly within the 15- to 18-year-old group of soccer players in this study, 22.0% of females had either a contralateral ACL reconstruction (10.2%) or a revision surgery (11.8%) compared to only 9.8% of males (4.4% contralateral and 5.4% revision). At the collegiate level, female soccer athletes also had significantly higher rates of recurrent ACL ruptures than male soccer players (5.2 vs. 1.4 per 10,000 AEs, respectively) over a 10-year study period.[49] Additionally, Fältström et al.[50] compared 117 active soccer players after ACL reconstruction to 119 knee-healthy matched controls on the same team (average age of 20 years old). The ACL-reconstructed group experienced new ACL injury at five times the rate of the control group and other traumatic and nontraumatic knee injuries at two to four times the rate, but no rate difference between the groups was observed for injuries unrelated to the knee. Throughout the 2-year study period, only 38% of the ACL-reconstructed group continued to play soccer compared to 64% of the control group, and the ACL-reconstructed group also had a greater reduction of activity level as indicated by a greater decrease in average Tegner Activity Scale score. Among the 62% of the players who quit after their ACL reconstruction, the main reasons were because they had suffered a new injury or because they had a lack of trust in their affected knee and feared a new injury. Based on this information, the researchers noted the importance of individualized rehabilitation and peak functional performance before returning to play, as well as allowing a proper amount of time for recovery after an ACL reconstruction. Interestingly, the optimal recovery time for minimizing risk of further injury in soccer is returning to play after at least 9 months,[51] and 1 out of 4 players in this study returned to soccer within 9 months of their ACL reconstruction surgery.

Similar findings were also supported by an earlier study that compared the risk of a second ACL injury in female soccer players to nonsoccer athletes matched by age, activity level, and graft type over a 2-year follow-up period.[52] Each group contained 90 female subjects and the average age was 20 years, and the nonsoccer group included athletes participating in basketball, downhill skiing, volleyball, and track. Compared to the nonsoccer group, soccer players had a significantly higher rate of graft failures (11% vs. 1%; $P < .01$) and contralateral ACL tears (17% vs. 4%; $P < .01$). With respect to survival rates at 6, 12, 24, 60, and 120 months, the graft survival rate for soccer players at each time point saw a significantly greater and consistent decline compared with that for nonsoccer players ($P < .01$). Similarly, the difference in survival rates of the contralateral ACL at each time point had the same pattern, with the most notable difference observed at the 120-month time point, where the contralateral survival rate for soccer players was merely 53% compared to 93% in nonsoccer players. Overall, 28% of the soccer athletes suffered a second ACL injury compared to only 5% of the nonsoccer athletes. Interestingly, soccer players also sustained significantly more lateral meniscal injuries alongside their primary ACL rupture compared with nonsoccer athletes (40% vs. 23%; $P = .02$). Particularly within the soccer group, players who returned to soccer after their primary ACL reconstruction surgery (67/90) had significantly more graft failures than the initial soccer players who did not return (15.0% vs. 0%; $P = .04$). A difference in contralateral tears was also observed, but it was not found to be statistically significant (19% vs. 9%; $P = .34$). Overall,

34% of the soccer players who returned suffered a second ACL injury compared to 9% of those who did not. Regarding graft survival rates from 6 to 120 months, the players who returned to soccer had a consistent decline at each time point, whereas players who did not return remained at a 100% graft survival rate throughout the study period. Interestingly, almost half of the graft failures that occurred within this group happened within 12 months of returning to soccer, whereas contralateral ACL tears tended to occur later and the survival rates between returners and nonreturners were similar. An additional finding that was reported only within the soccer group was older age as a risk factor for graft failure. The risk increased by a factor of 1.5 with every year of age, keeping in mind that the entire cohort was under 25 years old, which is generally considered young in age.

In a separate study, Bourne et al.[53] reported knee flexor weakness in 84 elite female soccer players who underwent an ACL reconstruction procedure in the previous 10 years. Within this group, 12 subjects had a history of a unilateral ACL reconstruction and their peak eccentric knee flexor force was compared to 72 subjects who did not have a history of an ACL reconstruction in the past 10 years. Values were measured during a Nordic hamstring exercise, where the participants knelt on a pad with their ankles secured and as they gradually leaned forward toward the ground, the force generated by their knee flexors was measured. It was found that those with a history of ACL reconstruction were weaker in their affected limb than their uninjured contralateral limb, represented by a 20% between-limb imbalance. In addition, the two-limb average peak eccentric knee flexor strength was weaker in the reconstructed group than the control group, and when hamstring-injured players were removed from analysis, the observed differences in strength were even greater. Notably, no difference was observed between the uninjured contralateral limbs of the ACL-reconstructed group and the healthy limbs of the control group. Additionally, among the ACL-reconstructed players, no correlation was found between the time since ACL reconstruction and a change in knee flexor strength or imbalance between limbs. Based on their study, the authors proposed that the postreconstruction knee flexor weakness may be explained by medial hamstring atrophy and reduced activation, which are known risk factors of primary ACL injury, although the mechanisms remain unclear. An additional noteworthy finding in this study was that 25% of the ACL-reconstructed players suffered a hamstring strain injury after reconstruction compared to only 2.8% of the uninjured players. Therefore it can be said that the further consequences of ACL injury and reconstruction and the strength imbalances that occur are an increased risk of sustaining a hamstring strain.[53] Worth mentioning as well is the consequence of developing osteoarthritis in the injured knee, where the likelihood has been reported to be as high as 80% within 15 years of an ACL injury.[4]

Despite the consistent findings of the high ACL reinjury risk in female soccer players, there is little understanding of the mechanisms and the reasons for the difference in rates compared to males. One possible mechanism is a further decrease in quadriceps and hamstring strength and inferior performance, particularly with jumping, of ACL-reconstructed athletes compared to healthy controls.[52] Additionally, increased risk in female soccer players compared with males may be explained by altered kinetics and neuromuscular control, a decrease in lower extremity agility, and consequent stiffening, which are all found after reconstruction predominantly in females. Also potentially affecting reinjury risk are influences of whether the injured limb is the player's dominant or nondominant leg, the increased demand placed on the contralateral limb after an injury, and the incomplete development of the athlete's original biomechanics, among other intrinsic factors specific to the individual.[54-58] Awareness of the epidemiologic data and risk factors associated with both primary and secondary ACL injuries further signifies the importance of implementing effective prevention programs to reduce injury in female soccer players.

CONCLUSIONS

With the continually increasing involvement and enhancement of athleticism in female soccer players, it is of utmost importance that athletes, coaches, and those involved in their healthcare are aware of the predominance of ACL injuries in this population. Additionally, knowledge of the severity of this injury and its consequences should not be overlooked when considering the high risks associated with sustaining an ACL injury. A better understanding of the specific risk factors and mechanisms involved is crucial for the development of effective injury prevention programs and for athletes to be able to protect themselves. Finally, great emphasis should be placed on the importance of implementing these programs in order to minimize risk exposure and reduce injury rates in this high-risk population.

REFERENCES

1. Acosta R, Carpenter L. *Women in Intercollegiate Sport. A Longitudinal, National Study, Thirty Seven Year Update. 1977-2014.* 2014.
2. Ladd AL. The sports bra, the ACL, and title IX — the game in play. *Clin Orthop Relat Res.* 2014;472(6):1681-1684.
3. Janssen KW, Orchard JW, Driscoll TR, Van Mechelen W. High incidence and costs for anterior cruciate ligament reconstructions performed in Australia from 2003-2004 to 2007-2008: time for an anterior cruciate ligament register by Scandinavian model? *Scand J Med Sci Sports.* 2012; 22(4):495-501.
4. Lin CY, Casey E, Herman DC, Katz N, Tenforde AS. Sex differences in common sports injuries. *PM R.* 2018;10(10): 1073-1082.
5. Agel J, Arendt EA, Bershadsky B. Anterior cruciate ligament injury in national collegiate athletic association basketball and soccer: a 13-year review. *Am J Sports Med.* 2005;33(4): 524-531.
6. Agel J, Rockwood T, Klossner D. Collegiate ACL injury rates across 15 sports: national collegiate athletic association injury surveillance system data update (2004-2005 through 2012-2013). *Clin J Sport Med.* 2016;26(6): 518-523.
7. Arendt E, Dick R. Knee injury patterns among men and women in collegiate basketball and soccer. *Am J Sports Med.* 1995;23(6):694-701.
8. Prodromos CC, Han Y, Rogowski J, Joyce B, Shi K. A meta-analysis of the incidence of anterior cruciate ligament tears as a function of gender, sport, and a knee injury—reduction regimen. *Arthrosc J Arthrosc Relat Surg.* 2007;23(12): 1320-1325.e6.
9. Hootman JM, Dick R, Agel J. Epidemiology of collegiate injuries for 15 sports: summary and recommendations for injury prevention initiatives. *J Athl Train.* 2007;42(2): 311-319.
10. Joseph AM, Collins CL, Henke NM, Yard EE, Fields SK, Comstock RD. A multisport epidemiologic comparison of anterior cruciate ligament injuries in high school athletics. *J Athl Train.* 2013;48(6):810-817.
11. Larruskain J, Lekue JA, Diaz N, Odriozola A, Gil SM. A comparison of injuries in elite male and female football players: a five-season prospective study. *Scand J Med Sci Sports.* 2018;28(1):237-245.
12. Faude O, Junge A, Kindermann W, Dvorak J. Injuries in female soccer players. *Am J Sports Med.* 2005;33(11): 1694-1700.
13. Giza E, Mithofer K, Farrell L, Zarins B, Gill T. Injuries in women's professional soccer. *Br J Sports Med.* 2005; 39(4):212-216.
14. Le Gall F, Carling C, Reilly T. Injuries in young elite female soccer players. *Am J Sports Med.* 2008;36(2):276-284.
15. Brant JA, Johnson B, Brou L, Comstock RD, Vu T. Rates and patterns of lower extremity sports injuries in all gender-comparable US high school sports. *Orthop J Sports Med.* 2019;7(10), 232596711987305.

16. Rechel JA, Collins CL, Comstock RD. Epidemiology of injuries requiring surgery among high school athletes in the United States, 2005 to 2010. *J Trauma.* 2011;71(4): 982–989.

17. Hewett TE. Neuromuscular and hormonal factors associated with knee injuries in female athletes. *Sports Med.* 2000;29(5):313–327.

18. Takahashi S, Nagano Y, Ito W, Kido Y, Okuwaki T. A retrospective study of mechanisms of anterior cruciate ligament injuries in high school basketball, handball, judo, soccer, and volleyball. *Medicine (Baltim).* 2019; 98(26):e16030.

19. Sutton KM, Bullock JM. Anterior cruciate ligament rupture: differences between males and females. *J Am Acad Orthop Surg.* 2013;21(1):41–50.

20. Ryman Augustsson S, Ageberg E. Weaker lower extremity muscle strength predicts traumatic knee injury in youth female but not male athletes. *BMJ Open Sport Exercise Med.* 2017;3(1):e000222.

21. Hannon JP, Wang-Price S, Garrison JC, Goto S, Bothwell JM, Bush CA. Normalized hip and knee strength in two age groups of adolescent female soccer players. *J Strength Cond Res.* 2019. https://doi.org/10.1519/JSC.0000000000003420. Epub ahead of print. PMID: 31868812.

22. Hansen M, Kjaer M. *Sex Hormones and Tendon.* Springer International Publishing; 2016:139–149.

23. Ford KR, Shapiro R, Myer GD, Van Den Bogert AJ, Hewett TE. Longitudinal sex differences during landing in knee abduction in young athletes. *Med Sci Sports Exerc.* 2010;42(10):1923–1931.

24. Marotta N, Demeco A, de Scorpio G, Indino A, Iona T, Ammendolia A. Late activation of the vastus medialis in determining the risk of anterior cruciate ligament injury in soccer players. *J Sport Rehabil.* 2019:1–4.

25. Huston LJ, Wojtys EM. Neuromuscular performance characteristics in elite female athletes. *Am J Sports Med.* 1996; 24(4):427–436.

26. Alentorn-Geli E, Myer GD, Silvers HJ, et al. Prevention of non-contact anterior cruciate ligament injuries in soccer players. Part 1: mechanisms of injury and underlying risk factors. *Knee Surg Sports Traumatol Arthrosc.* 2009;17(7): 705–729.

27. Hewett TE, Myer GD, Ford KR, et al. Biomechanical measures of neuromuscular control and valgus loading of the knee predict anterior cruciate ligament injury risk in female athletes: a prospective study. *Am J Sports Med.* 2005;33(4):492–501.

28. Fukuda Y, Woo SLY, Loh JC, et al. A quantitative analysis of valgus torque on the ACL: a human cadaveric study. *J Orthop Res.* 2003;21(6):1107–1112.

29. Stijak L, Kadija M, Djulejić V, et al. The influence of sex hormones on anterior cruciate ligament rupture: female study. *Knee Surg Sports Traumatol Arthrosc.* 2015;23(9): 2742–2749.

30. Balachandar V, Marciniak JL, Wall O, Balachandar C. Effects of the menstrual cycle on lower-limb biomechanics, neuromuscular control, and anterior cruciate ligament injury risk: a systematic review. *Muscles Ligaments Tendons J.* 2017;7(1):136–146.

31. Hewett TE, Zazulak BT, Myer GD. Effects of the menstrual cycle on anterior cruciate ligament injury risk. *Am J Sports Med.* 2007;35(4):659–668.

32. Florini JR. Hormonal control of muscle growth. *Muscle Nerve.* 1987;10(7):577–598.

33. Lebrun CM. The effect of the phase of the menstrual cycle and the birth control pill on athletic performance. *Clin Sports Med.* 1994;13(2):419–441.

34. Posthuma BW, Bass MJ, Bull SB, Nisker JA. Detecting changes in functional ability in women with premenstrual syndrome. *Am J Obstet Gynecol.* 1987;156(2):275–278.

35. Sarwar R, Niclos BB, Rutherford OM. Changes in muscle strength, relaxation rate and fatiguability during the human menstrual cycle. *J Physiol.* 1996;493(1):267–272.

36. Dragoo JL, Padrez K, Workman R, Lindsey DP. The effect of relaxin on the female anterior cruciate ligament: analysis of mechanical properties in an animal model. *Knee.* 2009;16(1):69–72.

37. Dragoo JL, Castillo TN, Braun HJ, Ridley BA, Kennedy AC, Golish SR. Prospective correlation between serum relaxin concentration and anterior cruciate ligament tears among elite collegiate female. *Athletes.* 2011; 39(10):2175–2180.

38. Snyder BJ, Hutchison R, Mills CJ, Parsons SJ. Effects of two competitive soccer matches on landing biomechanics in female division I soccer players. *Sports.* 2019;7(11):237.

39. Mercer TH, Gleeson NP, Wren K. Influence of prolonged intermittent high-intensity exercise on knee flexor strength in male and female soccer players. *Eur J Appl Physiol.* 2003; 89(5):506–508.

40. Myrick KM, Voss A, Feinn RS, Martin T, Mele BM, Garbalosa JC. Effects of season long participation on ACL volume in female intercollegiate soccer athletes. *J Exp Orthop.* 2019;6(1).

41. Hauser RA, Dolan EE, Phillips HJ, Newlin AC, Moore RE, Woldin BA. Ligament injury and healing: a review of current clinical diagnostics and therapeutics. *Open Rehabil J.* 2013;6(1):1–20.

42. Kosaka M, Nakase J, Numata H, et al. Psychological traits regarding competitiveness are related to the incidence of anterior cruciate ligament injury in high school female athletes. *Knee.* 2016;23(4):681–685.

43. Brooks MA, Peterson K, Biese K, Sanfilippo J, Heiderscheit B, Bell DR. Concussion increases odds of sustaining a lower extremity musculoskeletal injury after return to play among collegiate athletes. *Am J Sports Med.* 2016;44.

44. Gilbert FC, Burdette GT, Joyner AB, Llewellyn TA, Buckley TA. Association between concussion and lower extremity injuries in collegiate athletes. *Sports Health.* 2016; 8(6):561–567.

45. Houston MN, Hoch JM, Cameron KL, Abt JP, Peck KY, Hoch MC. Sex and number of concussions influence the association between concussion and musculoskeletal injury history in collegiate athletes. *Brain Inj.* 2018; 32(11):1353–1358.

46. Mørtvedt AI, Krosshaug T, Bahr R, Petushek E. I spy with my little eye … a knee about to go "pop"? Can coaches and sports medicine professionals predict who is at greater risk of ACL rupture? *Br J Sports Med.* 2020;54(3):154−158.

47. Sandon A, Engström B, Forssblad M. High risk of further anterior cruciate ligament injury in a 10-year follow-up study of anterior cruciate ligament-reconstructed soccer players in the Swedish national knee ligament registry. *Arthrosc J Arthrosc Relat Surg.* 2020;36(1):189−195.

48. Ahlden M, Samuelsson K, Sernert N, Forssblad M, Karlsson J, Kartus J. The Swedish National Anterior Cruciate Ligament Register: a report on baseline variables and outcomes of surgery for almost 18,000 patients. *Am J Sports Med.* 2012;40(10):2230−2235.

49. Gans I, Retzky JS, Jones LC, Tanaka MJ. Epidemiology of recurrent anterior cruciate ligament injuries in national collegiate athletic association sports: the injury surveillance program, 2004-2014. *Orthop J Sports Med.* 2018; 6(6), 232596711877782.

50. Fältström A, Kvist J, Gauffin H, Hägglund M. Female soccer players with anterior cruciate ligament reconstruction have a higher risk of new knee injuries and quit soccer to a higher degree than knee-healthy controls. *Am J Sports Med.* 2019;47(1):31−40.

51. Grindem H, Snyder-Mackler L, Moksnes H, Engebretsen L, Risberg MA. Simple decision rules can reduce reinjury risk by 84% after ACL reconstruction: the Delaware-Oslo ACL cohort study. *Br J Sports Med.* 2016;50(13):804−808.

52. Allen MM, Pareek A, Krych AJ, et al. Are female soccer players at an increased risk of second anterior cruciate ligament injury compared with their athletic peers? *Am J Sports Med.* 2016;44(10):2492−2498.

53. Bourne MN, Bruder AM, Mentiplay BF, Carey DL, Patterson BE, Crossley KM. Eccentric knee flexor weakness in elite female footballers 1−10 years following anterior cruciate ligament reconstruction. *Phys Ther Sport.* 2019; 37:144−149.

54. Pollard CD, Stearns KM, Hayes AT, Heiderscheit BC. Altered lower extremity movement variability in female soccer players during side-step cutting after anterior cruciate ligament reconstruction. *Am J Sports Med.* 2015;43(2): 460−465.

55. Stearns KM, Pollard CD. Abnormal frontal plane knee mechanics during sidestep cutting in female soccer athletes after anterior cruciate ligament reconstruction and return to sport. *Am J Sports Med.* 2013;41(4):918−923.

56. Lyle MA, Valero-Cuevas FJ, Gregor RJ, Powers CM. Control of dynamic foot-ground interactions in male and female soccer athletes: females exhibit reduced dexterity and higher limb stiffness during landing. *J Biomech.* 2014; 47(2):512−517.

57. Brophy R, Silvers HJ, Gonzales T, Mandelbaum BR. Gender influences: the role of leg dominance in ACL injury among soccer players. *Br J Sports Med.* 2010; 44(10):694−697.

58. Brophy RH, Schmitz L, Wright RW, et al. Return to play and future ACL injury risk after ACL reconstruction in soccer athletes from the multicenter orthopaedic outcomes network (MOON) group. *Am J Sports Med.* 2012;40(11): 2517−2522.

Anterior Cruciate Ligament Injury Prevention

KIRSTEN D. GARVEY, MS • NATALIE A. LOWENSTEIN, BS •
ELIZABETH G. MATZKIN, MD

INTRODUCTION

Anterior cruciate ligament (ACL) injury is of major concern in the field of sports medicine and orthopedics. From 2002 to 2014 the rate of ACL reconstructions has increased by 22%.[1] Those who experience ACL injury experience significant deficits in sports-related movement, including cutting, pivoting, decelerating, jumping, landing, and other functional movements. Concomitant injuries such as meniscal tear, chondral injuries, avulsion fractures, and collateral ligament injuries are common with ACL injury. ACL injuries primarily occur in young individuals who participate it cutting and pivoting sports such as soccer, basketball, football, and lacrosse.[2,3] Among adolescents and children, the rates of isolated ACL reconstruction and ACL reconstruction with a concomitant meniscal procedure increased noticeably from 2002 to 2014.[1] Individuals aged 13−17 years experienced 37% increase in isolated ACL reconstruction, 107% increase in ACL reconstruction with meniscal repair, and 63% increase in ACL reconstruction with meniscectomy.[1] The economic burden to society is significant, as one ACL injury (including long-term sequelae) currently costs approximately $38,000.[4]

Although ACL reconstruction surgery has a high success rate, younger and more active patients have a higher likelihood of reinjury.[5] Deficits in quadriceps strength, decreased postural control, and altered kinematics and abnormal joint loading contribute to the risk of reinjury.[6−8] Additionally, the risk for a second ACL injury is significant (about 10%), and this risk doubles if the athlete returns to his/her competitive sport.[9−11] In addition to reinjury, there is a risk of long-term complications that stem from ACL injury and reconstruction. Specifically, the risk for posttraumatic osteoarthritis, total knee replacement, and impaired knee quality of life 5−25 years after injury is high.[12−14] In a systematic review, a prevalence rate of 48% for osteoarthritis 10 years following reconstruction surgery was reported.[15]

It is well known that female athletes are four to six times more likely than their male counterparts to withstand a noncontact ACL injury.[16,17] Noncontact ACL injuries typically occur when the athlete is either landing from a jump or making a lateral pivot. Quadriceps dominance, leg dominance, and/or ligament dominance may contribute to the increased dynamic knee instability in females compared with males.[16] The recovery time for ACL reconstruction is significant, approximately 1 year, and among the athletes who do eventually return to their competitive sport (i.e., 55%),[18] their level of performance is likely to decrease.[19]

These trends are worrisome and a focus on implementing ACL prevention programs among young athletes, especially females, is critical. For over two decades, investigators have developed a variety of ACL injury prevention programs as well as neuromuscular training (NMT) programs to address this problem. We know that injury-preventing NMT programs indeed reduce the risk of ACL injury by roughly 50% in female athletes[20−23]; however, there are many variations of NMT programs that differ greatly in their individual components. In this chapter, we aim to synthesize and present the most recent meta-analyses and systematic reviews to aid coaches, athletic trainers, team physicians, and parents understand and implement the most effective components of prevention programs for their young female athletes.

NEUROMUSCULAR TRAINING PROGRAMS

Overview

Neuromuscular control is defined as an unconscious trained response of a muscle to stimuli regarding dynamic joint stability. It is a complex system of muscle activities including contraction, coordination, stabilization, postural control, and balance.[24] In sports, neuromuscular control is crucial to perform jumping, landing, and pivoting tasks correctly and without injury.[25] Neuromuscular control has been identified as an important factor when considering the differences in ACL injury risk and knee stability between males and females. Differences in muscle control, muscle activation, and movement patterns in male and female athletes have been implicated in the increased risk for ACL injury in female atheltes.[26,27] There have been many studies that describe these kinematic and biomechanical variations in sport movement patterns among males and females. For example, Chappell et al.[26] investigated the "stop-jump" maneuver in particular and found that female athletes prepared for landing with decreased hip and knee flexion, increased quadriceps activation, and decreased hamstring activation, leading to increased ACL loading during landing when compared with males. Additionally, Ford et al.[28] found that in middle- and high-school basketball players, females demonstrated greater knee valgus than males during a "jump-stop unanticipated cut" maneuver (Fig. 5.1).

It has been shown that neuromuscular risk factors are modifiable through NMT, which can lead to decreased risk for injury and increased sport performance. In a study by Myer et al., NMT protocols that utilized both plyometric and dynamic balance tasks were studied in high-school female athletes. The investigators measured power, balance, strength, and landing force before and after training. The female athletes were all able to decrease their standard deviation of center of pressure during hop landing tests, as well as increased hamstring strength and vertical jump measurements, after a three times per week NMT program for 7 weeks.[29]

The kinematic demands of sports differ and thus may be an important consideration when implementing NMT programs. As the majority of female ACL injuries stem from noncontact movements (i.e., cutting and pivoting maneuvers or jump landings), the frequency of these movements in their respective sports should be taken into account. For example, in a study by Cowley et al.[30] the researchers assessed differences in cutting and landing tasks among high-school female basketball and soccer players and concluded that sport-specific NMT may be warranted with soccer players focusing on training for pivot and cutting movements

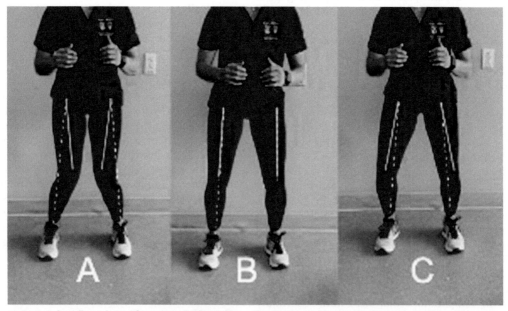

FIG. 5.1 Landings from "Stop-jump" Maneuver. The load-bearing axis (indicated in white) on the lower limbs in this maneuver can be represented by a line extending from the center of the femoral head to the center of the ankle joint. **(A)** Landing with knee valgus. Here the load-bearing axis passes laterally to the knee increasing force in the lateral compartment. **(B)** Neutral landing where patient's load-bearing axis passes directly through the center of the knee. **(C)** Landing with knee varus. Here the load-bearing axis passes medially to the knee increasing force in the medial compartment. In varus landing, knees lie outside the hip and ankle line.

and basketball players on jumping and landing mechanics. In a 2014 systematic review by Michaelidis et al.[31] ACL injury prevention programs were assessed on their effectiveness in different sports. The authors concluded that training programs for soccer and handball athletes require sport-specific agility training, while jump-focused sports, such as basketball, should involve high-intensity plyometrics.

Historically, NMT programs have included a mix of strength training, plyometrics, balance exercises, and stretching to address muscle imbalances and develop control over muscle activation. Many studies have confirmed that NMT and injury prevention programs are a cost-effective strategy. In a 2018 study by Lewis et al., ACL injury prevention programs prevented 3764 lifetime ACL ruptures per 100,000 individuals (i.e., a 40% reduction in ACL injuries). Subsequent cases of osteoarthritis and total knee replacement procedures are also averted through the utilization of ACL prevention programs.[32] Marshall et al. also investigated the economic impact of NMT programs compared to traditional warm-up strategies in youth soccer. A 38% reduction in injury risk and a 43% reduction in healthcare costs was found in the NMT group compared to the control. The authors projected that in 58,100 youth soccer players, an estimated $2.7 million in healthcare

costs could be avoided over the duration of one season of implementation of an NMT program.[33] Although NMT programs have been determined cost-effective, there is still considerable variation among programs, warranting an analysis of the most common and effective components of these prevention strategies. In the following section, common and effective components of ACL injury prevention programs will be reviewed.

Neuromuscular Training Program Characteristics

In 2018, the American Academy of Sports Physical Therapy published clinical practice guidelines for exercise-based knee and ACL injury prevention.[34] They recommend a number of specific programs for reducing ACL injuries in athletes, including but not limited to HarmoKnee,[35] Prevent Injury and Enhance Performance (PEP) program,[36] and Sportsmetrics (Table 5.1).[37] These exercise-based prevention programs employ numerous intervention strategies, including proprioceptive training, NMT, strengthening exercises, stretching, agility, and plyometric exercises. Additionally, many programs employ instructors or coaches to give feedback to athletes on their performance of specific movements and exercises, particularly jump landing movements.[38,39]

TABLE 5.1
Injury Prevention Program Characteristics.

Program	Study Type	Participants	Duration	Effect	Activities
PEP[58]	RCT	NCAA division I female soccer players: control, n = 852; intervention, n = 583	12 Weeks through soccer season (15–20 min, 3 times per week)	Intervention group had lower ACL injury rate in practices ($P = 0.01$), in late season ($P = 0.03$), and in noncontact ACL injuries in those with a history of ACL injury ($P = 0.05$)	*Flexibility* • Calf stretch • Quadriceps stretch • Figure-of-four hamstring stretch • Inner thigh stretch • Hip flexor stretch *Running* • Jog from line to line of soccer field (cone to cone) • Shuttle run (side to side) • Backward running • Shuttle run with forward/backward running (40 yds) • Diagonal runs (40 yds) • Bounding run (45–50 yds) *Strength* • Walking lunges, 20 yds × 2 sets • Russian hamstring, 3 sets × 10 repetitions or 30 s • Single toe raises, 30 repetitions each side

Continued

TABLE 5.1
Injury Prevention Program Characteristics.—cont'd

Program	Study Type	Participants	Duration	Effect	Activities
					Plyometrics • Lateral hops over cone • Forward/backward hops over cone • Single-leg hops over cone • Vertical jumps with headers • Scissors jump
HarmoKnee[35]	Cohort	Female soccer players aged 13–17 years: intervention, n = 777; control, n = 729	4 Months (approx. 20–25 min, 2× per week, during preseason, and 1× per week in regular season)	Knee injury intervention: adjusted RR for compliance 0.17 (95% CI: 0.04, 0.64) Noncontact knee injury intervention: RR adjusted for compliance 0.06 (95% CI: 0.01, 0.46)	*Flexibility* • Standing calf stretch • Standing quadriceps stretch • Half-kneeling hamstring stretch • Half-kneeling hip flexor stretch • Butterfly adductor stretch • Modified figure-of-four stretch *Running* • Jogging (4–6 min) • Backward jogging on toes (1 min) • High-knee skipping (30 s) • Defensive pressure technique: sliding slowly, zigzag backward (30 s) • Alternating forward zigzag running and pressure technique: zigzag backward (2 min) *Strength* • Lunges in place (alternating anterior lunges) • Nordic hamstring eccentric strengthening • Single-leg squat with toe raise *Core stability* • Sit-ups • Plank on elbows • Bridging *Plyometrics* • Forward and backward double-leg jumps • Lateral single-leg jumps • Forward and backward single-leg jumps • Double-leg jumps with or without ball
Sportsmetrics[43]	Cohort	High-school soccer, basketball, and volleyball players: female, intervention, n = 366; male, control, n = 434; female,	6 Weeks during preseason (60–90 min, 3 times per week)	Intervention females had lower rate of severe knee injury than control females ($P = 0.05$) Intervention females had lower rate of noncontact	*Flexibility* • Gastrocnemius • Soleus • Quadriceps • Hamstrings • Hip flexors • Iliotibial band/lower back • Posterior deltoids • Latissimus dorsi • Pectorals/bicep *Running* • Skipping

TABLE 5.1
Injury Prevention Program Characteristics.—cont'd

Program	Study Type	Participants	Duration	Effect	Activities
		control, n = 463		knee injuries than control females ($P = 0.01$) and control males ($P = 0.01$)	• Side shuffle • Cool-down walk (2 min) *Strength* • Back hyperextension • Leg press • Calf raise • Pullover • Bench press • Latissimus dorsi pulldown • Forearm curl *Core stability* • Abdominal curl *Plyometrics* • Wall jumps (20 s, progressing to 30 s) • Tuck jumps (20 s, progressing to 30 s) • Broad jumps, stick (hold) landing (5−10 repetitions) • Squat jumps (10 s, progressing to 25 s) • Double-legged cone jumps (30 s/30 s side to side and back to front) • 180-degree jumps (20−25 s) • Bounding in place (20−25 s) • Jump, jump, jump, vertical jump (5−8 repetitions) • Bounding for distance (1−2 runs) • Scissors jump (30 s) • Hop, hop, stick landing (5 repetitions per leg) • Step, jump up, down, vertical (5−10 repetitions) • Mattress jumps (30 s/30 s side to side and back to front) • Single-legged jumps for distance (5 repetitions per leg) • Jump into bounding (3−4 runs)

ACL, anterior cruciate ligament; *CI*, confidence interval; *PEP*, Prevent Injury and Enhance Performance; *RCT*, randomized controlled trial; *RR*, relative risk.

In the 2019 meta-analysis and systematic review on ACL prevention programs for female athletes, the authors utilized robust quantitative and statistical methods to develop best-practice guidelines and elucidate the most effective components of various prevention programs.[4] A total of 18 studies were included in the final analysis. Investigators determined that all NMT programs included some form of implementer training (i.e., brochure or workshop) to ensure proper implementation of the NMT program. Almost every program in the analysis included proper exercise instruction, exercise progression, and trainer or coach feedback.[4] Importantly, programs that taught proper movement technique and

knee stability during landing and other dynamic maneuvers during each training session were most effective.[4] Surprisingly, some exercise components were found to be irrelevant (i.e., these programs were no more effective than those that did not include these exercise components), including balance, core strengthening, agility, and stretching. Although these components may be helpful in preventing other types of injuries (i.e., ankle sprains and muscle strains), they may be an ineffective use of time if the primary goal is ACL injury prevention.[4] Some of these findings are consistent with those from other studies in the literature; for example, the prospective randomized intervention study by Söderman et al.[40] which found no

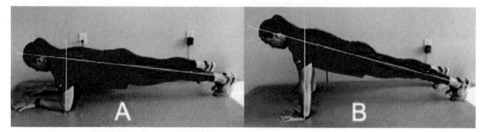

FIG. 5.2 **Plank Exercise.** A patient demonstrates proper spine alignment. The patient stabilizes that position by activating glutes, quadriceps, and core. Pelvis and neck should also be in a neutral position with gaze down at the floor. **(A)** Elbows should be directly underneath your shoulders. **(B)** Wrists planted directly underneath shoulders.

reduction in ACL injury in performing balancing exercises alone. However, Sugimoto et al.[23] found a significant association in the reduction of ACL injury in programs that included core-strengthening/proximal control exercises. The authors discovered a recent trend for NMT programs to incorporate proximal control exercises, including plank, side plank, sit-ups/abdominal curl, push-ups, and upper body weight training.[35,41–43] There have been many laboratory-controlled studies that investigated the influence of proximal control on lower extremity muscle function and found associations among trunk, hip strength, and dynamic knee stability.[44,45] This finding is also consistent with the clinical practice guidelines that found level I evidence that female athletes, in particular, benefit from prevention programs that include trunk/core strengthening and stability exercises (Fig. 5.2).[34] Therefore incorporation of core strengthening and trunk stabilization appears to increase the effectiveness of ACL injury prevention programs.

According to the systematic review by Petushek et al.[4] NMT programs that included landing stabilization maneuvers, hamstring-strengthening exercises (Fig. 5.3), vs. lunges (Fig. 5.4), and heel-calf raises reduced the risk of ACL injury more so than programs without these exercises, and several past studies reinforce this conclusion. For example, the 2015 study conducted by Sugimoto et al.[22] showed that programs that included strengthening exercises showed a significant reduction in ACL injury than programs without strengthening exercises. Additionally, the most recent clinical practice guidelines by Arundale et al.[34] emphasize this by summarizing level II evidence that shows increased effectiveness in reducing ACL injuries in females who trained in programs that included strengthening exercises.

Target Population

In female athletes, risk of sports-related injuries to the ACL increases in adolescence and peaks in the mid-teens to late

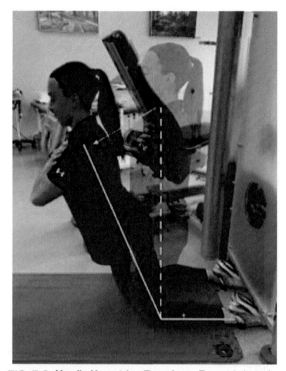

FIG. 5.3 **Nordic Hamstring Exercise.** Eccentric lowering of the upper body to the floor from a kneeling position. This movement is followed by a return to the starting position to increase hamstring strength in athletes.

teens.[20] To explain this age-related risk of ACL injury, studies have shown that the altered mechanics that predispose females to great risk of ACL injury emerges after puberty.[46,47] Some female pubertal changes are nonmodifiable, including anatomic and hormonal changes.[48,49] However, strength and coordination are two modifiable factors that have been demonstrated to increase in males undergoing puberty, yet not in females (Table 5.2).[50]

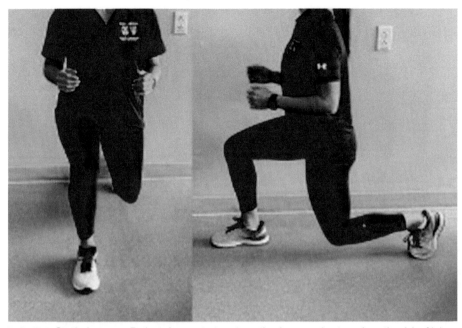

FIG. 5.4 **Static Lunge.** Patient demonstrates strengthening exercise to reduce the risk of injury.

TABLE 5.2
Nonmodifiable and Modifiable Risk Factors.

Nonmodifiable	Modifiable
Pubertal anatomic changes	Strength (proximal muscles and core)
Pubertal hormonal changes	Coordination (neuromuscular control)

The differing landing strategies between young females and young males, with young females landing with a more valgus stress over the knee and with less control in the lower extremity, explain the gender difference in injury risk. The postpubertal female may lack a proper landing technique owing to less coordination and strength compared to the postpubertal male. NMT that targets hip abductor strength (Fig. 5.5) and trunk stability to improve landing mechanics addresses the divergence in ACL injury risk between male and female athletes.[51,52] Based on this, many studies have investigated the efficacy of NMT programs on this particularly vulnerable young female population.

A 2013 meta-analysis by Myer et al.[20] studied the optimal timing for the initiation of NMT programs in young female athletes. After pooling data from 14 clinical trials, the authors found that there was a significant decrease in ACL injury risk in female athletes who were in their mid-teens compared with those in their late teens and early adulthood.[20] Interestingly, an additional study by Sugimoto et al.[23] broke down age even further and found that female athletes aged 14–18 years had a greater reduction in ACL injury compared with those younger than 14 years, aged 18–20 years, and those older than 20 years. Similarly, in a meta-analysis by Yoo et al.[53] a subgroup analysis demonstrated that an NMT program that emphasized plyometric and strengthening exercises was particularly effective in preventing ACL injury in female athletes under 18 years of age. Therefore implementing NMT programs for female athletes in early adolescence may have an optimal effect on decreasing the risk of ACL injury.

Aside from age and gender, another important factor when considering a target population for NMT programs is the sport of choice. For example, soccer has one of the highest incidences of ACL injury for both males and females.[54] In a meta-analysis of randomized controlled trials (RCTs) by Grimm et al.[55] a reduction in knee injury incidence was found in both male and female soccer players who underwent injury prevention programs. Additionally, they found a reduction in ACL injuries, although this was not statistically significant. Some individual prevention programs, including PEP and Sportsmetrics, have studied their individual effect on ACL injury rates in soccer players. A prospective

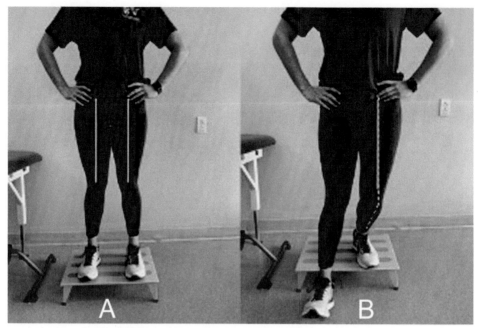

FIG. 5.5 Single-leg Step Down.   **(A)** The patient begins in a neutral standing position on an elevated step with legs shoulder width apart. **(B)** Keeping one leg on the step, the patient uses the other leg to touch down on the floor with their heel and return back up to the step. Note: hip abductor and external rotator strength are used to stabilize the supporting knee and maintain neutral position.

study by Hewett et al.[56] evaluating the Sportsmetrics program, found that injury incidence in soccer players was 0.56 in untrained female athletes and 0 in trained female athletes. Additionally, two studies have evaluated the efficacy of the PEP program in preventing ACL injury in female soccer players. One study, by Mandelbaum et al.[57] investigated the effect of the PEP program in female soccer players between the ages of 14 and 18 years. The players either participated in a traditional warm-up or the intervention before play over a 2-year period. The PEP intervention program consisted of education, strengthening exercises, stretching, plyometrics, and agility drills. Mandelbaum et al. found an 88% decrease in ACL injury in the intervention group compared with the control group. When matching for age and skill, there was a 74% reduction in ACL injury. In contrast to the study by Mandelbaum et al., an RCT by Gilchrist et al.[58] examined the effectiveness of the PEP program in division 1 collegiate female soccer players. Various National Collegiate Athletic Association (NCAA) teams were randomized to either PEP intervention or a control. Intervention teams performed the PEP program three times per week during the season. The overall ACL injury rate in the intervention teams was 1.7 times less than that of the control

teams, and noncontact ACL injuries in the intervention teams were 3.3 times less likely than those in controls; however, neither of these findings reached statistical significance. Interestingly, intervention athletes with a history of ACL injury were significantly less likely to undergo another ACL injury than controls with a similar history.

Basketball is another high-risk sport for ACL injury, as it involves a significant amount of jumping, landing, and pivoting maneuvers. There has been conflicting evidence on the efficacy of NMT programs in female basketball players. A 2-year prospective study conducted by Pfeiffer et al.[59] examined the effect of a knee ligament injury prevention program on the incidence of noncontact ACL injury. The authors split the cohort into treatment group and control group. The treatment group participated in a plyometrics-based injury prevention program twice a week throughout the season. Both groups were followed over the duration of two consecutive seasons. Pfeiffer et al. recorded three noncontact ACL injuries in the treatment group and three in the control group, suggesting a lack of effect of the prevention program in reducing noncontact ACL injuries in female basketball players. In contrast, Hewett et al.[43] found there were significantly less number of noncontact knee injuries in female basketball players who underwent their injury prevention program.

Several studies investigated the effect of NMT programs in handball athletes. For example, Olsen et al.[60] conducted a cluster RCT and found significant reductions in knee ligament injuries in 16- and 17-year-old male and female handball athletes, following implementation of an injury prevention program. The intervention tested included a structured warm-up to improve running, pivoting, and landing techniques as well as to improve neuromuscular control, increase strength, and improve balance. In contrast, Myklebust et al.[61] did not find a significant decrease in ACL injury after implementation of an exercise-based knee injury prevention program over two seasons in female handball players. Although when compliance with the program was controlled for (i.e., performed the NMT program at least 15 times throughout the season), they found a significant decrease in ACL injuries among compliant female handball athletes. Lastly, no conclusion on the efficacy of NMT programs in volleyball players can be made. Two studies have included volleyball players in their respective cohorts but neither study observed any serious knee injury or ACL injury in any volleyball players.[56,59]

In summary, for ideal target populations, clinicians, coaches, parents, and athletes should implement NMT injury prevention programs in female athletes, especially in female athletes under the age of 18 years to reduce the risk of ACL injury. Additionally, female soccer, basketball, and handball athletes should utilize prevention programs such as PEP and Sportsmetrics to prevent severe knee injury.

Training Duration and Timing

Several studies have investigated the impact of duration and timing on the efficacy of NMT injury prevention programs. A 2013 meta-analysis by Gagnier et al.[39] indicated that NMT programs that had a longer duration (i.e., greater than 14 months), higher hours of training per week, greater compliance, and no participant drop-out were most effective at decreasing the incidence of ACL injury in both males and females than NMT programs that did not have these characteristics.

Another important factor when considering the timing of NMT programs is whether or not the injury prevention training occurs in preseason versus preseason plus in-season. Donnell-Fink et al.[38] considered this factor and found that there was a lower risk for knee injuries in males and females when NMT programs were included in preseason. However, when looking at ACL injury alone, they did not find an association between preseason and preseason plus in-season timing of NMT injury prevention programs. However, the meta-analysis by Yoo et al.[53] that investigated NMT programs on ACL prevention in female athletes found that there was a significant effect of timing on risk reduction. In female athletes, they concluded that programs that were preseason only were not effective in reducing ACL injury rates. Programs that were conducted in-season only had a lesser effect on ACL injury reduction than programs that were conducted in the preseason and continued throughout the season.

Sugimoto et al.[62] investigated potential dosage effects and found that NMT ACL injury prevention programs with a high volume during the season (i.e., 30 min or more per week) has a greater risk reduction than programs with moderate to low volumes during the season (i.e., 15–30 min per week and up to 15 min per week). Sugimoto et al.[62] also looked into the dosage of specific sessions and found that programs whose sessions lasted 20 min or less had an odds ratio (OR) of 0.61 compared to sessions lasting longer than 20 min that had an OR of 0.35 in reducing ACL injury. Lastly, Sugimoto et al. studied the dosage effect of the number of sessions per week. NMT ACL injury prevention programs that were performed multiple times per week were more effective at reducing ACL injury risk than the programs that were performed only once per week (OR of 0.35 vs. OR of 0.62).[62]

The 2016 meta-regression analysis by Sugimoto et al.[23] investigated critical components of NMT to reduce ACL injury risk and evaluated the "synergistic effects" of these components that optimize ACL injury reduction in female athletes. The age of participants, NMT dosage, exercise variations within the NMT program, and utilization of verbal feedback were considered key predictors of ACL injury. For the analyses, the authors grouped age in tertiles (14–18 years of age, 18–20 years of age, and 20 years or older), grouped dosage in two categories (20 min or less per session and 20 min or greater per session), grouped frequency in two categories (once per week or multiple times per week), and grouped exercise variation in two categories (one exercise component or multiple exercise components).[23] They assigned points to groups based on ORs and found that the groups with the highest points were those aged 14–18 years, with sessions greater than 20 min in duration, programs that were performed multiple times per week, and programs with multiple exercise components. Finally, they concluded that the most common aspect in the highest scoring studies was dosage (i.e., longer than 20-min sessions and at least two times per week in frequency).[23] Evidently, dosage is a critical component to consider when implementing and developing an NMT program for ACL injury reduction.

Compliance

Compliance is likely an important factor when considering efficacy of NMT injury prevention programs. Compliance provides an indication for the number of athletes that actually completed the injury prevention program to reveal the actual impact of the training.[63] A 2012 meta-analysis by Sugimoto et al.[63] investigated the role of compliance on ACL injury reduction in female soccer, basketball, volleyball, and handball athletes undergoing an NMT program. The authors hypothesized that higher compliance would lead to lower ACL injury rates in female athletes. A total of six studies were included in their analysis and they found that ACL injury rates were lower in studies with high NMT program compliance compared with those in studies with low program compliance. The authors investigated compliance rates further and divided compliance rates into tertiles (i.e., low compliance = 33.3% or less, moderate compliance = 33.3%–66.6%, and high compliance = 66.6% or higher). Compliance rate was defined as the number of sessions completed in the study divided by the maximum number of sessions offered to the intervention group. Attendance rate was defined as the number of participants who completed the minimum amount of session criteria in the study divided by the total number of participants in the intervention group. Finally, the overall compliance rate was defined as the attendance rate multiplied by the compliance rate. The high-compliance groups had an 82% lower chance of ACL injury than the low- and moderate-compliance groups.

In studies of female soccer players, authors found less knee injury incidence in players who were compliant with their exercise-based prevention programs.[35,42] Waldén et al.[42] investigated the effectiveness of NMT in reducing the rate of acute knee injury in youth female soccer athletes. In this study, coaches monitored compliance by keeping attendance sheets of their players and therapists were instructed to make two unannounced visits to each intervention team to monitor compliance and proper execution of the exercise program. The authors found an overall 64% decrease in ACL injury incidence in their intervention group compared with controls. When controlling for compliance (i.e., they examined only compliant players who performed the intervention at least once per week), they found an 83% reduction in the ACL injury rate. In addition, compliant athletes had an 82% reduction in severe knee injuries and a 47% reduction in acute knee injuries.

Hägglund et al.[64] performed a subanalysis on the RCT by Waldén et al.[42] Teams and athletes were stratified into tertiles of compliance (i.e., low compliance, medium compliance, and high compliance). There were 184 teams and 2471 athletes in the intervention group. Compliance was measured by their mean number of weekly injury prevention program training sessions during the season. A high player compliance (89% compliance rate) resulted in an 88% reduction in ACL injury rate when comparing to low player compliance (63% compliance rate). Intermediate compliance (82% compliance rate) and high compliance reduced acute knee injury by 72% and 90%, respectively, when compared to low compliance. Interestingly, players with low compliance had higher rates of ACL injuries than control players.

A study by Kiani et al.[35] also adjusted for compliance rate when studying the effect of an exercise-based injury prevention program. Kiani et al. specifically utilized the HarmoKnee program to assess the prevention of soccer-related knee injuries in teenaged girls. The HarmoKnee program was specifically designed for female soccer players and was combined with the education of athletes, coaches, and parents on injury risk. The physical exercise program was aimed to improve body control, muscle activation, and motor skills and the main outcome measure was acute knee injuries diagnosed by a physician. Kiani et al. found a 77% lower incidence of knee injuries and a 90% lower incidence of noncontact knee injuries. Interestingly, the reductions in knee injury risk were further decreased when they were adjusted for compliance. In this study, coaches provided information on compliance at two time points, once at the end of preseason training and again at the end of the regular season. The compliance rate for these periods was estimated by the coaches to be less than 50%, at least 50%, at least 75%, or 100%. Of the 48 teams in the intervention group, 3 teams reported 50% adherence, 36 teams reported 75% adherence and 9 teams reported 100% adherence at the end of preseason training. For a regular season, one team reported less than 50% compliance with the program, whereas the rest of the teams reported 100% compliance. The authors explain that because the specific exercises in the program incorporate well into regular practice, little extra time is needed to implement the additional training. This makes the exercise program well received by coaches and athletes and does explain the high compliance rate found in this study. Finally, athletes who were compliant with the HarmoKnee program had an 83% reduction in knee injury incidence and a 94% decrease in noncontact knee injury rates.

Feedback

Recently, some studies have focused specifically on how feedback impacts the overall effectiveness of injury prevention training programs. Most ACL injury prevention programs utilize explicit instructions and feedback regarding desired landing positions. Benjaminse et al. described how these motor skills can be learned with an internal focus of attention (a focus on the movements themselves, i.e., 'land with your knees bent') or with an external focus of attention (a focus on the movement effect, i.e., 'touch target as you land').[65,66] Learning strategies with an internal focus have been shown to be less effective for the acquisition of complex motor skills required for sports, whereas external focus of attention facilitates automaticity in motor control and improves movement efficiency.[66] Compared to internal focus of attention or no instruction, an external focus of attention has shown superior results on a jump landing performance and improved transfer to sport.[66,67] In a study by Benajminse et al.[68] they assessed how learned movement patterns in training programs are carried over to the field. The authors assessed a jump landing task in three different groups (control, visual, verbal internal focus, and verbal external focus). The athletes performed the jump landing task at baseline, then underwent training, and finally took a post-test to assess the transfer of their learned skill. This post-test consisted of an unanticipated sidestep cutting task. The authors found that those in the visual learning and verbal external focus groups had greater knee flexion range of motion compared with the verbal internal focus group.

There have been a few ACL injury prevention studies that incorporated verbal feedback into their programs.[60,69] In a study by Olsen et al.[60] the incorporation of feedback demonstrated greater prophylactic effect. Specifically, players were encouraged to be focused on the quality of their movements and to emphasize core stability and the position of the hip and knee in relation to the foot (i.e., "knee over toe" position). Additionally, athletes were instructed to closely watch each other and give verbal feedback to their teammates during the training. Similarly, in a study by LaBella et al.[69] verbal cues and feedback enhanced the effectiveness of their training programs. In this study, 1492 athletes from Chicago public high schools were randomized to intervention and control groups. The authors trained the intervention coaches to implement a 20-min neuromuscular warm-up and control coaches used their usual warm-up. Coaches then reported weekly athlete exposures and lower extremity injuries that caused a missed practice or game. Interventional athletes were instructed to avoid dynamic knee valgus and to land jumps with flexed hips and knees. Coaches were taught how to distinguish between proper and improper forms and how to use verbal cues to promote proper form in the athletes (i.e., 'land softly' and 'don't let your knees cave inward'). Interventional athletes had lower rates per 1000 athlete exposures for acute noncontact lower extremity injuries, gradual onset lower extremity injuries, and lower extremity injuries treated surgically. In addition to reduction in injury rates, studies have reported more favorable biomechanical

TABLE 5.3 NMT Program Tips for ACL Injury Prevention.	
NMT programs combining proximal control, strength, and plyometric exercises	Focus on quality of movements, emphasizing core stability and hip, knee, and foot alignment
Training programs should begin in preseason and should continue throughout season[53]	NMT programs should be longer than 30 min at least 2× per week

ACL, anterior cruciate ligament; *NMT*, neuromuscular training.

alterations to movement when a feedback mechanism was added to an NMT program.[70–72] In a study by Myer et al.[71] the authors assessed the effect of augmented feedback on improving an athlete's biomechanics during a drop vertical jump task. They found that the augmented feedback supported the transfer of skills and reduced injury risk across different tasks.

DISCUSSION

There is substantial evidence that exercise-based knee injury prevention programs reduce the risk for knee and/or ACL injuries, carry little risk for adverse events, and have minimal cost. The most effective ACL injury prevention programs for females incorporate multiple components, proximal control exercises, and a combination of strength and plyometric exercises. The target population for NMT injury prevention programs should focus on female athletes. In female athletes, the risk of sports-related injuries to the ACL increases in adolescence and peaks in the mid-teens to late teens. ACL injury prevention programs should be implemented particularly in early adolescence, as this may have an optimal effect of decreasing ACL injury risk. Additionally, injury prevention programs should involve multiple training sessions per week, training sessions that last longer than 20 min per session, and training volumes that are longer than 30 min per week. Coaches, team physicians, parents, and athletes must ensure that they achieve high compliance with knee injury prevention programs to ensure the greatest efficacy. Finally, there is evidence that incorporating feedback in the form of verbal and visual instructions will increase the effectiveness of many NMT programs (Table 5.3).

CONCLUSION

There is rich evidence that NMT programs are very effective in preventing ACL injuries, particularly in the female athlete. Prevention programs are particularly beneficial for adolescent female athletes; however, there is no harm in performing prevention programs in athletes who are not deemed high risk. Cost may minimally increase as more athletes participate in injury prevention programs; however, the small increase in costs will likely be far outweighed by reduction in the long-term healthcare costs associated with ACL injuries. To prevent ACL injuries and future cases of osteoarthritis and total knee replacements, physicians, coaches, parents, and athletes should encourage the implementation of ACL injury prevention programs in all athletes who are involved in sports with a high risk of ACL injury.

REFERENCES

1. Herzog MM, Marshall SW, Lund JL, Pate V, Mack CD, Spang JT. Trends in incidence of ACL reconstruction and concomitant procedures among commercially insured individuals in the United States, 2002-2014. *Sports Health*. 2018;10(6):523–531. https://doi.org/10.1177/1941738118803616.
2. Bahr R, Holme I. Risk factors for sports injuries–a methodological approach. *Br J Sports Med*. 2003;37(5):384–392. https://doi.org/10.1136/bjsm.37.5.384.
3. Gornitzky AL, Lott A, Yellin JL, Fabricant PD, Lawrence JT, Ganley TJ. Sport-specific yearly risk and incidence of anterior cruciate ligament tears in high school athletes: a systematic review and meta-analysis. *Am J Sports Med*. 2016;44(10):2716–2723. https://doi.org/10.1177/0363546515617742.
4. Petushek EJ, Sugimoto D, Stoolmiller M, Smith G, Myer GD. Evidence-based best-practice guidelines for preventing anterior cruciate ligament injuries in young female athletes a systematic review and meta-analysis. *Am J Sports Med*. 2018. https://doi.org/10.1177/0363546518782460.
5. Kaeding CC, Pedroza AD, Reinke EK, Huston LJ, Consortium M, Spindler KP. Risk factors and predictors of subsequent ACL injury in either knee after ACL reconstruction: prospective analysis of 2488 primary ACL reconstructions from the MOON cohort. *Am J Sports Med*. 2015;43(7):1583. https://doi.org/10.1177/0363546515578836.
6. Greenberg EM, Greenberg ET, Ganley TJ, Lawrence JTR. Strength and functional performance recovery after anterior cruciate ligament reconstruction in preadolescent athletes. *Sports Health*. 2014;6(4):309–312. https://doi.org/10.1177/1941738114537594.
7. Paterno MV, Schmitt LC, Ford KR, et al. Biomechanical measures during landing and postural stability predict second anterior cruciate ligament injury after anterior cruciate ligament reconstruction and return to sport. *Am J Sports Med*. 2010;38(10):1968–1978. https://doi.org/10.1177/0363546510376053.
8. Elias ARC, Hammill CD, Mizner RL. Changes in quadriceps and hamstring cocontraction following landing instruction in patients with anterior cruciate ligament reconstruction. *J Orthop Sports Phys Ther*. 2015;45(4):273–280. https://doi.org/10.2519/jospt.2015.5335.
9. Wiggins AJ, Grandhi RK, Schneider DK, Stanfield D, Webster KE, Myer GD. Risk of secondary injury in younger athletes after anterior cruciate ligament reconstruction: a systematic review and meta-analysis. *Am J Sports Med*. 2016;44(7):1861–1876. https://doi.org/10.1177/0363546515621554.
10. Wright RW, Magnussen RA, Dunn WR, Spindler KP. Ipsilateral graft and contralateral ACL rupture at five years or more following ACL reconstruction. *J Bone Jt Surg*. 2011;93(12):1159–1165. https://doi.org/10.2106/JBJS.J.00898.
11. Magnussen RA, Meschbach NT, Kaeding CC, Wright RW, Spindler KP. ACL graft and contralateral ACL tear risk within ten years following reconstruction: a systematic review. *JBJS Rev*. 2015;3(1):1. https://doi.org/10.2106/JBJS.RVW.N.00052.
12. Lohmander LS, Östenberg A, Englund M, Roos H. High prevalence of knee osteoarthritis, pain, and functional limitations in female soccer players twelve years after anterior cruciate ligament injury. *Arthritis Rheum*. 2004;50(10):3145–3152. https://doi.org/10.1002/art.20589.
13. Suter LG, Smith SR, Katz JN, et al. Projecting lifetime risk of symptomatic knee osteoarthritis and total knee replacement in individuals sustaining a complete anterior cruciate ligament tear in early adulthood. *Arthritis Care Res*. 2017;69(2):201–208. https://doi.org/10.1002/acr.22940.
14. Filbay SR, Culvenor AG, Ackerman IN, Russell TG, Crossley KM. Quality of life in anterior cruciate ligament-deficient individuals: a systematic review and meta-analysis. *Br J Sports Med*. 2015;49(16):1033–1041. https://doi.org/10.1136/bjsports-2015-094864.
15. Øiestad BE, Engebretsen L, Storheim K, Risberg MA. Knee osteoarthritis after anterior cruciate ligament injury: a systematic review. *Am J Sports Med*. 2009;37(7):1434–1443. https://doi.org/10.1177/0363546509338827.
16. Hewett TE, Myer GD, Ford KR, Slauterbeck JR. Dynamic neuromuscular analysis training for preventing anterior cruciate ligament injury in female athletes. *Instr Course Lect*. 2007;56:397–406. http://www.ncbi.nlm.nih.gov/pubmed/17472323. Accessed July 24, 2019.
17. Hootman JM, Dick R, Agel J. Epidemiology of collegiate injuries for 15 sports: summary and recommendations for injury prevention initiatives. *J Athl Train*. 2007;42(2):311–319. http://www.ncbi.nlm.nih.gov/pubmed/17710181. Accessed July 24, 2019.
18. Ardern CL, Taylor NF, Feller JA, Webster KE. Fifty-five per cent return to competitive sport following anterior cruciate ligament reconstruction surgery: an updated systematic review and meta-analysis including aspects of physical functioning and contextual factors. *Br J Sports Med*. 2014;48(21):1543–1552. https://doi.org/10.1136/bjsports-2013-093398.
19. Ardern CL, Webster KE, Taylor NF, Feller JA. Return to the preinjury level of competitive sport after anterior cruciate ligament reconstruction surgery: two-thirds of patients have not returned by 12 months after surgery. *Am J Sports Med*. 2011;39(3):538–543. https://doi.org/10.1177/0363546510384798.

20. Myer GD, Sugimoto D, Thomas S, Hewett TE. The influence of age on the effectiveness of neuromuscular training to reduce anterior cruciate ligament injury in female athletes. *Am J Sports Med.* 2013;41(1):203–215. https://doi.org/10.1177/0363546512460637.

21. Soomro N, Sanders R, Hackett D, et al. The efficacy of injury prevention programs in adolescent team sports a meta-analysis. *Am J Sports Med.* 2015. https://doi.org/10.1177/0363546515618372.

22. Sugimoto D, Myer GD, Barber Foss KD, Hewett TE. Specific exercise effects of preventive neuromuscular training intervention on anterior cruciate ligament injury risk reduction in young females: meta-analysis and subgroup analysis. *Br J Sports Med.* 2015. https://doi.org/10.1136/bjsports-2014-093461.

23. Sugimoto D, Myer GD, Barber Foss KD, Pepin MJ, Micheli LJ, Hewett TE. Critical components of neuromuscular training to reduce ACL injury risk in female athletes: meta-regression analysis HHS public access. *Br J Sports Med.* 2016;50(20):1259–1266. https://doi.org/10.1136/bjsports-2015-095596.

24. Zech A, Hübscher M, Vogt L, Banzer W, Hänsel F, Pfeifer K. Balance training for neuromuscular control and performance enhancement: a systematic review. *J Athl Train.* 2010;45(4):392–403. https://doi.org/10.4085/1062-6050-45.4.392.

25. Hewett TE, Paterno MV, Myer GD. Strategies for enhancing proprioception and neuromuscular control of the knee. *Clin Orthop Relat Res.* 2002;402(402):76–94. https://doi.org/10.1097/00003086-200209000-00008.

26. Chappell JD, Creighton RA, Giuliani C, Yu B, Garrett WE. Kinematics and electromyography of landing preparation in vertical stop-jump. *Am J Sports Med.* 2007;35(2):235–241. https://doi.org/10.1177/0363546506294077.

27. Ford KR, Myer GD, Hewett TE. Valgus knee motion during landing in high school female and male basketball players. *Med Sci Sports Exerc.* 2003;35(10):1745–1750. https://doi.org/10.1249/01.MSS.0000089346.85744.D9.

28. Ford KR, Myer GD, Toms HE, Hewett TE. Gender differences in the kinematics of unanticipated cutting in young athletes. *Med Sci Sports Exerc.* 2005;37(1):124–129. http://www.ncbi.nlm.nih.gov/pubmed/15632678. Accessed July 24, 2019.

29. Myer GD, Ford KR, Brent JL, Hewett TE. The effects of plyometric vs. dynamic stabilization and balance training on power, balance, and landing force in female athletes. *J Strength Cond Res.* 2006;20(2):345. https://doi.org/10.1519/R-17955.1.

30. Cowley HR, Ford KR, Myer GD, Kernozek TW, Hewett TE. Differences in neuromuscular strategies between landing and cutting tasks in female basketball and soccer athletes. *J Athl Train.* 2006;41(1):67–73. http://www.ncbi.nlm.nih.gov/pubmed/16619097. Accessed July 24, 2019.

31. Michaelidis M, Koumantakis GA. Effects of knee injury primary prevention programs on anterior cruciate ligament injury rates in female athletes in different sports: a systematic review. *Phys Ther Sport.* 2014;15(3):200–210. https://doi.org/10.1016/j.ptsp.2013.12.002.

32. Lewis DA, Kirkbride B, Vertullo CJ, Gordon L, Comans TA. Comparison of four alternative national universal anterior cruciate ligament injury prevention programme implementation strategies to reduce secondary future medical costs. *Br J Sports Med.* 2018;52(4):277–282. https://doi.org/10.1136/bjsports-2016-096667.

33. Marshall DA, Lopatina E, Lacny S, Emery CA. Economic impact study: neuromuscular training reduces the burden of injuries and costs compared to standard warm-up in youth soccer. *Br J Sports Med.* 2016;50(22):1388–1393. https://doi.org/10.1136/bjsports-2015-095666.

34. Arundale AJH, Bizzini M, Airelle G, et al. Clinical practice guidelines exercise-based knee and anterior cruciate ligament injury prevention summary of recommendations. *J Orthop Sports Phys Ther.* 2018;48(9):1–42. https://doi.org/10.2519/jospt.2018.0303.

35. Kiani A, Hellquist E, Ahlqvist K, Gedeborg R, Byberg L. Prevention of soccer-related knee injuries in teenaged girls. *Arch Intern Med.* 2010;170(1):43. https://doi.org/10.1001/archinternmed.2009.289.

36. PEP Program | USF Health. https://health.usf.edu/medicine/orthopaedic/smart/pep. (Accessed 24 July 2019).

37. Noyes FR, Barber-Westin SD. Sportsmetrics ACL intervention training program: components, results. In: *ACL Injuries in the Female Athlete.* Berlin, Heidelberg: Springer; 2012:275–308. https://doi.org/10.1007/978-3-642-32592-2_14.

38. Donnell-Fink LA, Klara K, Collins JE, et al. Effectiveness of knee injury and anterior cruciate ligament tear prevention programs: a meta-analysis. *PLoS One.* 2015;10(12):144063. https://doi.org/10.1371/journal.pone.0144063.

39. Gagnier JJ, Morgenstern H, Chess L. Interventions designed to prevent anterior cruciate ligament injuries in adolescents and adults a systematic review and meta-analysis. *Am J Sports Med.* 2012. https://doi.org/10.1177/0363546512458227.

40. Söderman K, Werner S, Pietilä T, Engström B, Alfredson H. Balance board training: prevention of traumatic injuries of the lower extremities in female soccer players? *Knee Surg Sports Traumatol Arthrosc.* 2000;8(6):356–363. https://doi.org/10.1007/s001670000147.

41. Steffen K, Myklebust G, Olsen OE, Holme I, Bahr R. Preventing injuries in female youth football - a cluster-randomized controlled trial. *Scand J Med Sci Sports.* 2008;18(5):605–614. https://doi.org/10.1111/j.1600-0838.2007.00703.x.

42. Walden M, Atroshi I, Magnusson H, Wagner P, Hagglund M. Prevention of acute knee injuries in adolescent female football players: cluster randomised controlled trial (May 03 1) *BMJ.* 2012;344:e3042. https://doi.org/10.1136/bmj.e3042.

43. Hewett TE, Lindenfeld TN, Riccobene JV, Noyes FR. The effect of neuromuscular training on the incidence of knee injury in female athletes. *Am J Sports Med.* 1999;27(6):699–706. https://doi.org/10.1177/03635465990270060301.

44. Baldon R de M, Lobato DFM, Carvalho LP, Wun PYL, Santiago PRP, Serrão FV. Effect of functional stabilization training on lower limb biomechanics in women. *Med Sci Sports Exerc.* 2012;44(1):135−145. https://doi.org/10.1249/MSS.0b013e31822a51bb.

45. Earl JE, Hoch AZ. A proximal strengthening program improves pain, function, and biomechanics in women with patellofemoral pain syndrome. *Am J Sports Med.* 2011;39(1):154−163. https://doi.org/10.1177/0363546510379967.

46. Myer GD, Ford KR, Divine JG, Wall EJ, Kahanov L, Hewett TE. Longitudinal assessment of noncontact anterior cruciate ligament injury risk factors during maturation in a female athlete: a case report. *J Athl Train.* 2009;44(1):101−109. https://doi.org/10.4085/1062-6050-44.1.101.

47. Hewett TE, Myer GD, Ford KR, et al. Biomechanical measures of neuromuscular control and valgus loading of the knee predict anterior cruciate ligament injury risk in female athletes: a prospective study. *Am J Sports Med.* 2005;33(4):492−501. https://doi.org/10.1177/0363546504269591.

48. Alentorn-Geli E, Myer GD, Silvers HJ, et al. Prevention of non-contact anterior cruciate ligament injuries in soccer players. Part 2: a review of prevention programs aimed to modify risk factors and to reduce injury rates. *Knee Surg Sports Traumatol Arthrosc.* 2009;17(8):859−879. https://doi.org/10.1007/s00167-009-0823-z.

49. Hewett TE, Myer GD, Ford KR. Anterior cruciate ligament injuries in female athletes. *Am J Sports Med.* 2006;34(2):299−311. https://doi.org/10.1177/0363546505284183.

50. Beunen G, Malina RM. Growth and physical performance relative to the timing of the adolescent spurt. *Exerc Sport Sci Rev.* 1988;16:503−540. http://www.ncbi.nlm.nih.gov/pubmed/3292266. Accessed July 25, 2019.

51. Hewett TE, Myer GD. The mechanistic connection between the trunk, knee, and ACL injury. *Exerc Sport Sci Rev.* 2011;39(4):1. https://doi.org/10.1097/JES.0b013e3182297439.

52. Myer GD, Brent JL, Ford KR, Hewett TE. A pilot study to determine the effect of trunk and hip focused neuromuscular training on hip and knee isokinetic strength. *Br J Sports Med.* 2008;42(7):614−619. https://doi.org/10.1136/bjsm.2007.046086.

53. Yoo JH, Lim BO, Ha M, et al. A meta-analysis of the effect of neuromuscular training on the prevention of the anterior cruciate ligament injury in female athletes. *Knee Surg Sports Traumatol Arthrosc.* 2010;18(6):824−830. https://doi.org/10.1007/s00167-009-0901-2.

54. Shea KG, Grimm NL, Ewing CK, Aoki SK. Youth sports anterior cruciate ligament and knee injury epidemiology: who is getting injured? In what sports? When? *Clin Sports Med.* 2011;30(4):691−706. https://doi.org/10.1016/j.csm.2011.07.004.

55. Grimm NL, Jacobs Jr JC, Kim J, Denney BS, Shea KG. Anterior cruciate ligament and knee injury prevention programs for soccer players a systematic review and meta-analysis. *Am J Sports Med.* 2014. https://doi.org/10.1177/0363546514556737.

56. Hewett TE, Lindenfeld TN, Riccobene JV, Noyes FR. The effect of neuromuscular training on the incidence of knee injury in female athletes a prospective study. *Am J Sports Med;* 1999. https://journals.sagepub.com/doi/pdf/10.1177/03635465990270060301. Accessed July 25, 2019.

57. Mandelbaum BR, Silvers HJ, Watanabe DS, et al. Effectiveness of a neuromuscular and proprioceptive training program in preventing anterior cruciate ligament injuries in female athletes. *Am J Sports Med.* 2005;33(7):1003−1010. https://doi.org/10.1177/0363546504272261.

58. Gilchrist J, Mandelbaum BR, Melancon H, et al. A randomized controlled trial to prevent noncontact anterior cruciate ligament injury in female collegiate soccer players. *Am J Sports Med.* 2008;36(8):1476−1483. https://doi.org/10.1177/0363546508318188.

59. Pfeiffer RP, Shea KG, Roberts D, Grandstrand S, Bond L. Lack of effect of a knee ligament injury prevention program on the incidence of noncontact anterior cruciate ligament injury. *J Bone Jt Surg.* 2006;88(8):1769−1774. https://doi.org/10.2106/JBJS.E.00616.

60. Olsen O-E, Myklebust G, Engebretsen L, Holme I, Bahr R. Exercises to prevent lower limb injuries in youth sports: cluster randomised controlled trial. *BMJ.* 2005;330(7489):449. https://doi.org/10.1136/bmj.38330.632801.8F.

61. Myklebust G, Engebretsen L, Braekken IH, Skjølberg A, Olsen O-E, Bahr R. Prevention of anterior cruciate ligament injuries in female team handball players: a prospective intervention study over three seasons. *Clin J Sport Med.* 2003;13(2):71−78. http://www.ncbi.nlm.nih.gov/pubmed/12629423. Accessed July 25, 2019.

62. Sugimoto D, Myer GD, Foss KDB, Hewett TE. Dosage effects of neuromuscular training intervention to reduce anterior cruciate ligament injuries in female athletes: meta-and sub-group analyses. *Sports Med.* 2014;44(4):551−562. https://doi.org/10.1007/s40279-013-0135-9.

63. Sugimoto D, Myer GD, Bush HM, Klugman MF, McKeon JMM, Hewett TE. Compliance with neuromuscular training and anterior cruciate ligament injury risk reduction in female athletes: a meta-analysis. *J Athl Train.* 2012;47(6):714−723. https://doi.org/10.4085/1062-6050-47.6.10.

64. Hägglund M, Atroshi I, Wagner P, Waldén M. Superior compliance with a neuromuscular training programme is associated with fewer ACL injuries and fewer acute knee injuries in female adolescent football players: secondary analysis of an RCT. *Br J Sports Med.* 2013;47(15):974−979. https://doi.org/10.1136/bjsports-2013-092644.

65. Benjaminse A, Otten B, Gokeler A, Diercks RL, Lemmink KAPM. Motor learning strategies in basketball players and its implications for ACL injury prevention: a randomized controlled trial. *Knee Surg Sports Traumatol Arthrosc.* 2017;25(8):2365−2376. https://doi.org/10.1007/s00167-015-3727-0.

66. Wulf G, Shea C, Lewthwaite R. Motor skill learning and performance: a review of influential factors. *Med Educ.* 2010;44(1):75−84. https://doi.org/10.1111/j.1365-2923.2009.03421.x.

67. Benjaminse A, Gokeler A, Dowling AV, et al. Optimization of the anterior cruciate ligament injury prevention paradigm: novel feedback techniques to enhance motor learning and reduce injury risk. *J Orthop Sports Phys Ther.* 2015;45(3):170−182. https://doi.org/10.2519/jospt.2015.4986.

68. Benjaminse A, Welling W, Otten B, Gokeler A. Transfer of improved movement technique after receiving verbal external focus and video instruction. *Knee Surg Sports Traumatol Arthrosc.* 2018;26(3):955–962. https://doi.org/10.1007/s00167-017-4671-y.

69. LaBella CR, Huxford MR, Grissom J, Kim K-Y, Peng J, Christoffel KK. Effect of neuromuscular warm-up on injuries in female soccer and basketball athletes in urban public high schools. *Arch Pediatr Adolesc Med.* 2011; 165(11):1033. https://doi.org/10.1001/archpediatrics.2011.168.

70. Parsons JL, Alexander MJL. Modifying spike jump landing biomechanics in female adolescent volleyball athletes using video and verbal feedback. *J Strength Cond Res.* 2012;26(4):1076–1084. https://doi.org/10.1519/JSC.0b013e31822e5876.

71. Myer GD, Stroube BW, DiCesare CA, et al. Augmented feedback supports skill transfer and reduces high-risk injury landing mechanics. *Am J Sports Med.* 2013;41(3): 669–677. https://doi.org/10.1177/0363546512472977.

72. Stroube BW, Myer GD, Brent JL, Ford KR, Heidt RS, Hewett TE. Effects of task-specific augmented feedback on deficit modification during performance of the tuck-jump exercise. *J Sport Rehabil.* 2013;22(1):7–18. http://www.ncbi.nlm.nih.gov/pubmed/23238301. Accessed August 12, 2019.

CHAPTER 6

Meniscus and Articular Cartilage Injuries

CLAIRE D. ELIASBERG, MD • SABRINA M. STRICKLAND, MD

INTRODUCTION

Meniscal tears and cartilage injuries are common issues in the knee of a female athlete. As female athletes are significantly more likely to suffer anterior cruciate ligament (ACL), tears they are also prone to associated injuries to their meniscus and articular cartilage. The incidence of high-grade chondral injuries ranges from 5% to 10% in patients over 40 years old,[1,2] and cartilage lesions may be even higher in athletes.[3] Additionally, the incidence of chondral lesions in patients with recurrent patellofemoral instability may be as high as 63.2%−96%.[4,5] Meniscal tears are also more common in female athletes in gender-comparable sports.[6] Making an accurate diagnosis of these injuries in the primary care setting can be crucial to patient care, as untreated meniscal and articular cartilage injuries can lead to progressive degenerative changes, pain, and functional limitation. This chapter will review the anatomy, clinical and radiographic presentation, and treatment of meniscal tears and cartilage pathology in the female athlete.

MENISCUS INJURIES

Meniscus Structure and Function

Anatomy

The gross shape of the meniscus can be divided into two parts: the medial meniscus and the lateral meniscus. The medial meniscus is C-shaped with a triangular cross section, whereas the lateral meniscus is more circular and covers more of the articular cartilage surface area.[7] The medial and lateral menisci are connected by the transverse (intermeniscal) ligament anteriorly. While there are variants of the meniscal bony attachments,[8] the menisci are connected to the tibia peripherally by the coronary ligaments and posteriorly to the femur by the meniscofemoral ligaments. The anterior meniscofemoral ligament is often referred to as the ligament of Humphrey and runs from the posterior horn of the lateral meniscus anterior to the posterior cruciate ligament (PCL) and inserts on the femur. The posterior meniscofemoral ligament is referred to as the ligament of Wrisberg. This ligament attaches to the posterior aspect of the lateral meniscus and crosses the PCL superiorly and medially to insert onto the medial femoral condyle.[7]

The anatomy of the meniscus allows it to perform its two primary roles: modulating force transmission and acting as a secondary knee stabilizer. Owing to the elastic nature of the meniscus, it allows for more shock absorption than articular cartilage alone. The shape of the meniscus allows for increased contact area with the femoral condyles, thus increasing the congruency at the interface of the femur, meniscus, and tibia. Additionally, the shape of meniscus allows it to functionally deepen the tibial surface, which provides stability. The posterior horn of the medial meniscus acts as the main secondary stabilizer to anterior translation. The lateral meniscus is more mobile. Therefore it confers less stability than the medial meniscus, but in the setting of an ACL-deficient knee, the menisci become the primary knee stabilizers.[9]

Composition

The meniscus is composed of fibroelastic cartilage, which contains collagen, proteoglycans, glycoproteins, and cells. Water comprises 65%−75% of the total meniscal contents and collagen constitutes the majority (60%−70%) of the dry weight of the meniscus.[10] The majority of collagen in the meniscus is type I collagen. The meniscus also contains cells called fibrochondrocytes, which help synthesize the fibrocartilaginous matrix. An important point regarding the composition and structure of the meniscus is the orientation of its fibers. The meniscus contains both radially and longitudinally oriented fibers, which allow the meniscus to

The Female Athlete. https://doi.org/10.1016/B978-0-323-75985-4.00001-5

expand under compression and this is important for its functions of increasing contact area and providing shock absorption.[11]

Blood supply and healing potential

The blood supply to the meniscus is by the middle genicular artery, which supplies the posterior horns; the medial inferior genicular artery, which supplies the peripheral 10%–30% of the medial meniscus; and the lateral inferior genicular artery, which supplies the peripheral 10%–25% of the lateral meniscus.[12] In general, the innate healing potential of the meniscus is limited, largely because of its limited blood supply. Peripheral meniscal tears are considered to have healing potential because of their proximity to the vascular supply. It is believed that tears in the peripheral 25% of the meniscus can heal via fibrocartilage formation but that tears in the central 75% of the meniscus likely have limited to no intrinsic healing ability. Therefore identifying the location of meniscal tears is crucial, as the location of the tear is very important in determining the treatment plan.

Types of Injury
Epidemiology

Meniscal tears are very common and are one of the most frequent causes of knee pain in active patients. The mean annual incidence of meniscal tears is approximately 60 per 100,000.[13,14] The majority of meniscal tears affect the medial meniscus in the posterior horn, and meniscal tears are most common in the third, fourth, and fifth decades of life.[13] Meniscal tears are more common in males than in females in a ratio of 3:1 and are commonly associated with ACL injuries.[15] Isolated medial meniscal tears in females younger than 30 years and with stable knees are uncommon.[16] Injuries that are often concomitant with meniscal tears and should therefore raise the index of suspicion for a meniscal injury include tibial plateau fractures, femoral shaft fractures, and the presence of a hemarthrosis.[17,18]

Classification/types of meniscal injury

There are several methods for classifying meniscal tears. Important factors to consider when evaluating meniscal tears include chronicity, location, pattern, and size of the tear. Chronicity (acute vs. degenerative) can be determined from a combination of clinical history and imaging and is a very important factor in determining the treatment plan. Location of the meniscal tear is also important for decision-making regarding management. The "red-red zone" of the meniscus is often referred to as the outer third, which is considered to be the region of the meniscus that has adequate

blood supply and more intrinsic healing potential. The "red-white zone" refers to the middle third of the meniscus, and the "white-white zone" refers to the inner third of the meniscus. These areas do not have a direct blood supply and therefore their healing potential is limited. The pattern of meniscal tears is also variable and may include vertical/longitudinal, bucket handle, oblique/parrot beak, radial, horizontal, complex, and/or root tears (Fig. 6.1).[19] Finally, the size of the tear may be difficult to quantify, but it is also important in determining treatment. While no strict guidelines exist, understanding the percentage of the meniscus involved in the tear can be crucial to determine whether the patient needs a meniscectomy (partial removal of the torn meniscal segment) or a meniscal repair.

Special Considerations
Meniscal cysts

Meniscal cysts are also common and represent 1%–10% of meniscal pathology.[20] While patients may present with an isolated meniscal cyst, meniscal cysts are very commonly associated with meniscal tears. Patients may present with symptoms similar to those found with meniscal tears or meniscal cysts may be encountered incidentally on a magnetic resonance imaging (MRI). Meniscal cysts can be perimeniscal (within the meniscus itself) or parameniscal (extruded fluid outside the meniscus). Typically, cysts form because the meniscal tear functions as a one-way valve, and synovial fluid is extruded and forms a discrete collection. Symptomatic cysts are more common laterally.

Discoid meniscus

A discoid meniscus is a congenital abnormality in which the meniscus does not have its typical anatomic shape. The incidence of discoid meniscus is 3.5%–5% of the general population.[10] It typically involves the lateral meniscus and can be bilateral in 25% of cases. Although not always symptomatic, the presence of a discoid meniscus often presents in adolescence with symptoms including pain, clicking, and mechanical locking. In a retrospective review of adolescent patients undergoing arthroscopy for isolated lateral meniscal pathology, 75% had a discoid meniscus.[21] However, if patients are not symptomatic and the presence of a discoid meniscus is found only incidentally, surgical intervention is not recommended.

Clinical Presentation and Workup
Presentation

The clinical presentation of patients with isolated meniscal tears may be variable. If the tear is isolated

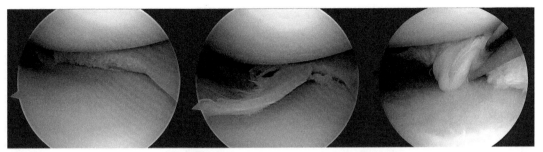

FIG. 6.1 Intraoperative arthroscopic images demonstrating examples of meniscal tears.

to the medial or lateral aspect of the meniscus, there may be pain, which localizes to the medial or lateral aspect of the knee. A careful history should be taken to elicit this. Additionally, patients should be asked whether or not they have mechanical symptoms, such as locking, catching, or clicking. They may also report delayed or intermittent knee swelling. Patients may or may not report a history of acute injury, but patients should always be asked if there were any inciting events that they can identify, as well as the mechanism of the injury. Typically, acute meniscal tears occur due to a twisting or hyperflexion injury and may present with acute pain and swelling subsequently. Degenerative tears, on the other hand, may occur in older patients who may report an atraumatic history of chronic pain and joint swelling.

Physical examination
A careful and thorough physical examination should be performed for any patient presenting with knee pain. To begin with, general alignment and gait should be observed and documented. Any swelling or joint effusion should be noted, and range of motion should be tested. It should be noted if there are mechanical blocks to motion at this time. Thorough palpation should be performed, and joint line tenderness is the single most sensitive physical examination finding for a meniscal tear.[22]

There are several provocative tests that can be used to help identify a meniscal injury on physical examination. The McMurray test consists of flexing the knee, placing one hand on the joint line and the other holding the foot. The leg should be rotated as it is brought from flexion to extension. A palpable click with associated pain is considered a positive test result. The Thessaly test consists of having the patient stand with the knee at 20 degrees of flexion and twisting the knee into internal and external rotation. Any clicking or discomfort elicited is considered a positive test result. Lastly, the Apley compression test involves having the

patient lie prone with the knee flexed. The examiner then applies an axial load and internally and externally rotates the tibia, again in an attempt to elicit any discomfort or a click in the knee. Although these tests may be helpful, they each have low sensitivity, specificity, and diagnostic accuracy, and therefore, advanced imaging is still recommended if the clinical suspicion for a meniscal tear is high.[23] Finally, additional ligamentous testing and a thorough neurovascular examination should be performed to rule out any concomitant injury. Other diagnoses that may be confused with a meniscal tear include symptomatic plica, fat pad impingement, chondral lesions, and synovitis.

Imaging
Plain radiographs should be obtained in patients presenting with knee pain, especially in the traumatic setting, to rule out fracture or gross abnormalities. Standard knee series should include anteroposterior, true lateral, and Merchant views. In addition to ruling out acute fractures and gross abnormalities, plain radiographs can help in evaluating overall alignment, degenerative changes, abnormal widening of the lateral compartment or squaring of the femoral condyles (commonly seen in the setting of a discoid meniscus), and meniscal calcifications (may be present in the setting of crystalline arthropathy). Thus other helpful views may include a posteroanterior flexion weight-bearing view to evaluate early joint space wear involving the posterior femoral condyles and standing hip-to-ankle images to evaluate overall alignment.

Although plain radiographs may be helpful in ruling out additional pathology, the mainstay imaging modality of choice for evaluating meniscal tears is MRI. If there is no acute pathology on plain radiographs and the patient continues to complain of symptoms consistent with a meniscal injury, an MRI should be considered (Fig. 6.2). Although MRI is the most sensitive test for identifying meniscal pathology, there are also high

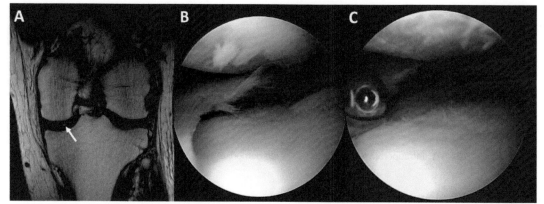

FIG. 6.2 **(A)** Coronal proton density magnetic resonance image of a left knee demonstrating small central medial meniscal tear (*arrow*). **(B)** Intraoperative arthroscopic image demonstrating the same central medial meniscal tear. **(C)** Intraoperative arthroscopic image taken status post partial meniscectomy.

false-positive rates, so results should be interpreted with caution.[24] Other important findings to identify on MRI are a "double PCL" sign or a "double anterior horn" sign that can represent a bucket handle meniscus tear and often requires surgical intervention.

Treatment
Nonoperative
After a thorough evaluation is performed as described earlier, treatment of the meniscal tear can be determined. Nonoperative treatment is typically indicated for physiologically older patients with degenerative tears and for patients without the presence of mechanical symptoms. Nonoperative treatment can consist of a combination of activity modification, antiinflammatory agents, and physical therapy as first-line treatment. Occasionally, intra-articular injection may be offered in the setting of a chronic meniscal tear refractory to the aforementioned nonoperative measures for symptomatic relief.

Surgical options
Surgery may be indicated for patients with mechanical symptoms and/or patients who have had acute tears. Surgical options for meniscal tears include partial meniscectomy, meniscal repair, and, in limited cases, meniscal substitution or transplantation. Overall, indications for surgical intervention are highly patient- and surgeon-dependent, but they typically include a combination of symptoms that affect activities of daily living, work, or sports; positive physical examination findings consistent with a meniscal tear; failure to respond to conservative measures; and an absence of other causes of knee pain.[10]

Partial meniscectomy is typically indicated for patients who have complex or degenerative tears that are not amenable to repair. Meniscal repair is best utilized for patients with tears in the "red-red zone"; those with vertical, longitudinal, or bucket handle tears; and those with root tears. Often the decision of whether to perform a partial meniscectomy or a meniscal repair is made intraoperatively after a more complete assessment of the tear pattern and tissue quality can be made under direct visualization. The decision to perform partial meniscectomy versus meniscal repair can be complex. Only approximately 20% of meniscal tears are considered reparable. Indications for meniscal repair are widely variable but may include a combination of the following: a complete vertical longitudinal tear >10 mm long, a tear in the peripheral 10%–30% of the meniscus, a tear that is unstable, a tear without secondary degeneration, a tear in an active patient, or a tear associated with concurrent ligamentous injury.[10] In younger patients with borderline tear patterns, a concerted effort is typically made to save the meniscus and perform a meniscus repair, particularly when it is a lateral meniscal tear.

Meniscus allograft transplantation (MAT) is an advanced procedure that has become more commonly practiced over the last decade. MAT is typically utilized for young, symptomatic patients who have undergone a near-total meniscectomy previously. These patients typically have limited alternative surgical options and are at risk for developing early degenerative changes over the course of their lifetime without the stabilizing and shock-absorbing properties present of the meniscus. Although MAT is not considered a definitive treatment option for these patients, it may help prevent rapid progression of degenerative changes. In addition, on the medial side, medial MAT may be a useful adjunct to stabilize a knee undergoing ACL reconstruction in the setting of medial meniscus deficiency, particularly in the young patient population. There are some contraindications to perform MAT, which include inflammatory arthritis, ligamentous instability, obesity, grade III-IV chondral wear, diffuse arthritis, and malalignment. Results at a minimum of 10-year postoperative follow-up have demonstrated survivorship rates of 73.5% at 10 years and 60.3% at 15 years, with improved functional outcomes compared to preoperative scores.[25]

ARTICULAR CARTILAGE INJURIES
Structure and Function
Types of cartilage
Articular (hyaline) cartilage is a specific type of cartilage that lines joint surfaces. Other types of cartilage in the human body include fibroelastic cartilage, fibrocartilage, elastic cartilage, and physeal cartilage. While articular cartilage injuries may occur on any articular surface, this chapter will focus on the articular cartilage injuries in the knee.

Composition
Articular cartilage is composed primarily of water, which accounts for approximately 75% of its overall mass.[26] The remainder of articular cartilage consists of collagen (of which 90% is type II), proteoglycans, noncollagenous proteins, and cells. The cells within articular cartilage are primarily chondrocytes, which help produce collagen, proteoglycans, and enzymes. The composition of articular cartilage is essential to its function, as its high water content and structural organization help decrease friction and evenly distribute force.

Layers of articular cartilage
Normal articular cartilage is composed of several layers, which also inform its function. There are three distinct zones that have been identified based on chondrocyte cell morphology and type II collagen fiber orientation.[26] The superficial zone is composed of type II collagen fibrils, which are oriented parallel to the joint line. This zone has the highest concentration of collagen and the highest cellular density. It contains flattened chondrocytes and sparse proteoglycans and is responsible for resisting shear forces. The next zone is the intermediate or transitional zone. This zone consists of type II collagen fibrils, which are oriented in an oblique and

less organized fashion. This is the thickest layer within the articular cartilage, and this layer contains round chondrocytes and abundant proteoglycans. The final zone is the deep or basal layer. This layer is composed of type II collagen fibrils, which are oriented perpendicular to the joint. This layer contains round chondrocytes arranged in columns, has the highest concentration of proteoglycans, and is responsible for resisting compressive forces. Deep to the basal layer is the tidemark, which separates the true articular cartilage from the deep, calcified cartilage.[26]

Stress response and injury
Articular cartilage is able to respond to various forms of stress and injury over time. Physiologic stress can stimulate matrix synthesis and inhibit chondrolysis; however, excess stress on articular cartilage can suppress matrix synthesis and promote chondrolysis.[27] It has been proposed that primary chondrocyte cilia act as mechanosensory organelles, which can help modulate the adaptive signaling mechanisms in response to various levels and durations of mechanical loads.[28]

Injury to articular cartilage can arise acutely as a result of a single mechanical load or multiple repetitive loads over time. Injury types can be categorized into microdamage (which typically results from repetitive blunt trauma with no gross disruption of the articular cartilage), chondral fractures (which consist of articular cartilage disruption ranging from surface disruption to lesions that reach the tidemark), and osteochondral fractures (which involve lesions that penetrate through the subchondral bone).[26]

Innate repair and healing potential
Owing to its avascular nature, articular cartilage has limited healing potential, which makes management of articular cartilage injuries particularly challenging. With very limited inherent blood supply, articular cartilage relies primarily on synovial fluid for oxygen and nutrients. Superficial cartilage lesions (those that do not pass through the tidemark) do not typically result in true "healing," as mature articular cartilage chondrocytes have limited proliferative potential.[29] In contrast, deep cartilage lesions (those that do pass through the tidemark) can result in fibrocartilage healing. A deep laceration that penetrates the subchondral bone allows for hematoma formation and mesenchymal stem cell migration. However, the resultant fibrocartilage has distinct characteristics from native hyaline cartilage. In general, fibrocartilage has poor wear characteristics compared with normal hyaline articular cartilage.

Types of Injury
Epidemiology
The spectrum of cartilage injuries is wide, ranging from acute focal defects to more chronic, diffuse injuries. Overall, the incidence of true articular cartilage injuries is unclear, but it is estimated that the incidence of high-grade chondral injuries ranges from 5% to 10% in people over 40 years old.[1,2] However, this likely underestimates the true incidence of articular cartilage injuries, as these estimates were obtained from arthroscopic studies and therefore likely more accurately reflect the incidence of symptomatic articular cartilage injuries. The incidence of asymptomatic articular cartilage injuries may be as high as 14%—59% in athletes.[3]

Classification
The first step of classification for articular cartilage injuries should be descriptive and should focus on the location of the lesion. For the knee in particular, the location is essential, especially with regard to whether or not the lesion is in a weight-bearing region of the knee, as this is important for management. Lesions located in the femoral condyles afford the widest variety of treatment options, whereas lesions located in the patella and trochlea can be more difficult to treat, in large part due to the variable topography of these regions.[30] Tibial cartilage defects can also be challenging to manage, given the relatively thin cartilage in this area and the difficulty in accessing the mid-tibia to posterior tibia through arthroscopic techniques.

Defect size is also pivotal in determining the treatment plan for patients with articular cartilage injuries. While the absolute size of a lesion is often referenced when making surgical decisions, it is important to remember that the lesion size relative to the size of patient's bony anatomy is likely more clinically relevant.[30] In general, small symptomatic lesions can be treated with a variety of procedures, whereas the options for the treatment of larger, more extensive articular cartilage defects are more limited.

There are two main classification systems commonly utilized to describe the severity of an articular cartilage lesion. The Outerbridge grading system was developed for arthroscopic evaluation of articular cartilage and includes ranges from grade 0 to grade IV. Grade 0 represents normal cartilage, grade I represents cartilage softening and swelling, grade II represents superficial fissures, grade III represents deep fissures without exposed bone, and grade IV represents exposed subchondral bone. The International Cartilage Repair Society (ICRS) also developed a grading system that consists of five different grades, ranging from 0 to 4. Grade 0 is

normal cartilage. Grade 1 is nearly normal cartilage with only superficial lesions. Grade 2 is abnormal cartilage with lesions that extend to <50% of the cartilage depth. Grade 3 is severely abnormal cartilage with lesions that extend to >50% of the cartilage depth. Grade 4 is severely abnormal cartilage that has lesions that extend through the subchondral bone (Fig. 6.3).[31]

Special Considerations
Osteochondritis dissecans
Osteochondritis dissecans is a specific pathologic entity that should be considered distinct from other articular cartilage injuries, which are often referred to as osteochondral defects. Osteochondritis dissecans is primarily a bony disease that affects the subchondral bone and the overlying cartilage. The disease was originally described in the 1880s and named "osteochondritis," as the underlying pathophysiology was thought to be due to an inflammatory disease process. Today, the specific underlying pathophysiology of osteochondritis dissecans remains unknown, but it is thought to be due to repetitive microtrauma.[32] It most commonly occurs in the knee, specifically on the posterolateral aspect of the medial femoral condyle as well as the posterior aspect of the lateral femoral condyle. Osteochondritis dissecans commonly presents in skeletally immature, adolescent patients and is often approached differently from a treatment perspective than traumatic osteochondral lesions in adults.

Clinical Presentation and Workup
Presentation
The mechanism of articular cartilage injuries is variable. Acute trauma may be responsible for impaction or shear injuries, whereas chronic repetitive loading may lead to cartilage softening, fissuring, and delamination over time. Patients who present with acute articular cartilage injuries of the knee typically report a history of trauma, but a careful history should be elicited to identify any other inciting factors. At times, cartilage lesions may be identified incidentally on imaging, but these findings should be clinically correlated to the patient's symptoms. Patients who are symptomatic may complain of effusions; restricted range of motion; mechanical symptoms such as clicking, catching, or locking; and localized knee pain. Pain may be exacerbated by weight-bearing or by knee flexion for lesions that are located more posteriorly on the femoral condyles.

Physical examination
Physical examination for suspected articular cartilage injuries should include a thorough knee examination.

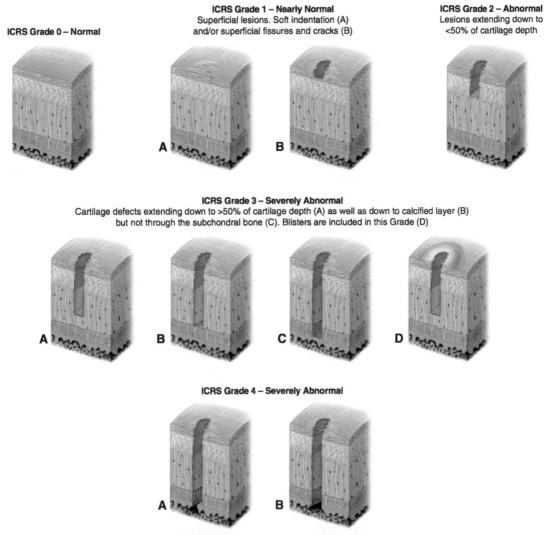

FIG. 6.3 The International Cartilage Repair Society (ICRS) classification of cartilage lesions. (Adapted with permission from the International Cartilage Repair Society. *ICRS Cartilage Injury Evaluation Page*; 2000.)

Starting with inspection, the patient should be examined for any malalignment, rotational deformity, abnormal gait, or joint effusion. Additionally, overall ligamentous laxity should be evaluated. Knee range of motion should be assessed to evaluate for any mechanical blocks to motion. Hip range of motion, hamstring tightness, and foot alignment should also be assessed, as rotational deformity and muscular imbalances in the lower extremities can contribute to altered biomechanics in the knee.[30,33] Extensive palpation should be performed to determine if the site of pain can be localized to a specific area. Finally, a thorough

ligamentous and neurovascular examination should be performed with particular attention paid to examine the ACL, PCL, medial collateral ligament, lateral collateral ligament, posterolateral corner, and posteromedial corner. Wilson's sign, originally described in 1967 as a test to identify osteochondritis dissecans, can be performed, but its clinical utility has been questioned. This test involves internally rotating the patient's tibia during knee extension from 90 to 30 degrees that produces pain, and the pain is then alleviated by externally rotating the tibia. While one study found that the sensitivity of this test was 90.9%,[34] a more recent study found that 75% of patients with radiographically evident osteochondritis dissecans had negative Wilson's sign at their initial visit.[35]

Imaging

Plain radiographs should be obtained in all patients presenting with knee pain to rule out degenerative changes and bony defects. Standard knee radiographs include standing anteroposterior, lateral, and Merchant views. Additional views may include a posteroanterior flexion weight-bearing view to evaluate early joint space wear involving the posterior femoral condyles and standing hip-to-ankle images to evaluate overall alignment.

Computed tomographic scans may be utilized if there is a concern for extensive bone loss; however, MRI is the most sensitive imaging modality for evaluating focal cartilage defects. MRI can be used to identify the specific location and size of the cartilage defects (Fig. 6.4). Fluid-sensitive sequences can be utilized to evaluate for underlying bone marrow edema.

Treatment

Nonoperative

The treatment for articular cartilage injuries is highly dependent on many patient- and injury-specific factors. Patient factors to consider include age,[36–38] activity level, body mass index,[39] number of prior surgeries, smoking status, and gender.[40] Female gender has been associated with greater cartilage loss and defect progression in patients with articular cartilage injuries.[40,41] Additionally, lesion location, defect severity, and clinical symptoms should be considered. Nonoperative treatment is indicated for patients with mild symptoms.

Conservative treatment methods include activity modification, antiinflammatory agents, physical therapy, weight loss, viscosupplementation, corticosteroid injections, and bracing. Biologic injections, including platelet-rich plasma, can be utilized, though there is limited research supporting any injection for the treatment of focal chondral defects. If there is a focal lesion in the medial or lateral compartment of the knee, a medial or lateral unloader brace, respectively, may help alleviate symptoms. However, none of these modalities is thought to reverse the underlying pathology of the articular cartilage defect.

Surgical treatment

Surgical indications for patients with articular cartilage defects are variable, but, in general, surgery should be considered for patients who have symptomatic, focal, and severe lesions as well as for patients who have failed conservative measures. There are many surgical options for articular cartilage injuries, which we will describe in the following sections. They include chondroplasty, fragment fixation, marrow stimulation techniques, matrix-associated autologous chondrocyte implantation (MACI), osteochondral autograft transfer (OATS), and osteochondral allograft (OCA) transplantation. In general, determining which technique to use depends on many variables including patient factors, lesion characteristics, and surgeon-specific preferences.

Chondroplasty. Chondroplasty or debridement involves the surgical shaping of articular cartilage. This is typically performed arthroscopically, and therefore it has an additional benefit of simultaneously joint irrigation to remove any intra-articular proinflammatory

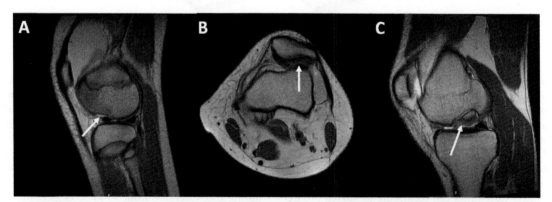

FIG. 6.4 Representative magnetic resonance images demonstrating cartilage defects. **(A)** Sagittal proton density (PD) image demonstrating cartilage defect in lateral femoral condyle (*arrow*). **(B)** Axial PD image demonstrating patellofemoral chondromalacia (*arrow*). **(C)** Sagittal PD image demonstrating large osteochondral defect (*arrow*).

mediators (Fig. 6.5). The primary goal of chondroplasty is to help alleviate mechanical symptoms by debriding loose chondral fragments and removing unstable, degenerative cartilage flaps. This is a relatively simple procedure that can provide patients with expeditious symptomatic relief if the cause of their symptoms is truly mechanical in nature. However, this procedure does not address the resultant cartilage defect and may leave the underlying layers of cartilage and/or subchondral bone exposed depending on the extent of the lesion. Additionally, patients with extensive degenerative cartilage wear are unlikely to be good candidates for isolated chondroplasty procedures.

Unstable fragment fixation. Unstable fragment fixation is controversial and rarely indicated in the adult patient with a true articular cartilage injury. In younger patients who have osteochondral defects with substantial subchondral bone attached to the cartilage fragment, arthroscopic versus open reduction and internal fixation should be considered. This method has been most successfully utilized for young patients with open physes who have osteochondral fragments with adequate subchondral bone. For these patients, the technique consists of debriding the underlying nonviable tissues, drilling the underlying subchondral bone, and fixing the fragment to the underlying bone with metal implants and/or absorbable sutures, screws, or tacks (Fig. 6.6).

Marrow stimulation. The concept of marrow stimulation, often referred to as "microfracture," was initially developed in the early 1980s as a treatment method for full-thickness chondral lesions in an effort to regenerate cartilage.[42] The technique involves utilizing an awl or a drill to create multiple small holes in the subchondral bone and allowing regenerative elements

FIG. 6.5 Intraoperative arthroscopic image demonstrating a large patellar cartilage defect.

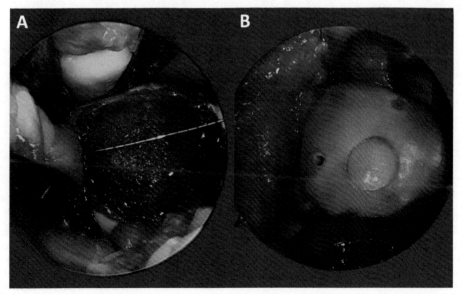

FIG. 6.6 **(A)** Intraoperative image demonstrating large lateral femoral condyle cartilage defect after a patellar dislocation. **(B)** Image of the same patient status post open reduction internal fixation of the cartilage defect.

from the bone marrow to develop into fibrocartilage. Because the resultant effect of microfracture is the development of fibrocartilage and not hyaline cartilage, the utility of the method for large defects, as well as the durability even for small defects, has been called into question. Therefore, today, microfracture is primarily used only for very small cartilage defects. While mid- to long-term follow-up of patients who have undergone microfracture has demonstrated satisfactory results,[37,43,44] the heterogeneity of the patients analyzed in these studies calls into question the validity of these results.

Matrix-associated autologous chondrocyte implantation. Autologous chondrocyte implantation (ACI) is another technique being used with increasing frequency for the treatment of full-thickness, symptomatic chondral defects. This is a cell-based therapy used to treat cartilage defects with the goal of restoring hyalinelike cartilage. Current ACI techniques utilize a matrix associated with the implant, and thus the procedure is now referred to as MACI. This type of

restorative cartilage restoration technique involves a two-staged approach (two surgeries) in which cartilage is first harvested from the patient from a non-weight-bearing area of the articular surface during an initial arthroscopic surgery, followed by implantation in a subsequent surgery. Between procedures, chondrocytes are expanded in culture for approximately 4–6 weeks and are grown on a matrix (MACI). In the second, open procedure, the bed of the chondral defect is debrided thoroughly down through the calcified layer to the subchondral bone, as full-thickness cartilage margins must be developed for the graft to sit within. The cell matrix is then placed in the debrided bed of the cartilage defect and is secured into place with fibrin glue (see Fig. 6.7 for representative intraoperative images). The benefits of this procedure include the regeneration of the patient's own tissue and the fact that this technique can be used for relatively large defects or multiple defects. Follow-up studies have demonstrated that the cartilage produced from MACI procedures is more similar to native cartilage than the fibrocartilage produced from

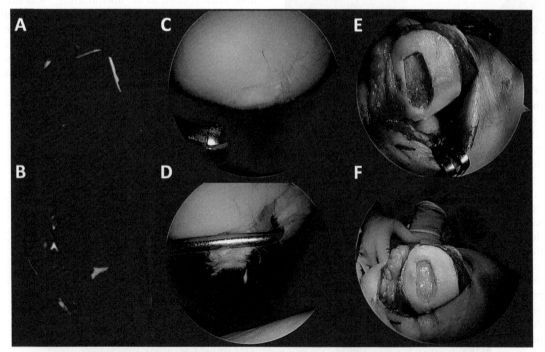

FIG. 6.7 Representative images from patient with patellar articular cartilage defect. **(A,B)** Inversion recovery (IR) magnetic resonance imaging representative images demonstrating subchondral bony edema. **(C,D)** Intraoperative arthroscopic images from the first-stage matrix-associated autologous chondrocyte implantation (MACI) procedure, demonstrating the lateral patellar facet chondral defect. **(E,F)** Intraoperative images obtained during the second-stage MACI procedure, demonstrating the debrided chondral defect and matrix-associated autologous chondrocyte implant secured with fibrin glue.

microfracture procedures.[45] However, MACI does involve two procedures spaced several weeks apart, is costly, and includes open as opposed to arthroscopic surgery.

Osteochondral autograft transfer. OATS or mosaic-plasty is utilized for patients with small to medium osteochondral cartilage defects. The goal of this procedure is to replace the cartilage defect in a high-weight-bearing area with normal autologous hyaline cartilage from a non-weight-bearing area. This procedure utilizes the patient's own cartilage to restore hyaline cartilage in the area of the previous defect. The chondrocytes residing in the transplanted portion of the cartilage are thought to remain viable, and the underlying subchondral bone becomes incorporated into the subchondral bone at the base of the defect. Typically, donor plugs are less than 10 mm in diameter, but several plugs can be used to fill a single defect. Sites for obtaining donor plugs include the intercondylar notch and the peripheral medial and lateral edges of the femoral condyle articular surfaces. While grafts can be harvested either arthroscopically or via a mini-open approach, there is some evidence that the mini-open approach may be preferred to obtain optimal graft perpendicularity.[46]

Osteochondral allograft transplantation. OCA transplantation involves utilizing a fresh allograft to replace the cartilage defect. An advantage of OCAs is that they can be used to treat a wide spectrum of pathologies, and their use eliminates the morbidity of osteochondral autograft procedures by preserving the patient's native tissue. OCAs are typically recommended for large chondral defects or as a salvage procedure option when the other procedures listed earlier have failed. The fresh grafts retain chondrocyte viability for up to 28 days and are matched to the size of the recipient's bone. A recipient socket is drilled at the site of the defect and an osteochondral graft matching the size of the defect is then cut and press-fit into place. This technique has been utilized with good to excellent results at up to 20 years' follow-up.[47-49] While OCA may not be considered the definitive treatment for many patients, it has utility as a viable option to help delay the need for arthroplasty in a young, active patient population.[49]

Outcomes

Cartilage restoration outcomes as a function of gender are not entirely understood, as relatively few authors have examined patient gender as an independent variable. Frank et al.[50] evaluated the outcomes following fresh OCA on the basis of age and gender and found that while overall outcomes and failure rates were similar among males and females, in patients <40 years of age, female patients who failed following OCA tended to fail earlier than male patients ($P = .039$). In contrast, in patients >40 years of age, male patients who failed following OCA tended to fail more quickly than female patients ($P = .046$).

REFERENCES

1. Alford JW, Cole BJ. Cartilage restoration, part 1: basic science, historical perspective, patient evaluation, and treatment options. *Am J Sports Med.* 2005;33(2):295–306. https://doi.org/10.1177/0363546504273510.
2. Åroøen A, Løken S, Heir S, et al. Articular cartilage lesions in 993 consecutive knee arthroscopies. *Am J Sports Med.* 2004;32(1):211–215. https://doi.org/10.1177/0363546503259345.
3. Flanigan DC, Harris JD, Trinh TQ, Siston RA, Brophy RH. Prevalence of chondral defects in athletes' knees: a systematic review. *Med Sci Sports Exerc.* 2010;42(10):1795–1801. https://doi.org/10.1249/MSS.0b013e3181d9eea0.
4. Nomura E, Inoue M. Cartilage lesions of the patella in recurrent patellar dislocation. *Am J Sports Med.* 2004;32(2):498–502. https://doi.org/10.1177/0095399703258677.
5. Franzone JM, Vitale MA, Shubin Stein BE, Ahmad CS. Is there an association between chronicity of patellar instability and patellofemoral cartilage lesions? An arthroscopic assessment of chondral injury. *J Knee Surg.* 2012. https://doi.org/10.1055/s-0032-1313747.
6. Mitchell J, Graham W, Best TM, et al. Epidemiology of meniscal injuries in US high school athletes between 2007 and 2013. *Knee Surg Sports Traumatol Arthrosc.* 2016;24(3):715–722. https://doi.org/10.1007/s00167-015-3814-2.
7. Pagnani M, Warren R, Arnoczky SP, Wickiewicz TL. Anatomy of the knee. In: Nichloas J, Hershman E, eds. *The Lower Extremity and Spine in Sports Medicine.* St. Louis: Mosby; 1996:581–614.
8. Berlet GC, Fowler PJ. The anterior horn of the medial meniscus. An anatomic study of its insertion. *Am J Sports Med.* 1998;26(4):540–543. https://doi.org/10.1177/03635465980260041201.
9. Thompson WO, Fu FH. The meniscus in the cruciate-deficient knee. *Clin Sports Med.* 1993;12(4):771–796.
10. Greis PE, Bardana DD, Holmstrom MC, Burks RT. Meniscal injury: I. Basic science and evaluation. *J Am Acad Orthop Surg.* 2002;10(3):168–176. http://www.ncbi.nlm.nih.gov/pubmed/12041938. Accessed July 8, 2019.
11. Bullough PG, Munuera L, Murphy J, Weinstein AM. The strength of the menisci of the knee as it relates to their fine structure. *J Bone Joint Surg Br.* 1970;52:564–567.

12. Arnoczky SP, Warren RF. Microvasculature of the human meniscus. *Am J Sports Med.* 1982;10(2):90–95. https://doi.org/10.1177/036354658201000205.

13. Hede A, Jensen DB, Blyme P, Sonne-Holm S. Epidemiology of meniscal lesions in the knee: 1,215 open operations in copenhagen 1982-84. *Acta Orthop.* 1990;61: 435–437. https://doi.org/10.3109/17453679008993557.

14. Nielsen AB, Yde J. Epidemiology of acute knee injuries: a prospective hospital investigation. *J Trauma.* 1991;31: 1644–1648.

15. Poehling GG, Ruch DS, Chabon SJ. The landscape of meniscal injuries. *Clin Sports Med.* 1990;9:539–549.

16. Haviv B, Bronak S, Thein R. Low prevalence of isolated medial meniscal tears in young females with stable knees. *Orthopedics.* 2015;38(3):e196–e199. https://doi.org/10.3928/01477447-20150305-56.

17. Vangsness C, Ghaderi B, Hohl M, Moore T. Arthroscopy of meniscal injuries with tibial plateau fractures. *J Bone Joint Surg Br.* 1994;76:488–490. https://doi.org/10.1302/0301-620x.76b3.8175862.

18. Vangsness CT, DeCampos J, Merritt PO, Wiss DA. Meniscal injury associated with femoral shaft fractures. An arthroscopic evaluation of incidence. *J Bone Joint Surg Br.* 1993; 75:207–209.

19. Ciccotti M, Shields C, El Attrache N. Meniscectomy. In: Fu F, Harner C, Vince K, eds. *Knee Surgery.* Baltimore: Williams & Wilkins; 1994:591–613.

20. Lantz B, Singer K. Meniscal cysts. *Clin Sport Med.* 1990;9: 707–725.

21. Ellis HB, Wise K, LaMont L, Copley L, Wilson P. Prevalence of discoid meniscus during arthroscopy for isolated lateral meniscal pathology in the pediatric population. *J Pediatr Orthop.* 2017;37(4):285–292. https://doi.org/10.1097/BPO.0000000000000630.

22. Weinstabl R, Muellner T, Vécsei V, Kainberger F, Kramer M. Economic considerations for the diagnosis and therapy of meniscal lesions: can magnetic resonance imaging help reduce the expense? *World J Surg.* 1997;21:363–368. https://doi.org/10.1007/PL00012254.

23. Blyth M, Anthony I, Francq B, et al. Diagnostic accuracy of the thessaly test, standardised clinical history and other clinical examination tests (Apley's, mcmurray's and joint line tenderness) for meniscal tears in comparison with magnetic resonance imaging diagnosis. *Health Technol Assess.* 2015. https://doi.org/10.3310/hta19620.

24. Reicher MA, Hartzman S, Duckwiler GR, Bassett LW, Anderson LJ, Gold RH. Meniscal injuries: detection using MR imaging. *Radiology.* 1986;159(3):753–757. https://doi.org/10.1148/radiology.159.3.3754645.

25. Novaretti JV, Patel NK, Lian J, et al. Long-term survival analysis and outcomes of meniscal allograft transplantation with minimum 10-year follow-up: a systematic review. *Arthroscopy.* 2019;35(2):659–667. https://doi.org/10.1016/j.arthro.2018.08.031.

26. Ulrich-Vinther M, Maloney M, Schwarz E, Rosier R, O'Keefe RJ. Articular cartilage biology. *J Am Acad Orthop Surg.* 2003;11(6):685–692. https://doi.org/10.1007/978-3-642-15630-4_91.

27. Visser NA, De Koning MHMT, Lammi MJ, Häkkinen T, Tammi M, Van Kampen GPJ. Increase of decorin content in articular cartilage following running. *Connect Tissue Res.* 1998;37:295–302. https://doi.org/10.3109/03008209809002446.

28. McGlashan SR, Knight MM, Chowdhury TT, et al. Mechanical loading modulates chondrocyte primary cilia incidence and length. *Cell Biol Int.* 2010;34(5):441–446. https://doi.org/10.1042/CBI20090094.

29. Carballo CB, Nakagawa Y, Sekiya I, Rodeo SA. Basic science of articular cartilage. *Clin Sports Med.* 2017;36(3): 413–425. https://doi.org/10.1016/j.csm.2017.02.001.

30. Mall NA, Harris JD, Cole BJ. Clinical evaluation and preoperative planning of articular cartilage lesions of the knee. *J Am Acad Orthop Surg.* 2015;23(10):633–640. https://doi.org/10.5435/JAAOS-D-14-00241.

31. International Cartilage Repair Society. *ICRS Clinical Cartilage Injury Evaluation System.* 2000.

32. Crawford DC, Safran MR. Osteochondritis dissecans of the knee. *J Am Acad Orthop Surg.* 2006;14(2):90–100. http://www.ncbi.nlm.nih.gov/pubmed/16467184. Accessed July 11, 2019.

33. Collado H, Fredericson M. Patellofemoral pain syndrome. *Clin Sport Med.* 2010;29(3):379–398.

34. Kocher MS, Dicanzio J, Zurakowski D, Micheli LJ. Diagnostic performance of clinical examination and selective magnetic resonance imaging in the evaluation of intraarticular knee disorders in children and adolescents. *Am J Sports Med.* 2001;29(3):292–296. https://doi.org/10.1177/03635465010290030601.

35. Conrad JM, Stanitski CL. Osteochondritis dissecans: Wilson's sign revisited. *Am J Sports Med.* 2003;31(5): 777–778. https://doi.org/10.1177/03635465030310052301.

36. Bekkers JEJ, Inklaar M, Saris DBF. Treatment selection in articular cartilage lesions of the knee: a systematic review. *Am J Sports Med.* 2009;37(Suppl. 1):148S–155S. https://doi.org/10.1177/0363546509351143.

37. Steadman JR, Briggs KK, Rodrigo JJ, Kocher MS, Gill TJ, Rodkey WG. Outcomes of microfracture for traumatic chondral defects of the knee: average 11-year follow-up. *Arthrosc J Arthrosc Relat Surg.* 2003;19(5):477–484. https://doi.org/10.1053/jars.2003.50112.

38. Knutsen G, Isaksen V, Johansen O, et al. Autologous chondrocyte implantation compared with microfracture in the knee: a randomized trial. *J Bone Jt Surg Ser A.* 2004; 86(3):455–464. https://doi.org/10.2106/00004623-200403000-00001.

39. Mithoefer K, Mcadams T, Williams RJ, Kreuz PC, Mandelbaum BR. Clinical efficacy of the microfracture technique for articular cartilage repair in the knee: an evidence-based systematic analysis. *Am J Sports Med.* 2009;37(10):2053–2063. https://doi.org/10.1177/0363546508328414.

40. Behery O, Siston RA, Harris JD, Flanigan DC. Treatment of cartilage defects of the knee: expanding on the existing algorithm. *Clin J Sport Med*. 2014;24(1):21–30. https://doi.org/10.1097/JSM.0000000000000004.

41. Gille J, Schuseil E, Wimmer J, Gellissen J, Schulz AP, Behrens P. Mid-term results of Autologous Matrix-Induced Chondrogenesis for treatment of focal cartilage defects in the knee. *Knee Surg Sports Traumatol Arthrosc*. 2010. https://doi.org/10.1007/s00167-010-1042-3.

42. Steadman JR, Rodkey WG, Briggs KK. Microfracture: its history and experience of the developing surgeon. *Cartilage*. 2010;1(2):78–86. https://doi.org/10.1177/194760351036 5533.

43. Weber AE, Locker PH, Mayer EN, et al. Clinical outcomes after microfracture of the knee: midterm follow-up, 2325967117753572 *Orthop J Sport Med*. 2018;6(2). https://doi.org/10.1177/2325967117753572.

44. Kraeutler MJ, Belk JW, Purcell JM, McCarty EC. Microfracture versus autologous chondrocyte implantation for articular cartilage lesions in the knee: a systematic review of 5-year outcomes. *Am J Sports Med*. 2018. https://doi.org/10.1177/0363546517701912.

45. Grawe B, Burge A, Nguyen J, et al. Cartilage regeneration in full-thickness patellar chondral defects treated with particulated juvenile articular allograft cartilage: an MRI analysis. *Cartilage*. 2017. https://doi.org/10.1177/1947603517710308.

46. Epstein DM, Choung E, Ashraf I, et al. Comparison of mini-open versus arthroscopic harvesting of osteochondral autografts in the knee: a cadaveric study. *Arthroscopy*. 2012;28(12):1867–1872. https://doi.org/10.1016/j.arthro.2012.06.014.

47. Wang T, Wang DX, Burge AJ, et al. Clinical and MRI outcomes of fresh osteochondral allograft transplantation after failed cartilage repair surgery in the knee. *J Bone Joint Surg Am*. 2018;100(22):1949–1959. https://doi.org/10.2106/JBJS.17.01418.

48. Cavendish PA, Everhart JS, Peters NJ, Sommerfeldt MF, Flanigan DC. Osteochondral allograft transplantation for knee cartilage and osteochondral defects: a review of indications, technique, rehabilitation, and outcomes. *JBJS Rev*. 2019;7(6):e7. https://doi.org/10.2106/JBJS.RVW.18.00123.

49. Abolghasemian M, León S, Lee PTH, et al. Long-term results of treating large posttraumatic tibial plateau lesions with fresh osteochondral allograft transplantation. *J Bone Joint Surg Am*. 2019;101(12):1102–1108. https://doi.org/10.2106/JBJS.18.00802.

50. Frank Rachel M, Cotter Eric J, Lee Simon, Poland Sarah, Cole Brian J. Do outcomes of osteochondral allograft transplantation differ based on age and sex? A comparative matched group analysis. *Am J Sports Med*. 2018;46(1):181–191.

CHAPTER 7

Patellofemoral Pain in the Female Athlete

HEATHER R. CICHANOWSKI, MD, CAQ • CAITLIN C. CHAMBERS, MD

INTRODUCTION

Patellofemoral pain is one of the most common sports-related knee conditions.[1,2] Patellofemoral pain is characterized by pain around or behind the patella during activities that load the patellofemoral joint, such as squatting, stair ambulation, running, jumping, and prolonged sitting with knees in a flexed position.[3] Patellofemoral pain is particularly prevalent in younger, active populations,[2,4,5] with females twice as likely to develop patellofemoral pain as males (29.2% vs. 15.5%, respectively).[5,6]

As the pathogenesis of patellofemoral pain remains largely unknown, it continues to be a complex and challenging problem to treat. While once thought as a benign, self-limiting condition, research has shown that patellofemoral pain can be recurrent and can persist for years[7-10]. Patellofemoral pain can negatively affect sports participation in adolescent female athletes.[10] Notably, single-sport specialization was found to increase the risk of patellofemoral pain incidence by 1.5-fold compared to multiple-sport adolescent female athletes.[4] Patellofemoral pain may also be a contributing factor to the development of patellofemoral osteoarthritis.[11-13] In addition, young females with patellofemoral pain may have risk factors that increase the risk of future ACL injury as they mature.[14] Emerging research is allowing for better understanding of gender-specific risk factors that will lead to better treatment and, more importantly, prevention strategies. Here, patellofemoral anatomy, patellofemoral pain causes, risk factors, diagnoses, and both nonsurgical and surgical treatments will be reviewed.

ANATOMY
Bony Anatomy

The patella is the largest sesamoid bone in the body, coupling the quadriceps tendon to the patellar tendon and acting to optimize the extensor mechanism's mechanical advantage by increasing its moment arm. The patella has seven articular facets, but it can largely be referred to by its medial and lateral facets with interposing central ridge. Articular cartilage is present on the superior two-thirds of the patella, with the inferior pole remaining as an extra-articular attachment point for the patellar tendon.[15] The size of the patella relative to the trochlea has been tied to patellofemoral pain, with increased patellar to trochlear width and volume ratios observed in adolescent females with patellofemoral pain.[16]

The femoral trochlea is complementary to the patella, composed of medial and lateral facets of the femoral sulcus, allowing a congruent surface for patellar tracking throughout knee flexion, with increasing engagement due to a deeper groove more distally.[15] In cases of trochlear dysplasia, the trochlea is shallow to flattened or even convex with increasing degrees of medial facet hypoplasia and supratrochlear spur formation. Trochlear dysplasia represents one of the most impactful anatomic variants in cases of patellar instability, but it should not be overlooked in patients with patellofemoral pain without instability. Dejour et al.[17] described Potential Patellar Instability as occurring in patients with anatomic instability factors but without a history of patellar dislocations. Within this group, there is a high incidence of patellofemoral cartilage damage. Particularly in females with trochlear dysplasia, the incidence of chondromalacia patella and structural cartilage damage is elevated.[18] In patients with end-stage patellofemoral osteoarthritis at the time of patellofemoral arthroplasty, 78% of patients had high-grade trochlear dysplasia, whereas only 33% had a history of patellar instability.[19] These findings highlight the role that trochlear dysplasia plays not only in patellar instability but also in patellofemoral pain and arthrosis.

The Female Athlete. https://doi.org/10.1016/B978-0-323-75985-4.00017-9

Limb Alignment

Frontal plane limb alignment plays an essential role in patellofemoral mechanics. The quadriceps angle (Q-angle) is commonly used as a means of quantifying the quadriceps' summative force vector on the patellofemoral joint. This is assessed by measuring the angle formed by lines drawn (1) from the anterior superior iliac spine to the center of the patella and (2) from the tibial tubercle to the center of the patella. The mean Q-angle is 15 degrees, but on average the Q-angle is 3−6 degrees larger in females than males, attributable largely to females' wider pelvis.[20,21] Q-angle greater than 20 degrees is generally considered abnormal. While elevated Q-angle theoretically increases lateral displacement forces across the patellofemoral joint,[21] current literature does not support static Q-angle as a risk factor for patellofemoral pain, but rather emphasizes the impact of alterations in dynamic quadriceps force vector.[22−24]

Axial alignment, namely, lateral patellar tilt, is another important consideration in evaluating the female athlete with patellofemoral pain. Excessive lateral patellar tilt increases contact stresses on the lateral patellar facet and lateral trochlea, with resultant pain and chondral wear. Contributors to lateral patellar tilt include tight lateral retinaculum, weak vastus medialis, medial ligamentous laxity, and bony alignment.[25] While more commonly pathologic in those with patellofemoral instability, relative lateralization of the tibial tubercle is also seen with increased frequency in adolescent females with patellofemoral pain without instability.[26] Excessive femoral anteversion and tibial external torsion each function to increase lateralization of the quadriceps vector and likely play a role in some cases of patellofemoral pain when significantly altered; however, their exact role in patellofemoral pain is not yet fully understood.[27]

Patellar height is also implicated in patellofemoral pain. The inferior patellar position in patella baja allows contact with the trochlea earlier in a range of flexion and has been shown to result in lower patellofemoral contact stresses.[28,29] Patella baja can be secondary to severe quadriceps inhibition, postoperative arthrofibrosis, patellar tendon scarring, or congenital growth disorders. Thus anterior knee pain associated with patella baja may be attributable to poor parapatellar soft tissue mobility rather than alterations in joint loading patterns.[15] Patella alta, on the other hand, allows a greater arc of flexion prior to patellar engagement in the trochlear groove, which can result in instability as well as smaller patellar contact area. Patella alta has been shown to correlate with significantly increased contact force and contact pressure[29,30] and can yield inferior-predominant patellar chondrosis and pain.[31]

There is some evidence that an overpronated foot posture, measured using navicular drop, may represent a minor component of the multifactorial cause for patellofemoral pain development.[32] Conflicting studies debate the magnitude of this impact, which does not appear to be gender-specific.[22,33] Despite inconclusive evidence to support foot alignment as the risk factor for patellofemoral pain development, there is likely a subset of persons in which this is a contributory factor.

PATHOPHYSIOLOGY

Pain Pathogenesis

The mechanisms that cause patellofemoral pain remain poorly understood, and the prevailing theory is that patellofemoral pain is the result of excessive joint loading and elevated joint stress.[23,34−36] Although the local tissue structures and specific pain pathways involved with the pain associated with patellofemoral pain are unknown,[23,37] it is thought that the abnormal loading causes strain to innervated structures within the patellofemoral joint. These structures include the infrapatellar fat pad, medial and lateral retinacula, synovium, and subchondral bone.[23,36,38] Furthermore, those with persistent patellofemoral pain can exhibit altered nociceptive processing such as generalized hyperalgesia and increased perceived pain through sensitization of both peripheral and central pain mechanisms.[23,37,39] Generalized hyperalgesia has been reported more frequently in females with patellofemoral pain,[40] with evidence from a meta-analysis suggesting the presence of altered pain processing and sensitization in individuals with patellofemoral pain, particularly in females.[41] Pain sensitization and other nonmechanical influences on symptoms, such as psychologic factors, may play roles in patellofemoral pain pathogenesis and are current research focus areas.[42]

Altered Lower Extremity Joint Kinematics

The theorized biomechanical risk factors for patellofemoral pain include lower extremity structural malalignment as discussed earlier in this chapter as well as altered lower extremity joint kinematics, decreased muscle strength, altered neuromuscular recruitment, and muscle tightness.[23,43] In particular, altered hip[44] and knee[14,45] frontal plane dynamic alignment have been reported as potential risk factors for patellofemoral pain development in females. Excessive activity leading to overuse or overload is also considered a potential contributor.[34,46] With its multifactorial cause, patellofemoral pain appears to be the result of multiple interactive underlying conditions and/or impairments that challenge the load-bearing capacity of the joint, leading to symptom onset and contributing to its persistence.[47,48]

Evidence suggests that under weight-bearing conditions, patellofemoral maltracking is the result of femoral internal rotation generating a relative lateral displacement of the patella with respect to the femur.[49] This lateralized patellar tracking reduces patellofemoral contact area, which increases focal joint stress and can ultimately contribute to the development of patellofemoral pain[36]. This suggests that the control of femoral rotation, especially during weight-bearing activities, may be important for optimal patellofemoral joint function, highlighting the influence that proximal factors have on knee biomechanics. Elevated dynamic Q-angle describes altered lower extremity kinematics, which increases laterally directed forces on the patellofemoral joint and may contribute to patellofemoral pain development, especially in females[36]. The altered kinematic factors considered to have greatest influence on the dynamic Q-angle, or dynamic functional valgus, include increased hip adduction affecting knee frontal plane motion through excessive knee valgus and increased hip internal rotation affecting transverse plane knee motion.[36] Even 5 degrees of excessive femoral internal rotation has been shown to increase patella cartilage stress during a squatting task in females.[50]

It should be noted that the available data is not consistent regarding an association between altered lower extremity kinematics and patellofemoral pain development.[23] However, evidence is mounting that, especially in females, impaired control of the hip can adversely impact patellofemoral mechanics. Specifically, increased hip adduction, hip internal rotation, contralateral hip drop, and reduced peak hip flexion are seen in both female and mixed-gender patellofemoral pain populations.[44,51] These unfavorable proximal kinematics are most influential during running, jump landing, and single-leg squat activities. In particular, increased hip adduction angles are seen in female but not male runners with patellofemoral pain as well as decreased peak hip flexion angles.[52] Increased hip internal rotation during a single-leg squat has also been reported in females with patellofemoral pain.[53] In regard to jump landing, increased dynamic knee valgus as well as hip adduction and knee internal rotation have significant correlation with the development of patellofemoral pain in females.[22,45,54] In one study, two-dimensional measures of knee valgus displacement ≥ 10.6 degrees during a jump landing task predicted patellofemoral pain in adolescent females, with a sensitivity of 0.75 and specificity of 0.85, and appeared to represent a manifestation of altered motions at the

hip.[54] As knee valgus displacement is also considered a risk factor associated with ACL injury in females, Myer et al.[14] concluded that young girls with patellofemoral pain may have risk factors that increase their odds of future ACL injury as they mature. In summary, for active females, altered hip kinematics significantly affect patellofemoral biomechanics, causing abnormal joint stress and likely represent a contributing factor to patellofemoral pain development.

Muscle Strength, Neuromuscular Recruitment, and Muscle Tightness

While retrospective studies have found that females with patellofemoral pain have decreased hip abduction, external rotation, and extension strength on the affected side as compared with asymptomatic controls,[55] these studies cannot determine whether muscle weakness is a cause or an effect of patellofemoral pain.[43,56] To this point, prospective studies have not found an association between isometric hip strength and the risk of developing patellofemoral pain.[24,57] Reduced hip strength is more likely a result of patellofemoral pain, not the cause.[23,57] Of note, in adults with patellofemoral pain, larger hip strength deficits are found in females than in males and mixed-gender populations, indicating the importance of hip strengthening in female adults and possibly less so in male adults and adolescents of either sex.[57] Conversely, one large prospective study found that female adolescent basketball athletes with greater hip abduction strength were at an increased risk for patellofemoral pain development. The authors theorized that this could be a result of increased eccentric loading of the hip abductors due to higher peak hip adduction during landing to correct for dynamic valgus biomechanics.[56] This highlights the need for different treatment strategies between female and male adolescent and adult populations.

Individuals with patellofemoral pain often exhibit altered trunk kinematics in the sagittal and frontal planes, which can contribute to added strain to the patellofemoral joint.[23] Specifically, those with patellofemoral pain more often exhibit an ipsilateral trunk lean during a jump landing task[58] and single-leg squat,[53] which can increase the potential for a knee valgus moment by shifting the center of mass of the body toward the stance limb.[23] Abnormal motions of the trunk, including ipsilateral trunk lean, may be a compensatory strategy for weak hip strength, especially of the hip abductors.[23,53,58]

Altered neuromuscular function of the knee extensor and gluteal muscles has been investigated as a potential contributor to patellofemoral pain. Increased neural drive to the vastus lateralis as compared to the vastus medialis is seen in females with patellofemoral pain[59] and may represent a risk factor in a subgroup of individuals with patellofemoral pain, but the larger role of this altered activation and its effect on patellar function remains uncertain.[23] In regard to gluteal muscle activity and patellofemoral pain, studies have found delayed and shorter duration of gluteus medius activity in those with patellofemoral pain during climbing stairs,[60] in females while performing single-leg squats,[53] and in female runners.[51]

Decreased flexibility of the quadriceps, hamstrings, gastrocnemius, and soleus has been implicated as risk factors for patellofemoral pain theorized to increase patellar compression.[23,43,61] Those with patellofemoral pain can also exhibit a tighter and thicker iliotibial band, which can affect patellar alignment and increase lateral patellar forces.[23] However, there are inconsistent findings among prospective studies linking muscle tightness to patellofemoral pain development, so no direct relationship is currently delineated.[23]

Several systematic reviews from the past decade have consistently found only decreased knee extension strength as a consistent risk factor for patellofemoral pain development in both adult female and male populations.[24,62,63] Unique to adolescent populations, quadriceps weakness was not found to be a risk factor for patellofemoral pain development, but stronger hip abductors were.[24] Despite the many variables that have been investigated in relation to the development of patellofemoral pain, clearly identified risk factors are not evident. This is in comparison to the structural, biomechanical, pain-processing, and certain psychologic factors found in those *with* patellofemoral pain.[47] As patellofemoral pain pathogenesis is believed to be complex and multifaceted, future studies investigating interactions of multiple variables as predictive of patellofemoral pain are warranted.[24]

Overuse/Overload

As with other overuse injuries, training errors and overactivity can contribute to patellofemoral pain. Any increase in frequency, duration, or intensity without proper rest and adaptation can push the knee outside its "load acceptance capacity" through loss of tissue homeostasis that can ultimately lead to pain and injury.[34] For some active individuals with patellofemoral pain, there is lack of significant findings on physical examination, suggesting a role of overuse and training errors.[46] This is highlighted by the fact that the most common overuse running injury is patellofemoral pain.[2] Education on load management is thus recommended as an important treatment strategy.[39,42,64]

IMAGING

Assessment of static anatomic factors contributing to patellofemoral pain is best achieved through a combination of physical examination with critical analysis of orthogonal radiographs and, when indicated, magnetic resonance imaging (MRI) and/or computed tomographic (CT) scan. Standard knee radiographs including weight-bearing anteroposterior (AP) and true lateral views, as well as an axial view of the patellofemoral compartment should be obtained in all patients with anterior knee pain. A summary of measurements and findings on orthogonal radiographic views pertinent to patellofemoral pain is provided in Table 7.1.

The AP view is useful for identifying tibiofemoral degenerative changes and can also demonstrate bipartite patella if present.

Lateral radiographs allow assessment of patellar height and classification of trochlear morphology. Patellar

TABLE 7.1
Radiographic Assessments for Patellofemoral Pain.
ANTEROPOSTERIOR VIEW
Bipartite patella
Tibiofemoral degenerative changes
TRUE LATERAL VIEW
Caton-Deschamps index   Normal: 0.6–1.2
Trochlear dysplasia findings (supratrochlear spur, crossing sign, double contour)
AXIAL (MERCHANT OR LAURIN) VIEW
Sulcus angle   Normal: 138 ± 6 degrees
Congruence angle   Normal: −6 ± 6 degrees
Lateral patellofemoral angle   Normal: ≥8 degrees
Patellofemoral index   Normal: 1.6
Signs of lateral overload (subchondral sclerosis, lateral patellar spur)
STANDING LONG-LEG ALIGNMENT VIEW
Limb mechanical axis
Frontal plane malalignment
Signs of malrotation (hidden lesser trochanters, squinting patellae)

height can be measured by several ratios including the Insall-Salvati ratio, Caton-Deschamps index (CDI), and Blackburne-Peel index.[65–67] Among patellofemoral surgeons, the CDI is generally preferred because of its independence from both degree of knee flexion and tibial tubercle position, maintaining the index's reliability after tibial tubercle osteotomy.[68] The CDI is measured as the ratio between the patellar articular surface length and the distance from the inferior articular surface to the anterosuperior tibial border (Fig. 7.1). Normal CDI is defined as 0.6 to 1.2, with values less than 0.6 denoting patella baja and greater than 1.2 denoting patella alta.[69] The lateral view is also useful in identifying findings of trochlear dysplasia, including the crossing sign, a supratrochlear spur, and the double contour sign.[15] Radiographic and MRI findings consistent with trochlear dysplasia are discussed in greater depth in Chapter 8.

Axial views in low degrees of flexion, 30 degrees or less, provide an optimal view of patellofemoral articular congruence, lateral tilt, subluxation, and trochlear dysplasia. Axial radiographs in greater flexion allow for increased trochlear capture and can obscure patellar subluxation present at lesser degrees of flexion.[70] The sulcus angle (Fig. 7.2), discussed in further detail in Chapter 8, is increased in the setting of trochlear

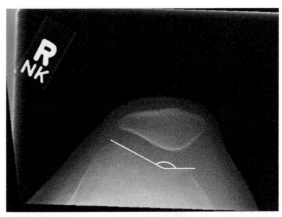

FIG. 7.2 The sulcus angle is the angle formed by a line along the medial and lateral aspects of the trochlea and is elevated above 145 degrees in trochlear dysplasia.

dysplasia. The congruence angle is measured as the angle between a line bisecting the sulcus angle and a line from the deepest point of the sulcus to the retropatellar apex (Fig. 7.3). A patellar apex line located medial to the bisector line is considered a negative value, with normal congruence angles averaging −6 ± 6 degrees.[70] The lateral patellofemoral angle is formed between a line connecting the anterior medial to lateral condyle and a line along the lateral patellar facet (Fig. 7.4). In normal knees, this opens laterally (≥8 degrees) with smaller angles signifying increased lateral tilt.[70,71] Patellofemoral index is a ratio between the smallest distance from the median ridge to medial femoral condyle and the smallest distance between the lateral facet and lateral condyle (Fig. 7.5). Normal patellofemoral index is 1.6 or less, with smaller values seen in the setting of increased lateral tilt.[70] Subtle signs of lateral overload can also be visualized on axial views even in the absence of any grossly abnormal values as earlier, with lateral facet subchondral sclerosis or cyst formation, lateralization of the patellar trabecular pattern, and lateral patellar facet traction spur formation (Fig. 7.6).[70]

A scanogram, or bilateral standing long-leg lower extremity alignment radiograph, allows the identification of the lower extremity mechanical axis and quantification of frontal plane malalignment. Significant valgus alignment is associated with greater incidence of patellofemoral pain and instability.[72] Scanogram can also demonstrate qualitative indicators of femoral malversion, with decreased visualization of the lesser trochanters and squinting patellae suggesting increased femoral anteversion. Although the sensitivity for malrotation identification on scanogram is poor, these findings can hint at a need for formal analysis of limb rotation.

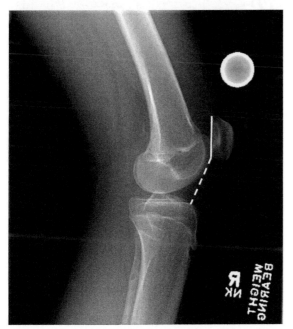

FIG. 7.1 The Caton-Deschamps index is the ratio between the patellar articular surface length (*solid line*) and the distance from the inferior articular surface to the anterosuperior tibial border (*dashed line*), with normal values ranging from 0.6 to 1.2.

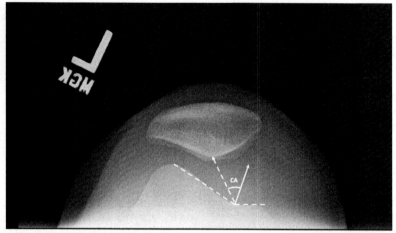

FIG. 7.3 The congruence angle is formed by a line (*solid arrow*) bisecting the sulcus angle (*dashed lines*) and a line from the deepest point of the sulcus to the retropatellar apex (*dashed arrow*). The patellar apex line located medial to the bisector line is given a negative value, with normal congruence angles averaging −6 ± 6 degrees, and increasingly positive values seen in the setting of lateral patellar subluxation.

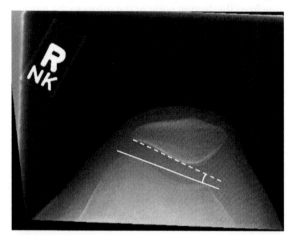

FIG. 7.4 The lateral patellofemoral angle is formed between a line connecting the anterior medial to the lateral condyle (*solid line*) and a line along the lateral patellar facet (*dashed line*). Normal knees open laterally with values ≥8 degrees; smaller angles are seen in the setting of increased lateral patellar tilt.

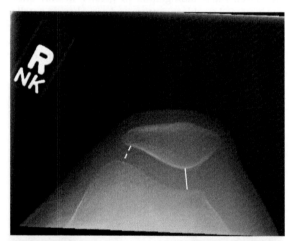

FIG. 7.5 The patellofemoral index is the ratio between the smallest distance from the median ridge to the medial femoral condyle (*solid line*) and the smallest distance between the lateral facet and the lateral condyle (*dashed line*). Normal patellofemoral index is 1.6 or less, with smaller values seen with increasing lateral tilt.

MRI has become a common adjunct to traditional radiographs in the workup of patients with patellofemoral pain. MRI allows for visualization of cartilaginous and bony surfaces as well as the soft tissues intimately involved with the patellofemoral joint. This can reveal parapatellar causes of pain, such as quadriceps or patellar tendinopathy, fat pad hypertrophy, edema, or scarring, and lateral retinacular thickening. MRI is limited in its provision of a static view of the

joint in knee extension and thus should not be regarded as a substitution for appropriate orthogonal radiographs and physical examination. MRI should be considered in cases of significant effusion, mechanical symptoms, or failure of nonoperative care, but it should not represent the first-line imaging study in a majority of patients with patellofemoral pain. Outerbridge grade 3−4 chondral defects can be seen in the patellofemoral

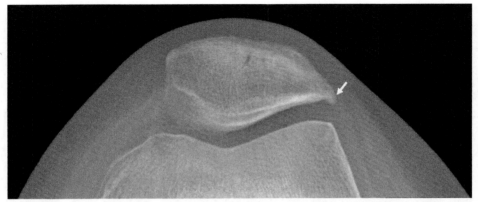

FIG. 7.6 Signs of lateral patellofemoral overload can be seen on this axial radiograph, with subchondral sclerosis of the lateral patellar facet, lateral patellofemoral joint space narrowing, increased trabeculation of the lateral patella, and lateral patellar traction osteophyte formation (*arrow*).

joint in up to 45% of knee arthroscopies, representing the most frequently compromised compartment of the knee when considering high-grade cartilage injury.[73] MRI is highly sensitive and specific in identifying patellofemoral cartilage defects, but it is important to recognize that these lesions are often asymptomatic incidental findings[74] and structural abnormalities are seen on MRI imaging of the patellofemoral compartment with similar frequency in patients with and without patellofemoral pain.[75] Lateral patellofemoral chondral lesions are more often symptomatic than those located medially, and defects with subjacent bone marrow edema either medially or laterally are frequently symptomatic.[76]

Lateral patellofemoral overload is commonly involved in cases of patellofemoral pain and has several indicators on MRI. Generally, this involves lateral chondral lesions and subchondral marrow edema, thickening of the lateral retinaculum, and lateral tilt or translation of the patella. Lateral patellar tilt can be measured on MRI axial series as the angle between a lie drawn along the transverse axis of the patella (on the cut with the greatest patellar width) and a line tangent to the posterior femoral condyles on axial MRI (Fig. 7.7). Normal patellar tilt is on average 2–5 degrees, but is most predictive of full-thickness chondral defect when in excess of 15 degrees.[68,77] Bisect offset (Fig. 7.8) is another indicator of lateral patellar malalignment, measured as the percentage of the patella lateral to the midline of the trochlea (with the trochlear midline transposed from the axial slice with the widest posterior condylar line to the slice with the widest patella). Bisect offset greater than 61.5% is strongly predictive of full-thickness lateral

patellofemoral cartilage defect and pain with stairs.[77] Elevated tibial tubercle to trochlear groove (TT-TG) distance has been found to correlate with Q-angle and is linked to patellar instability, chondrosis, effusion, and pain.[26,78,79] TT-TG distance is the horizontal distance between the tibial tubercle and the trochlear groove, parallel to the posterior intercondylar line, on superimposed axial MRI images (Fig. 7.9). TT-TG distance greater than 15–20 mm is considered abnormal.

Patellar height can also be assessed on sagittal MRI images. The patellar articular overlap provides a means of assessing functional patellar engagement on MRI and has been found to correlate well with radiologic indices such as CDI.[80] This is assessed by looking at the patellar articular length, which aligns with the trochlear cartilage on a sagittal view as a percentage of total patellar articular surface length (Fig. 7.10).

In cases of suspected malrotation, a CT scanogram can help quantify femoral version and tibial torsion. Cuts should be taken through the femoral neck, the mid-trochlear region of the knee, the proximal tibia, and the distal tibiofibular joint to provide a complete limb rotational profile.[72] CT scan can also be used to make axial-cut measurements such as TT-TG distance, sulcus angle, patellar offset, and trochlear inclination, as on MRI.

PATIENT PRESENTATION

Patients with patellofemoral pain classically present with anterior knee pain. The differential diagnosis of patients complaining of anterior knee pain is extensive (Table 7.2), and identification of those with patellofemoral pain central to their symptomatology depends

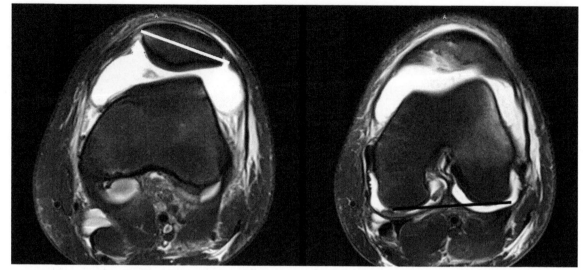

FIG. 7.7 The lateral patellar tilt is measured on magnetic resonance imaging as the angle between a line drawn along the transverse axis of the patella on axial cut with the greatest patellar width (*white line*) and a line tangent to the posterior femoral condyles (*black line*) on the cut with maximum posterior condylar width. Normal patellar tilt is 2–5 degrees.

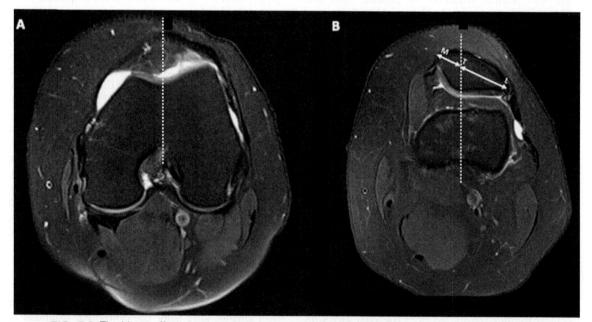

FIG. 7.8 The bisect offset measures the percentage of the patella lateral to the midline of the trochlea (TL/ML), transposing the trochlear midline point (*dotted line*) from **(A)** the axial slice with the widest posterior condylar line onto **(B)** the axial slice with maximum patellar width.

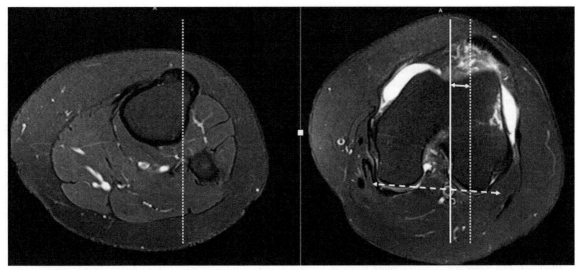

FIG. 7.9 The tibial tubercle-trochlear groove (TT-TG) distance (*double-headed arrow*) is the distance between the tibial tubercle (*dotted line*) and the deepest portion of the trochlear groove (*solid line*), parallel to the posterior intercondylar line (*dashed double-headed arrow*), on superimposed axial magnetic resonance images. TT-TG distance greater than 15–20 mm is considered abnormal.

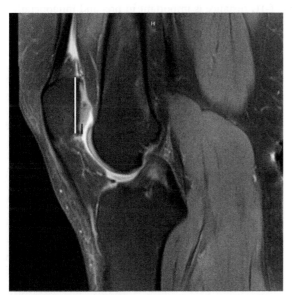

FIG. 7.10 Patellar articular overlap is the patellar articular length aligned with trochlear cartilage (*black line*) as a percentage of total patellar articular surface length (*white line*).

on careful consideration of the history, physical examination, and imaging findings. Patients should be asked about the onset of pain, noting the presence of any antecedent trauma or change in training activities. While patellofemoral pain is classically a problem of overuse, direct trauma to the anterior knee can cause crush-type injuries to the articular cartilage and subchondral bone. Patients should be asked to point with one finger to the location of their pain, as this can help discern anterior knee pain located within the patellofemoral joint (deep to the patella) versus along the patellar or quadriceps tendons. Symptoms of patellofemoral pain are often worst with activities requiring prolonged or repetitive knee flexion, such as squats, stair climbing, and prolonged sitting. Depending upon the underlying pathophysiology, patients may also complain of swelling, crepitus, locking, and weakness or giving way in the affected limb. The position of mechanical locking can be helpful in determining the underlying cause. A knee locked in full extension with hesitancy to flex is due to avoidance of engaging the patella within the trochlear groove and thus typically relates to the patellofemoral joint.[81] Loose body or meniscal pathology conversely locks the knee in some degree of flexion.

Although patients with patellar instability may also complain of pain, typically this occurs for an acute period after an instability episode; however, between instability events, patients remain relatively pain-free. Those patients with a primary complaint of pain should be considered an entirely separate entity from patients with instability, as interventions targeting patellofemoral instability do not reliably improve chronic baseline pain.

TABLE 7.2
Differential Diagnoses of Anterior Knee Pain.

Muscle/Tendon	Soft Tissue
Quadriceps tendinopathy	Patellofemoral instability/subluxation
Patellar tendinopathy	Lateral patellofemoral overload
Quadriceps atrophy/deconditioning	Potential patellofemoral instability
Hamstring contracture	Fat pad impingement
Bone	Prepatellar bursitis
Patellar stress fracture	Pes anserine bursitis
Symptomatic bipartite patella	Iliotibial band syndrome
Loose body	**Synovial**
Osteochondritis dissecans	Symptomatic synovial plica
Bone tumor	Pigmented villonodular synovitis
Frontal plane malalignment (genu valgum)	**Inflammatory**
Rotational malalignment (femoral or tibial)	Rheumatologic/autoimmune arthropathy
Apophyseal	Lyme disease
Sinding-Larsen-Johansson syndrome	Septic joint
Osgood-Schlatter disease	**Neurologic**
Cartilage	Lumbar radiculopathy
Articular cartilage injury	Saphenous neuritis
Chondromalacia	Neuroma
Osteoarthritis	Complex regional pain syndrome
	Referred
	Hip pathology

PHYSICAL EXAMINATION

Gait pattern should always be evaluated in patients with anterior knee pain. In cases of acute knee injury or chronic patellofemoral pain, a quadriceps avoidance gait can be observed, with hesitance to flex the knee throughout the stance phase. In-toeing can be seen with increased femoral anteversion, while out-toeing is seen with external tibial torsion. Clinical observation of more advanced dynamic movement patterns, such as a single-leg squat or jump landing mechanics (i.e., drop landing), can be very helpful in identifying biomechanical contributors to patellofemoral pain.

Inspection of the knee should be performed both standing and supine. Frontal, sagittal, and rotational malalignment can be screened for by looking at patients standing with their feet parallel. Significant genu valgum or recurvatum can predispose to patellofemoral pain, and increased femoral anteversion with squinting patellae can also be identified with observation. Q-angle can be measured utilizing a goniometer on a supine patient with knees in full extension. Supine measurement eliminates the confounding impact of hip rotation and quadriceps activation seen with standing Q-angle measurements.[79] The tubercle sulcus angle (TSA), or "sitting Q-angle," provides information on the quadriceps vector in the setting of increased tibial internal rotation during knee flexion. TSA is measured as the amount of lateral deviation of the tibial tubercle relative to the trochlear groove with the knee at 90 degrees, and in normal knees, it measures 0 degree. Consideration of TSA in combination with the Q-angle and imaging-based measurements such as TT-TG distance is important in pre- and intraoperative planning to avoid overmedialization with extensor mechanism realignment procedures.[79] Supine inspection should additionally assess for the presence of an effusion and any quadriceps atrophy.

Palpation can be positive for pain along the medial or lateral facets of the patella, or at the insertion point of the quadriceps or patellar tendons, depending on the underlying pathology. Range of motion is most often maintained in patients with patellofemoral pain syndrome, although end-range flexion can be painful because of the increased patellofemoral contact stresses in this position.

Patellar mobility is quantified by diving the patella into four equally sized quadrants from medial to lateral and assessing passive patellar glide in each direction. Two quadrants of mobility both medially and laterally from the midline is considered normal, with more quadrants of passive translation seen in the setting of laxity (i.e., three quadrants of lateral translation with medial ligamentous laxity) and less with tightness (i.e., one quadrant of medial translation with lateral retinacular tightness).[82] Passive medial patellar tilt is tested by centering the patella within the trochlear groove then pressing downward on the medial aspect of the patella, lifting upward on its lateral aspect. Inability to tilt the lateral border of the patella upward to at least neutral is considered abnormal, with females typically displaying an average of 5 degrees more tilt than males.[82] Decreased medial patellar translation and tilt is seen in the setting of lateral retinacular tightness with resultant lateral patellofemoral overload. Clarke's grind test is performed by using the examiner's hand to place distally directed pressure proximal to the superior pole of the patella as the patient activates his/her quadriceps muscle isometrically. A positive test result is seen with pain due to compression of the patella against the trochlea with quadriceps activation during this maneuver. Assessment of lower extremity limb rotational profile with bilateral comparison of passive hip rotation and thigh-foot angle can be helpful in identifying malversion or tibial torsion, respectively, which can alter quadriceps vector and contribute to patellofemoral pain.

TREATMENT

With its complex and multifactorial causes, patellofemoral pain remains a challenging diagnosis to manage, requiring a comprehensive and individualized treatment approach focusing on risk factors unique to each individual.[48,64] This may be of particular importance as longer term follow-up data (5–8 years) indicates that more than half of those with patellofemoral pain report continued symptoms and unfavorable outcomes, especially in those with longer symptom duration.[9] The mainstay of management is nonsurgical with exercise therapy, incorporating both hip and knee exercises, as the cornerstone treatment strategy to reduce pain and improve function, based on the current and consistent evidence.[83] However, other treatment strategies such as movement and gait retraining, education, and addressing psychologic factors are emerging as potential ways to enhance treatment success.[47]

Multimodal Approach

A multimodal approach is recommended when treating patellofemoral pain.[64,83] This should include exercise therapy targeting hip and knee musculature plus the addition of other interventions, based on individual needs, including patellar taping, foot orthoses, and patellar mobilizations.[64,83] Patient education discussing patellofemoral pain contributing factors, managing rehabilitation expectations, counseling on activity modification, emphasizing the importance of active exercise participation, and addressing any fear-avoidant behaviors is also highly encouraged.[42,64] See Table 7.3 for a summary of "Best Practice Guide to Conservative Management of Patellofemoral Pain" based on level 1 evidence and expert opinion.[64]

Exercise Therapy

Traditionally, rehabilitation protocols for patellofemoral pain treatment have focused on quadriceps strengthening, which continues to be an important part of treatment.[39,43] As previously discussed, altered hip kinematics and its subsequent effects on patellofemoral biomechanics and abnormal joint stress is likely a contributing factor to patellofemoral pain development, especially in active females. Current evidence supports a combination of hip and knee strengthening exercises to reduce pain and improve function in those with patellofemoral pain, and these exercises should be performed in preference to knee exercises alone.[83–85] Furthermore, initial hip strengthening prior to functional weight-bearing exercises may reduce pain sooner than initial quadriceps strengthening in females.[84] This may be of particular importance in those individuals who have symptom flares with quadriceps-focused exercises during the beginning stages of rehabilitation.[39,47,85] Adding to the robust body of work in support of proximal rehabilitation in patellofemoral pain treatment, a 2018 systematic review provided evidence that hip and knee strengthening is effective and superior to knee strengthening alone for decreasing pain and improving activity in individuals with patellofemoral pain. Benefits were maintained beyond the intervention period, even despite insignificant changes in strength, with these proximally targeted protocols.[86] With the average duration of strength training being 6 weeks in this review, it is likely that the study interventions were not of sufficient duration and/or intensity to improve muscle strength,[86] and the initial symptomatic improvements could be explained by the neural adaptations that occur in the beginning stages of resistance training.[39] Considering adult females with patellofemoral pain have reduced hip strength[55,57] and deficits in hip muscle power,[87] fully addressing the muscle function deficits takes time, much longer than 6 weeks. The resistance exercise training program prescribed, tailored to each individual's needs, should be progressive in nature and must be of appropriate strength load, quantity of repetitions, and duration of muscular tension to achieve the desired response.[39,88] The absence of significant pain during the exercises (up to 2–3 out of 10 in severity) and of significant symptomatic flare can be used to help guide the exercise progression.[47] See Fig. 7.11 for resistance exercise prescription principles. For those who desire to return to activities with higher joint forces, advancing to a gym-based rehabilitation program, a minimum of 2 days per week,[88] is recommended to achieve further progressive strength and power gains.[39]

TABLE 7.3
Best Practice Guide to Conservative Management of Patellofemoral Pain.

Education	Active Rehabilitation	Passive Interventions
1. *Ensure the patients understand potential contributing factors to their condition and treatment options* 2. *Advise of appropriate activity modification* 3. *Manage the patients' expectations regarding rehabilitation* 4. *Encourage and emphasize the importance of participation in active rehabilitation*	**Principles** 1. *Give preference to CKC exercises to replicate function* 2. *Consider OKC exercises in early stages of rehabilitation to target specific strength deficits and movements* 3. *Provide adequate supervision in the early stages to ensure correct exercise techniques, but progress to independence as soon as possible* 4. *When independent limit the number of exercises to 3 or 4 to aid compliance* 5. *Use biofeedback such as mirrors and videos to improve exercise quality* **Specifics** 1. Incorporate quadriceps and gluteal strengthening 2. *Target distal and core muscles where deficits exist* 3. *Consider stretching, particularly of the calf and hamstrings, based on assessment findings* 4. *Incorporate movement pattern retraining, particularly of the hip*	**Pain reduction** 1. Provide tailored patellar taping to reduce pain in the immediate term 2. Provide PFJ braces where taping is inappropriate (e.g., skin irritation) 3. Consider foot orthoses **Optimizing biomechanics** 1. *Consider foot orthoses based on assessment findings (i.e. presence of excessive dynamic pronation)* 2. *Consider massage and acupuncture/ dry needling to improve the flexibility of tight muscle and fasciae structures, particularly laterally* 3. *Consider PFJ mobilization but only in the presence of hypomobility* 4. *Consider mobilization of the ankle and first ray in the presence of sagittal plane joint restriction*

Texts in italics are based on expert opinion without supporting level 1 evidence.
CKC, closed kinetic chain; *OKC*, open kinetic chain; *PFJ*, patellofemoral joint.
Reprinted with permission from Barton CJ, Lack S, Hemmings S, Tufail S, Morrissey D. The 'Best Practice Guide to Conservative Management of Patellofemoral Pain': incorporating level 1 evidence with expert clinical reasoning. Br J Sports Med. 2015;49(14):923–934.

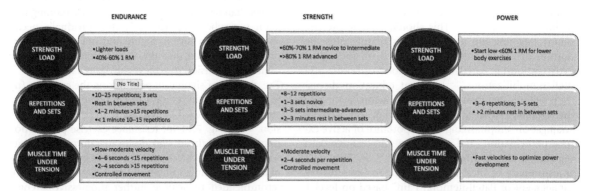

FIG. 7.11 Resistance exercise principles. *RM*, Repetition maximum. (Summarized from American College of Sports Medicine Position Stand. Progression models of resistance training for healthy adults. Med Sci Sports Exerc. 2009;41(3):687–708.)

In summary, exercise therapy, combining both hip and knee exercises, remains the intervention of choice for patellofemoral pain.[83] Hip exercises should target the posterolateral hip musculature,[42] and core strengthening should be incorporated when deficits exist.[64] Most importantly, the exercise therapy prescribed, driven by the individual's goals and desired activity level, must be of adequate progression in load and intensity and of appropriate duration to adequately target strength and power deficits seen in active females with patellofemoral pain.

Foot Orthoses

Prefabricated foot orthoses are recommended to reduce patellofemoral pain in the short term (6 weeks) and should be combined with exercise therapy; there is no evidence supporting the use of custom foot orthoses.[64,83] Not all individuals with patellofemoral pain benefit from foot orthoses. Those likely to benefit have greater midfoot mobility, less ankle dorsiflexion, and immediate improvements in patellofemoral pain while wearing the foot orthoses during a single-leg squat.[8]

Taping and Bracing

Patellar taping is frequently used to treat patellofemoral pain and is popular with athletic populations. A variety of taping techniques exist, with the tailored McConnell taping technique widely used. This technique reduces patellar lateral glide, tilt, and rotation to achieve pain reduction during functional activity.[89] Patellar taping has been shown to shift the patella inferiorly likely leading to increased patellofemoral contact area,[90] with pain reduction likely attributable to the distribution of joint forces over a greater surface area and shifting the contact away from more sensitive areas.[91] Current evidence supports the use of tailored patellar taping for immediate pain reduction in combination with exercise therapy for patellofemoral pain.[64,83] Patellar taping utilized in isolation for patellofemoral pain is not recommended.[92]

Patellar bracing may also provide immediate pain reduction[93] and can be helpful where taping produces skin irritation.[64] Similar to patellar taping, the primary mechanism of pain reduction may be increasing contact area rather than changes in patellar alignment.[91] While there is no convincing evidence supporting the use of patellofemoral braces with exercise therapy as compared to exercise therapy alone, the overall quality of evidence is very low and this warrants further investigation to effectively inform treatment strategies.[94]

Modalities and Manual Therapy

Current evidence does not support electrophysical and biophysical agents, such as ultrasound, iontophoresis, phonophoresis, electrical stimulation, cryotherapy, and laser therapy, as the primary interventions for patellofemoral pain.[42,83,95] Evidence does support the use of patellar mobilization as a component of a combined intervention approach with exercise therapy, but only in the presence of hypomobility.[64,83]

Blood Flow Restriction Therapy

In blood flow restriction (BFR) therapy, the individual performs lower load-strengthening exercises with a tourniquet around the proximal thigh, encouraging anaerobic anabolic effects. For those whose strengthening program progression is limited secondary to pain, this can be a useful treatment strategy. In one randomized controlled trial, BFR reduced pain with daily activity more effectively than standard quadriceps strengthening exercises over 8 weeks in subjects with patellofemoral pain; however, the between-group differences failed to exceed the minimal clinically important difference for pain using a visual analog scale.[96] Those with painful resisted knee extension had greater improvement in quadriceps strength using BFR therapy. Considering this is a new treatment approach to exercise therapy in those with patellofemoral pain, further research is needed to make any evidence-based recommendations regarding its use.[83]

Gait/Movement Retraining

Especially in females, altered hip kinematics, primarily excessive hip adduction and internal rotation, can result in a dynamic valgus movement pattern at the knee, contributing to either the development or the persistence of patellofemoral pain. Evidence suggests that exercises targeting hip strength may be insufficient to correct abnormal movement patterns during functional activities such as running,[97] even despite improved pain and function with the strengthening intervention.[51] Furthermore, a movement retraining program to successfully help control a single-leg squat did not carry over into a more functional task such as running.[97] Movement pattern and gait retraining have thus been receiving more attention[39] and are recommended by expert opinion as a treatment strategy.[64] Running retraining including visual (video or mirror) and verbal ("point your knees straight ahead") feedback help reduce hip adduction in females with patellofemoral pain.[98] Increasing step rate also reduces patellofemoral joint stress and load[98] and improves hip and pelvis kinematics and function in runners with patellofemoral pain.[99,100] Valgus control instruction exercises have produced positive results in female volleyball players by reducing knee valgus angles and pain during functional dynamic tasks in those with patellofemoral pain.[101]

Education

Education focusing on managing expectations, counseling on activity management, emphasizing the importance of active rehabilitation, and addressing any fear-avoidant behaviors is vital to the successful treatment of patellofemoral pain.[64] Highlighted as a primary target for future research,[64] the results of a study looking at runners with patellofemoral pain emphasize how important education can be. Runners who targeted isometric strength and running mechanics had no more additional benefits in improving symptoms and function than those who only received education on the appropriate management of training loads according to symptoms.[102] Furthermore, this strategy of activity modification and load management is associated with high rates of successful outcomes among adolescent populations with patellofemoral pain.[103] Education on activity modification may be of particular importance in patellofemoral treatment of adolescent populations, as research has shown less successful outcomes at 12 months after exercise therapy in adolescents as compared with adults.[37] Education on weight management strategies may also be beneficial. A higher body mass index (BMI) is present in those with patellofemoral pain in mixed-gender adult populations with patellofemoral pain compared with pain-free individuals, but this is not seen in adolescents.[104]

Psychologic Factors

As previously discussed, patellofemoral pain has proven not to be the benign, self-limiting entity it was once thought, with increasing recognition of poor long-term outcomes.[9] Like other painful chronic musculoskeletal conditions, psychologic features may play a role contributing to pain chronicity and barriers to recovery. Anxiety, depression, catastrophizing, and fear of movement (kinesiophobia) may be heightened in those with patellofemoral pain.[105] This highlights that for certain individuals with patellofemoral pain, these nonphysical, psychologic features need to be recognized and addressed, as these factors can influence severity and chronicity of symptoms.[39]

SURGICAL TREATMENT

In cases of patellofemoral pain recalcitrant to the above-mentioned nonoperative care, surgery can be considered. Determination of appropriate surgical recommendations demands an understanding of all pathoanatomic contributions to the patient's pain. As discussed previously within this chapter, the cause of anterior knee pain is not always truly the patellofemoral joint and can be attributed to abnormalities within the adjacent (i.e., Hoffa's fat pad, quadriceps and patellar tendons) or distant (i.e., lumbar or hip) structures. Additionally, abnormal lower extremity alignment, particularly in the frontal and axial (rotational) planes, can alter patellofemoral kinematics and loading, leading to symptoms. An appropriate surgical plan must take all these factors into account. Within the patellofemoral joint proper, the most common pathology leading to patellofemoral pain includes lateral patellofemoral overload and chondral defect.

Lateral Patellofemoral Overload

Surgical correction of lateral patellofemoral overload should be considered in patients with convincing radiographic and physical examination findings, who have failed to see lasting relief with appropriate conservative care. Importantly, medial glide and medial tilt McConnell taping should be trialed during physical therapy for these patients. Improvement in symptoms or function with taping can not only proves therapeutic but also serves as a helpful preoperative prognostic tool in predicting the likelihood of pain relief after lateral unloading procedures. Poor pain relief with medial taping techniques may implicate lesser functional improvements postoperatively, and consideration should be given to other sources of pain before proceeding with a lateral unloading procedure.

Lateral retinacular release or lengthening

Lateral retinacular release (LRR) or lateral retinacular lengthening (LRL), initially used indiscriminately for anterior knee pain, have now been better defined as appropriate options for patients with intractable anterior knee pain and patellar malalignment, as denoted by a tight lateral retinaculum and lateral patellar tilt. The International Patellofemoral Study Group (IPSG) agrees that LRR and LRL prove a useful treatment option, but expert members very rarely perform this procedure in isolation, representing only 2% of their annual cases.[106] The procedure can serve as a useful adjunct to medial patellofemoral ligament (MPFL) reconstruction and/or tibial tubercle osteotomy for patellar instability and to lateral facetectomy for lateral patellofemoral osteoarthritis, or it can be used to improve patellar tracking during patellofemoral or total knee arthroplasty.

LRR can be performed arthroscopically or open. This should not extend higher than the proximal pole of the patella, and the vastus lateralis obliquus attachment should remain intact to reduce the risk of iatrogenic medial instability and quadriceps atrophy.[107] Alternatively, LRL requires an open approach but allows for more exact correction of the degree of lateral retinacular relaxation. This is done through a lateral parapatellar incision, with Z-plasty lengthening between the superficial and deep layers of the lateral retinaculum and subsequent end-to-end or pants-over-vest closure at 60 degrees of flexion.[108,109] In both LRR and LRL, care must be taken to ligate the lateral geniculate vessels to avoid postoperative hematoma from unrecognized bleeding.

Although LRR is appealing owing to its technical ease, decreased operative time, and arthroscopic option, it does carry the unique risks of creating iatrogenic medial instability, severe quadriceps atrophy due to muscular detachment, and synovial herniation.[107] Improved clinical outcomes as well as decreased medial instability and quadriceps atrophy have been demonstrated after LRL when compared to LRR in randomized controlled trials.[110,111]

Outcomes of isolated LRR are poor in the setting of patellar instability, high Q-angle (>20 degrees), Outerbridge grade 3 or 4 chondral damage, and patellofemoral osteoarthritis.[108] A majority of experts agree that generalized joint hypermobility represents an additional contraindication to LRR.[106] Because generalized joint hypermobility is seen in up to 36.7% of young females, this exclusion criterion can present a problem for female athletes with patellofemoral pain due to both lateral overload and hypermobility.[112] This contraindication is due to concerns of medial instability after lateral release and is abated with retinacular closure during LRL.

In cases of lateral patellofemoral overload caused by patellar instability or otherwise incompetent medial patellofemoral checkrein, MPFL reconstruction can be performed concurrent with LRR or LRL. A discussion of MPFL reconstruction techniques is beyond the scope of this chapter, and they are discussed more thoroughly in Chapter 8.

Partial lateral facetectomy

The lateral facet is the most commonly involved portion of the patella in isolated patellofemoral osteoarthritis.[113] Chondral wear in this location can arise due to chronic lateral patellofemoral overload, due to instability, or as idiopathic degenerative changes. Partial lateral facetectomy can be performed as an arthroscopic or open procedure in patients with lateral-predominant isolated patellofemoral degenerative changes with an overhanging lateral osteophyte, anterior knee pain refractory to conservative care, and no history of patellar instability. Removal of the lateral osteophyte in itself creates more lateral tissue laxity, but in cases of continued lateral tilt or retinacular tightness, this can be combined with an LRR or LRL. This procedure yields significant clinical improvements in appropriately indicated patients but performs poorly in those with tibiofemoral pain, tibiofemoral osteoarthritis, or flexion contracture.[114]

Chondral Defect

A normal patellofemoral joint sees up to 6.5 times body weight, with these forces further increased when factoring in malalignment, lateral tilt, trochlear dysplasia, or chondral defects, which decrease contact area.[115] Patellofemoral chondral injury is incredibly common, but is not always associated with pain. Cartilage restoration techniques should be considered in patellofemoral joints with full-thickness (Outerbridge grade 3 or 4) cartilage lesions with functionally limiting anterior knee pain despite appropriate conservative care. Contraindications include diffuse patellofemoral or tibiofemoral osteoarthritis, inflammatory arthropathy, low-grade cartilage lesions, patients unable to comply with the necessary rehabilitation, and those with medical contraindications to the procedure.[115] While not an absolute contraindication to patellofemoral cartilage restoration, bipolar lesions may have lesser clinical improvements as compared with unipolar lesions.[116] Notably, off-loading tibial tubercle osteotomy via anteromedialization and/or anteriorization should be considered when performing patellofemoral cartilage restoration. The techniques for these cartilage restoration procedures are beyond the scope of this chapter, but information specific to their use in the patellofemoral joint is discussed in this section.

Chondroplasty

Chondroplasty is best utilized for debridement of incidentally found patellofemoral cartilage flaps less than $1-2$ cm^2 in size.[117] The goal of this debridement is to achieve stable borders to eliminate mechanical irritants. Overaggressive debridement should be avoided, as converting partial thickness lesions to full-thickness lesions and disrupting the subchondral plate can create bone marrow edema and subchondral cysts, with increase in pain.[118]

Marrow stimulation

Marrow stimulation techniques such as microfracture, represent a simple cartilage restoration method, but come with flaws. They can be considered for patients with small lesions (<2 cm^2), and they have been shown to work best in those who are younger (<40 years), with less than 12 months of symptom duration, and who are not obese.[119] While short-term benefits may be seen, deterioration in follow-up beyond 5 years has been demonstrated, and subsequent cartilage restoration procedures have demonstrated worse outcomes when performed after prior microfracture.[119,120] At best, marrow stimulation results in fibrocartilaginous fill of defects.

Autologous and allogeneic cell-based scaffolds

Cell-based treatments for focal chondral defects can be considered in the case of moderate- to large-sized defects, >2 cm^2, with an intact subchondral bony surface. The best studied technique in current use is matrix-induced autologous chondrocyte implantation (MACI). This represents the third generation of the technique, utilizing the patient's own harvested chondrocytes, which are propagated in the laboratory then transferred onto a porcine collagen membrane for implantation in t second stage of surgery. MACI has replaced autologous chondrocyte implantation (ACI), which initially required water-tight suturing of a periosteal patch to secure the liquid-suspended chondrocytes, the elimination of which has improved ease of the procedure. Within the patellofemoral compartment, MACI has demonstrated excellent durability of MRI cartilage fill, functional improvement, and high patient satisfaction at up to 5-year follow-up in current studies, exceeding results seen after microfracture when compared in a randomized controlled trial.[121,122] These improvements both clinically and on imaging after patellofemoral MACI are comparable to those seen after MACI in the tibiofemoral compartment.[123] MACI, therefore, represents an excellent treatment option for patients with symptomatic full-thickness cartilage defects, with excellent results even in the face of large or bipolar patellofemoral lesions.[124]

Other commercially available products such as micronized allogeneic cartilage or juvenile particulated cartilage have recently been suggested as a single-stage means of treating focal chondral lesions by creating a cell-based scaffold for cartilage regeneration in combination with microfracture. These heal with "hyaline-like" cartilage, which is an improvement from the fibrocartilage seen after microfracture alone.[125] Mid- and long-term data on these products is scarce and requires further study before widespread adoption.

Osteochondral autograft transfer and osteochondral allograft transplantation

Because both osteochondral autograft and allograft replace the subchondral bone, these represent reasonable salvage options after failed microfracture, whereas cartilage-only procedures such as MACI have demonstrated increased failure rates in the setting of compromised subchondral bone.[120]

The benefit of osteochondral autograft over allograft is the direct transfer of viable hyaline cartilage and the lack of need for a donor eliminating both wait times and risks specific to cadaveric tissue use. Downsides include the risk for donor site morbidity, which significantly increases when harvest sites exceed 4 cm^2 in size.[126] Osteochondral autograft transfer is therefore best utilized for osteochondral lesions exceeding 1 cm^2, but less than 4 cm^2, in size. Patellofemoral joint contour matching can be difficult, as the typical autologous harvest sites including the far peripheral femoral condyles and intercondylar notch do not provide a matched radius of curvature for trochlear or patellar lesions. Additionally, the patella has the most robust articular cartilage in the body, measuring up to 7 mm in thickness centrally, while the periphery of the femoral condyles from which autograft plugs are harvested can be as thin as 2 mm.[127] This can result in a step off between transferred and native subchondral bone plates, with increase in local contract stresses, stress riser formation, fibrous union or nonunion of the subchondral bone, subchondral cystic formation, and graft failure.[117] This in combination with the high shear stresses seen by the patellofemoral joint may explain why osteochondral autograft transfer has shown good to excellent results with 10-year follow-up of 79% of patellofemoral transfers as compared to 92% of femoral condyle and 87% of tibial osteochondral autograft transfers.[126]

Osteochondral allograft transplantation, on the other hand, allows for closer contour- and cartilage thickness-matching, although significant variability in patellar morphology can also create an imperfect match. Osteochondral allografts can be used for focal defects or thin shell allografts can be used for large, irregular defects in young patients with compromised subchondral bone. Shell allografts can be performed in a bipolar nature on both patella and trochlea and are secured with screw fixation outside the main articulating surface. Unfortunately, the results of osteochondral allograft in the patellofemoral compartment are inferior to those of osteochondral allograft of the femoral condyles, as well as to patellofemoral ACI or MACI and patellofemoral arthroplasty.[117,128] The indications for osteochondral allograft are therefore very limited and best reserved for young patients with large full-thickness cartilage defects and compromised subchondral bone.

Tibial tubercle osteotomy

One of the reasons for more recent improvements in outcomes after patellofemoral cartilage restoration procedures may be the increasing recognition and correction of patellofemoral malalignment. Anteromedialization and/or distalization of the tibial tubercle can be utilized in isolation or in combination with cartilage procedures to offload the newly repaired site. Anterior shift of the tibial tubercle results decreased contact stresses through the patellofemoral joint, which is favorable in the setting of patellofemoral pain.[129,130] Pure anteriorization as in the Maquet osteotomy yielded symptomatic improvements in patellofemoral arthrosis at the cost of significant complications, including nonunion, fracture, and skin necrosis, and is thus no longer a commonly used technique.[131] In 1983, John Fulkerson[132] introduced the anteromedialization tibial tubercle osteotomy, with modifications of this procedure remaining the most commonly used now for both patellofemoral pain and instability. The degree of anteriorization is increased with a steeper cut, while a flatter cut allows more medialization; determination of optimal osteotomy trajectory is based on preoperative measurements of tibial tubercle lateralization (TT-TG). Distalizing tibial tubercle osteotomy is useful in the face of patella alta with distal pole chondral pathology or subchondral bony edema.

Isolated osteotomy of the tibial tubercle yields the most favorable results in patients with cartilage lesions located on the lateral facet or distal pole of the patella and the lateral trochlea, whereas those with medial and proximal patellar lesions, central trochlear lesions, or diffuse wear do poorly.[133] More studies of anteromedialization tibial tubercle osteotomy in combination with ACI for proximal or panpatellar full-thickness cartilage lesions have demonstrated significant clinical improvements, with 75%–80% reporting good to excellent results, as compared to previous studies of osteotomy alone showing 0%–20% good to excellent with lesions in this location.[134] Tibial tubercle osteotomy for diffuse patellofemoral osteoarthritis has variable results reported in the literature and should be used sparingly for this indication, with a frank discussion of the uncertainty of clinical benefit.[131]

Patellofemoral arthroplasty

Patellofemoral arthroplasty is an appropriate treatment for patients with symptomatic diffuse patellofemoral osteoarthritis recalcitrant to conservative care or for those with failed previous cartilage restoration attempts. Patellofemoral arthroplasty with first-generation implants had distressingly poor clinical outcomes with high revision surgery rates, but newer implants with improved trochlear design boast excellent survivorship and good to excellent outcomes in 66%–100% of patients at both short- and long-term follow-up.[135–137]

Peripatellar soft tissue problems

Problems outside the patellofemoral joint itself can cause anterior knee pain and should be recognized and treated appropriately. These can include impingement of Hoffa's fat pad, saphenous neuroma, and patellar or quadriceps tendinosis. Additionally, significant frontal or axial plane malalignment, namely, genu valgum, excessive femoral anteversion, and tibial external torsion, act to increase the Q-angle and are increasingly recognized as a likely contributor to anterior knee pain, although evidence of their direct and independent role in anterior knee pain pathogenesis is lacking.[27] Recognition is key, and in the case of failed nonoperative care, surgical treatment for these problems should be targeted at the underlying pathology.

REFERENCES

1. Baquie P, Brukner P. Injuries presenting to an Australian sports medicine centre: a 12-month study. *Clin J Sport Med*. 1997;7(1):28–31.
2. Taunton JE, Ryan MB, Clement DB, McKenzie DC, Lloyd-Smith DR, Zumbo BD. A retrospective case-control analysis of 2002 running injuries. *Br J Sports Med*. 2002;36(2):95–101.
3. Crossley KM, Stefanik JJ, Selfe J, et al. 2016 Patellofemoral pain consensus statement from the 4th International Patellofemoral Pain Research Retreat, Manchester. Part 1: terminology, definitions, clinical examination, natural history, patellofemoral osteoarthritis and patient-reported outcome measures. *Br J Sports Med*. 2016;50(14):839–843.
4. Hall R, Barber Foss K, Hewett TE, Myer GD. Sport specialization's association with an increased risk of developing anterior knee pain in adolescent female athletes. *J Sport Rehabil*. 2015;24(1):31–35.
5. Smith BE, Selfe J, Thacker D, et al. Incidence and prevalence of patellofemoral pain: a systematic review and meta-analysis. *PLoS One*. 2018;13(1):e0190892.

6. Boling M, Padua D, Marshall S, Guskiewicz K, Pyne S, Beutler A. Gender differences in the incidence and prevalence of patellofemoral pain syndrome. *Scand J Med Sci Sports.* 2010;20(5):725−730.

7. Collins NJ, Bierma-Zeinstra SM, Crossley KM, van Linschoten RL, Vicenzino B, van Middelkoop M. Prognostic factors for patellofemoral pain: a multicentre observational analysis. *Br J Sports Med.* 2013;47(4): 227−233.

8. Crossley KM, van Middelkoop M, Callaghan MJ, Collins NJ, Rathleff MS, Barton CJ. 2016 Patellofemoral pain consensus statement from the 4th International Patellofemoral Pain Research Retreat, Manchester. Part 2: recommended physical interventions (exercise, taping, bracing, foot orthoses and combined interventions). *Br J Sports Med.* 2016;50(14):844−852.

9. Lankhorst NE, van Middelkoop M, Crossley KM, et al. Factors that predict a poor outcome 5-8 years after the diagnosis of patellofemoral pain: a multicentre observational analysis. *Br J Sports Med.* 2016;50(14):881−886.

10. Rathleff MS, Rathleff CR, Olesen JL, Rasmussen S, Roos EM. Is knee pain during adolescence a self-limiting condition? Prognosis of patellofemoral pain and other types of knee pain. *Am J Sports Med.* 2016; 44(5):1165−1171.

11. Collins NJ, Oei EHG, de Kanter JL, Vicenzino B, Crossley KM. Prevalence of radiographic and magnetic resonance imaging features of patellofemoral osteoarthritis in young and middle-aged adults with persistent patellofemoral pain. *Arthritis Care Res.* 2019;71(8): 1068−1073.

12. Hinman RS, Lentzos J, Vicenzino B, Crossley KM. Is patellofemoral osteoarthritis common in middle-aged people with chronic patellofemoral pain? *Arthritis Care Res.* 2014;66(8):1252−1257.

13. Utting MR, Davies G, Newman JH. Is anterior knee pain a predisposing factor to patellofemoral osteoarthritis? *Knee.* 2005;12(5):362−365.

14. Myer GD, Ford KR, Di Stasi SL, Foss KD, Micheli LJ, Hewett TE. High knee abduction moments are common risk factors for patellofemoral pain (PFP) and anterior cruciate ligament (ACL) injury in girls: is PFP itself a predictor for subsequent ACL injury? *Br J Sports Med.* 2015; 49(2):118−122.

15. Tecklenburg K, Dejour D, Hoser C, Fink C. Bony and cartilaginous anatomy of the patellofemoral joint. *Knee Surg Sports Traumatol Arthrosc.* 2006;14(3):235−240.

16. Smith RM, Boden BP, Sheehan FT. Increased patellar volume/width and decreased femoral trochlear width are associated with adolescent patellofemoral pain. *Clin Orthop Relat Res.* 2018;476(12):2334−2343.

17. Dejour H, Walch G, Nove-Josserand L, Guier C. Factors of patellar instability: an anatomic radiographic study. *Knee Surg Sports Traumatol Arthrosc.* 1994;2(1):19−26.

18. Duran S, Cavusoglu M, Kocadal O, Sakman B. Association between trochlear morphology and chondromalacia patella: an MRI study. *Clin Imaging.* 2017;41:7−10.

19. Grelsamer RP, Dejour D, Gould J. The pathophysiology of patellofemoral arthritis. *Orthop Clin N Am.* 2008; 39(3):269−274. v.

20. Earl JE, Vetter CS. Patellofemoral pain. *Phys Med Rehabil Clin N Am.* 2007;18(3):439−458 (viii).

21. Aglietti P, Insall JN, Cerulli G. Patellar pain and incongruence. I: measurements of incongruence. *Clin Orthop Relat Res.* 1983;176:217−224.

22. Boling MC, Nguyen AD, Padua DA, Cameron KL, Beutler A, Marshall SW. Gender-specific risk factor profiles for patellofemoral pain. *Clin J Sport Med.* 2021;31(1): 49−56. https://doi.org/10.1097/JSM.0000000000000719.

23. Powers CM, Witvrouw E, Davis IS, Crossley KM. Evidence-based framework for a pathomechanical model of patellofemoral pain: 2017 patellofemoral pain consensus statement from the 4th International Patellofemoral Pain Research Retreat, Manchester, UK: part 3. *Br J Sports Med.* 2017;51(24):1713−1723.

24. Neal BS, Lack SD, Lankhorst NE, Raye A, Morrissey D, van Middelkoop M. Risk factors for patellofemoral pain: a systematic review and meta-analysis. *Br J Sports Med.* 2019;53(5):270−281.

25. Balcarek P, Jung K, Ammon J, et al. Anatomy of lateral patellar instability: trochlear dysplasia and tibial tubercle-trochlear groove distance is more pronounced in women who dislocate the patella. *Am J Sports Med.* 2010;38(11):2320−2327.

26. Carlson VR, Boden BP, Sheehan FT. Patellofemoral kinematics and tibial tuberosity-trochlear groove distances in female adolescents with patellofemoral pain. *Am J Sports Med.* 2017;45(5):1102−1109.

27. Erkocak OF, Altan E, Altintas M, Turkmen F, Aydin BK, Bayar A. Lower extremity rotational deformities and patellofemoral alignment parameters in patients with anterior knee pain. *Knee Surg Sports Traumatol Arthrosc.* 2016;24(9):3011−3020.

28. Meyer SA, Brown TD, Pedersen DR, Albright JP. Retropatellar contact stress in simulated patella infera. *Am J Knee Surg.* 1997;10(3):129−138.

29. Singerman R, Davy DT, Goldberg VM. Effects of patella alta and patella infera on patellofemoral contact forces. *J Biomech.* 1994;27(8):1059−1065.

30. Luyckx T, Didden K, Vandenneucker H, Labey L, Innocenti B, Bellemans J. Is there a biomechanical explanation for anterior knee pain in patients with patella alta?: influence of patellar height on patellofemoral contact force, contact area and contact pressure. *J Bone Joint Surg Br.* 2009;91(3):344−350.

31. Ward SR, Terk MR, Powers CM. Patella alta: association with patellofemoral alignment and changes in contact area during weight-bearing. *J Bone Jt Surg Am.* 2007; 89(8):1749−1755.

32. Neal BS, Griffiths IB, Dowling GJ, et al. Foot posture as a risk factor for lower limb overuse injury: a systematic review and meta-analysis. *J Foot Ankle Res.* 2014;7(1):55.

33. Boling MC, Padua DA, Marshall SW, Guskiewicz K, Pyne S, Beutler A. A prospective investigation of

biomechanical risk factors for patellofemoral pain syndrome: the Joint Undertaking to Monitor and Prevent ACL Injury (JUMP-ACL) cohort. *Am J Sports Med.* 2009; 37(11):2108−2116.

34. Dye SF. The pathophysiology of patellofemoral pain: a tissue homeostasis perspective. *Clin Orthop Relat Res.* 2005;(436):100−110.

35. Farrokhi S, Keyak JH, Powers CM. Individuals with patellofemoral pain exhibit greater patellofemoral joint stress: a finite element analysis study. *Osteoarthritis Cartilage.* 2011;19(3):287−294.

36. Powers CM, Bolgla LA, Callaghan MJ, Collins N, Sheehan FT. Patellofemoral pain: proximal, distal, and local factors, 2nd International Research Retreat. *J Orthop Sports Phys Ther.* 2012;42(6):A1−A54.

37. Rathleff MS, Vicenzino B, Middelkoop M, et al. Patellofemoral pain in adolescence and adulthood: same same, but different? *Sports Med.* 2015;45(11):1489−1495.

38. Post WR, Dye SF. Patellofemoral pain: an enigma explained by homeostasis and common sense. *Am J Orthoped.* 2017;46(2):92−100.

39. Lack S, Neal B, De Oliveira Silva D, Barton C. How to manage patellofemoral pain - understanding the multifactorial nature and treatment options. *Phys Ther Sport.* 2018;32:155−166.

40. van der Heijden RA, Rijndertse MM, Bierma-Zeinstra SMA, van Middelkoop M. Lower pressure pain thresholds in patellofemoral pain patients, especially in female patients: a cross-sectional case-control study. *Pain Med.* 2018;19(1):184−192.

41. Bartholomew C, Lack S, Neal B. Altered pain processing and sensitisation is evident in adults with patellofemoral pain: a systematic review including meta-analysis and meta-regression. *Scand J Pain.* 2019;20.

42. Willy RW, Hoglund LT, Barton CJ, et al. Patellofemoral pain. *J Orthop Sports Phys Ther.* 2019;49(9):Cpg1−cpg95.

43. Bolgla LA, Boling MC, Mace KL, DiStefano MJ, Fithian DC, Powers CM. National athletic trainers' association position statement: management of individuals with patellofemoral pain. *J Athl Train.* 2018;53(9):820−836.

44. Noehren B, Hamill J, Davis I. Prospective evidence for a hip etiology in patellofemoral pain. *Med Sci Sports Exerc.* 2013;45(6):1120−1124.

45. Myer GD, Ford KR, Barber Foss KD, et al. The incidence and potential pathomechanics of patellofemoral pain in female athletes. *Clin Biomech.* 2010;25(7):700−707.

46. Fredericson M, Powers CM. Practical management of patellofemoral pain. *Clin J Sport Med.* 2002;12(1):36−38.

47. Crossley KM, van Middelkoop M, Barton CJ, Culvenor AG. Rethinking patellofemoral pain: prevention, management and long-term consequences. *Best Pract Res Clin Rheumatol.* 2019;33(1):48−65.

48. Dutton RA, Khadavi MJ, Fredericson M. Patellofemoral pain. *Phys Med Rehabil Clin N Am.* 2016;27(1):31−52.

49. Souza RB, Draper CE, Fredericson M, Powers CM. Femur rotation and patellofemoral joint kinematics: a weight-bearing magnetic resonance imaging analysis. *J Orthop Sports Phys Ther.* 2010;40(5):277−285.

50. Liao TC, Yang N, Ho KY, Farrokhi S, Powers CM. Femur rotation increases patella cartilage stress in females with patellofemoral pain. *Med Sci Sports Exerc.* 2015;47(9): 1775−1780.

51. Neal BS, Barton CJ, Gallie R, O'Halloran P, Morrissey D. Runners with patellofemoral pain have altered biomechanics which targeted interventions can modify: a systematic review and meta-analysis. *Gait Posture.* 2016;45: 69−82.

52. Neal BS, Barton CJ, Birn-Jeffery A, Morrissey D. Increased hip adduction during running is associated with patellofemoral pain and differs between males and females: a case-control study. *J Biomech.* 2019;91:133−139.

53. Nakagawa TH, Moriya ET, Maciel CD, Serrao FV. Trunk, pelvis, hip, and knee kinematics, hip strength, and gluteal muscle activation during a single-leg squat in males and females with and without patellofemoral pain syndrome. *J Orthop Sports Phys Ther.* 2012;42(6):491−501.

54. Holden S, Boreham C, Doherty C, Delahunt E. Two-dimensional knee valgus displacement as a predictor of patellofemoral pain in adolescent females. *Scand J Med Sci Sports.* 2017;27(2):188−194.

55. Prins MR, van der Wurff P. Females with patellofemoral pain syndrome have weak hip muscles: a systematic review. *Aust J Physiother.* 2009;55(1):9−15.

56. Herbst KA, Barber Foss KD, Fader L, et al. Hip strength is greater in athletes who subsequently develop patellofemoral pain. *Am J Sports Med.* 2015;43(11):2747−2752.

57. Rathleff MS, Rathleff CR, Crossley KM, Barton CJ. Is hip strength a risk factor for patellofemoral pain? A systematic review and meta-analysis. *Br J Sports Med.* 2014; 48(14):1088.

58. Boling M, Padua D. Relationship between hip strength and trunk, hip, and knee kinematics during a jump-landing task in individuals with patellofemoral pain. *Int J Sports Phys Ther.* 2013;8(5):661−669.

59. Gallina A, Hunt MA, Hodges PW, Garland SJ. Vastus lateralis motor unit firing rate is higher in women with patellofemoral pain. *Arch Phys Med Rehabil.* 2018;99(5): 907−913.

60. Barton CJ, Lack S, Malliaras P, Morrissey D. Gluteal muscle activity and patellofemoral pain syndrome: a systematic review. *Br J Sports Med.* 2013;47(4):207−214.

61. Piva SR, Goodnite EA, Childs JD. Strength around the hip and flexibility of soft tissues in individuals with and without patellofemoral pain syndrome. *J Orthop Sports Phys Ther.* 2005;35(12):793−801.

62. Lankhorst NE, Bierma-Zeinstra SM, van Middelkoop M. Risk factors for patellofemoral pain syndrome: a systematic review. *J Orthop Sports Phys Ther.* 2012;42(2):81−94.

63. Pappas E, Wong-Tom WM. Prospective predictors of patellofemoral pain syndrome: a systematic review with meta-analysis. *Sports Health.* 2012;4(2):115−120.

64. Barton CJ, Lack S, Hemmings S, Tufail S, Morrissey D. The 'Best Practice Guide to Conservative Management of Patellofemoral Pain': incorporating level 1 evidence with expert clinical reasoning. *Br J Sports Med.* 2015; 49(14):923−934.

65. Blackburne JS, Peel TE. A new method of measuring patellar height. *J Bone Joint Surg Br.* 1977;59(2):241–242.

66. Caton J, Deschamps G, Chambat P, Lerat JL, Dejour H. Patella infera. Apropos of 128 cases. *Revue de chirurgie orthopedique et reparatrice de l'appareil moteur.* 1982; 68(5):317–325.

67. Insall J, Salvati E. Patella position in the normal knee joint. *Radiology.* 1971;101(1):101–104.

68. Sherman SL, Plackis AC, Nuelle CW. Patellofemoral anatomy and biomechanics. *Clin Sports Med.* 2014;33(3): 389–401.

69. Seil R, Muller B, Georg T, Kohn D, Rupp S. Reliability and interobserver variability in radiological patellar height ratios. *Knee Surg Sports Traumatol Arthrosc.* 2000;8(4): 231–236.

70. Merchant AC. Patellofemoral imaging. *Clin Orthop Relat Res.* 2001;389:15–21.

71. Gulati A, McElrath C, Wadhwa V, Shah JP, Chhabra A. Current clinical, radiological and treatment perspectives of patellofemoral pain syndrome. *Br J Radiol.* 2018; 91(1086):20170456.

72. Beaconsfield T, Pintore E, Maffulli N, Petri GJ. Radiological measurements in patellofemoral disorders. A review. *Clin Orthop Relat Res.* 1994;(308):18–28.

73. Widuchowski W, Lukasik P, Kwiatkowski G, et al. Isolated full thickness chondral injuries. Prevalance and outcome of treatment. A retrospective study of 5233 knee arthroscopies. *Acta Chir Orthop Traumatol Cech.* 2008;75(5):382–386.

74. Harris JD, Brophy RH, Jia G, et al. Sensitivity of magnetic resonance imaging for detection of patellofemoral articular cartilage defects. *Arthroscopy.* 2012;28(11): 1728–1737.

75. van der Heijden RA, de Kanter JL, Bierma-Zeinstra SM, et al. Structural abnormalities on magnetic resonance imaging in patients with patellofemoral pain: a cross-sectional case-control study. *Am J Sports Med.* 2016; 44(9):2339–2346.

76. Stefanik JJ, Gross KD, Guermazi A, et al. The relation of MRI-detected structural damage in the medial and lateral patellofemoral joint to knee pain: the Multicenter and Framingham Osteoarthritis Studies. *Osteoarthritis Cartilage.* 2015;23(4):565–570.

77. Macri EM, Felson DT, Zhang Y, et al. Patellofemoral morphology and alignment: reference values and dose-response patterns for the relation to MRI features of patellofemoral osteoarthritis. *Osteoarthritis Cartilage.* 2017; 25(10):1690–1697.

78. Thakkar RS, Del Grande F, Wadhwa V, et al. Patellar instability: CT and MRI measurements and their correlation with internal derangement findings. *Knee Surg Sports Traumatol Arthrosc.* 2016;24(9):3021–3028.

79. Graf KH, Tompkins MA, Agel J, Arendt EA. Q-vector measurements: physical examination versus magnetic resonance imaging measurements and their relationship with tibial tubercle-trochlear groove distance. *Knee Surg Sports Traumatol Arthrosc.* 2018;26(3):697–704.

80. Munch JL, Sullivan JP, Nguyen JT, et al. Patellar articular overlap on MRI is a simple alternative to conventional measurements of patellar height. *Orthop J Sports Med.* 2016;4(7), 2325967116656328.

81. Gorman McNerney ML, Arendt EA. Anterior knee pain in the active and athletic adolescent. *Curr Sports Med Rep.* 2013;12(6):404–410.

82. Kolowich PA, Paulos LE, Rosenberg TD, Farnsworth S. Lateral release of the patella: indications and contraindications. *Am J Sports Med.* 1990;18(4):359–365.

83. Collins NJ, Barton CJ, van Middelkoop M, et al. 2018 Consensus statement on exercise therapy and physical interventions (orthoses, taping and manual therapy) to treat patellofemoral pain: recommendations from the 5th International Patellofemoral Pain Research Retreat, Gold Coast, Australia, 2017. *Br J Sports Med.* 2018; 52(18):1170–1178.

84. Dolak KL, Silkman C, Medina McKeon J, Hosey RG, Lattermann C, Uhl TL. Hip strengthening prior to functional exercises reduces pain sooner than quadriceps strengthening in females with patellofemoral pain syndrome: a randomized clinical trial. *J Orthop Sports Phys Ther.* 2011;41(8):560–570.

85. Lack S, Barton C, Sohan O, Crossley K, Morrissey D. Proximal muscle rehabilitation is effective for patellofemoral pain: a systematic review with meta-analysis. *Br J Sports Med.* 2015;49(21):1365–1376.

86. Nascimento LR, Teixeira-Salmela LF, Souza RB, Resende RA. Hip and knee strengthening is more effective than knee strengthening alone for reducing pain and improving activity in individuals with patellofemoral pain: a systematic review with meta-analysis. *J Orthop Sports Phys Ther.* 2018;48(1):19–31.

87. Nunes GS, Barton CJ, Serrao FV. Hip rate of force development and strength are impaired in females with patellofemoral pain without signs of altered gluteus medius and maximus morphology. *J Sci Med Sport.* 2018;21(2): 123–128.

88. American College of Sports Medicine position stand. Progression models in resistance training for healthy adults. *Med Sci Sports Exerc.* 2009;41(3):687–708.

89. Barton C, Balachandar V, Lack S, Morrissey D. Patellar taping for patellofemoral pain: a systematic review and meta-analysis to evaluate clinical outcomes and biomechanical mechanisms. *Br J Sports Med.* 2014;48(6): 417–424.

90. Derasari A, Brindle TJ, Alter KE, Sheehan FT. McConnell taping shifts the patella inferiorly in patients with patellofemoral pain: a dynamic magnetic resonance imaging study. *Phys Ther.* 2010;90(3):411–419.

91. Powers CM, Ward SR, Chan LD, Chen YJ, Terk MR. The effect of bracing on patella alignment and patellofemoral joint contact area. *Med Sci Sports Exerc.* 2004;36(7): 1226–1232.

92. Logan CA, Bhashyam AR, Tisosky AJ, et al. Systematic review of the effect of taping techniques on patellofemoral pain syndrome. *Sports Health.* 2017;9(5):456–461.

93. Warden SJ, Hinman RS, Watson Jr MA, Avin KG, Bialocerkowski AE, Crossley KM. Patellar taping and bracing for the treatment of chronic knee pain: a systematic review and meta-analysis. *Arthritis Rheum.* 2008; 59(1):73−83.

94. Smith TO, Drew BT, Meek TH, Clark AB. Knee orthoses for treating patellofemoral pain syndrome. *Cochrane Database Syst Rev.* 2015;(12):Cd010513.

95. Lake DA, Wofford NH. Effect of therapeutic modalities on patients with patellofemoral pain syndrome: a systematic review. *Sports Health.* 2011;3(2):182−189.

96. Giles L, Webster KE, McClelland J, Cook JL. Quadriceps strengthening with and without blood flow restriction in the treatment of patellofemoral pain: a double-blind randomised trial. *Br J Sports Med.* 2017;51(23): 1688−1694.

97. Willy RW, Davis IS. The effect of a hip-strengthening program on mechanics during running and during a single-leg squat. *J Orthop Sports Phys Ther.* 2011;41(9):625−632.

98. Barton CJ, Bonanno DR, Carr J, et al. Running retraining to treat lower limb injuries: a mixed-methods study of current evidence synthesised with expert opinion. *Br J Sports Med.* 2016;50(9):513−526.

99. Bramah C, Preece SJ, Gill N, Herrington L. A 10% increase in step rate improves running kinematics and clinical outcomes in runners with patellofemoral pain at 4 weeks and 3 months. *Am J Sports Med.* 2019;47(14):3406−3413.

100. Neal BS, Barton CJ, Birn-Jeffrey A, Daley M, Morrissey D. The effects & mechanisms of increasing running step rate: a feasibility study in a mixed-sex group of runners with patellofemoral pain. *Phys Ther Sport.* 2018;32:244−251.

101. Emamvirdi M, Letafatkar A, Khaleghi Tazji M. The effect of valgus control instruction exercises on pain, strength, and functionality in active females with patellofemoral pain syndrome. *Sports Health.* 2019;11(3):223−237.

102. Esculier JF, Bouyer LJ, Dubois B, et al. Is combining gait retraining or an exercise programme with education better than education alone in treating runners with patellofemoral pain? A randomised clinical trial. *Br J Sports Med.* 2018;52(10):659−666.

103. Rathleff MS, Graven-Nielsen T, Holmich P, et al. Activity modification and load management of adolescents with patellofemoral pain: a prospective intervention study including 151 adolescents. *Am J Sports Med.* 2019; 47(7):1629−1637.

104. Hart HF, Barton CJ, Khan KM, Riel H, Crossley KM. Is body mass index associated with patellofemoral pain and patellofemoral osteoarthritis? A systematic review and meta-regression and analysis. *Br J Sports Med.* 2017; 51(10):781−790.

105. Maclachlan LR, Collins NJ, Matthews MLG, Hodges PW, Vicenzino B. The psychological features of patellofemoral pain: a systematic review. *Br J Sports Med.* 2017;51(9): 732−742.

106. Fithian DC, Paxton EW, Post WR, Panni AS. Lateral retinacular release: a survey of the International Patellofemoral Study Group. *Arthroscopy.* 2004;20(5):463−468.

107. Fulkerson JP. Diagnosis and treatment of patients with patellofemoral pain. *Am J Sports Med.* 2002;30(3): 447−456.

108. Unal B, Hinckel BB, Sherman SL, Lattermann C. Comparison of lateral retinaculum release and lengthening in the treatment of patellofemoral disorders. *Am J Orthoped.* 2017;46(5):224−228.

109. Hinckel BB, Arendt EA. Lateral retinaculum lengthening/release. *Operat Tech Orthop.* 2015;23:100−106.

110. Pagenstert G, Wolf N, Bachmann M, et al. Open lateral patellar retinacular lengthening versus open retinacular release in lateral patellar hypercompression syndrome: a prospective double-blinded comparative study on complications and outcome. *Arthroscopy.* 2012;28(6): 788−797.

111. O'Neill DB. Open lateral retinacular lengthening compared with arthroscopic release. A prospective, randomized outcome study. *J Bone Jt Surg Am.* 1997; 79(12):1759−1769.

112. Russek LN, Errico DM. Prevalence, injury rate and, symptom frequency in generalized joint laxity and joint hypermobility syndrome in a "healthy" college population. *Clin Rheumatol.* 2016;35(4):1029−1039.

113. Iwano T, Kurosawa H, Tokuyama H, Hoshikawa Y. Roentgenographic and clinical findings of patellofemoral osteoarthrosis. With special reference to its relationship to femorotibial osteoarthrosis and etiologic factors. *Clin Orthop Relat Res.* 1990;(252):190−197.

114. Paulos LE, O'Connor DL, Karistinos A. Partial lateral patellar facetectomy for treatment of arthritis due to lateral patellar compression syndrome. *Arthroscopy.* 2008;24(5):547−553.

115. Brophy RH, Wojahn RD, Lamplot JD. Cartilage restoration techniques for the patellofemoral joint. *J Am Acad Orthop Surg.* 2017;25(5):321−329.

116. Mestriner AB, Ackermann J, Gomoll AH. Patellofemoral cartilage repair. *Curr Rev Musculoskelet Med.* 2018;11(2): 188−200.

117. Mosier BA, Arendt EA, Dahm DL, Dejour D, Gomoll AH. Management of patellofemoral arthritis: from cartilage restoration to arthroplasty. *J Am Acad Orthop Surg.* 2016;24(11):e163−e173.

118. Galloway MT, Noyes FR. Cystic degeneration of the patella after arthroscopic chondroplasty and subchondral bone perforation. *Arthroscopy.* 1992;8(3):366−369.

119. Mithoefer K, McAdams T, Williams RJ, Kreuz PC, Mandelbaum BR. Clinical efficacy of the microfracture technique for articular cartilage repair in the knee: an evidence-based systematic analysis. *Am J Sports Med.* 2009;37(10):2053−2063.

120. Pestka JM, Bode G, Salzmann G, Sudkamp NP, Niemeyer P. Clinical outcome of autologous chondrocyte implantation for failed microfracture treatment of full-thickness cartilage defects of the knee joint. *Am J Sports Med.* 2012;40(2):325−331.

121. Meyerkort D, Ebert JR, Ackland TR, et al. Matrix-induced autologous chondrocyte implantation (MACI) for

chondral defects in the patellofemoral joint. *Knee Surg Sports Traumatol Arthrosc.* 2014;22(10):2522–2530.

122. Brittberg M, Recker D, Ilgenfritz J, Saris DBF. Matrix-applied characterized autologous cultured chondrocytes versus microfracture: five-year follow-up of a prospective randomized trial. *Am J Sports Med.* 2018;46(6): 1343–1351.

123. Ebert JR, Schneider A, Fallon M, Wood DJ, Janes GC. A comparison of 2-year outcomes in patients undergoing tibiofemoral or patellofemoral matrix-induced autologous chondrocyte implantation. *Am J Sports Med.* 2017; 45(14):3243–3253.

124. Gomoll AH, Gillogly SD, Cole BJ, et al. Autologous chondrocyte implantation in the patella: a multicenter experience. *Am J Sports Med.* 2014;42(5):1074–1081.

125. Albright JC, Daoud AK. Microfracture and microfracture plus. *Clin Sports Med.* 2017;36(3):501–507.

126. Hangody L, Fules P. Autologous osteochondral mosaicplasty for the treatment of full-thickness defects of weight-bearing joints: ten years of experimental and clinical experience. *J Bone Jt Surg Am.* 2003;85-A(Suppl 2): 25–32.

127. Gallo RA, Feeley BT. Cartilage defects of the femoral trochlea. *Knee Surg Sports Traumatol Arthrosc.* 2009; 17(11):1316–1325.

128. Assenmacher AT, Pareek A, Reardon PJ, Macalena JA, Stuart MJ, Krych AJ. Long-term outcomes after osteochondral allograft: a systematic review at long-term follow-up of 12.3 years. *Arthroscopy.* 2016;32(10): 2160–2168.

129. Lewallen DG, Riegger CL, Myers ER, Hayes WC. Effects of retinacular release and tibial tubercle elevation in patellofemoral degenerative joint disease. *J Orthop Res.* 1990;8(6):856–862.

130. Maquet P. Advancement of the tibial tuberosity. *Clin Orthop Relat Res.* 1976;115:225–230.

131. Sherman SL, Erickson BJ, Cvetanovich GL, et al. Tibial tuberosity osteotomy: indications, techniques, and outcomes. *Am J Sports Med.* 2014;42(8):2006–2017.

132. Fulkerson JP. Anteromedialization of the tibial tuberosity for patellofemoral malalignment. *Clin Orthop Relat Res.* 1983;177:176–181.

133. Pidoriano AJ, Weinstein RN, Buuck DA, Fulkerson JP. Correlation of patellar articular lesions with results from anteromedial tibial tubercle transfer. *Am J Sports Med.* 1997;25(4):533–537.

134. Farr J. Autologous chondrocyte implantation improves patellofemoral cartilage treatment outcomes. *Clin Orthop Relat Res.* 2007;463:187–194.

135. Walker T, Perkinson B, Mihalko WM. Patellofemoral arthroplasty: the other unicompartmental knee replacement. *J Bone Jt Surg Am.* 2012;94(18):1712–1720.

136. Dy CJ, Franco N, Ma Y, Mazumdar M, McCarthy MM, Gonzalez Della Valle A. Complications after patellofemoral versus total knee replacement in the treatment of isolated patello-femoral osteoarthritis. A meta-analysis. *Knee Surg Sports Traumatol Arthrosc.* 2012; 20(11):2174–2190.

137. Kazarian GS, Tarity TD, Hansen EN, Cai J, Lonner JH. Significant functional improvement at 2 years after isolated patellofemoral arthroplasty with an onlay trochlear implant, but low mental health scores predispose to dissatisfaction. *J Arthroplasty.* 2016;31(2):389–394.

CHAPTER 8

Patellar Instability

JACQUELINE M. BRADY, MD • WARREN NIELSEN, MD • BETH E. SHUBIN STEIN, MD

INTRODUCTION

Patellar instability remains a problematic entity in the athletic patient population. Most studies agree that adolescent females represent the highest risk group of patients for first-time patellofemoral dislocation. Treatment of patellar instability must be individualized, with care taken to identify both historical and anatomic risk factors. First-time instability that results in a loose chondral or osteochondral body should be addressed with both attention to the loose piece and the stabilization of the joint, most commonly in the form of medial patellofemoral ligament (MPFL) reconstruction. Treatment of recurrent instability begins with MPFL reconstruction and involves the addition of realignment procedures and/or reshaping of the dysplastic trochlea, according to the limited available literature and surgeon judgment. This chapter will focus on the recognition and treatment of patellar instability in the female athlete.

PATIENT POPULATION AND PREDICTORS OF RECURRENCE

Most studies agree that adolescent females are the highest risk group of patients for first-time patellofemoral dislocation. Other risk factors include family history, history of contralateral instability, and a number of anatomic factors.

The most predictive anatomic risk factor for patellar instability is trochlear dysplasia. Several different classification systems and strategies have been employed to describe an abnormally shaped trochlea, including the Dejour classification, sulcus angle, trochlear depth, and trochlear facet ratio. Others focus simply on the anterior height of any supratrochlear "spur," or "boss" as predictive of recurrence. A complete understanding of the three-dimensional nature of a dysplastic trochlea can prove elusive, but many studies have concluded

that trochlear dysplasia, no matter its definition, emerges as the most predictive of the risk factors for recurrence following a first-time patellofemoral dislocation.[1] Thus many surgeons discard the precise quantification of dysplasia and classify it on a lateral X-ray or cross-sectional imaging simply as mild, moderate, or severe (Fig. 8.1).

Patella alta has also been described as a risk factor for recurrent instability. This risk factor has also been measured in several ways, some of which reference either the joint line (Blackburne-Peel) or the tibia (Insall-Salvati, modified Insall-Salvati, and Caton-Deschamps). Others have focused on the relationship of the patella to the femur and/or femoral trochlea, including simple articular overlap, Biedert's patellotrochlear index, and/or Dejour's sagittal patellofemoral index. The latter strategy is attractive because the relationship of the patella to the trochlea seems most relevant in the measurement of patellar height. However, these measurements require magnetic resonance imaging (MRI) and can be confounded by a laterally tracking patella and difficulty identifying the precise distal location of the transition from trochlear groove to femoral condyle. In principle, patella alta indicates that a higher riding patella requires more knee flexion to engage and stabilize the patella in its trochlear groove. This places more stress on the soft tissue restraints of the knee during early flexion until bony congruity and its inherent stability take over. An axial MRI can provide clues that patella alta is present, when the patellar chondral surface is visualized without the corresponding trochlear cartilage in view (Fig. 8.2).

Coronal alignment also plays a role in patellar stability. Significant genu valgum is useful to recognize during skeletal immaturity, as guided growth or hemiepiphysiodesis can be a simple intervention to resolve this problem, rather than a more invasive distal femoral osteotomy if correction is required in a

The Female Athlete. https://doi.org/10.1016/B978-0-323-75985-4.00007-6
Copyright © 2022 Elsevier Inc. All rights reserved.

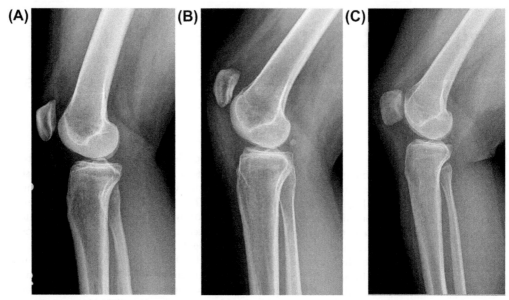

FIG. 8.1 Trochlear dysplasia. **(A)** Mild dysplasia: the trochlear groove line reaches the anterior femur before the anterior femoral cortical line intersects with it ("crossing sign"). **(B)** Moderate dysplasia: crossing sign plus small prominence of the supratrochlear bone. **(C)** Severe dysplasia: crossing, large supratrochlear prominence and evidence of a hypoplastic medial trochlear facet ("double contour").

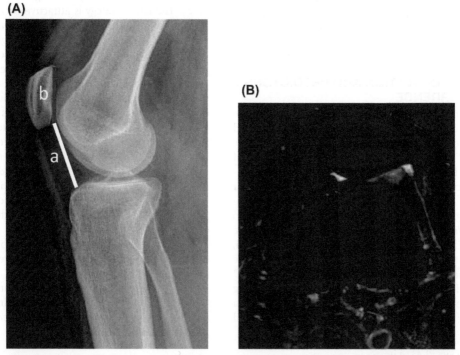

FIG. 8.2 Patella alta. **(A)** Patella altaon X-ray as demonstrated by the Caton-Deschamps measurement technique (alta = a/b > 1.2). **(B)** Patella altaas viewed on an axial magnetic resonance imaging. The majority of the patellar chondral surface is demonstrated with no corresponding trochlear cartilage in view.

(A)   (B)

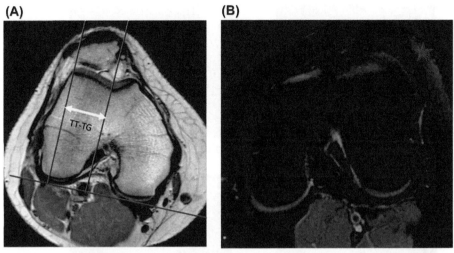

FIG. 8.3 Extensor mechanism malalignment. **(A)** The distance between the tibial tubercle (TT) and the deepest portion of the trochlear groove (TG) as measured on magnetic resonance imaging. **(B)** The patellar tendon (star) overlaps the lateral femoral condyle of the left knee, indicating a pathologic trajectory toward its attachment on the tibial tubercle.

skeletally mature patient. More complicated is the understanding of the path taken by the extensor mechanism as it crosses the knee. Arthroplasty surgeons often use the tibial tubercle-to-posterior cruciate ligament (PCL) distance (TT-PCL), a measure of the lateralization of the tibial tubercle relative to the PCL origin on the tibia. For patellar stability, this has not been shown to be as predictive as the tibial tubercle-to-trochlear groove (TT-TG, Fig. 8.3A) distance, a measure of the distance from the trochlear groove nadir to the midpoint of the tibial tubercle. The difference indicates that something about the dynamic rotation of the tibia with knee flexion and extension contributes to patellar stability. More recently, attention has been paid to the location of the patellar tendon relative to the lateral trochlea (Fig. 8.3B). One group even found this factor to be more predictive of patellar instability than the TT-TG.[2]

Perhaps the most poorly understood risk factor of all is femoral anteversion, in part because it is not always routinely measured in the process of evaluating an unstable patellofemoral joint. Average femoral anteversion is 15 degree, and some authors have demonstrated that even at 20 degrees, the patellofemoral joint exhibits abnormal lateral forces.[3] Many different methods of measuring femoral anteversion have been suggested, rendering comparison of studies difficult (Fig. 8.4). Literature guidance for correction of femoral anteversion in patellofemoral instability is limited, but surgeons who commonly perform

derotational femoral osteotomy procedures cite a margin of error of 10–15 degrees during the procedure and therefore do not intervene unless the femoral neck is 30–35 degrees or more anteverted relative to the shaft.

Other factors such as ligamentous laxity and lower extremity motion patterns with jumping and landing have been implicated in patellar instability, but little is known precisely about how they should affect surgical management or factor into rehabilitation protocols.

APPROACH TO THE FIRST-TIME DISLOCATION

After a first-time patellar dislocation, the patella should be relocated as expeditiously as possible. Gentle extension of the knee, sometimes combined with pressure on the lateral patella, generally allows the patellofemoral joint to reduce. Some patients require sedation to permit relief of muscle spasm that is preventing relocation, but more commonly, the patella relocates on its own. The knee often develops a rapid hemarthrosis, resulting in quadriceps inhibition in the early postinjury period. For this reason, a brief period of immobilization is useful to prevent buckling of the knee with ambulation, and some physicians aspirate the hemarthrosis in the hopes of a faster quadriceps recovery. Prolonged immobilization should be avoided, however, as the resultant quadriceps atrophy affects the vastus medialis most quickly (due to a higher proportion of

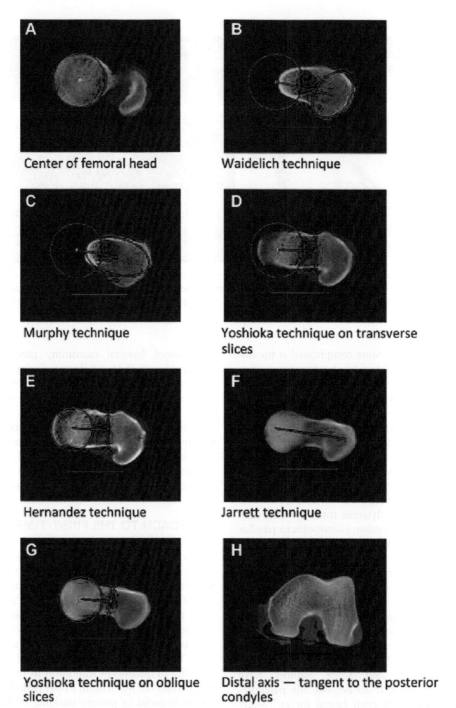

FIG. 8.4 Femoral anteversion. The various methods of measurement of the femoral neck for use in quantification of femoral anteversion. (Kaiser et al. Arch Orthop Trauma Surg. 2016.)

Type 1 muscle fibers), potentially worsening patellar tracking and therefore predisposing the patient to future injury. Physical therapy should focus on normalizing gait, restoring motion, and engaging the extensor mechanism without aggravating the knee pain.

Bracing an unstable patellofemoral joint can provide symptomatic relief and help control swelling by way of compression. Many different types of braces have been developed, but no studies have supported the ability of a patellofemoral brace to effectively prevent recurrent instability. This is unsurprising, given the amount of shear force experienced by the patellofemoral joint with daily activities (up to nine times body weight, depending on the activity). Likewise, a specific method of applying therapeutic tape has been developed by Jenny McConnell, a physical therapist in Australia, to help reduce symptoms of patellofemoral pain in the setting of patellar instability.[4] When patients have a mixed picture of instability and anterior knee pain, some surgeons look to the symptomatic response to McConnell taping as predictive of any pain relief that might result from surgical stabilization of the joint.

Physical Examination

Physical examination of an unstable patellofemoral joint begins with direct inspection. The quadriceps muscles are visually examined in standing, seated, and supine positions. Subtle atrophy can be revealed with straight leg raises or active knee extension in the sitting position. Occasionally, patients cannot actively extend due to severe maltracking or apprehension (see later discussion) but can complete a straight leg raise in a supine position. Quadriceps atrophy is important to recognize because it can be a driver of persistent symptoms, due to either buckling from muscular weakness or true recurrent subluxations of the patellofemoral joint.

Effusion is often present in the immediate aftermath of a patellar dislocation. Pathoanatomic findings such as patella alta can occasionally be identified upon inspection and palpation of the joint lines relative to the poles of the patella but are more often subtle and identified on imaging. Palpation can reveal tenderness over the medial facet of the patella and lateral aspect of the trochlea (sites of typical bony contusion) and/or at the femoral original of the MPFL between the medial epicondyle and the adductor tubercle. Crepitus can be palpated or reported subjectively and is often an indicator of chondral injury. Crepitus may be elicited during active knee range of motion during seated knee extension and/or standing squat. The compression test, during which the examiner places pressure on the patella during active knee range of motion, has been described to give some clue as to the location of a chondral injury.

Maltracking indicative of instability can be seen on physical examination by the J-sign, which is a pathologic lateral shift of the patella as the knee moves from flexion into full extension. Palpation during range of motion can also reveal deviation of the patella from the trochlear groove with more subtle instability. The pathoanatomic implications of J-sign are still under investigation but suspected contributors include high-grade trochlear dysplasia, an increased TT-TG, and patella alta. Patella alta in particular may play a role in the J-sign, as dynamic studies of patella alta have shown greater lateral displacement of the patella with the knee in increased extension.[5]

The apprehension sign is a valuable physical examination tool in assessing the patient with patellar instability. With the knees in full extension the 'normal' or contralateral knee is examined first and then the 'affected knee.' The patella is translated medially and laterally, and the test result is considered positive if the patient develops an impending sense of instability or fear that the patella may dislocate. The test is often more sensitive for apprehension if the knee is moved from full extension through 60 degrees of flexion while placing the lateral force on the patella: the so-called 'moving patella apprehension test.'

Patellar glide can assess for degree of instability by utilizing quadrants of lateral and medial patellar translation in a fully extended position. During tibiofemoral extension to flexion, the medial and lateral displacement is about 3 mm in each direction in a normal setting. Both sides should be examined whenever possible, as hypermobility can be detected with symmetric translation of three or more quadrants. When one knee is unaffected, lateral translation is generally found to be asymmetrically high on the injured side. In patients with a history of lateral retinacular release (LRR), medial translation can be increased and sometimes can even correlate with iatrogenic medial instability. If the patient is able to tolerate it, a dynamic examination of patellar glide can also be informative, to determine how much knee flexion is required to minimize the translation of the patella as it is stabilized within the bony confines of the trochlear groove. The dynamic patellar glide test can aid in understanding the contribution of patella alta to overall patellar instability: if the patella is still able to be subluxated laterally when the knee is flexed to 45 degrees, for instance, distalization of the tibial tubercle will likely aid in earlier patellofemoral engagement (see later discussion).

During examination of apprehension and patellar glide, the medial and lateral poles of the patella can be assessed to determine the resting or passive patellar tilt. In patients with lateral patellar tilt, the patella is gently manually everted to assess tightness of the lateral retinaculum. If the patella is fixed in a laterally tilted position, and/or excessive correction is required to reduce it to a normal position relative to the trochlea, a tight lateral retinaculum may be addressed at the time of any planned stabilization surgery (see later discussion). If the patella is easily everted to neutral on physical examination, especially in the setting of a ligamentously lax patient, the lateral retinaculum is not considered tight and should not be released or lengthened at the time of surgery.

Historically, coronal plane alignment was assessed on physical examination using the quadriceps angle (Q-angle). However, the Q-angle varies based on patient positioning, quadriceps contraction, etc. Thus cross-sectional MRI or computed tomography has become the gold standard in assessing extensor mechanism alignment using measurements such as the TT-TG distance or the TT-PCL distance, and more recently the position of the patellar tendon relative to the lateral trochlea (see later discussion).

Clinical identification of genu valgum can also be accomplished on physical examination. Supine and/or prone rotation of the hips can reveal pathologic internal rotation indicative of femoral anteversion. Observation of gait can lend clues to rotational and coronal plane alignment due to in-toeing or out-toeing, and examination of the prone thigh-foot angle can give the examiner an idea of tibial torsion, in addition to the femoral rotation maneuvers.

Imaging Studies

Imaging after an acute patellar dislocation should include radiographic evaluation to determine whether the patient has an osteochondral injury. If at all possible, standing anteroposterior and lateral views should be obtained, along with an axial view or Merchant view X-ray in early flexion. A true lateral X-ray can be difficult to obtain in patients with anatomic variabilities such as femoral anteversion or genu valgum, and radiographic technicians should be counseled to repeat an attempt if needed as the lateral X-ray is critical for assessing trochlear dysplasia and patellar height. A standing tunnel or "Salt Lake" view can help identify additional injuries in the posterior aspect of the tibiofemoral compartment. Standing bilateral hip-to-ankle radiographs can quantify coronal plane deformity, and in skeletally immature patients, they can give an idea of a leg length discrepancy at baseline, which can be useful for later comparison if surgery is undertaken around open physes. Skeletal maturity can be quantified using the traditional left-hand "bone age" X-ray and/or the recently produced atlas of physeal growth about the knee as viewed on MRI.[6]

Most osseous abnormalities following patellar dislocation are in the form of avulsion fractures of the medial patella. Less commonly, radiography and/or MRI demonstrate an osteochondral fracture. The rate of chondral and osteochondral injury has been shown to be 70% in first-time dislocations, so routine MRI evaluation is recommended following an instability event.

SURGICAL MANAGEMENT OF PATELLOFEMORAL INSTABILITY

If a loose body or osteochondral fracture is discovered in the workup of patellofemoral instability, surgical intervention is indicated to either remove a small fragment or repair a larger one. A consensus statement from the International Patellofemoral Study Group indicates that concomitant stabilization of the patellofemoral joint should be undertaken with any surgery to address a loose chondral or osteochondral fragment in the high-risk, young patients with first-time patellar dislocation (Liu et al. AJSM 2018). This is supported by a clinical study of patients treated for osteochondral injury, who showed a recurrence rate of 60% when the fragment was addressed without stabilization of the joint.[7] Fig. 8.5 shows MRI images of a 15-year-old patient who dislocated and injured LFC, which was fixed without stabilization of the joint. After 8 months, the dislocation recurred and injured the osteochondral surface of the patella.

Other than the patient with a loose fragment, controversy persists regarding which first-time dislocations are suitable for surgical stabilization. Historical and current standard-of-care treatment for first-time dislocation is still nonoperative treatment, but several studies have defined a high-risk population for recurrence. Thus many authors have begun to more precisely risk-stratify patients and offer surgical intervention to those who are at high risk—most notably young patients with trochlear dysplasia. In cases of recurrent instability (subluxation or dislocation), surgical intervention is indicated without significant controversy.

Although surgery is clearly indicated in the recurrent dislocation, the decision regarding the appropriate specific surgical intervention(s) remains elusive. The MPFL is the primary restraint to lateral translation of the patella. It is injured in nearly all cases of patellar

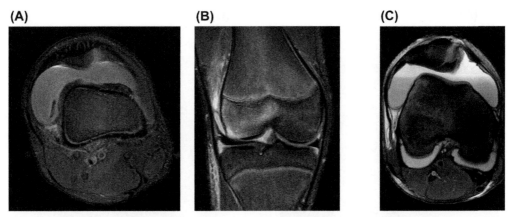

FIG. 8.5 Osteochondral injury in patellofemoral instability. **(A,B)** A 15-year-old patient has dislocation for the first time and sustained an osteochondral injury to the lateral femoral condyle. The lesion was repaired, but the joint was not stabilized in any way. **(C)** After 8 months, the patient sustained a recurrent dislocation and an associated osteochondral injury to the patella.

instability, and most surgeons therefore agree that it is necessary to address the MPFL with any stabilizing procedure. Primary repair of the MPFL has been shown to have a high rate of failure and is not indicated in recurrent or chronic instability. There may be a role for repair in first-time dislocation, but the rate of recurrence is higher after MPFL repair than MPFL reconstruction. There are many techniques described for MPFL reconstruction, and each has specific risks and potential complications, including patellar fracture, femoral tunnel malposition, graft overtensioning, loss of range of motion, and pain.

A common approach for reconstructing the MPFL is to use a free hamstring tendon. Studies regarding graft choice (autograft vs. allograft) are few, but they indicate that graft choice does not drive outcomes for MPFL reconstruction in the same way as it does for ACL reconstruction. Thus either autograft or allograft is considered to be an acceptable choice. The graft is typically anchored to the femur and to the patella by bony sockets/tunnels or anchors. The selection of the femoral attachment is the most subject to error, with points that are too superior or too anterior both carrying risk for anisometry of the graft and/or capture of the knee in flexion. Some surgeons prefer to anchor the graft to the distal aspect of the quadriceps tendon (as opposed to the patella), as the medial patellofemoral complex of ligamentous/retinacular structures in most cases does exhibit a reflection onto the quadriceps tendon in anatomic dissection. Other surgeons anchor one limb of a graft to the patella and the other to the quad tendon. When concerns arise regarding skeletal maturity, the technique can be modified to spare the growing

distal femoral physis: a standard bony socket can be directed just distal to the physis (Fig. 8.6), the graft can be secured by soft tissue alone to the adductor tendon and/or MCL, or the adductor tendon itself can be harvested as a graft and reflected up to the patella/quad tendon in order to avoid bony femoral injury altogether. In the latter two cases, the isometry of the graft must be carefully scrutinized before it is secured because anchoring the graft to the adductor tendon/tubercle is more proximal than the anatomic origin. If placed too proximally on the femur, the reconstructed ligament will tighten in knee flexion, resulting in pain, loss of flexion, and eventual graft stretching and failure leading to recurrent instability. A final graft option for MPFL reconstruction is either the central portion or the medial portion of the quadriceps tendon itself. No matter the technique used, setting the correct tension on the graft is of paramount importance. As mentioned earlier, the MPFL serves as a checkrein and should not be under resting tension. Several techniques can and should be used during surgery to determine the appropriate graft length before final fixation. Important principles include allowing the knee full range of motion and ensuring good patellar translation in full extension and early flexion prior to fixation without overconstraint.

Other surgical strategies for addressing instability focus on realignment of a malaligned joint. Tibial tubercle osteotomy is a mainstay for realigning the extensor mechanism. Currently, it remains unclear as to which patients will be successfully treated with an isolated soft tissue reconstruction (MPFL) and which patients will need a bony realignment, in addition to

(A)   **(B)**

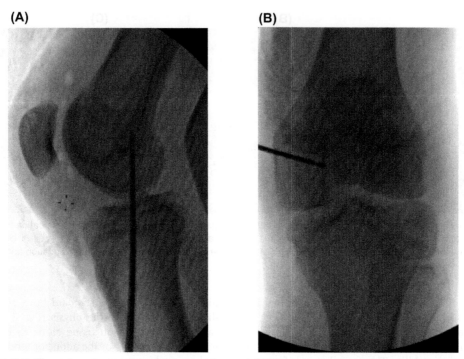

FIG. 8.6 Physeal sparing medial patellofemoral ligament (MPFL) reconstruction. **(A)** A guidepinis started in the anatomic origin of the MPFL on the lateral fluoroscopic view. **(B)** An anteroposterior view is utilized to direct the guidepindistal to the physis.

the MPFL. Studies are underway to help create a patellar instability severity index score (much like the Instability Severity Index Score, or the ISIS score, in the shoulder literature) that will help guide us in terms of which patients have a high risk of failure with an isolated soft tissue ligament reconstruction. Such a score will likely not be based on any single factor but a combination of many variables that, when present together in the same patient, indicate a high likelihood of failure and thus indicate which patients will be more successfully treated by adding a bony realignment (tibial tubercle osteotomy, varus-producing or derotational femoral osteotomy, and/or trochleoplasty). Currently, many surgeons use the TT-TG distance measurement as a guide, and a cutoff of 20 mm has been recommended but not robustly proven as an indication. Other surgeons simply use the presence of a J-sign on physical examination. Biomechanical literature indicates that the various anatomic factors act synergistically to affect the isometry of any MPFL reconstruction, so a lower TT-TG distance may affect tracking in the setting of patella alta, for instance. In a typical tibial tubercle osteotomy, the tubercle is left attached by a distal periosteal hinge and rotated medially (Fig. 8.7). A component of

anteriorization can be incorporated into the direction of the osteotomy to unload a joint with injured cartilage. When this intervention is employed via a freehand technique, the amount of medialization and anteriorization can be customized based on the patient's anatomy and the degree of chondral injury.

If patella alta is identified as a risk factor, the distal portion of the tibial tubercle can be removed to permit distalization of the structure and earlier engagement of the patella with flexion (Fig. 8.8). This disrupts the periosteal hinge and increases the chances of complications such as fracture and nonunion, so most surgeons do not undertake this intervention for mild patella alta, saving it instead for patients with significantly high riding patellae requiring approximately 1 cm of correction to shift into a normal range.

If genu valgum is identified as a contributor, a distal femoral osteotomy is added, most commonly a lateral opening wedge osteotomy, to address a hypoplastic lateral femoral condyle. Likewise, if excessive femoral anteversion is confirmed, derotational osteotomy can be employed at the proximal, midshaft, or distal femur.

In severe cases of trochlear dysplasia, trocheoplasty, or reshaping of the dysplastic trochlea, can be

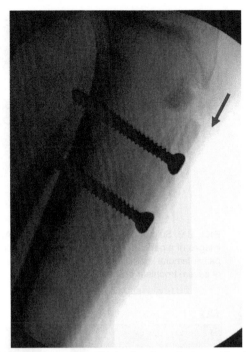

FIG. 8.8 Distalizing tibial tubercle osteotomy. To treat patella alta, the distal portion of a tibial tubercle osteotomy can be removed in order to permit sliding of the shingle distally (in this example, the removed segment is replaced in the proximal gap created by the distalization). Arrow indicates direction of tubercle shift (distal) prior to fixation.

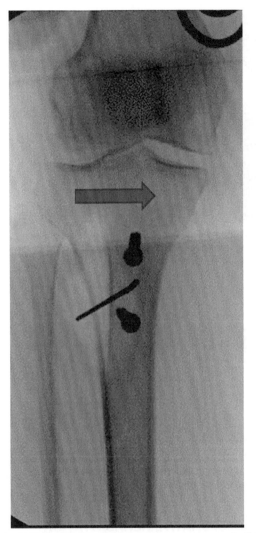

FIG. 8.7 Medializing tibial tubercle osteotomy. A tibial tubercle osteotomy fragment is rotated medially on its distal periosteal hinge to realign the extensor mechanism for more central tracking of the patella. Arrow indicates direction of tubercle shift (anteromedial) prior to fixation.

undertaken. Several strategies have been described, including a sulcus-deepening wedge (Fig. 8.9), a flattening of the surface using a thinner flap in the same location to reduce the height of the supratrochlear boss, or a simple removal of the supratrochlear spur (Fig. 8.10). These interventions are most often used in cases of extreme anatomy and/or salvage situations in the United States, although sulcus deepening and thin flap trochleoplasty have a more routine role in patellofemoral stabilization surgery in other countries. Concerns remain regarding the health of the trochlear cartilage after such procedures and deciphering the existing studies can be difficult because of limited follow-up and/or such aberrant anatomy that chondral overload and eventual breakdown seem inevitable even when not addressed surgically. The literature is clear, however, that trochleoplasty for severe trochlear dysplasia is an effective means of stabilizing the joint.

LRR was historically utilized with the goal of allowing the patella to track more medially, assisting with joint stability. However, biomechanical studies have demonstrated that while this can improve patellar tilt, LRR performed in isolation actually increases instability, as the lateral retinaculum contributes 10% to resisting lateral patellar translation. In addition, as mentioned earlier, excessive lateral release, combined with aggressive medialization of the tibial tubercle, can cause iatrogenic medial patellar instability. For these reasons, many surgeons who recognize the concomitant existence of lateral patellar overload with instability employ lateral retinacular lengthening, typically performed in conjunction with a realignment

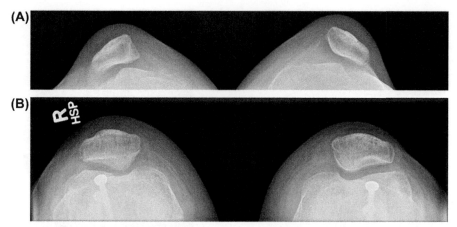

FIG. 8.9 Sulcus-deepening trochleoplasty. **(A)** Preoperative and **(B)** postoperative merchant axial X-rays images of a patient who underwent bilateral sulcus-deepening trochleoplasty (along with medial patellofemoral ligament reconstruction and tibial tubercle osteotomy) for patellofemoral instability in the setting of severe trochlear dysplasia.

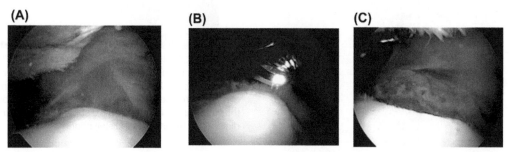

FIG. 8.10 Peterson trochleoplasty ("bumpectomy"). **(A–C)** A prominent supratrochlear boss is removed using an arthroscopic burr in order to permit improved patellar tracking into the trochlear groove entrance. Note the patellar chondral wear corresponding to its interface with the supratrochlear boss.

procedure such as tibial tubercle osteotomy, in order to avoid excessive release. In patients with a history of extensive LRR that is thought to be contributing to their instability, the lateral retinaculum can either be primarily repaired or reconstructed with a graft.

A multicenter effort is underway to provide the orthopedic community with evidence-based guidance on the treatment for both first-time and recurrent patellofemoral instabilities. Using the acronym JUPITER (Justifying Patellar Instability Treatment by Early Results), the group hopes to contribute to the patellofemoral literature in the same way that the MOON (Multicenter Orthopaedic Outcomes Network) and MARS (Multicenter ACL Revision Study) cohorts have expanded other aspects of orthopedic sports knowledge.

POSTOPERATIVE REHABILITATION

Postoperative rehabilitation involves first protecting the knee, then pursuing range of motion, strength, and proprioception/sports-specific training. Bracing and taping have not been proven specifically to stabilize the joint, but they may be employed for aid with proprioception and confidence as the patient recovers. Blood flow restriction therapy can serve a helpful role in this patient population, whose rehabilitation depends so heavily on quadriceps rehabilitation. In this tourniquet-based technique, low-resistance exercise can minimize exacerbation of painful symptoms while prompting muscle recovery and development via anaerobic metabolism. Return to sport for simple ligament reconstruction has been shown to take 6–8 months, and 8–10 months when tibial tubercle osteotomy is added.

SUMMARY

Treatment of patellar instability must be individualized, with care taken to identify both historical and anatomic risk factors. First-time instability that results in a loose chondral or osteochondral body should be addressed with both attention to the loose piece and the stabilization of the joint, most commonly in the form of MPFL reconstruction. Treatment of recurrent instability begins with MPFL reconstruction and involves the addition of realignment procedures and/or reshaping of the dysplastic trochlea, according to the limited available literature and surgeon judgment. Postoperative rehabilitation is key to regain motion and normalize muscle function, particularly that of the extensor mechanism. Studies are underway in an effort to examine patients in larger groups and capture more elusive factors, such as ligamentous laxity and femoral anteversion, so that we can standardize treatment for this difficult problem.

REFERENCES

1. Arendt EA, Askenberger M, Agel J, Tompkins MA. *Risk of Redislocation After Primary Patellar Dislocation A Clinical Prediction Model Based on Magnetic Resonance Imaging Variables.* 2018:3385−3390. https://doi.org/10.1177/036354651880 3936.

2. Mistovich RJ, Urwin JW, Fabricant PD, Lawrence JTR. *Patellar Tendon − Lateral Trochlear Ridge Distance A Novel Measurement of Patellofemoral Instability.* 2018:3400−3406. https://doi.org/10.1177/0363546518809982.

3. Kaiser P, Schmoelz W, Schoettle P, Zwierzina M, Heinrichs C, Attal R. Increased internal femoral torsion can be regarded as a risk factor for patellar instability — a biomechanical study. June *Clin BioMech.* 2017;47: 103−109. https://doi.org/10.1016/j.clinbiomech.2017. 06.007.

4. Crossley KM, Bennell KL, Cowan SM, Green S. Analysis of outcome measures for persons with patellofemoral pain: which are reliable and valid? *Arch Phys Med Rehabil.* 2004; 85(5):815−822.

5. Ward BSR, Terk MR, Powers CM. *Patella Alta : Association with Patellofemoral Alignment and Changes in Contact Area During Weight-Bearing.* 2007:1749−1755. https://doi.org/ 10.2106/JBJS.F.00508.

6. Pennock AT, Bomar JD, Manning JD. The creation and validation of a knee bone age atlas utilizing MRI. *J Bone Jt Surg Am.* 2018;100(4):e20. https://doi.org/10.2106/JBJS.17. 00693.

7. Pedowitz JM, Edmonds EW, Chambers HG, Dennis MM, Bastrom T, Pennock AT. Recurrence of patellar instability in adolescents undergoing surgery for osteochondral defects without concomitant ligament reconstruction. *Am J Sports Med.* 2019;47(1):66−70. https://doi.org/10.1177/0363 546518808486.

CHAPTER 9

Hip Anatomy and Biomechanics

ELISE B.E. RANEY, MD • ANDREA M. SPIKER, MD

INTRODUCTION

The human hip consists of a stable but very mobile skeletal framework for the surrounding capsule, ligaments, muscles, nerves, and vasculature. Understanding the anatomy and the development of intra- and extra-articular pathologies is critical in any patient population, and careful consideration must go into the evaluation of a painful hip in the female athlete. The anatomy, biomechanics, and pathologies specific to the female athlete are explored in this chapter.

The hip is a ball-and-socket joint that is formed by the articulation of the femoral head and the acetabulum, between which there is a high level of congruence. The joint's configuration allows for multiplanar movement; however, due to the joint being an integral part of lower limb motions such as walking, running, jumping, and kicking, a high degree of stability is also required.[1] It is markedly stable because of not only its osseous and articular architecture but also the encompassing soft tissues. Numerous structures provide stability to the joint. The capsule is one of these essential structures, and it is reinforced by the embedded capsular ligaments. The labrum helps stabilize the joint by deepening the socket, while the ligamentum teres acts to tether the femur to the acetabulum. Furthermore, the musculature surrounding the joint provides both static and dynamic stability. This chapter explores how each of these structures contributes to the function of the hip joint and its physical implications, with a focus on the female athletic population.

ANATOMY
Basic Anatomy
Bony and articular anatomy

The hip joint is a synovial joint that can be further categorized as a ball-and-socket-type of joint. The hip joint is composed of the femoral head and the acetabulum, and these two components are in high congruence with one another. The acetabulum is formed by the junction of three bones, namely, the ilium, the ischium, and the pubis, that intersect to form the triradiate zone.[2] The ilium is a broad, fanlike bone that expands superiorly from the acetabulum. The ischium extends posteroinferiorly from the acetabulum, while the pubis does so anteroinferiorly. These bones expand peripherally during growth to give the acetabulum its depth, and the concavity of the acetabulum develops around the sphericity of the head of the femur.[3] The acetabulum is a relatively deep cavity, which contributes significantly to the stability of the joint; its depth has been measured to be approximately 30 mm.[4] The articular cartilage of the acetabulum varies throughout the cavity, and it typically ranges between 1.3 and 3.0 mm in thickness, with the greatest thickness in the superolateral quadrant.[5] Although the acetabulum is commonly described as a hemisphere, it is devoid of cartilage in the central-inferior portion, with an opening at its inferior aspect spanned by the transverse acetabular ligament. The bare area is where the ligamentum teres originates.

The diameter of a native femoral head can range from 40 to 54 mm, with smaller sizes usually found in females.[6] All areas of the femoral head that articulate with the acetabulum are covered with hyaline cartilage, therefore covering 60%–70% of the spherical head.[7] The articular cartilage of the femoral head can be between 0.8 and 2.8 mm in thickness.[5] The inferomedial part of the head, the fovea capitis, lacks cartilage, as that is where the ligamentum teres inserts.

Capsular and ligamentous anatomy

The capsule consists of dense fibers that are cylindrically arranged around the joint to form a sleeve; they insert proximally along the acetabular periosteum, just proximal to the labrum, and distally to the anterior aspect of the femur, along the intertrochanteric line.[8] The capsule functions to both constrain the hip joint and maintain congruence. Posteriorly, the capsule is composed mainly of the ischiofemoral ligament

The Female Athlete. https://doi.org/10.1016/B978-0-323-75985-4.00027-1

proximally and the zona orbicularis (ZO) distally.[8] The ZO forms an arched free border that partially covers the femoral neck; it attaches just medial to the intertrochanteric crest.[9]

Most fibers of the capsule are longitudinally oriented, as is the strongest of the capsular ligaments, the iliofemoral ligament, also known as the Y-ligament of Bigelow. This ligament is located anteriorly and lies between the anterior inferior iliac spine and the ilial portion of the acetabular rim and the intertrochanteric line. It fans across the front of the joint, dividing into superior and inferior bands, taking the shape of an inverted Y. Its fibers are taut in extension and external rotation and lax in flexion, thus this ligament is thought to be essential in maintaining erect posture and reducing the requirement for active muscle contribution.[8,10]

The ischiofemoral ligament lies posterior to the joint and is spiral in shape. The fibers of the ligament are oblique, but the ischiofemoral ligament is less defined than the pubofemoral and iliofemoral ligaments.[8] The ischiofemoral ligament extends from the ischial rim of the acetabulum to the posterior aspect of the femoral neck, at the base of the greater trochanter. The literature describes two distinct bands in this ligament: the superior and the inferior bands.[8,10] The superior band inserts at the base of the greater trochanter, where it intermingles with the fibers of the ZO. The inferior band spreads downward to insert more posteriorly on the intertrochanteric crest.[8,9] The ischiofemoral ligament is thought to be at maximal tautness primarily during internal rotation, and also during adduction when the hip is flexed, thus limiting the extent of these actions.[9,11]

The pubofemoral ligament is slinglike in appearance; it originates proximally at the obturator crest and the superior pubic ramus. Distally, it blends anteriorly with the inferior part of the iliofemoral ligament and wraps posteriorly to insert inferior to the ischiofemoral ligament. It works in conjunction with the iliofemoral ligament to control external rotation of the hip and has been found to be maximally taut in hip abduction and lax in adduction.[9]

The fibers of the ZO are circular and resist distraction of the hip.[12] It is primarily a posterior and inferior structure, forming the free border of the posterior capsule. Recent studies indicate that the ZO has a role in synovial fluid circulation within the joint; it has been postulated that it acts as a bellow to unidirectionally force fluid from the peripheral compartment to the central compartment when the hip moves in flexion and extension.[13]

Neurovascular anatomy

Vascular anatomy (blood supply). The primary source of blood to the hip joint is the medial femoral circumflex artery (MFCA). It arises as a branch of the deep femoral artery, and its superficial branch supplies the adductor musculature. Direct branches of the MFCA and the lateral femoral circumflex artery (LFCA), which also arises from the deep femoral artery, predominantly supply the anterior capsule; they enter from the femoral aspect and run superficially along the capsule, encircling it from distal to proximal. The superior and inferior gluteal arteries divide into supra-acetabular and acetabular branches that terminate as capsular vessels; these run from proximal to distal to form anastomoses with the MFCA and LFCA and are the major supply to the posterior capsule.[14]

The vascular supply of the labrum is formed by branches of the medial and lateral circumflex arteries, the superior and inferior gluteal arteries, and the vascular system within the pelvis. The primary blood supply to the labrum is postulated to be the connective tissue interposed between the capsule and the capsular region of the labrum; therefore the capsular side is more vascular than the articular region (Fig. 9.1).[15] The bone adjoining the labrum is also a major contributor of blood to the structure. In one study, vascular channels originating in the osseous acetabulum were found to cross into the labrum, demonstrating that the bone-adjacent labrum has greater vascularity than its more peripheral aspects.[16] This can have significant implications in labral healing and repair.

The blood supply to the femoral head is variable. A minor branch off of the posterior division of the obturator artery supplies the ligamentum teres and thus plays a small role in vascularizing the proximal part of the head. Ascending cervical branches that arise from the extracapsular arterial ring perforate the capsule to form retinacular arteries; these are the main supply to the femoral head. The retinacular arteries have classically been divided into three main groups: posterosuperior, posteroinferior, and anterior.[17] The posterosuperior and posteroinferior arteries are supplied primarily by the MFCA, with the anterior most commonly from the LFCA. However, Ganz et al. determined that the deep branch of the MFCA can give rise to two to four superior retinacular vessels and, occasionally,

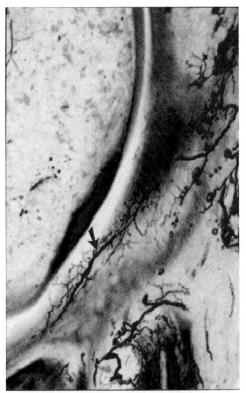

FIG. 9.1 Capsular blood supply (*arrow*) as shown on a high-power sagittal section. (Reprinted from Kelly BT, Shapiro GS, Digiovanni CW, Buly RL, Potter HG, Hannafin JA. Vascularity of the hip labrum: a cadaveric investigation. *Arthroscopy* 2005;21(1):3–11. https://doi.org/10.1016/j.arthro.2004.09.016, Copyright (2005), with permission from Elsevier.)

to inferior retinacular vessels (Fig. 9.2). The head can be completely perfused by the superior retinacular vessels alone.[18] This can have significant consequences in the development of avascular necrosis of the femoral head, particularly after dislocation or during surgical management of femur fractures.

Nerve anatomy. The obturator nerve is considered to be the primary source of innervation to the hip joint; however, the femoral nerve and the sciatic nerve also contribute sensory and motor innervation. The hip capsule is believed to be regionally innervated; the anterior region of the hip capsule receives innervation from the femoral and obturator nerves, while the posterior region receives innervation from the superior gluteal nerve, the nerve to the quadratus femoris, and direct branches of the sciatic nerve.[19]

The labrocapsular complex receives innervation from the sciatic, inferior gluteal, and femoral nerves, but more substantially from the nerve to the quadratus femoris and the obturator nerve.[20] Sensory end organs, such as Pacinian, Golgi-Mazzoni, Ruffini, and Krause corpuscles, in addition to free nerve endings, have been found in the hip labrum. Pacinian, Golgi-Mazzoni, and Ruffini corpuscles aid in proprioception, and the free nerve endings sense pain. The highest concentration of nociceptive and proprioceptive fibers is found along the attachment site of the labrum to the acetabulum. There is also a fair amount of these fibers in the center of the ligamentum teres.[21]

As for muscular innervations, the femoral nerve provides innervation to the psoas, iliacus, pectineus, sartorius, and quadriceps muscles and provides sensory innervation to the anterior thigh via cutaneous branches. The sciatic nerve arises from spinal nerves L4 through S3 to form part of the sacral plexus and consolidates to course through the greater sciatic foramen, just inferior to the piriformis. It then divides into the tibial and the peroneal branches; the tibial branch supplies the semitendinosus, the semimembranosus, and the long head of the biceps femoris. The peroneal branch of the sciatic nerve innervates the short head of the biceps femoris. The sciatic nerve does not have any direct sensory functions.

The obturator nerve, originating from L2-4, provides innervation to the obturator externus, gracilis, and adductor muscle group. It provides sensory innervation to the inferomedial thigh via its cutaneous branches. The superior and inferior gluteal nerves arise from the ventral rami of the L4-S1 and L5-S2 sacral spinal nerves, respectively, and transverse through the greater sciatic foramen from the sacral plexus. The superior gluteal nerve exits the pelvis at or just above the piriformis and innervates the gluteus medius, gluteus minimus, and tensor fascia latae. The gluteus maximus receives its innervation from the inferior gluteal nerve, which exits the greater sciatic foramen just inferior to the piriformis muscle. Neither nerve has a sensory role.

The short external rotators, with the exception of the obturator externus, receive innervation from the sacral plexus that descends from the ventral rami of the L4-S2.

Muscular anatomy

The muscular anatomy of the hip joint can be categorized by regions. The regions include the gluteal muscles and the muscles of the anterior, posterior, and medial thigh. The gluteal region can be further divided into the superficial and deep groups. The following section

(A)

(B)

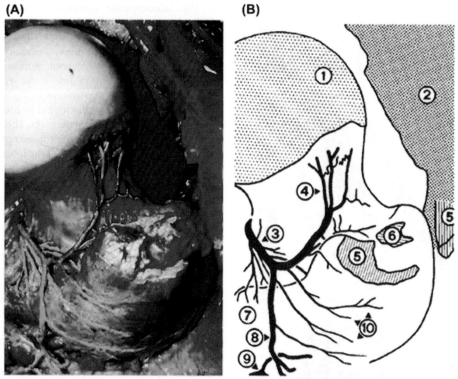

FIG. 9.2 **(A)** The perforation of the terminal branches into the bone (right hip, posterosuperior view). The terminal subsynovial branches are located on the posterosuperior aspect of the neck of the femur and penetrate the bone 2–4 mm lateral to the bone-cartilage junction. **(B)** A diagram showing (1) the head of the femur, (2) the gluteus medius, (3) the deep branch of the medial femoral circumflex artery (MFCA), (4) the terminal subsynovial branches of the MFCA, (5) insertion of and the tendon of gluteus medius, (6) insertion of the tendon of piriformis, (7) the lesser trochanter with nutrient vessels, (8) the trochanteric branch, (9) the branch of the first perforating artery, and (10) the trochanteric branches. (Republished with permission of Gautier E, Ganz K, Krügel N, Ganz R. Anatomy of the medial femoral circumflex artery and its surgical implications. *J Bone Joint Surg Br* 2000;82-B(5):679–683; permission conveyed through Copyright Clearance Center, Inc.)

provides a detailed summary of these muscle groups and individual muscles as they relate to the function and pathoanatomy of the hip.

Gluteal muscles (superficial and deep). The superficial gluteal group is composed of the gluteus maximus, gluteus medius, gluteus minimus, and tensor fascia latae. The gluteus maximus originates from a broad area that includes the external surface of the ilium behind the posterior gluteal line, the fascia of the gluteus medius, the fascia of the erector spinae, the dorsal surface of the sacrum, the lateral margin of the coccyx, and the sacrotuberal ligament.[22] The majority of the muscle inserts on the iliotibial (IT) band at its aponeurotic origin on the greater trochanter; the inferior segment inserts on the gluteal tuberosity of the femur.[22] The main function of the muscle is to act as a hip extensor, primarily when the hip is in flexed position, such as when rising from a seated position. The gluteus maximus also functions as an external rotator and abductor of the hip. The gluteus medius originates from the ilium, from the anterior to the posterior gluteal lines. It then inserts onto the lateral aspect of the greater trochanter.[23] The gluteus medius is considered the main abductor of the hip. Gluteus minimus, another abductor, originates from the external ilium, from the anterior gluteal line to the inferior gluteal line, covering the posterosuperior acetabulum.[23] It inserts with the gluteus medius on the greater trochanter of the femur, notably on the anterior aspect. The gluteus minimus is also thought to insert onto the anterosuperior hip joint capsule; as a result, it may stabilize the femoral head in the acetabulum by tightening the capsule and thus putting pressure on the head of the femur.[24] In addition to being an abductor, it can function as a hip flexor, internal rotator, and external rotator, depending on the position of the hip. The tensor fascia latae is the last muscle of the superficial gluteal group; it originates from the anterolateral portion of the iliac crest and the lateral aspect of the anterior superior iliac spine (ASIS). Its attachment is on the fascia lata, and continuing debate exists regarding whether this attachment is just inferior to the muscle belly where it attaches on the IT band or if the fibers of the attachment run with the IT band and the actual attachment is on Gerdy's tubercle. This muscle primarily abducts the hip.

The deep group of the gluteal region includes the six short external rotators. These consist of the piriformis, the superior and inferior gemellus muscles, the obturator externus and internus muscles, and the quadratus femoris. The piriformis originates on the anterior surface of the second through fourth sacral vertebrae and emerges from the greater sciatic foramen of the pelvis. Its distal attachment is typically defined as anterosuperior to the trochanteric fossa.[25] A common anatomic variant of the piriformis is for it to be split by the sciatic nerve into inferior and superior muscle bellies. However, typically, the sciatic nerve passes completely under the piriformis, through a canal formed by the piriformis and the superior gemellus.[26] The superior gemellus, the smaller of the two gemelli, originates on the ischial spine. Inferior to that, the obturator internus arises from the medial surface of the obturator membrane as it spans the obturator foramen and the surrounding bone. The inferior gemellus originates just superior to the ischial tuberosity. The gemelli insert into the tendon of the obturator internus, creating a conjoint tendon that then inserts into the greater trochanter anteriorly.[27] The quadratus femoris originates from the lateral aspect of the ischial tuberosity and has its muscular insertion on the posterior femur partially overlying the inferior margin of the intertrochanteric crest.

Thigh muscles (anterior, posterior, and medial compartments). The anterior compartment of the thigh is composed of the sartorius, rectus femoris, iliopsoas, pectineus, and the lesser known iliocapsularis muscle. Together these muscles contribute to the flexion of the hip. The origin of the sartorius is on the ASIS; the muscle courses downward to insert medially to the tibial tuberosity via the pes anserinus. The rectus femoris has two heads: the anterior/direct head originates on the anterior inferior iliac spine and the posterior/

indirect head originates just superior to the acetabulum. The two heads unite to form an aponeurosis that joins the muscle belly; the muscle then inserts into the base of the patella. The pectineus arises from the pectineal line of the superior ramus of the pubis; it is a flat quadrangular muscle that is the most anterior hip adductor. However, it also acts to flex the hip joint, and it is classified in the anterior compartment because of its innervation, which is primarily via the femoral nerve. It inserts onto the pectineal line of the femur, distal to the lesser trochanter.[28] Due to its unique composition, origin, and insertion, the iliopsoas is the only periarticular hip muscle that is able to contribute to the stability of the trunk, pelvis, and leg. It has two muscle bellies that are separately innervated, allowing them to act in conjunction or separately from one another. The muscle complex originates from the transverse processes of the T12-L5 vertebrae, the anterior surface of the iliac crest, and the anterior sacrum; they merge distally to insert on the lesser trochanter.[29] Both the iliacus and the psoas are involved in hip flexion and maximal thigh abduction; however, the iliacus can be selectively activated to control movement between the hip and pelvis, whereas the psoas is selectively activated for stabilizing the lumbar spine in standing when an axial load is applied to the contralateral hip.[30] As a result of the psoas tendon's position in relation to the anterior capsule, it serves as both a dynamic and a static stabilizer of the hip; it may be displaced laterally during hip flexion and medially during extension. The iliocapsularis, also called iliacus minor or iliotrochantericus, is a lesser known muscle that overlies the anterior hip capsule. It originates mostly from the anteromedial hip capsule and in part from the anterior inferior iliac spine; its insertion is located just distal to the lesser trochanter.[31] Research suggests that contraction of the iliocapsularis results in tightening of the hip capsule, thus aiding in dynamic stabilization of the joint. Several studies have found that the iliocapsularis is hypertrophied in dysplastic hips, suggesting that it is particularly important for stabilizing the femoral head in a deficient acetabulum.[31,32]

The posterior compartment of the thigh is composed of the hamstring muscles; these include the semitendinosus, semimembranosus, and the biceps femoris. The semitendinosus lies superficial to the semimembranosus in the posteromedial aspect of the thigh. It arises from the superomedial aspect of the ischial tuberosity and shares a common tendon with the long head of the biceps femoris. It courses distally to insert as part of the pes anserinus with the sartorius and gracilis. The

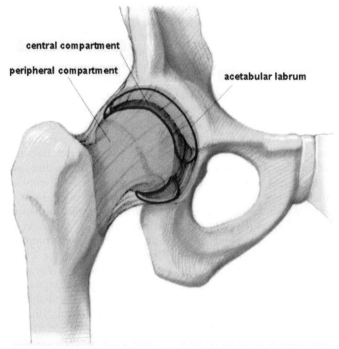

central compartment

peripheral compartment

acetabular labrum

FIG. 9.3 The central and peripheral arthroscopic compartments of the hip. (Reprinted from Wettstein M, Dienst M. Arthroscopy of the peripheral compartment of the hip. *Operat Tech Orthop* 2005;15(3):225–230. https://doi.org/10.1053/j.oto.2005.07.003, Copyright (2005), with permission from Elsevier.)

semimembranosus arises on the superolateral aspect of the ischial tuberosity and inserts on the medial condyle of the tibia. The biceps femoris arises via two heads. As described earlier, the long head originates with the semitendinosus on the ischial tuberosity. The short head arises from the lateral lip of the linea aspera along the posterior femur, between the adductor magnus and vastus lateralis. It then terminates primarily on the lateral head of the fibula; however, a small, separate insertion is also found on the lateral condyle of the tibia.[33]

The medial compartment of the thigh is made up of the adductor brevis, adductor longus, adductor magnus, and gracilis muscles; they are the primary adductors of the thigh and also contribute to flexion and internal rotation. The adductor brevis is the most superior, and it arises from the inferior pubic ramus. The adductor longus originates from the anterior aspect of the pubis, under the pubic tubercle. The origin of the adductor magnus is from the inferior pubic ramus and the ischial tuberosity; the gracilis originates solely from the inferior pubic ramus. The adductors then all insert on the medial lip of the linea aspera, with the exception of the adductor magnus, which also inserts on the adductor tubercle, and the gracilis, which inserts solely as part of the pes anserinus on the tibia.

Functional Anatomy: Central and Peripheral Compartments

Arthroscopically, the hip can be divided into two compartments: the central and the peripheral compartments (Figs. 9.3 and 9.4). These compartments are demarcated by the labrum.

Central compartment

The central compartment, also known as the iliofemoral joint, includes the lunate cartilage of the acetabulum, the acetabular fossa, the ligamentum teres, and the loaded articular surface of the femoral head.[34,35] This part of the joint can only be visualized arthroscopically with hip distraction.

The labrum is a fibrocartilaginous structure composed of types I, II, and III collagen that attaches to both the perimeter of the bony acetabulum and the articular cartilage within the cavity. It courses along the acetabular rim to attach to the transverse acetabular ligament anteriorly and posteriorly, forming a contiguous structure around the acetabulum.[36] The labrum increases the total acetabular surface area coverage by more than 25% and acetabular volume by approximately 20%, as found by Tan et al.[37] Furthermore, stability is augmented by a vacuum force of about

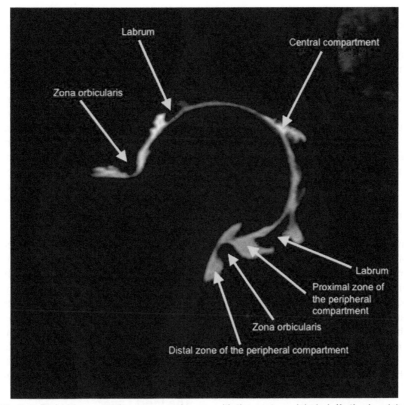

FIG. 9.4 Right hip magnetic resonance image, with the anatomy labeled. (Author's original.)

120 200 N created by the labrum, which seals the joint space between the lunate cartilage and the femoral head and maintains the femoral head within the socket.[38,39]

The type I collagen fibers of the labrum are oriented in different directions depending on the region. Anteriorly, the fibers are attached parallel to the bony edge of the acetabulum, making them susceptible to shear forces. Posteriorly, they attach perpendicular to the bony edge, allowing them to be more resistant to these forces.[36] In the sagittal plane, the labrum appears to have a horseshoe shape. As the labrum extends peripherally from its bony attachment, the structure tapers. This gives it a triangular shape in cross-section, with the apex creating the free edge closest to the joint center. It maintains joint fluid in the central compartment, which reduces friction and supplies chondral nutrition.[40] The labrum can be divided into two regions when observed under light microscopy: the capsular region and the articular region. The articular region attaches to the bony rim of the acetabulum through a zone of calcified cartilage, while the capsular region attaches without this zone.[40] The thickness of the labrum varies by location; however, the average thickness is reported as approximately 5.3 mm.[37]

Historically, the ligamentum teres was considered to be an embryonic remnant; however, with the advent of hip arthroscopy, recent investigations indicate that it may play a role in hip stabilization and may also participate in fine coordination by transmitting somatosensory afferent signals.[41] It originates along the transverse acetabular ligament, as well as from the pubic and ischial aspects of the acetabulum. The structure then inserts onto the fovea capitis of the femur. It is enveloped in its own synovial membrane and is surrounded by a synovial fat pad, also known as the pulvinar. Additionally, the ligament carries within it an anterior branch of the posterior division of the obturator artery.[41] Studies indicate that it may be an important stabilizer in hip adduction, flexion, and external rotation.[42]

Peripheral compartment

The peripheral compartment of the hip includes the unloaded articular surface of the femoral head; the femoral neck; the medial, anterior, and posterolateral synovial folds; and the articular capsule with its intrinsic ligaments, including the ZO.[35] Arthroscopically, the peripheral hip compartment can be divided into seven zones: anterior neck area, medial neck area, medial head area, anterior head area, lateral head area, lateral neck area, and posterior area.[43] This allows for a systematic approach to view the hip so as to accurately and thoroughly view the joint space.

The retinacula of Weitbrecht (Weitbrecht ligaments) are three synovial folds that appear medial, anterior, and posterolateral in relation to the femoral neck. They overlie the retinacular branches of the femoral circumflex artery that supplies the femoral head and can be helpful landmarks during arthroscopic review of the joint. The medial synovial fold, which does not adhere to the femoral neck, can be found consistently and is a helpful landmark, especially if visibility within the peripheral compartment is poor.[43]

The capsule inserts directly onto the acetabulum immediately proximal to the labrum, creating a capsulolabral recess that contains vascularized connective tissue and fat. After hip arthroscopy, patients who develop scarring in the region between the capsule and the labrum can have symptoms of pain and limited motion, lending to the theory that this recess is important for hip motion.[44]

LAYERED APPROACH TO THE HIP

The layered approach to the hip compartmentalizes the anatomy to aid in diagnostic evaluation. In doing so, an examiner can perform a comprehensive and systematic evaluation of the hip. Four layers are described, each progressing from deep to superficial: the osteochondral layer, the inert layer, the contractile layer, and the neurokinetic layer. These are also referred to as the osseous, capsulolabral, musculotendinous, and neurovascular layers, respectively.[45]

The Osteochondral Layer

The osteochondral layer encompasses the pelvis, acetabulum, and femur. Structural pathologies within this compartment can be further classified into three groups: static overload, dynamic impingement, and dynamic instability.[46] Static mechanical factors occur either in standing or axially loading of the joint. Static overload can be caused by several anatomic variants, including acetabular protrusio, excessive femoral anteversion/retroversion, excessive acetabular retroversion/anteversion, lateral or anterior acetabular undercoverage, and coxa vara/valga. These deviations change the mechanics

of the hip joint and thus can predispose the hip to abnormal stress and eccentric loading, leading to accelerated cartilage degeneration.

Dynamic impingement can be caused by variants such as femoroacetabular impingement (FAI), relative femoral anteversion, and coxa vara. Pain often presents during terminal hip motion as a result of these variations. FAI is becoming increasingly documented not only in the athletic population but also in the general population. It is characterized by abnormal contact between the femoral head and the acetabulum during terminal hip movement, with associated pain, and labral and articular cartilage damage. FAI can be categorized as cam type (femoral based), pincer type (acetabular based), or combined impingement, which is the most common.

When the range of motion required for normal function of the hip starts to exceed the limits of an individual's physiologic range as set by his/her anatomy, there can be compensatory stresses and dynamic instability, in addition to the pain previously described. Instability is in the form of small, repetitive posterior hip subluxations as the femoral head shifts out of the acetabulum.[46] As the periarticular musculature attempts to stabilize the incongruent anatomy, layers 2 and 3 are subsequently affected, as discussed later in this chapter.

The Inert Layer

The inert layer consists of the labrum, capsule, ligamentous complex, and ligamentum teres. This layer not only does provides stability to the hip joint but also serves as protection for the cartilage and as a scaffold for the vascular supply to the joint. As such, mismatched anatomy described in layer 1 has a direct effect on this layer. The underlying abnormalities can result in pathologies such as labral injury, capsular injury, ligamentum teres tears, adhesive capsulitis, and instability.

The labrum increases the intra-articular hydrostatic pressure and load distribution; therefore biomechanical studies have shown that progressive labral wear correlates with an increase in hip instability.[47] As previously described, the labrum also contains free nerve endings that carry both nociceptive and proprioceptive fibers, which corroborates the findings of decreased proprioception and pain in athletes with torn labrums.[21,48]

The Contractile Layer

The contractile layer is composed of the periarticular musculature, the lumbosacral musculature, and the pelvic floor. This layer plays a crucial role in balance and dynamic stability of the hip. Abnormal morphologies in layer 1, particularly dynamic impingement such as

FAI, can lead to increased mechanical stresses in the sacroiliac joint, pubic symphysis, and ischium, and this strains the muscles that are attached to these structures, leading to muscle dysfunction. Patients with FAI have been found to have decreased maximal voluntary contraction levels in all the major muscle groups surrounding the hip joint, when compared with the control group. The authors of this study concluded that this anatomic pathology in layer 1 can lead to hip muscle malfunction, and as a result, the risk of compensatory injuries in these muscles is increased.[49]

Enthesopathy, a general term for pathology in tendons or ligaments as they attach to bones, in the musculature around the joint can result in numerous muscular injuries. Because of the myriad muscles that surround the joint, injuries in this layer are categorized based on the muscles' location relative to the hip joint; thus injuries are classified as anterior, posterior, medial, and lateral. Anterior enthesopathy includes hip flexor strains, psoas impingement, and subspine impingement. Posterior enthesopathies consist of proximal hamstring strains, piriformis injuries, and the pain syndrome known as "deep gluteal syndrome," which involves posterior soft tissue injury and entrapment of the sciatic nerve.[50] Medial enthesopathy is composed of adductor and rectus abdominus tendinopathies; these have been historically referred to as athletic pubalgia, or "sports hernias," and are now often referred to as core muscle injuries.

Lateral enthesopathies include gluteus medius and minimus strains and injuries within the peritrochanteric space. Lateral enthesopathies of both gluteus medius and gluteus minimus play a role in greater trochanteric pain syndrome (GTPS), and recalcitrant GTPS has been shown to be successfully treated with surgical gluteus medius repairs.[51,52] Medius tears are much more common than minimus tears, and medius tendinopathy and tears can lead to the Trendelenburg gait and difficulty ascending stairs.

As previously described, the psoas can be displaced laterally during hip flexion and medially during extension; this motion may explain the pain that can be generated in "snapping hip." This pathology is likely related to the psoas snapping over the femoral head or iliopectineal eminence.[53] Fabricant et al.[54] observed that patients with femoral anteversion greater than 25 degrees had inferior clinical outcomes when they underwent arthroscopic psoas lengthening for refractory symptomatic internal snapping hip; this further demonstrates the critical interactions between layers 1 and 3.

The hamstring tendons can tear with and without underlying layer 1 pathology. The classic mechanism of injury for a proximal hamstring tear occurs when the knee is extended and the hip is forced into flexion. However, proximal hamstring injuries can also occur during sports with rapid acceleration and deceleration.[55] It has been hypothesized that proximal hamstring tendinopathy can also arise due to increased stress on the tendon, secondary to FAI.[56] The decreased rotation of the hip places undue stress on the hamstring tendons, subsequently causing degeneration of the tendon. This restricted range of motion may also play a role in the development of athletic pubalgia, as well as pain at other sites, such as the lumbar spine, pubic symphysis, sacroiliac joint, and posterior acetabulum, as they increase their motion to compensate. Hammoud and colleagues reported on a series of professional athletes with recalcitrant athletic pubalgia; 32% had undergone surgery to solely address the symptoms, without undergoing treatment for the underlying FAI. After surgery to subsequently correct the underlying FAI, 95% of the athletes were finally able to return to their previous level of play, indicating the role FAI hip pathology has in developing neighboring pain syndromes.[57]

The Neurokinetic Layer

The thoracolumbosacral nerve plexus, lumbopelvic tissue, and lower extremity structures and mechanics compose layer 4, the neurokinetic layer. From a purely reductionist view, this layer supplies blood and innervation to the joint. To expand upon this, the nerves contain nociceptive and proprioceptive receptors, which are responsible for pain and stability felt in and around the joint. This layer serves as the neuromuscular link, thus controlling how this segment of the body functions and moves, and dictates posture.

Thus the pathology seen in this layer includes neuromuscular dysfunction, nerve compression and pain syndromes, spinal radicular symptoms, and myelopathies. The more common peripheral nerve conditions around the hip include sciatic neuropathy (piriformis syndrome), superior and inferior gluteal neuropathies, lateral femoral cutaneous neuropathy (meralgia paresthetica), femoral neuropathy, obturator neuropathy, and pudendal, ilioinguinal, iliohypogastric, and genitofemoral neuropathies.[45] The lateral femoral cutaneous nerve is a branch of the lumbar plexus, arising from the dorsal divisions on L2 and L3. It runs along the lateral edge of the psoas and then passes beneath the iliac fascia and the inguinal ligament, close to the ASIS. Owing to its location, the nerve can be subject to external compression or injury.

The sciatic nerve is commonly compressed at the level of the piriformis, resulting in a constellation of symptoms known as the piriformis syndrome. This entails buttock pain, posterior muscular tension, and radicular symptoms down the length of the leg.

The obturator nerve, as stated previously, innervates the medial muscular compartment of the leg and the inferomedial thigh via cutaneous branches; injury to the nerve has been reported from retractor placement on the transverse acetabular ligament during open approaches to the hip. Although radiculopathies and myelopathies are less common causes of hip pain, they should be kept in mind when evaluating a painful hip.

BIOMECHANICS OF THE HIP

There can be significant variability in the morphologies of the femur and acetabulum, with a few that have been elucidated over the years to have substantial clinical relevance. Regarding the femur, the angle of inclination, or the neck-shaft angle, and the amount of femoral version can significantly impact the function of the joint. The neck-shaft angle is measured as the angle formed from the bisection of the line drawn through the axis of the femoral neck and the line drawn through the axis of the shaft of the femur.

The neck-shaft angle of the femur, normally approximately 125 degrees, determines the offset (Fig. 9.5).

The femoral offset is found by measuring the perpendicular line from the center of rotation of the femoral head to where it intersects with the line drawn down the center of the shaft. The greater the value of offset, the more lateralized the muscular attachments are, which decreases the chances of impingement and creates greater tension in the abductor mechanism and enhances stability. This occurs in femurs with decreased neck-shaft angles; these are termed *coxa vara*.

The femoral version, or torsion, is measured in the axial plane in relation to the knee joint and is approximately 15−20 degrees (Fig. 9.6).[58] Decreased angles of version can be classified as relative retroversion or retroversion. An increase in torsion causing excessive anteversion places the greater trochanter in a more posterior position, thus decreasing the lever arm of the gluteus medius, which in turn decreases its strength and efficiency.

The orientation of the acetabulum in the axial plane is called acetabular version. Reikeras et al.[59] found that normal acetabular version is approximately 17 (±6) degrees of anteversion. Females, on average, have higher acetabular version than males; in one study the average central anteversion in males was 16.46 (±4.42) degrees and in females was 19.31 (±5.04) degrees.[60] Acetabular dysplasia describes an acetabulum that is too shallow or

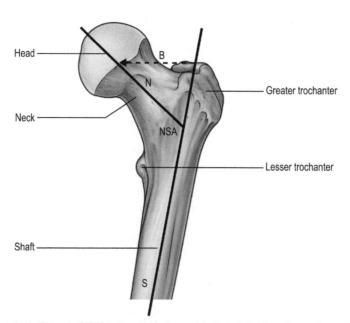

FIG. 9.5 The neck-shaft angle (NSA) is the angle formed between the line drawn through the axis of the femoral neck (N) and the line drawn through the long axis of the shaft of the femur (S). In most hips, a line perpendicular to the long axis of the femur from the tip of the greater trochanter (B) passes through the center of the femoral head. (Reprinted from Standring S, Gray H. Chapter 81: Hip. In: *Gray's Anatomy: the Anatomical Basis of Clinical Practice.* 41st ed:1376−1382, Copyright (2016), with permission from Elsevier.)

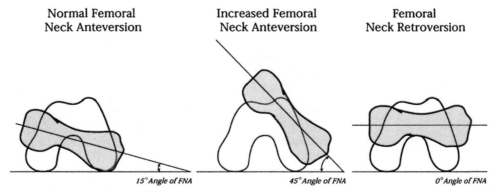

Normal Femoral Neck Anteversion   Increased Femoral Neck Anteversion   Femoral Neck Retroversion

15° Angle of FNA   *45° Angle of FNA*   *0° Angle of FNA*

FIG. 9.6 Depictions of normal femoral neck version, increased femoral neck anteversion, and femoral neck retroversion. The femoral neck angle is determined by drawing a line posterior to the distal femoral condyles and through the femoral neck. *FNA*, femoral neck anteversion. (From Cibulka MT. Determination and significance of femoral neck anteversion. *Phys Ther* 2004;84(6):550–558.[96] https://doi.org/10.1093/ptj/84.6.550 by permission of Oxford University Press and The American Physical Therapy Association.)

is deformed in such a way that it does not adequately cover the femoral head. Although it is commonly thought that hip dysplasia is associated with excessive acetabular anteversion, it can also occur with retroversion. Tonnis[61] found that decreased acetabular anteversion (less than 10 degrees, or retroverted) was found in 29% of the dysplastic hips he examined.

The ball-in-socket structure allows the hip to move in the coronal, sagittal, and axial planes, with 6 degrees of freedom around these axes of motion. Therefore the osteokinematic motions associated with this include flexion and extension, abduction and adduction, and internal and external rotations. The arthrokinematic motions between the femoral head and the acetabulum encompass spinning and gliding. In flexion, the femoral head rolls anteriorly and glides posteriorly on the acetabulum. In extension, the opposite occurs—the femoral head rolls posteriorly and glides anteriorly. In abduction, the femoral head rolls laterally and glides medially, and vice versa in adduction. The active range of motion of the hip is greatest in the sagittal plane; on average, an individual can attain 120 degrees of flexion and 20 degrees of extension. Within the coronal plane, there is an anticipated 40 degrees of abduction; internal and external rotations are measured as both 30 degrees in the axial plane when measured in the seated position with the knee flexed at 90 degrees.[62]

The closed packed position of the hip is when the joint is at its greatest point of stability. The surfaces of the joints are maximally congruent at this point, which is found when the hip is in extension with some amount of adduction and internal rotation. This is because all the capsular ligaments are taut in this position. The hip is designed to tolerate large amounts of force. For example, the hip joint contact forces during level walking have been calculated to be approximately 1.5 times body weight, whereas running can produce loads between 4.5 and 6 times body weight.[63–65]

Gait

The principal role of the hip joint is lower extremity advancement during ambulation. The arc of motion of the hip during the walking cycle is typically between 40 and 50 degrees; this consists of 30–40 degrees of flexion and 5–10 degrees of extension.[66–68] The walking gait cycle consists of two phases: the stance phase, which makes up approximately 60% of the cycle, and the swing phase, which makes up the remaining 40% (Fig. 9.7).[69,70] The stance phase is the period during which the foot remains in contact with the ground, beginning with heel strike and ending at toe-off. The double support phase during stance is when both feet are in contact with the ground; this accounts for approximately 20% of the total gait cycle, and it is the part of the cycle that defines walking.[69] The percentage of time spent in double support decreases as the speed of walking increases.[71] Perry[69] further divided the stance phase into five subphases: initial contact, loading response, midstance, terminal stance, and preswing. The swing phase is the period during which the foot is in the air, beginning at toe-off and ending with heel strike. The swing phase can be subdivided into three secondary phases: initial swing, midswing, and terminal swing. External and internal rotations occur in the pelvis and femur during the walking cycle. Total pelvic rotation covers a 10-degree arc; internal rotation is

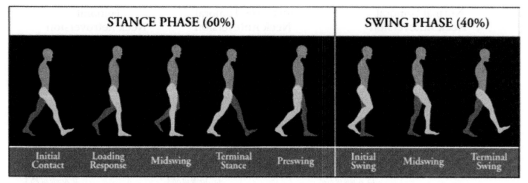

FIG. 9.7 The walking gait cycle. (Reprinted from Hughes PE, Hsu JC, Matava MJ. Hip anatomy and biomechanics in the athlete. *Sports Med Arthrosc* 2002;10(2):103–114. https://doi.org/10.1097/00132585-200210020-00002. https://journals.lww.com/sportsmedarthro, with permission from Wolters Kluwer Health, Inc.; Originally adapted from Perry J. *Gait Analysis: Normal and Pathological Function*. New York: McGraw-Hill; 1992.)

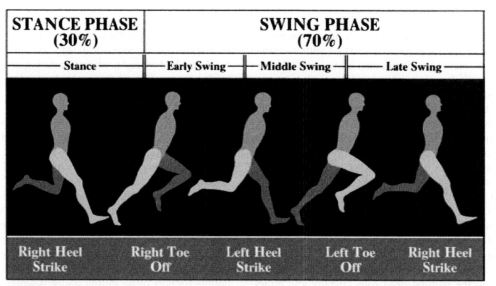

FIG. 9.8 The running gait cycle. (Reprinted from Hughes PE, Hsu JC, Matava MJ. Hip anatomy and biomechanics in the athlete. *Sports Med Arthrosc* 2002;10(2):103–114. https://doi.org/10.1097/00132585-200210020-00002; https://journals.lww.com/sportsmedarthro, with permission from Wolters Kluwer Health, Inc.; Originally adapted from Montgomery III WH, Pink M, Perry J. Electromyographic analysis of hip and knee musculature during running. *Am J Sports Med* 1994;22:272–278.)

maximized at initial ground contact. External rotation is greatest at toe-off.[72]

Running is defined as when the double-stance phase is lost from the gait cycle (Fig. 9.8).[73] Instead, a float phase develops; this is the period when both feet are off of the ground. This phase lasts for approximately 30% of the running gait cycle. The stance phase decreases to 30% of the gait cycle, while the swing phase increases to 70%.[74] In order for this sequence of events to occur, the hip muscles must work in concert with one another to smoothly transition between phases; when they are weak, it could have a considerable effect on athletic performance and could put the athlete at risk for injury.

Gait Differences Between Females and Males

Although the variances in gait are visually subtle between the genders, quantifiable differences exist. On average, females walk at a higher step frequency, or cadence, than males, and females have been found to have marginally shorter stride lengths, but this is likely related to females' shorter statures.[68,75,76] The higher cadence means females also perform greater mechanical work per unit time and unit distance.[77] However, there is no difference in velocity between genders.[75] Kerrigan et al.[61] found that females, when normalized for height and weight, have significantly greater hip flexion and less knee extension before initial contact, greater knee flexion moment in preswing, and greater peak mechanical joint power absorption at the knee in preswing.[77] They hypothesized that greater hip flexion is likely due to females' greater stride length when normalized for height, as well as females' tendencies toward greater hip power generation in loading response. The authors had anticipated that females would actually have greater knee extension before initial ground contact than their male counterparts, as that can increase stride length; however, the finding of decreased knee extension could be due to an intrinsic gender difference in walking. These differences have yet to be fully studied in regard to their clinical relevance, particularly regarding hip pathology.

THE FEMALE ATHLETE'S HIP

The female athletes are now of particular interest, as this population has exponentially grown since the passing of the Title IX civil rights law in 1972; between 1972 and 2018, the number of girls participating in high-school sports jumped from under 295,000 to over 3,415,000.[78] As the female athlete population has increased, so has the incidence of hip injury. This may result from the high stresses placed on the hip joint from repetitive axial loading and the wide ranges of motion required by sports activities, allowing underlying impingement or instability to reveal themselves. Furthermore, more females than males participate in flexibility sports that require extreme ranges of motion, such as dance, gymnastics (Fig. 9.9), cheerleading, and figure skating, which may contribute to the increasing prevalence of hip injuries. Depending on the specific activity, injuries in and around the hip make up between 6% and 12% of all injuries sustained from these sports.[79–82] A systematic review of musculoskeletal injury rates in dancers found that 17.2% of all injuries were hip or groin injuries.[83] Dancers in particular are subject to labral

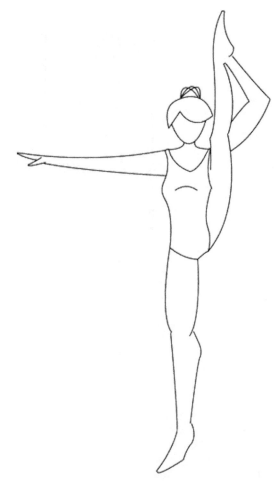

FIG. 9.9 An artist's depiction of a gymnast's side split with hand support. (Reprinted from Rutkowska-Kucharska A, Szpala A, Jaroszczuk S, Sobera M. Muscle coactivation during stability exercises in rhythmic gymnastics: a two-case study. *Appl Bionics Biomech* 2018;2018:8260402.[97] https://doi.org/10.1155/2018/8260402. Available in Creative Commons.)

pathology, coxa saltans ("snapping hip") syndrome, and piriformis syndrome. Furthermore, these athletes are at a risk for intra-articular FAI, and these movements also allow for extra-articular bony impingement to occur. Extreme hip flexion can lead to contact between anterior inferior iliac spine and the distal femoral neck, causing subspinous impingement (Fig. 9.10).[84] In ballet, the extreme range of motion required for some maneuvers can pinch the labrum between the femoral head and the acetabulum, leading to labral tears, as well. The extreme movements can also cause the piriformis muscle

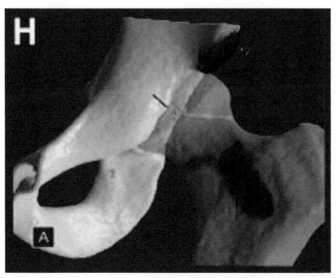

FIG. 9.10 Areas of impingement between the subspine and femoral neck are marked in blue on this three-dimensional computed tomographic image, which has been imported into a software program (software prototype; A2 Surgical). (Reprinted from Larson CM, Kelly BT, Stone RM. Making a case for anterior inferior iliac spine/subspine hip impingement: three representative case reports and proposed concept. *Arthroscopy* 2011; 27(12):1732–1737.[98] https://doi.org/10.1016/j.arthro.2011.10.004, Copyright (2011), with permission from Elsevier.)

to become tight, leading to sciatic nerve irritation. Female dancers may be at a higher risk for hip injury than their male counterparts, as they use their legs as levers for lifts, and typically the height of their gesturing leg is expected to be higher, which requires increased motion of the hip joint.

Hip dysplasia is much more common in females than in males, and in a series of 41 hips of professional dancers undergoing hip arthroscopy, 55% had radiographic and intraoperative evidence of hip dysplasia.[85,86] The high prevalence of dysplasia in this population may be due to the fact that dance and other flexibility sports select for athletes with greater range of motion, and dysplastic hips allow for exaggerated movements. When compared with patients with isolated FAI, patients with dysplastic hips were able to achieve significantly more internal rotation and abduction, even with concomitant FAI.[87] Of interest, females, particularly active, middle-aged women, tend to exhibit a higher prevalence of pincer-type FAI, compared with males, who predominantly display cam-type FAI.[88,89]

Furthermore, female athletes are predisposed to increased laxity compared with their male counterparts. Females may be more prone to instability inherently due to hormonal laxity; females have been found to have greater generalized joint laxity following puberty, as female sex hormones enable relaxation of pelvic

ligaments.[90] These hormones may affect ligament formation, degradation, and loading properties, but the biology is not yet fully understood. In one study of high-level athletes who underwent arthroscopic hip surgery, females were more likely to have hip instability that required capsular plication.[91]

Finally, female athletes have a higher incidence of stress injuries than males; pelvic and sacral stress injuries particularly occur with a greater female predominance.[92,93] This may in part be because of the high prevalence of what is known colloquially as the "female athlete triad," now also identified as "relative energy deficiency in sports," which consists of low energy availability with or without disordered eating, functional hypothalamic amenorrhea, and low bone density. Femoral neck stress fractures are associated with this condition; these patients often complain of anterior hip or groin pain.[94,95] These fractures must always be considered when evaluating a female hip, as their symptomology can overlap with those of joint pathology.

SUMMARY

The human hip is an integral part of ambulation, and its form and function allow it to handle tremendous amounts of stress and broad motions, while maintaining considerable stability. Knowledge of the anatomy and the relationships that exist between the different components and layers of this joint is essential in diagnosing and treating hip pathology. Furthermore, understanding how female anatomy differs, and how female athletes are prone to certain pathologies, is paramount in treating this ever-growing population. Hip pathology has important ramifications, for if not treated properly, it may also predispose patients to other injuries along the kinematic chain.

REFERENCES

1. Hughes PE, Hsu JC, Matava MJ. Hip anatomy and biomechanics in the athlete. *Sports Med Arthrosc.* 2002;10(2):103–114. https://doi.org/10.1097/00132585-200210020-00002.
2. Verbruggen SW, Nowlan NC. Ontogeny of the human pelvis. *Anat Rec.* 2017;300(4):643–652. https://doi.org/10.1002/ar.23541.
3. Ponseti IV. Growth and development of the acetabulum in the normal child. Anatomical, histological, and roentgenographic studies. *J Bone Joint Surg Am.* 1978;60(5):575–585.
4. Šalamon A, Šalamon T, Šef D, Jo-Osvatić A. Morphological characteristics of the acetabulum. *Coll Antropol.* 2004;28(2):221–226.
5. Wyler A, Bousson V, Bergot C, et al. Comparison of MR-arthrography and CT-arthrography in hyaline cartilage-thickness measurement in radiographically normal cadaver hips with anatomy as gold standard. *Osteoarthritis Cartilage.* 2009;17(1):19–25. https://doi.org/10.1016/j.joca.2008.05.015.
6. Affatato S. Chapter 4: Contemporary designs in total hip arthroplasty (THA). In: Affatato S, ed. *Perspectives in Total Hip Arthroplasty: Advances in Biomaterials and Their Tribological Interactions.* 1st ed. Woodhead Publishing; 2014:46–64. https://doi.org/10.1533/9781782420392.1.46.
7. Ulici V, Chen AF, Cheng AWM, Tuan RS. In: McCarthy JC, Noble PC, Villar RN, eds. *Hip Joint Restoration: Worldwide Advances in Arthroscopy, Arthroplasty, Osteotomy and Joint Preservation Surgery.* New York: Springer Science and Business Media; 2017:15–22. https://search.library.wisc.edu/catalog/9912285143602121.
8. Wagner FV, Negrão JR, Campos J, et al. Capsular ligaments of the hip: anatomic, histologic, and positional study in cadaveric specimens with MR arthrography. *Radiology.* 2012;263(1):189–198. https://doi.org/10.1148/radiol.12111320.
9. Martin HD, Savage A, Braly BA, Palmer IJ, Beall DP, Kelly B. The function of the hip capsular ligaments: a quantitative report. *Arthroscopy.* 2008;24(2):188–195. https://doi.org/10.1016/j.arthro.2007.08.024.
10. Fuss FK, Bacher A. New aspects of the morphology and function of the human hip joint ligaments. *Am J Anat.* 1991;192(1):1–13. https://doi.org/10.1002/aja.1001920102.
11. Hewitt JD, Glisson RR, Guilak F, Vail TP. The mechanical properties of the human hip capsule ligaments. *J Arthroplasty.* 2002;17(1):82–89. https://doi.org/10.1054/arth.2002.27674.
12. Ito H, Song Y, Lindsey DP, Safran MR, Giori NJ. The proximal hip joint capsule and the zona orbicularis contribute to hip joint stability in distraction. *J Orthop Res.* 2009;27(8):989–995. https://doi.org/10.1002/jor.20852.
13. Field RE, Rajakulendran K. The labro-acetabular complex. *J Bone Joint Surg Am.* 2011;93(Suppl. 2):22–27. https://doi.org/10.2106/JBJS.J.01710.
14. Kalhor M, Beck M, Huff TW, Ganz R. Capsular and pericapsular contributions to acetabular and femoral head perfusion. *J Bone Joint Surg Am.* 2009;91(2):409–418. https://doi.org/10.2106/JBJS.G.01679.
15. Kelly BT, Shapiro GS, Digiovanni CW, Buly RL, Potter HG, Hannafin JA. Vascularity of the hip labrum: a cadaveric investigation. *Arthroscopy.* 2005;21(1):3–11. https://doi.org/10.1016/j.arthro.2004.09.016.
16. McCarthy J, Noble P, Aluisio FV, Schuck M, Wright J, Lee J. Anatomy, pathologic features, and treatment of acetabular labral tears. *Clin Orthop Relat Res.* 2003;406:38–47. https://doi.org/10.1097/01.blo.0000043042.84315.17.
17. Tucker FR. Arterial supply to the femoral head and its clinical importance. *J Bone Joint Surg Br.* 1949;31-B(1):82–93. https://doi.org/10.1302/0301-620X.31B1.82.
18. Gautier E, Ganz K, Krügel N, Ganz R. Anatomy of the medial femoral circumflex artery and its surgical implications. *J Bone Joint Surg Br.* 2000;82-B(5):679–683.
19. Birnbaum K, Prescher A, Heßler S, Heller K-D. The sensory innervation of the hip joint - an anatomical study. *Surg Radiol Anat.* 1997;19(6):371–375. https://doi.org/10.1007/BF01628504.
20. Putz R, Schrank C. Anatomy of the labro-capsular complex. *Orthopade.* 1998;27(10):675–680. https://doi.org/10.1007/s001320050286.
21. Haversath M, Hanke J, Landgraeber S, et al. The distribution of nociceptive innervation in the painful hip. *Bone Joint J.* 2013;95-B(6):770–776. https://doi.org/10.1302/0301-620X.95B6.30262.
22. Barker PJ, Hapuarachchi KS, Ross JA, Sambaiew E, Ranger TA, Briggs CA. Anatomy and biomechanics of gluteus maximus and the thoracolumbar fascia at the sacroiliac joint. *Clin Anat.* 2014;27(2):234–240. https://doi.org/10.1002/ca.22233.
23. Flack NAMS, Nicholson HD, Woodley SJ. A review of the anatomy of the hip abductor muscles, gluteus medius, gluteus minimus, and tensor fascia lata. *Clin Anat.* 2012;25(6):697–708. https://doi.org/10.1002/ca.22004.
24. Beck M, Sledge JB, Gautier E, Dora CF, Ganz R. The anatomy and function of the gluteus minimus muscle. *J Bone Joint Surg Br.* 2000;82-B(3):358–363. https://doi.org/10.1302/0301-620X.82B3.0820358.
25. Roche JJW, Jones CDS, Khan RJK, Yates PJ. The surgical anatomy of the piriformis tendon, with particular reference to total hip replacement. *Bone Joint J.* 2013;95-B(6):764–769. https://doi.org/10.1302/0301-620X.95B6.30727.

26. Lewis S, Jurak J, Lee C, Lewis R, Gest T. Anatomical variations of the sciatic nerve, in relation to the piriformis muscle. *Transl Res Anat.* 2016;5:15–19. https://doi.org/10.1016/j.tria.2016.11.001.

27. Philippon MJ, Michalski MP, Campbell KJ, et al. Surgically relevant bony and soft tissue anatomy of the proximal femur, 2325967114535188 *Orthop J Sport Med.* 2014;2(6). https://doi.org/10.1177/2325967114535188.

28. Standring S. *Gray's Anatomy: The Anatomical Basis of Clinical Practice.* 2016.

29. Robbins CE. Anatomy and biomechanics. In: *Hip Handbook.* Boston, MA: Butterworth-Heinemann; 1998: 1–37.

30. Andersson E, Oddsson L, Grundstrom H, Thorstensson A. The role of the psoas and iliacus muscles for stability and movement of the lumbar spine, pelvis and hip. *Scand J Med Sci Sports.* 1995;5(1):10–16. https://doi.org/10.1111/j.1600-0838.1995.tb00004.x.

31. Babst D, Steppacher SD, Ganz R, Siebenrock KA, Tannast M. The iliocapsularis muscle: an important stabilizer in the dysplastic hip. *Clin Orthop Relat Res.* 2011; 469(6):1728–1734. https://doi.org/10.1007/s11999-010-1705-x.

32. Ward WT, Fleisch ID, Ganz R. Anatomy of the iliocapsularis muscle. Relevance to surgery of the hip. *Clin Orthop Relat Res.* 2000;374:278–285. https://doi.org/10.1097/00003086-200005000-00025.

33. Marshall JL, Girgis FG, Zelko RR. The biceps femoris tendon and its functional significance. *J Bone Joint Surg Am.* 1972;54(7):1444–1450.

34. Ilizaliturri VM, Mangino G, Valero FS, Camacho-Galindo J. Hip arthroscopy of the central and peripheral compartments by the lateral approach. *Tech Orthop.* 2005;20(1): 32–36. https://doi.org/10.1097/01.bto.0000152167.94084.94.

35. Dienst M. Chapter 11 - Peripheral compartment approach to hip arthroscopy. In: Sekiya JK, Safran MR, Ranawat AS, eds. *Leunig MBT-T in HA and JPS.* Philadelphia: W.B. Saunders; 2011:105–112. https://doi.org/10.1016/B978-1-4160-5642-3.00011-6.

36. Grant AD, Sala DA, Davidovitch RI. The labrum: structure, function, and injury with femoro-acetabular impingement. *J Child Orthop.* 2012;6(5):357–372. https://doi.org/10.1007/s11832-012-0431-1.

37. Tan V, Seldes RM, Katz MA, Freedhand AM, Klimkiewicz JJ, Fitzgerald RHJ. Contribution of acetabular labrum to articulating surface area and femoral head coverage in adult hip joints: an anatomic study in cadavera. *Am J Orthop (Belle Mead NJ).* 2001;30(11):809–812.

38. Weber W, Weber E. Ueber die Mechanik der menschlichen Gehwerkzeuge, nebst der Beschreibung eines Versuchs über das Herausfallen des Schenkelkopfs aus der Pfanne im luftverdünnten Raume. *Ann Phys.* 1837;116(1):1–13. https://doi.org/10.1002/andp.18371160102.

39. Wingstrand H, Wingstrand A, Krantz P. Intracapsular and atmospheric pressure in the dynamics and stability of the hip. A biomechanical study. *Acta Orthop Scand.* 1990; 61(3):231–235. https://doi.org/10.3109/17453679900 8993506.

40. Safran MR. The acetabular labrum: anatomic and functional characteristics and rationale for surgical intervention. *J Am Acad Orthop Surg.* 2010;18(6):338–345. https://doi.org/10.5435/00124635-201006000-00006.

41. Bardakos NV, Villar RN. The ligamentum teres of the adult hip. *J Bone Joint Surg Br.* 2009;91-B(1):8–15. https://doi.org/10.1302/0301-620X.91B1.21421.

42. Cerezal L, Kassarjian A, Canga A, et al. Anatomy, biomechanics, imaging, and management of ligamentum teres injuries. *Radiographics.* 2010;30(6):1637–1651. https://doi.org/10.1148/rg.306105516.

43. Wettstein M, Dienst M. Arthroscopy of the peripheral compartment of the hip. *Operat Tech Orthop.* 2005;15(3): 225–230. https://doi.org/10.1053/j.oto.2005.07.003.

44. Philippon MJ, Schenker ML, Briggs KK, Kuppersmith DA, Maxwell RB, Stubbs AJ. Revision hip arthroscopy. *Am J Sports Med.* 2007;35(11):1918–1921. https://doi.org/10.1177/0363546507305097.

45. Draovitch P, Edelstein J, Kelly BT. The layer concept: utilization in determining the pain generators, pathology and how structure determines treatment. *Curr Rev Musculoskelet Med.* 2012;5(1):1–8. https://doi.org/10.1007/s12178-011-9105-8.

46. Bedi A, Dolan M, Leunig M, Kelly BT. Static and dynamic mechanical causes of hip pain. *YJARS.* 2019;27(2): 235–251. https://doi.org/10.1016/j.arthro.2010.07.022.

47. Ferguson SJ, Bryant JT, Ganz R, Ito K. An in vitro investigation of the acetabular labral seal in hip joint mechanics. *J Biomech.* 2003;36(2):171–178. https://doi.org/10.1016/S0021-9290(02)00365-2.

48. Kim YT, Azuma H. The nerve endings of the acetabular labrum. *Clin Orthop Relat Res.* 1995;320:176–181.

49. Casartelli NC, Maffiuletti NA, Item-Glatthorn JF, et al. Hip muscle weakness in patients with symptomatic femoroacetabular impingement. *Osteoarthritis Cartilage.* 2011;19(7):816–821. https://doi.org/10.1016/j.joca.2011.04.001.

50. Martin HD, Reddy M, Gomez-Hoyos J. Deep gluteal syndrome. *J Hip Preserv Surg.* 2015;2(2):99–107. https://doi.org/10.1093/jhps/hnv029.

51. Torres A, Fernandez-Fairen M, Sueiro-Fernandez J. Greater trochanteric pain syndrome and gluteus medius and minimus tendinosis: nonsurgical treatment. *Pain Manag.* 2018; 8(1):45–55. https://doi.org/10.2217/pmt-2017-0033.

52. Kagan 2nd A. Rotator cuff tears of the hip. *Clin Orthop Relat Res.* 1999;368:135–140.

53. Allen, Cope. Coxa saltans: the snapping hip revisited. *J Am Acad Orthop Surg.* 1995;3(5):303–308. https://doi.org/10.5435/00124635-199509000-00006.

54. Fabricant PD, Bedi A, De La Torre K, Kelly BT. Clinical outcomes after arthroscopic psoas lengthening: the effect of femoral version. *Arthroscopy.* 2012;28(7):965–971. https://doi.org/10.1016/j.arthro.2011.11.028.

55. Orava S, Kujala UM. Rupture of the ischial origin of the hamstring muscles. *Am J Sports Med.* 1995;23(6):702−705. https://doi.org/10.1177/036354659502300612.

56. Talathi N, LaValva S, Lopez-Garib A, Kelly 4th JD, Khoury V. Correlation between femoroacetabular impingement and hamstring tendon pathology on magnetic resonance imaging and arthrography. *Orthopedics.* 2017;40(6):e1086−e1091. https://doi.org/10.3928/01477447-20171020-04.

57. Hammoud S, Bedi A, Magennis E, Meyers WC, Kelly BT. High incidence of athletic pubalgia symptoms in professional athletes with symptomatic femoroacetabular impingement. *Arthroscopy.* 2012;28(10):1388−1395. https://doi.org/10.1016/j.arthro.2012.02.024.

58. Fabry G, MacEwen GD, Shands ARJ. Torsion of the femur. A follow-up study in normal and abnormal conditions. *J Bone Joint Surg Am.* 1973;55(8):1726−1738.

59. Reikeras O, Bjerkreim I, Kolbenstvedt A. Anteversion of the acetabulum and femoral neck in normals and in patients with osteoarthritis of the hip. *Acta Orthop Scand.* 1983;54(1):18−23. https://doi.org/10.3109/17453678308992864.

60. Klasan A, Neri T, Sommer C, et al. Analysis of acetabular version: retroversion prevalence, age, side and gender correlations. *J Orthop Transl.* 2019;18:7−12. https://doi.org/10.1016/j.jot.2019.01.003.

61. Tonnis D, Heinecke A. Acetabular and femoral anteversion: relationship with osteoarthritis of the hip. *J Bone Joint Surg Am.* 1999;81(12):1747−1770. https://doi.org/10.2106/00004623-199912000-00014.

62. Roach KE, Miles TP. Normal hip and knee active range of motion: the relationship to age. *Phys Ther.* 1991;71(9):656−665. https://doi.org/10.1093/ptj/71.9.656.

63. Bergmann G, Deuretzbacher G, Heller M, et al. Hip contact forces and gait patterns from routine activities. *J Biomech.* 2001;34(7):859−871. https://doi.org/10.1016/S0021-9290(01)00040-9.

64. Rydell N. Biomechanics of the hip-joint. *Clin Orthop Relat Res.* 1973;92. https://journals.lww.com/clinorthop/Fulltext/1973/05000/Biomechanics_of_the_Hip_Joint.3.aspx.

65. Bergmann G, Graichen F, Rohlmann A. Hip joint loading during walking and running, measured in two patients. *J Biomech.* 1993;26(8):969−990. https://doi.org/10.1016/0021-9290(93)90058-m.

66. Kadaba MP, Ramakrishnan HK, Wootten ME, Gainey J, Gorton G, Cochran GV. Repeatability of kinematic, kinetic, and electromyographic data in normal adult gait. *J Orthop Res.* 1989;7(6):849−860. https://doi.org/10.1002/jor.1100070611.

67. Johnston RC, Smidt GL. Measurement of hip-joint motion during walking. Evaluation of an electrogoniometric method. *J Bone Joint Surg Am.* 1969;51(6):1082−1094.

68. Murray MP, Kory RC, Sepic SB. Walking patterns of normal women. *Arch Phys Med Rehabil.* 1970;51(11):637−650.

69. Perry J. *Gait Analysis: Normal and Pathological Function.* Thorofare, NJ: Slack, Incorporated.; 1992.

70. Nordin M, Frankel V. In: Nordin M, Frankel V, eds. *Biomechanics of the Hip.* Philadelphia, PA: Lippincott Williams and Wilkins; 2001.

71. Williams DS, Martin AE. Gait modification when decreasing double support percentage. *J Biomech.* 2019;92:76−83. https://doi.org/10.1016/j.jbiomech.2019.05.028.

72. Murray MP, Drought AB, Kory RC. Walking patterns of normal men. *J Bone Joint Surg Am.* 1964;46:335−360.

73. Mann RA, Hagy J. Biomechanics of walking, running, and sprinting. *Am J Sports Med.* 1980;8(5):345−350. https://doi.org/10.1177/036354658000800510.

74. Nicola T, Jewison D. The anatomy and biomechanics of running. *Clin Sports Med.* 2012;31:187−201. https://doi.org/10.1016/j.csm.2011.10.001.

75. Oberg T, Karsznia A, Oberg K. Basic gait parameters: reference data for normal subjects, 10-79 years of age. *J Rehabil Res Dev.* 1993;30(2):210−223.

76. Richard R, Weber J, Mejjad O, et al. Spatiotemporal gait parameters measured using the Bessou gait analyzer in 79 healthy subjects. Influence of age, stature, and gender. Study Group on Disabilities due to Musculoskeletal Disorders (Groupe de Recherche sur le Handicap de l'Appareil Locomoteu. *Rev Rhum Engl Ed.* 1995;62(2):105−114.

77. Kerrigan DC, Todd MK, Della Croce U. Gender differences in joint biomechanics during walking: normative study in young adults. *Am J Phys Med Rehabil.* 1998;77(1):2−7. https://doi.org/10.1097/00002060-199801000-00002.

78. Associations NF of SHS. *2017-18 High School Athletics Participation Survey;* 2018. https://www.nfhs.org/media/1020205/2017-18_hs_participation_survey.pdf.

79. Leanderson C, Leanderson J, Wykman A, Strender L-E, Johansson S-E, Sundquist K. Musculoskeletal injuries in young ballet dancers. *Knee Surg Sports Traumatol Arthrosc.* 2011;19(9):1531−1535. https://doi.org/10.1007/s00167-011-1445-9.

80. Evans RW, Evans RI, Carvajal S, Perry S. A survey of injuries among Broadway performers. *Am J Public Health.* 1996;86(1):77−80. https://doi.org/10.2105/ajph.86.1.77.

81. Ojofeitimi S, Bronner S, Woo H. Injury incidence in hip hop dance. *Scand J Med Sci Sports.* 2012;22(3):347−355. https://doi.org/10.1111/j.1600-0838.2010.01173.x.

82. Dubravcic-Simunjak S, Pecina M, Kuipers H, Moran J, Haspl M. The incidence of injuries in elite junior figure skaters. *Am J Sports Med.* 2003;31(4):511−517. https://doi.org/10.1177/03635465030310040601.

83. Trentacosta N, Sugimoto D, Micheli LJ. Hip and groin injuries in dancers: a systematic review. *Sports Health.* 2017;9(5):422−427. https://doi.org/10.1177/1941738117724159.

84. Weber AE, Bedi A, Tibor LM, Zaltz I, Larson CM. The hyperflexible hip: managing hip pain in the dancer and gymnast. *Sports Health.* 2015;7(4):346−358. https://doi.org/10.1177/1941738114532431.

85. Brown HC, Kelly BT, Padgett DE. Hip arthroscopy in the professional dancer. In: *AAOS Annu Meet.* Podium; 2011:642.

86. Loder RT, Skopelja EN. The epidemiology and demographics of hip dysplasia. *ISRN Orthop.* 2011;2011: 238607. https://doi.org/10.5402/2011/238607.

87. Kraeutler MJ, Garabekyan T, Pascual-Garrido C, Mei-Dan O. Hip instability: a review of hip dysplasia and other contributing factors. *Muscles Ligaments Tendons J.* 2016; 6(3):343—353. https://doi.org/10.11138/mltj/2016.6.3.343.

88. Pfirrmann CWA, Mengiardi B, Dora C, Kalberer F, Zanetti M, Hodler J. Cam and pincer femoroacetabular impingement: characteristic MR arthrographic findings in 50 patients. *Radiology.* 2006;240(3):778—785. https://doi.org/10.1148/radiol.2403050767.

89. Leunig M, Juni P, Werlen S, et al. Prevalence of cam and pincer-type deformities on hip MRI in an asymptomatic young Swiss female population: a cross-sectional study. *Osteoarthritis Cartilage.* 2013;21(4):544—550. https://doi.org/10.1016/j.joca.2013.01.003.

90. Quatman CE, Ford KR, Myer GD, Paterno MV, Hewett TE. The effects of gender and pubertal status on generalized joint laxity in young athletes. *J Sci Med Sport.* 2008;11(3): 257—263. https://doi.org/10.1016/j.jsams.2007.05.005.

91. Shibata KR, Matsuda S, Safran MR. Arthroscopic hip surgery in the elite athlete: comparison of female and male competitive athletes. *Am J Sports Med.* 2017;45(8): 1730—1739. https://doi.org/10.1177/0363546517697296.

92. Johnson AW, Weiss CBJ, Stento K, Wheeler DL. Stress fractures of the sacrum. An atypical cause of low back pain in the female athlete. *Am J Sports Med.* 2001;29(4):498—508. https://doi.org/10.1177/03635465010290042001.

93. Hosey RG, Fernandez MMF, Johnson DL. Evaluation and management of stress fractures of the pelvis and sacrum. *Orthopedics.* 2008;31(4):383—385. https://doi.org/10.3928/01477447-20080401-14.

94. Boden BP, Speer KP. Femoral stress fractures. *Clin Sports Med.* 1997;16(2):307—317. https://doi.org/10.1016/S0278-5919(05)70024-7.

95. Feingold D, Hame SL. Female athlete triad and stress fractures. *Orthop Clin.* 2006;37(4):575—583. https://doi.org/10.1016/j.ocl.2006.09.005.

96. Cibulka MT. Determination and significance of femoral neck anteversion. *Phys Ther.* 2004;84(6):550—558. https://doi.org/10.1093/ptj/84.6.550.

97. Rutkowska-Kucharska A, Szpala A, Jaroszczuk S, Sobera M. Muscle coactivation during stability exercises in rhythmic gymnastics: a two-case study. *Appl Bionics Biomech.* 2018; 2018:8260402. https://doi.org/10.1155/2018/8260402.

98. Larson CM, Kelly BT, Stone RM. Making a case for anterior inferior iliac spine/subspine hip impingement: three representative case reports and proposed concept. *Arthroscopy.* 2011;27 (12):1732—1737. https://doi.org/10.1016/j.arthro.2011.10.004.

CHAPTER 10

Nonarthritic Hip Pathology

HANNAH L. BRADSELL, BS • KATHERINE C. BRANCHE, MD •
RACHEL M. FRANK, MD

INTRODUCTION

Due to the high loads received by the hip joint during walking and running, the hip and its surrounding structures are prone to numerous pathologies with varying degrees of severity. In a population of participants 65 years and older, near 20% had self-reported hip pain that consequently impacted their overall health such that without these symptoms, their average general health status would be similar to people under 65 years of age.[1] Hip pathology is especially prominent in the athletic population due to the additional forces experienced by the hip during high-impact sports-related activities. According to a recent study by Kerbel et al.[2] athletes participating in soccer, ice hockey, and running are among the most at risk for hip injuries and disorders that can occur as a result of acute trauma or overuse or as gradual onsets.

The more widely researched conditions, and much of our understanding of hip pathologies, are associated with intra-articular pathologies and arthritic disorders. There are, however, many abnormalities that contribute to significant hip pain, which exist outside these types of lesions. An important part of treating patients with hip pain is to consider the local and surrounding factors, including nervous, osteoligamentous, tendinous, and muscular structures.[3] Properly diagnosing and understanding hip pathology can be difficult because of its complex nature and the tendency for conditions to be concomitant and symptoms to overlap, but it is crucial nonetheless. This chapter will focus on the recognition and management of extra-articular hip pathologies.

STRUCTURAL AND FUNCTIONAL ANATOMY

The hip joint plays a key role in movement, stability in facilitating weight-bearing, and dynamic support for the body. It is composed of a system of interactions between the skeleton and the surrounding soft connective tissue. A ball-and-socket joint is formed by the articulation of the femoral head and the acetabulum, which is formed by the ischium, ilium, and pubis bones. The acetabulum encompasses the entire head of the femur allowing for movement along three major axes.[4] For support, the hip labrum and a group of superficial and deep ligaments form a fibrous capsulolabral structure, which restricts translation at the femoroacetabular articulation while still allowing for complex rotation and planar movements.[5,6] The movements permitted by the hip are flexion, extension, adduction, abduction, external rotation, and internal rotation. Some of the major muscles that provide these movements include the iliopsoas (hip flexion), the hamstring muscles (extension), the adductor muscles (adduction), and the gluteus maximus (extension and external rotation), minimus (abduction and internal rotation), and medius (abduction) muscles.[7] Overall, there are 22 muscles providing stability and the forces necessary for movement, which can be divided by their anatomic positioning or their actions.[8]

Based on the pathways of nerves through the hip and thigh regions, most intra-articular pathologies elicit pain that radiates to the anterior and medial hip (i.e., groin), whereas extra-articular conditions typically cause pain rotating to the posterior and lateral aspect of the hip.[7] However, intra-articular pathology can certainly cause posterior and/or laterally based hip pain, and clinicians must be aware of atypical sources of hip pain when evaluating patients, particularly females.

Key anatomic structures within and around the hip and groin area include several bursae, which are fluid-filled sacs that function to cushion the joint area.[9] These bursae include the trochanteric bursa on the lateral side of the hip as well as the iliopsoas bursa, found in the anteromedial aspect of the hip and thigh. Inflammation of these sacs, called bursitis, can be caused by several different conditions and represents a common

The Female Athlete. https://doi.org/10.1016/B978-0-323-75985-4.00023-4

TABLE 10.1 Summary of Nonarthritic Pathologies.	
Anterior hip	• Internal snapping hip • Iliopsoas tendinitis • Rectus femoris tendinosis • Athletic pubalgia • Osteitis pubis • Femoral neck and pubic rami stress fractures • Femoral, obturator, iliolingual, and genitofemoral neuropathy
Lateral hip	• Greater trochanteric bursitis • Greater trochanteric pain syndrome • Gluteal tendinopathy • Gluteal tears (tendon and muscle) • Iliotibial band syndrome • External snapping hip • Meralgia paresthetica (lateral femoral cutaneous neuropathy) • Iliohypogastric neuropathy
Posterior hip	• Sacroiliac joint dysfunction • Sacral stress fracture • Hip extensor or rotator muscle strain • Proximal hamstring rupture • Proximal hamstring tendinopathy (proximal hamstring syndrome) • Avulsion fracture of the ischial tuberosity • Piriformis syndrome • Ischiofemoral impingement • Sciatic and pudendal compression (deep gluteal syndrome)

extra-articular pathology that is a source of hip pain. In addition, injuries to the thigh muscles that generate hip movement, including strains and tears, as well as lumbar spine conditions, can often be causes of the referred hip pain.[7] Furthermore, stress fractures about the hip and dysfunction in the surrounding joints, such as the sacroiliac (SI) joint, are all among the various nonarthritic hip pathologies that lead to hip pain.[7,9] Table 10.1 provides a summary of the nonarthritic and extra-articular hip pathologies to be discussed in the subsequent sections of this chapter, which are organized by anatomic location.

ANTERIOR HIP PATHOLOGY

Anterior hip pain tends to localize to the anteromedial thigh and can result from various nonarthritic and extra-articular pathologies within the surrounding areas. Internal snapping hip is a condition found more frequently in athletes and female patients that results in a deep pain and clicking sensation within the anterior groin during hip flexion and can be caused by either acute trauma or overuse.[10] It is characterized by

the iliopsoas tendon snapping over the iliopectineal eminence, femoral head, or the lesser trochanter due to repetitive flexion and external rotation.[10,11] Frequently associated with snapping hip, although relatively uncommon, is iliopsoas tendonitis and iliopsoas bursitis. As the affected regions are so close, these conditions are interrelated due to the observation that inflammation of one can result in inflammation of the other.[12] The key symptoms of iliopsoas tendonitis are anterior groin pain while climbing stairs and getting in and out of a car, and clinical indications include anterior groin pain during active hip flexion or passive hip extension.[13] The most frequent source of this condition appears to be after a total hip arthroplasty, although the exact cause is inconclusive. The psoas and iliac muscles join to form a strong flexor and weak external rotator of the hip, and the iliopsoas tendon inserts into the lesser trochanter and is bordered by the iliopsoas bursa overlying the hip joint capsule.[14] Along the tendon tract, prior to its insertion at the lesser trochanter, is the anterior edge of the acetabulum, the convex surface of the femoral head, and the overlying anterior capsule. As stated by O'Sullivan et al.[14] any deviation from this system can generate inflammation and thus tendonitis, which is one plausible explanation for iliopsoas tendonitis occurring from mechanical faults during a total hip arthroplasty. The authors also suggest that anatomic variations and osteophytes along the anterior femoral neck can be related factors that may cause this condition. In addition to the iliopsoas, the rectus femoris is a muscle responsible for hip flexion and can be a cause of anterior hip pain. Notably in 2018, Kaya et al.[15] studied the impact of extra-articular pathologies in a cohort of patients with anterior hip pain and found that tendinosis of the direct head of the rectus femoris muscle was common.

In a condition known as athletic pubalgia, also referred to as "inguinal disruption" or "sports hernia," the pubic symphysis is disrupted producing activity-related lower abdominal, deep inguinal, and/or groin pain.[3,16] This condition is a common extra-articular referral source of anterior hip pain and most often occurs as a result of injuries in athletes participating in activities that require rapid changes in direction and speed, specifically twisting at the waist while running and sideways movement.[3,16,17] As described by Battaglia et al.[3] the rectus abdominis and adductor longus tendons merge at the pubic symphysis and form an aponeurotic plate. The tearing of these tissues and the adjacent oblique aponeuroses, as well as the widening and erosion of the pubic symphysis, called osteitis pubis, produces athletic pubalgia. Furthermore, as summarized by Le and colleagues,[16] other proposed mechanisms leading to this condition include ilioinguinal or genitofemoral nerve entrapment, musculotendinous strain of the adductor, and other various involvements of the adductor muscles. Overall, the authors concluded that it is likely a multifactorial process caused by a combination of multiple anatomic and physiologic disruptions. Overlapping with athletic pubalgia is osteitis pubis, which is a chronic inflammatory state of the pubic symphysis and the surrounding soft tissue causing debilitating anterior and medial groin pain and is common in athletes.[18] This pain is exacerbated by rapid hip flexion from an extended position, such as kicking, or standing from a seated position.[18] It can result from microtrauma and altered biomechanics leading to instability, as seen in overuse injuries, caused by repetitive muscle strains and stress forces on the pubis symphysis from the rectus abdominis and adductor muscles that act antagonistically.[19] Distinguishing between athletic pubalgia and osteitis pubis can be difficult because of their many similarities, but as summarized by Dirkx and Vitale,[18] osteitis pubis can typically be separated by pain that is prompted by direct palpation over the pubis symphysis and by direct pressure laterally on the ramus. This condition may also be referred to as pubic symphysis stress injury owing to the overuse nature of the injury.[20]

In sports medicine, stress fractures are a common injury that are more often experienced by female patients, and a portion of these stress fractures occur in the hip region. Stress fractures that cause anteromedial hip and groin pain most frequently occur at the femoral neck and pubic rami.[9] As with all stress fractures, these are typically overuse injuries that are caused by repeated strain without proper recovery time. More specifically, as indicated by Paluska et al.[9] they can originate from abnormal forces on a normal bone (fatigue fracture) or from normal forces on an abnormal bone (insufficiency fracture). Femoral neck stress fractures cause pain that worsens with weight-bearing and motion, particularly internal rotation, and are common in runners. There are two types of femoral neck stress fractures: tension type and compression type.[21] Tension-type fractures are located on the superolateral aspect of the neck and have the highest risk for a complete fracture and other complications. Compression-type fractures involve the inferomedial aspect of the femoral neck, may be managed more conservatively, and tend to be common in younger athletes. Femoral neck stress fractures can be detected by pain, which is elicited with activity or at night.[3] Physical signs and symptoms, including swelling, may occur but are less common. These fractures must be recognized and quickly treated to avoid the disastrous outcome of a displaced femoral neck fracture. A pubic ramus stress fracture is also a low-risk fracture that occurs at the junction of the ischium and inferior pubic ramus and is most likely caused by excessive contraction of the muscles that attach at the pubis.[20,21] This type of stress fracture is characterized by a gradual onset and increase in pain that is worsened by activity and can lead to the pain persisting at rest.[20] Furthermore, point tenderness over the area is common and pain with standing on the fractured leg or the inability to stand unsupported on the affected side is frequently associated with stress fractures of the pubic rami.[20]

Anterior hip pain can also be a result of several neuropathies, with femoral nerve pathology being the most often described cause. In 2013, Martinoli and colleagues[22] provided descriptions of peripheral nerve paths based on diagnostic imaging in studying chronic hip pain and disability caused by neuropathies. The authors noted that neuropathic conditions occur as a result of mechanical or dynamic compression of a segment of a nerve within an osteofibrous tunnel, a fibrous structure opening, or a passageway close to a ligament or muscle.[22] The femoral nerve has both motor and sensory components and is the largest branch of the lumbar plexus, originating from L2 to L4. The nerve continues down through the psoas muscle to its lower lateral border where it passes down the iliacus muscle, exits the pelvis beneath the inguinal ligament, crosses a rigid osteofibrous tunnel next to the iliopsoas tendon, and then branches in the thigh.[22] Femoral neuropathy causes weakness in hip flexion and knee extension related to the iliopsoas and quadriceps femoris, respectively. Less studied are neuropathies of the obturator, iliolingual, and genitofemoral nerves as causes of anterior hip pain. However, their mechanisms of producing pain can be similar to the aforementioned description provided by Martinoli et al.[22] and are similarly related to their respective nerve tracts, with various causes typically revolved around concomitant injuries and postoperative complications.[23]

LATERAL HIP PATHOLOGY

Greater trochanteric bursitis (GTB) is a condition characterized by pain over the lateral aspect of the hip that may radiate to the lateral thigh and/or lower buttocks.[24] It is typically an aching, chronic pain triggered by various activities including prolonged standing, running, and external rotation and abduction of the hip. It can also present as a sharp pain that is directly related to pressure over the greater trochanteric bursa. This condition and its related symptoms can be caused by irritation of the bursae surrounding the greater trochanter, particularly the three constant bursae: the gluteus minimus bursa, the subgluteus medius bursa, and the subgluteus maximus bursa. Overall, GTB can be caused by acute trauma or, more frequently, repeated microtrauma related to active use of the muscles that insert on the greater trochanter, which cause degenerative changes in tendons, muscles, and fibrous tissue.[24] Interestingly, Zibis and colleagues[25] reported in 2018 that females were more likely to experience GTB than males. Related to GTB is the greater trochanteric pain syndrome (GTPS), which refers more generally to pain in the lateral hip caused by various structures, in addition to bursae, such as tendons.[26] Associated conditions include gluteus medius and minimus tendinopathy, gluteal tears, iliotibial band (ITB) syndrome, and external snapping hip.[3,26–28] In 2013, Long et al.[29] reported that in a population of 877 patients with GTPS, 49.9% had gluteal tendinopathy, 28.5% had ITB syndrome characterized by thickening, 20.2% had trochanteric bursitis, and 0.5% had gluteal tears.

Gluteal tendinopathy refers to tendinopathy of the gluteus medius and/or minimus tendons resulting in local tenderness and pain over the greater trochanter that may radiate into the lateral thigh to the level of the knee.[3,30] The pain may be described as a burning or deep, dull ache that is worsened by hip abduction, prolonged sitting, side-lying positons, and climbing stairs.[3] The most significant factors in the pathomechanics of this disorder include excessive static and dynamic hip adduction, which leads to a compressive tendon loading, combined with interactions between joint position and bone and muscle factors.[31] The most damaging effects on the tendon are high tensile loads and excessive compression, which results in a net catabolic effect on the tendon.[31]

As gluteal tendinopathy can coexist with other disorders and mimic the symptoms of other causes of lateral hip pain, Grimaldi et al.[30] performed a study in 2016 to determine valid clinical tests for the diagnosis gluteal tendinopathy. The authors found that patients who experienced both pain on palpation of the greater trochanter (80% sensitivity) and lateral hip pain within 30 s of single-leg standing (100% specificity) were likely to have gluteal tendinopathy. Combining these two types of clinical tests provided the greatest accuracy in properly diagnosing gluteal tendinopathy. Gluteal tendon tears have also been reported as a cause of lateral hip pathology and have similar symptoms as the aforementioned conditions. They more commonly occur from degenerative processes, similar to the development of a rotator cuff tear in the shoulder, but can happen after trauma and result in an aching pain that radiates down the outside of the thigh with tenderness over the greater trochanter, a positive result of Trendelenburg test, and/or pain on resisted external rotation or abduction.[32] Although less common, gluteus medius muscle (as opposed to tendon) tears can also cause lateral hip pain.[33]

The ITB is a key component in extension, abduction, and lateral rotation of the hip.[34] ITB syndrome is a common overuse injury that predominately causes pain in the lateral knee, but it can sometimes trigger lateral hip pain with or without snapping during activity.[35,36] It is also common at the lateral hip for abnormal ITB anatomy and kinematics to be associated with pain, tenderness, or weakness.[37] Similarly, proximal ITB thickening at the greater trochanter level has been frequently observed in patients with lateral hip pain correlated to GTPS.[3] Closely related to ITB syndrome is the external snapping hip syndrome, which occurs with the forward abrupt movement of the ITB over the greater trochanter with hip motion, particularly hip flexion or extension.[3,34] Often accompanying the sudden snapping, or the translocation of the ITB, is pain caused by repeated rubbing that may reflect tendonitis or bursitis.[34] It appears that hip weakness may cause increasing friction between the ITB and the greater trochanter, and ITB thickening contributes to the snapping hip syndrome.[37] Rarely, external snapping hip can occur via a different mechanism, when the distal gluteus maximus rolls over the greater trochanter, or from the passive movement of an adducted and internally rotated hip to flexion and external rotation.[34]

Peripheral neuropathy, particularly that involves the lateral femoral cutaneous and the iliohypogastric nerves, can also be a cause of lateral hip pain. Entrapment of the lateral femoral cutaneous nerve at the ilioinguinal ligament is called meralgia paresthetica and typically causes burning pain, muscle aches, paresthesias, and sensory loss within the tract of the lateral femoral cutaneous nerve, over the lateral or anterolateral aspect of the thigh.[3,38,39] According to Pearce,[39] it is distinguished from radiculopathy, as motor strength and the knee jerk reflex are preserved. Symptoms may be triggered by prolonged standing or sitting with the thigh extended due to the increased tension and angulation of the nerve. On the contrary, symptoms are improved with flexion of the thigh on the pelvis as this decreases the forces acting on the nerve.[39] The lateral femoral cutaneous nerve originates from L2 and L3 of the lumbar spine and emerges at the lateral border of the psoas major, crosses the iliacus to the anterior superior iliac spine, and then passes under the inguinal ligament and over the sartorius muscle, where it then enters the thigh.[38] Despite the reported variations in the course of the nerve after exiting the pelvis, the compression of the nerve observed in meralgia paresthetica most often occurs as it exits.[38] This condition can have a diverse set of causes that have been previously summarized by Cheatham and colleagues in a literature review.[38] They include mechanical factors, metabolic factors, and postsurgical complications after hip replacement and spine surgery. Iliohypogastric neuropathy is characterized by sensory abnormalities along the superolateral gluteal region, directly posterior to the greater trochanter, and tension occurs during extension and adduction of the hip, similar to the lateral femoral cutaneous nerve, with additional trunk extension and lateral bending.[3] Symptoms of iliohypogastric neuropathy are similar to those of other neuropathies and can produce pain that mimics GTPS.

POSTERIOR HIP PATHOLOGY

A common source of posterior hip pain is referred pain from pathologies of the SI joint. The SI joint and its intricate ligamentous system play a main role in stability and limiting motion in all planes of movement. The muscles that support the SI joint help deliver regional forces to the pelvic bones.[40] More specifically, the SI joint functions as a load-transferring junction between the spine and the pelvis, transmitting and dissipating truncal loads to the lower extremities while limiting rotation.[40,41] Dysfunction of this joint is not entirely understood but is described as an anatomic disruption resulting in abnormal positioning and movement (hyper- or hypomobility) of the SI joint structures, often associated with inflammation.[41,42] This pain is most commonly located near the posterior superior iliac spine and radiates to the buttock or thigh.[41] The mechanisms leading to SI joint dysfunction are typically idiopathic and can occur both acutely and gradually with cumulative trauma.[43]

Another source of posterior hip pathology is sacral stress fractures, which can be either insufficiency or fatigue fractures. Insufficiency fractures are often caused by osteoporosis, while fatigue fractures are more common in athletes who participate in prolonged periods of intense training.[44] In describing the pathophysiology of this condition, Urits et al.[45] explained that the SI joint normally relieves the torsional stress that is created around the sacrum during a normal gait as the lower extremities alternate between flexion and extension. However, pathology of the SI joint causes this mechanical load to be transferred to the sacrum, which becomes prone to injury in cases where it is unable to withstand the offloaded stress.[45] The symptoms of sacral stress fracture tend to overlap with those of SI joint dysfunction and other pathologies, making it a difficult condition to properly diagnose.[44] Sacral stress fractures often present with severe buttock, low-back, hip, groin, and/or pelvic pain with limited low-back range of motion and tenderness to palpation over the sacrum, which is reportedly the trademark physical finding of this condition.[46]

Attached at the posterior aspect of the hip are the hamstring muscles (biceps femoris, semimembranosus, and semitendinosus) responsible for extension, as well as the internal and external rotators. Tendinopathy and strains of these structures generally lead to posterior hip pain and can fall under posterior hip pathology.[7] Specific injuries involving the hamstring are known to result in posterior hip pain, including proximal hamstring ruptures and tendinopathy.[3,7] Proximal hamstring injuries are among the most common muscle and tendon injuries seen in athletes.[47] Proximal hamstring ruptures are typically caused via noncontact, high-energy injuries involving a rapid forceful hip flexion with the knee in extension and can result in one- to three-tendon avulsions.[48] A rupture may also occur after multiple repetitive incidents of hamstring strains or tendonitis, essentially the result of cumulative microtrauma.[7,48] Symptoms of a proximal hamstring rupture include a sudden onset of pain with a reported tearing or popping sensation near the ischial tuberosity region with associated ecchymoses down the thigh.[48] Furthermore, walking and sitting can be challenging due to tenderness and discomfort, and feelings of instability and muscle weakness may occur, as well as sciatica symptoms may occur in some cases.[48] Similar but less severe is proximal hamstring tendinopathy, also referred to as "proximal hamstring syndrome" or a "recurrent hamstring tear," which causes deep pain at the ischial tuberosity with or without sciatica radiating to the posterior thigh, accompanied by difficulty sitting for an extended period.[49] In addition, pain may be worsened during walking when the hamstring muscles control knee extension during hip flexion, as in the swing phase of gait.[49] Activity-related abrupt tension of the hamstring or long-term chronic strain can also lead to an avulsion fracture of the ischial tuberosity, the starting point of the hamstring muscle, in adolescent athletes.[50] The symptoms of this injury include the sudden onset of pain in the posterior thigh and hip, an abnormal gait, and an occasional "pop" sensation in the hip, with physical presentation similar to that of the aforementioned posterior hip pathologies.[50]

The piriformis muscle, primarily responsible for external rotation of the hip, runs laterally from the frontal surface of the sacrum and inserts at the greater trochanter. Piriformis syndrome is a condition caused by irritation of this muscle resulting in pain that radiates from the lower back to the buttock and thigh, mimicking sciatica symptoms because of its close proximity to the sciatic nerve.[51] As outlined by Hicks et al.[52] indications of piriformis syndrome include chronic pain in the buttock and hip area, pain when getting out of bed, inability to sit for an extended period, and pain that is worsened by hip movements. These symptoms can arise from an acute injury by forceful internal rotation of the hip, altered biomechanics due to a chronic condition, or excessive strain on the muscle from sports-related activities.[51,52] Several factors, including anatomic variations, may also increase the

risk of this condition and compression on the sciatic nerve.[51]

Other sources of posterior hip pain include disorders related to the ischiofemoral space (between the ischial tuberosity and lesser trochanter) and the quadratus femoris space (between the hamstring origin and lesser trochanter).[53] Ischiofemoral impingement is a condition characterized by posterior hip pain and quadratus femoris abnormalities caused by the narrowing of the aforementioned spaces.[54,55] The resulting pain is localized to the deep gluteal region and is typically greatest with hip extension and external rotation, particularly a worsening of pain during running or while taking larger steps due to the added narrowing between the ischial tuberosity and the lesser trochanter during extension.[54-56] Pathologies of the quadratus femoris muscle that may occur due to the impingement include edema, tears, or muscle atrophy.[54,55] Furthermore, symptoms related to sciatica are common as a result of the narrowing, and there can be tenderness directly over the ischiofemoral space.[57] Although nonspecific in relation to other posterior hip pathologies, pain may occur when in a seated position because of the posterior pressure and a snapping sensation may be felt while walking with an associated antalgic gait.[57] Interestingly, ischiofemoral impingement is considerably more common in females and occasionally occurs bilaterally.[53] Multiple studies have attempted to determine the cause of ischiofemoral impingement and quadratus femoris muscle abnormalities, but an exact cause has not been established. For example, a greater femoral neck-shaft angle has been previously reported as a factor leading to ischiofemoral or quadratus femoris space narrowing, but Gardner et al.[57] found that there is no correlation. On the other hand, Kheterpal and colleagues[53] reported a higher incidence of abductor tears and abductor muscle atrophy in patients with ischiofemoral impingement compared with controls, indicating its potential pathophysiologic role.

Encompassing many of the previously mentioned conditions is a more recently recognized disorder called deep gluteal syndrome, which is caused by sciatic or pudendal nerve compression (neuropathy) as a result of pelvic lesions.[56] In a systematic review by Park et al.[56] the authors noted that this syndrome is generally characterized by intermittent or persistent pain and/or dysaesthesia in the posterior hip, buttock, or thigh region in which pain is increased with activity involving flexion of the hip, such as walking or sitting. Other indications of deep gluteal syndrome include sustained external rotation when in a supine position and tenderness throughout the region, noting that the precise location of tenderness may suggest the specific pathology of deep gluteal syndrome that is causing the pain and other symptoms.[56] Based on the path of the sciatic nerve, its kinematic behavior, and tensions relative to knee and hip positioning, the authors denoted four main syndromes that impair the sciatic nerve, resulting in deep gluteal syndrome. The four conditions are piriformis syndrome, gemelli-obturator internus syndrome, ischiofemoral impingement syndrome, and proximal hamstring syndrome. The gemelli-obturator internus syndrome, the only disorder not previously discussed, is sciatic entrapment located at the gemelli-obturator internus complex.[56] The nerve is attached by connective tissue and runs posterior to the complex and the quadratus femoris muscle after passing the piriformis. In the variable paths of the piriformis prior to its insertion on the greater trochanter, impingement of the piriformis on the sciatic nerve can occur, especially during internal rotation, in the joining of the piriformis to differing tendons related to the gemelli-obturator internus complex.[56] Overall, posterior hip pain can be caused by impaired functioning of the structures associated with the conditions that lead to nerve entrapment, leading to deep gluteal syndrome.

SUMMARY

Numerous nonarthritic and extra-articular pathologies exist that affect the anterior, lateral, and posterior regions of the hip. The nature of these conditions includes all structures of the hip's complex anatomy, involving interactions between the nervous, muscular, and skeletal systems. Often times, multiple conditions occur simultaneously leading to frequent misdiagnoses and insufficient treatment management. Furthermore, separate pathologies can have overlapping symptoms, which emphasizes the importance of obtaining a wide range of understanding of various abnormalities in the structures of the hip. Ongoing research in imaging, testing, and treatment options allows clinicians to properly and adequately provide patients with the ability to recover and return to uninterrupted daily living.

REFERENCES

1. Dawson J, Linsell L, Zondervan K, et al. Epidemiology of hip and knee pain and its impact on overall health status in older adults. *Rheumatology*. 2004;43:497–504.
2. Kerbel YE, Smith CM, Prodromo JP, Nzeogu MI, Mulcahey MK. Epidemiology of hip and groin injuries in collegiate athletes in the United States. *Orthop J Sports Med*. 2018;6, 232596711877167.
3. Battaglia PJ, D'Angelo K, Kettner NW. Posterior, lateral, and anterior hip pain due to musculoskeletal origin: a narrative literature review of history, physical examination, and diagnostic imaging. *J Chiropr Med*. 2016;15: 281–293.
4. Gold M, Munjal A, Varacallo M. Anatomy, bony pelvis and lower limb, hip joint. In: *StatPearls*. Treasure Island (FL): StatPearls Publishing; 2020.
5. Grumet RC, Frank RM, Slabaugh MA, Virkus WW, Bush-Joseph CA, Nho SJ. Lateral hip pain in an athletic population: differential diagnosis and treatment options. *Sport Health*. 2010;2:191–196.
6. Hewitt JD, Glisson RR, Guilak F, Vail TP. The mechanical properties of the human hip capsule ligaments. *J Arthroplasty*. 2002;17:82–89.
7. Frank RM, Slabaugh MA, Grumet RC, Virkus WW, Bush-Joseph CA, Nho SJ. Posterior hip pain in an athletic population: differential diagnosis and treatment options. *Sport Health*. 2010;2:237–246.
8. Byrne DP, Mulhall KJ, Baker JF. Anatomy & biomechanics of the hip. *Open Sports Med J*. 2010;4:51–57.
9. Paluska SA. An overview of hip injuries in running. *Sports Med*. 2005;35:991–1014.
10. Khan M, Adamich J, Simunovic N, Philippon MJ, Bhandari M, Ayeni OR. Surgical management of internal snapping hip syndrome: a systematic review evaluating open and arthroscopic approaches. *Arthrosc J Arthrosc Relat Surg*. 2013;29:942–948.
11. Winston P, Awan R, Cassidy JD, Bleakney RK. Clinical examination and ultrasound of self-reported snapping hip syndrome in elite ballet dancers. *Am J Sports Med*. 2007; 35:118–126.
12. Johnston CAM, Wiley JP, Lindsay DM, Wiseman DA. Iliopsoas bursitis and tendinitis. *Sports Med*. 1998;25:271–283.
13. Ueno T, Kabata T, Kajino Y, Inoue D, Ohmori T, Tsuchiya H. Risk factors and cup protrusion thresholds for symptomatic iliopsoas impingement after total hip arthroplasty: a retrospective case-control study. *J Arthroplasty*. 2018;33:3288–3296.e3281.
14. O'Sullivan M, Tai CC, Richards S, Skyrme AD, Walter WL, Walter WK. Iliopsoas tendonitis. *J Arthroplasty*. 2007;22: 166–170.
15. Kaya M. Impact of extra-articular pathologies on groin pain: an arthroscopic evaluation. *PLoS One*. 2018;13: e0191091.
16. Le CB, Zadeh J, Ben-David K. Total extraperitoneal laparoscopic inguinal hernia repair with adductor tenotomy: a 10-year experience in the treatment of athletic pubalgia. *Surg Endosc*. 2021;35(6):2743–2749.
17. Zoga AC, Mullens FE, Meyers WC. The spectrum of MR imaging in athletic pubalgia. *Radiol Clin North Am*. 2010;48: 1179–1197.
18. Dirkx M, Vitale C. Osteitis pubis. In: *StatPearls*. Treasure Island (FL): StatPearls Publishing; 2020.
19. Angoules AG. Osteitis pubis in elite athletes: diagnostic and therapeutic approach. *World J Orthoped*. 2015;6:672.
20. Miller C, Major N, Toth A. Pelvic stress injuries in the athlete. *Sports Med*. 2003;33:1003–1012.
21. Kiel J, Kaiser K. Stress reaction and fractures. In: *StatPearls*. Treasure Island (FL): StatPearls Publishing; 2020.

22. Martinoli C, Miguel-Perez M, Padua L, Gandolfo N, Zicca A, Tagliafico A. Imaging of neuropathies about the hip. *Eur J Radiol.* 2013;82:17–26.

23. Kohan L, McKenna C, Irwin A. Ilioinguinal neuropathy. *Curr Pain Headache Rep.* 2020;24.

24. Mulford K. Greater trochanteric bursitis. *J Nurse Pract.* 2007;3:328–332.

25. Zibis AH, Mitrousias VD, Klontzas ME, et al. Great trochanter bursitis vs sciatica, a diagnostic–anatomic trap: differential diagnosis and brief review of the literature. *Eur Spine J.* 2018;27.

26. Mallow M, Nazarian LN. Greater trochanteric pain syndrome diagnosis and treatment. *Phys Med Rehabil Clin.* 2014;25:279–289.

27. Redmond JM, Chen AW, Domb BG. Greater trochanteric pain syndrome. *J Am Acad Orthop Surg.* 2016;24:231–240.

28. Lall AC, Schwarzman GR, Battaglia MR, Chen SL, Maldonado DR, Domb BG. Greater trochanteric pain syndrome: an intraoperative endoscopic classification system with pearls to surgical techniques and rehabilitation protocols. *Arthrosc Tech.* 2019;8:e889–e903.

29. Long SS, Surrey DE, Nazarian LN. Sonography of greater trochanteric pain syndrome and the rarity of primary bursitis. *Am J Roentgenol.* 2013;201:1083–1086.

30. Grimaldi A, Mellor R, Nicolson P, Hodges P, Bennell K, Vicenzino B. Utility of clinical tests to diagnose MRI-confirmed gluteal tendinopathy in patients presenting with lateral hip pain. *Br J Sports Med.* 2016;51:519–524.

31. Grimaldi A, Mellor R, Hodges P, Bennell K, Wajswelner H, Vicenzino B. Gluteal tendinopathy: a review of mechanisms, assessment and management. *Sports Med.* 2015;45:1107–1119.

32. Westacott DJ, Minns JI, Foguet P. The diagnostic accuracy of magnetic resonance imaging and ultrasonography in gluteal tendon tears - a systematic review. *Hip Int.* 2011;21:637–645.

33. Mehta P, Telhan R, Burge A, Wyss J. Atypical cause of lateral hip pain due to proximal gluteus medius muscle tear: a report of 2 cases. *PM&R.* 2015;7:1002–1006.

34. Flato R, Passanante GJ, Skalski MR, Patel DB, White EA, Matcuk GR. The iliotibial tract: imaging, anatomy, injuries, and other pathology. *Skeletal Radiol.* 2017;46:605–622.

35. Williams BS, Cohen SP. Greater trochanteric pain syndrome: a review of anatomy, diagnosis and treatment. *Anesth Analg.* 2009;108:1662–1670.

36. Fairclough J, Hayashi K, Toumi H, et al. The functional anatomy of the iliotibial band during flexion and extension of the knee: implications for understanding iliotibial band syndrome. *J Anat.* 2006;208:309–316.

37. Khoury AN, Brooke K, Helal A, et al. Proximal iliotibial band thickness as a cause for recalcitrant greater trochanteric pain syndrome. *J Hip Preserv Surg.* 2018;5:296–300.

38. Cheatham SW, Kolber MJ, Salamh PA. Meralgia paresthetica: a review of the literature. *Int J Sports Phys Ther.* 2013;8:883–893.

39. Pearce JMS. Meralgia paraesthetica (Bernhardt-Roth syndrome). *J Neurol Neurosurg Psychiatry.* 2006;77:84.

40. Cohen SP. Sacroiliac joint pain: a comprehensive review of anatomy, diagnosis, and treatment. *Anesth Analg.* 2005;101:1440–1453.

41. Prather H, Decker G, Bonnette M, et al. Hip radiograph findings in patients aged 40 years and under with posterior pelvic pain. *PM&R.* 2019;11.

42. Gusfa D, Bashir DA, Saffarian MR. Clinical pearl: diagnosing and managing sacroiliac joint pain. *Am J Phys Med Rehabil.* 2021;100(4):40–42.

43. Dreyfuss P, Dreyer SJ, Cole A, Mayo K. Sacroiliac joint pain. *J Am Acad Orthop Surg.* 2004;12:255–265.

44. Yoder K, Bartsokas J, Averell K, McBride E, Long C, Cook C. Risk factors associated with sacral stress fractures: a systematic review. *J Man Manip Ther.* 2015;23:84–92.

45. Urits I, Orhurhu V, Callan J, et al. Sacral insufficiency fractures: a review of risk factors, clinical presentation, and management. *Curr Pain Headache Rep.* 2020;24.

46. Zaman FM, Frey ME, Slipman CW. Sacral stress fractures. *Curr Sports Med Rep.* 2006;5:37–43.

47. Fouasson-Chailloux A, Menu P, Mesland O, Dauty M. Strength assessment after proximal hamstring rupture: a critical review and analysis. *Clin Biomech.* 2020;72:44–51.

48. Lempainen L, Banke IJ, Johansson K, et al. Clinical principles in the management of hamstring injuries. *Knee Surg Sports Traumatol Arthrosc.* 2015;23:2449–2456.

49. Martin RL, Schröder RG, Gomez-Hoyos J, et al. Accuracy of 3 clinical tests to diagnose proximal hamstrings tears with and without sciatic nerve involvement in patients with posterior hip pain. *Arthrosc J Arthrosc Relat Surg.* 2018;34:114–121.

50. Liu H, Zhang Y, Rang M, et al. Avulsion fractures of the ischial tuberosity: progress of injury, mechanism, clinical manifestations, imaging examination, diagnosis and differential diagnosis and treatment. *Med Sci Monit.* 2018;24:9406–9412.

51. Albayrak A, Ozcafer R, Balioglu MB, Kargin D, Atici Y, Ermis MN. Piriformis syndrome: treatment of a rare cause of posterior hip pain with fluoroscopic-guided injection. *HIP Int.* 2015;25:172–175.

52. Hicks BL, Lam JC, Varacallo M. Piriformis syndrome. In: *StatPearls.* Treasure Island (FL): StatPearls Publishing; 2020.

53. Kheterpal AB, Harvey JP, Husseini JS, Martin SD, Torriani M, Bredella MA. Hip abductor tears in ischiofemoral impingement. *Skeletal Radiol.* 2020;49.

54. Vicentini JRT, Martinez-Salazar EL, Simeone FJ, Bredella MA, Palmer WE, Torriani M. Kinematic MRI of ischiofemoral impingement. *Skeletal Radiol.* 2021;50(91):97–106.

55. Torriani M, Souto SC, Thomas BJ, Ouellette H, Bredella MA. Ischiofemoral impingement syndrome: an entity with hip pain and abnormalities of the quadratus femoris muscle. *AJR Am J Roentgenol.* 2009;193:186–190.

56. Park JW, Lee YK, Lee YJ, Shin S, Kang Y, Koo KH. Deep gluteal syndrome as a cause of posterior hip pain and sciatica-like pain. *Bone Joint J.* 2020;102-b:556–567.

57. Gardner SS, Dong D, Peterson LE, Park KJ, Harris JD. Is there a relationship between femoral neck-shaft angle and ischiofemoral impingement in patients with hip pain? *J Hip Preserv Surg.* 2020;7:43–48.

CHAPTER 11

Hip Disorders in the Female Athlete

STEPHANIE W. MAYER, MD • ALISON DITTMER FLEMIG, MD •
STEPHANIE S. PEARCE, MD

FEMOROACETABULAR IMPINGEMENT AND ASSOCIATED LABRAL TEARS

Femoroacetabular impingement syndrome (FAIS) refers to pathologic abutment between the femoral head-neck junction and the acetabular rim.[1] This generally occurs due to a combination of structural, soft tissue, and activity-related factors. Two main forms of FAIS include cam morphology and pincer morphology, and many people have both.[1] Cam morphology refers to an abnormally shaped femoral head and neck junction that causes either a convexity at this location or a flattening at this location on the bone (Fig. 11.1). This effectively causes a mismatch between the shape of the acetabulum and the femoral head, and the cam

lesion impinges on the acetabular rim and labrum, and as it moves farther into the joint with flexion, it impinges on the cartilage as well. Pincer morphology refers to an abnormality of the acetabulum in which the socket is deep and covering too far over the femoral head (Fig. 11.2). This causes the edge of the acetabulum and labrum to impinge upon the femoral neck with hip flexion. Many people have a combination of both these abnormalities.[2] FAIS can cause labral tears from the chronic impingement of the labrum between the bones.[2,3] Additionally, impingement between a prominent anterior inferior iliac spine (AIIS) and the femoral head-neck junction, also called subspine impingement, can occur.[4] Although all three types of FAIS are noted in

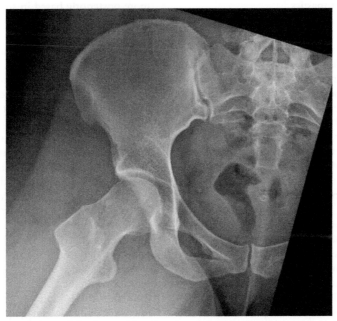

FIG. 11.1 Cam morphology of the femoral head and neck junction. Note the lack of offset between the superior aspect of the femoral head and the femoral neck.

The Female Athlete. https://doi.org/10.1016/B978-0-323-75985-4.00015-5

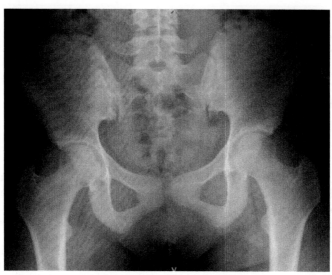

FIG. 11.2 Pincer morphology of the acetabulum. Note the deep acetabular coverage over the femoral head.

female athletes, pincer morphology is more common in females, while males generally have larger cam lesions. FAIS is most often seen in active adolescents and adults and in athletes, as the demand on the hip is higher than that in sedentary people. All types of female athletes can develop FAIS; however, it is commonly seen in soccer, lacrosse, dance, and gymnastics.[5]

Clinical Symptoms, Examination, Radiology, and Diagnosis

Most commonly, FAIS is described as a slow progression of pain over time rather than an acute injury. Classically, pain is in the groin or anterior hip and is described in a C-shaped location over the anterior and lateral groin crease, which is termed a "c-sign".[6] However, female patients may have pain patterns that are more laterally or even posteriorly based. Generally, pain is described as activity related, particularly with running or squatting, but it can also be associated with sitting for prolonged periods. Mechanical symptoms due to labral tears or cartilage injury in the hip may be present; however, most often a complaint of popping will be due to an associated internal or external snapping hip. Pain in certain muscle groups such as hip flexors, glutes, and short external rotators is commonly associated and should be considered as a source of pain, in addition to FAIS.[3,7]

Physical examination related to possible FAIS should include a gait assessment, palpation of periarticular muscles, range-of-motion testing, and strength testing to determine if an intra- or extra-articular source of pain is present.[8,9] Classically, FAIS will cause pain

with flexion, adduction, and internal rotation (FADIR) (Fig. 11.3). This places the most contact between the femur and acetabulum and places the most pressure on the labrum. However, the combination of flexion, abduction, and external rotation (FABER) can cause pain if a labral tear or the position of impingement is more posteriorly based in some cases (Fig. 11.4). Pain with flexion past 90 degrees may be associated with AIIS impingement.[4]

Radiographs including an anteroposterior (AP) pelvis view, lateral hip view, and often a false profile view are taken for assessment of femoroacetabular impingement (FAI) morphology including cam lesion, pincer lesion, and prominent AIIS.[10] The lateral center edge angle (LCEA) and the Tonnis angle are measured on an AP pelvis radiograph to evaluate the amount of coverage of the acetabulum and the slope of the acetabular roof, respectively (Fig. 11.5A and B). An LCEA between 25 and 40 degrees and a Tonnis angle between 0 and 10 degrees are considered normal.[11,12] The alpha angle is measured on a lateral view of the femur and measurements above 50–55 degrees indicate cam morphology.[11] (Fig. 11.5C) The AIIS should have approximately 1 cm of space between its base and the edge of the acetabulum.[4,13] A thorough assessment of any concomitant acetabular dysplasia should be performed, as this is more common in females than males. Magnetic resonance imaging (MRI) is useful to determine the presence and extent of labral pathology, cartilage injury, and possible associated psoas or rectus tendonitis (Fig. 11.6). Computed tomographic (CT)

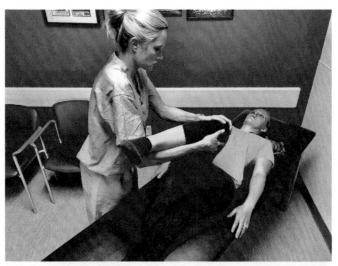

FIG. 11.3 The flexion, adduction, and internal rotation (FADIR) test. With the patient supine, the examiner brings affected leg into hip flexion, adduction, and internal rotation. Intra-articular pathology such as labral tears or chondral injury usually results in anterior groin pain.

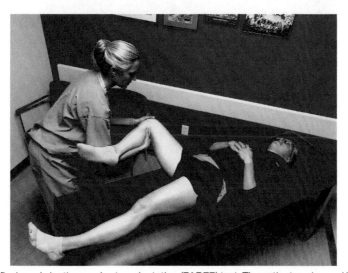

FIG. 11.4 The flexion, abduction, and external rotation (FABER) test. The patient supine and hip is placed into the flexed, abducted, and externally rotated position to elicit pain. The examiner should note if anterior, lateral, or posterior pain is reported.

scan is helpful to understand the three-dimensional anatomy of the cam or pincer lesion and evaluate the femoral torsion for any femoral retroversion that could be exacerbating the FAIS.[10]

Treatment

Initial treatment for FAIS includes conservative care including activity modification, physical therapy, and antiinflammatory medications. Therapy should focus on core strength, stability, and balancing of muscle groups including anterior and posterior chains.[7] Selective injections may be helpful in confirming a diagnosis of FAIS when a possible extra-articular source of pain is in question, such as psoas or rectus tendonitis. Female athletes have a higher incidence of psoas snapping and tendonitis than males, and this may be difficult

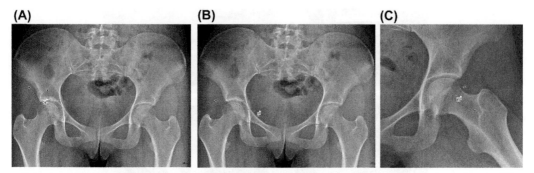

FIG. 11.5 **(A)** Measurement of lateral center edge angle, **(B)** measurement of the Tonnis angle, and **(C)** measurement of alpha angle.

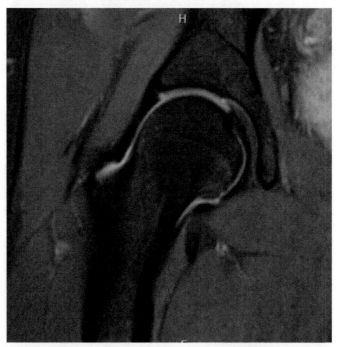

FIG. 11.6 Magnetic resonance image of the hip showing labral tearing due to femoroacetabular impingement.

to differentiate from FAIS.[14,15] Intra-articular injections may also be used as part of conservative treatment. A single injection may be an effective aide in pain relief and may facilitate a course of physical therapy or allow further athletic participation. There is evidence, however, that 2—3 months should pass between the injection of corticosteroid and surgical intervention to prevent an increase in perioperative infection rate.[16]

If nonoperative treatment fails to improve pain and mechanical symptoms, surgical intervention most commonly includes hip arthroscopy to perform labral repair (or reconstruction with a graft), femoroplasty and/or acetabuloplasty, and possible AIIS decompression. If a concomitant diagnosis of acetabular dysplasia is present, the surgeon should consider whether a periacetabular osteotomy for correction of dysplasia is necessary. Patients should be counseled that an associated snapping psoas or iliotibial band (ITB) may not be immediately corrected with hip arthroscopy. Rather, their soft tissues will benefit from a course of postoperative physical therapy after the underlying anatomic abnormalities have been addressed.

Outcomes

Outcomes of hip arthroscopy for FAIS show good improvement in functional scores and return to athletic participation in 50%–95% of female patients.[17–20] Some studies show that overall improvement is lower in females than males. Older females, especially, tend to show less improvement in functional scores and worse outcomes than their younger female counterparts.[17,21–23] There is evidence that arthroscopy in patients with combined borderline acetabular dysplasia and FAI can be successful, but arthroscopy for isolated dysplasia with a labral tear is not indicated.

HIP DYSPLASIA AND ASSOCIATED LABRAL TEARS

Acetabular dysplasia refers to an increasingly wide spectrum of pathologies that affect the acetabular and proximal femoral morphology.[24,25] The dysplastic acetabulum is typically shallow and low in volume, creating an abnormal articulation between it and the femoral head (Fig. 11.7). This mismatch can create intra-articular damage due to excessive stress on the labrum and cartilage and extra-articular stress on muscles and tendons, which are overloaded due to the abnormal hip joint.[26] Dysplasia is now recognized as a cause of primary osteoarthritis (OA) of the hip.[27–29] Various patterns of dysplasia can occur, and some can be subtle on radiographic examination. The undercoverage of the femoral head can be global, or it can be focal in the anterior, lateral, or even posterior acetabulum in cases of acetabular retroversion.[30,31] Each of these may cause a different location of labral or chondral injury, as well as a different pattern of symptoms. The concept of microinstability in the setting of dysplasia refers to the mismatch and undercoverage of the femoral head causing some laxity of the joint, which is sensed by the body.[32] The periarticular muscles such as gluteal muscles or hip flexors are then overloaded and can become a source of discomfort.[33] It is common to see a combination of ligamentous laxity and dysplasia in females.[32] This combination can exacerbate the microinstability due to the increased range of motion these athletes will have, in addition to increased capsular volume or incompetence.[34,35]

Clinical Symptoms, Examination, Radiology, and Diagnosis

Many female athletes presenting with symptoms from acetabular dysplasia will note an insidious onset of pain that is often activity related. If groin pain or a c-sign is a main complaint, intra-articular pathology or hip flexor tendonitis should be considered. If the pain is mainly laterally based, often a large component of pain is due to gluteal overload. If posterior pain is present, posterior undercoverage should be considered.[24,26] Anterior pain may be exacerbated with activities involving hip flexion and significant external rotation, as they place stress on the labrum and anterior capsule, respectively. Additionally, symptoms of psoas snapping may be a sign of anterior instability, as the psoas acts as a secondary stabilizer.[33] Long

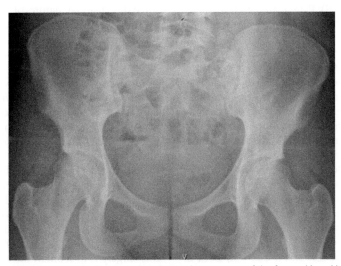

FIG. 11.7 Anteroposterior pelvis radiograph showing undercoverage of the femoral head by the acetabulum on the right hip consistent with acetabular dysplasia.

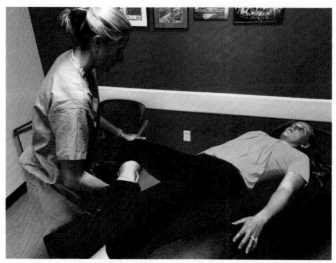

FIG. 11.8 Apprehension test. The examiner places the hip into flexion and external rotation and places a posteriorly directed force on the hip. Anterior pain or apprehension with a sense of instability is a positive test result.

periods of weight-bearing activity such as walking or running also place stress on the gluteal musculature and may exacerbate lateral pain.

Physical examination of a patient with possible acetabular dysplasia should include evaluation of gait, palpation of periarticular muscles, range of motion, and strength to determine locations of pain and intra- versus extra-articular sources of pain.[32] Examination maneuvers related to dysplasia include an anterior apprehension test in which the patient is placed in the position in Fig. 11.4 and the femur is forced into external rotation (Fig. 11.8). Pain or apprehension ante- riorly, which is improved with posteriorly directed force on the joint (similar to a shoulder apprehension test), can be a sign of anterior instability. FADIR or FABER test results may be positive for pain if there is a labral tear. Evaluation of abductor fatigue with the Trendelen- burg sign or trochanteric region pain with abductor strength testing indicates lateral overload. Internal and external rotation in flexion gives an idea of femoral tor- sion. Increased internal rotation indicates femoral ante- version, and increased external rotation indicates femoral retroversion. Both are seen in the setting of dysplasia and have treatment implications. Ligamen- tous laxity should be evaluated, as this also has treat- ment implications. The Beighton criteria is the most common way to qualify the level of general ligamen- tous laxity.[36] Laxity, specifically of the hip capsule, can be tested with a log roll test and a dial test, both of which evaluate the amount of rotation and the spring

back the capsule has in a neutral position of extension.[32]

Initial radiographic evaluation is similar to evalua- tion for FAIS with AP Pelvis, lateral, and false profile ra- diographs.[26] An LCEA below 25 degrees indicates dysplasia. Evaluation for increased alpha angle and combined dysplasia and FAI is important for treatment. MRI may show a labral tear, and it is important to eval- uate the quality of the labral tissue, as it can often appear degenerative.[37,38] CT scan with evaluation of femoral torsion also aides in the evaluation of the three-dimensional nature of the acetabular dysplasia and any contribution of femoral anteversion to an instability picture.[39]

Treatment

In most cases, treatment for dysplasia begins with con- servative management.[32] Activity modification, antiin- flammatory medications, and physical therapy are first-line treatment options. Physical therapy will focus on core strength, abductor strength, and balancing of anterior and posterior chain muscle groups. If the athlete is a dancer or other flexibility sport athlete, a thorough evaluation of compensatory movements dur- ing sport should be performed.

If nonsurgical management fails, treatment of dysplasia often requires periacetabular osteotomy for correction of the acetabular anatomy.[40,41] The goal of this surgery is to reorient the acetabulum such that the weight-bearing dome of the acetabulum is centered over the femoral head. Often this is combined with a hip arthroscopy if a labral tear or cam lesion is also present.

ILIOPSOAS TENDONITIS AND INTERNAL SNAPPING HIP SYNDROME

The iliopsoas muscle has been seen to be a source of a spectrum of hip symptoms, from debilitating mechanical hip pain to asymptomatic snapping of the hip.[14] Internal snapping hip, also known as coxa saltans interna, is defined as the iliopsoas musculotendinous junction snapping over the anterior pelvic structures deep to it, including the iliopectineal ridge, the iliopsoas bursa, the iliofemoral ligament, the superior pubic ramus, the anterior capsule, the femoral head, or the lesser trochanter of the femur, with the femoral head being the most common location.[14,15]

The psoas muscle originates from the lumbar spine (T12-L4), joins with the iliacus muscle at the levels of L5-S2, and inserts on the lesser trochanter as the iliopsoas tendon acting as one of the body's strongest hip flexors.[14,42] Additional movements of the iliopsoas muscle include abduction and external rotation of the femur, in addition to flexion. Philippon et al.[14] report in their anatomic study of cadaveric iliopsoas tendons that the majority of hips examined had iliopsoas tendons composed of more than two tendons and that the largest tendon usually was the psoas major, which tends to lie more medially and may not be the first tendon encountered endoscopically.

Clinical Symptoms, Examination, Radiology, and Diagnosis

Symptoms range from audible, nonpainful snapping to debilitating pain preventing athletic participation. Usually, pain is located anteriorly and is worsened with activities involving hip flexion to extension or hip circumduction.[15,43] It is more commonly seen in women and girls than in men and boys.[43] Other activities of daily life that may worsen the painful snapping of internal coxa saltans include rising from a chair or walking upstairs. Athletic activities commonly associated with internal snapping hip are ones that involve large hip range-of-motion movements and high hip flexion such as dance, soccer, football, running, and hockey.[43–45]

Physical examination maneuvers to detect internal snapping hip typically involve the hip moving from flexion to extension. The snap can be palpated or heard as the patient moves from hip flexion to extension at around 30 degrees of flexion.[43] Another method to detect internal coxa saltans is to begin with the patient supine with the involved hip flexed, abducted, and externally rotated (FABER) and to bring the patient's leg into an extended, adducted, and internal rotated position in a circumduction motion (Fig. 11.9). The author's preferred technique is to perform a "bicycle maneuver" where the patient laying supine cycles his/her legs as if riding a bicycle, with the hips alternating from flexion to extension bilaterally and the ipsilateral knee of the flexed hip also flexed to 90 degrees (Fig. 11.10). Finally, tenderness to palpation of the

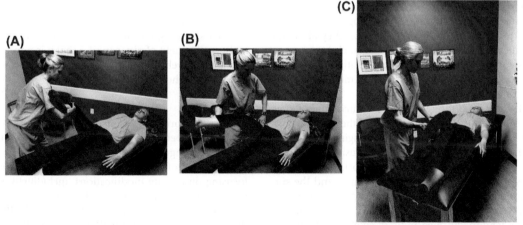

FIG. 11.9 **(A–C)** Internal snapping hip examination. The hip is first placed in a flexed, abducted, and externally rotated position and moves in a circumduction motion toward extension, adduction, and internal rotation. The iliopsoas tendon is palpated to detect a snap.

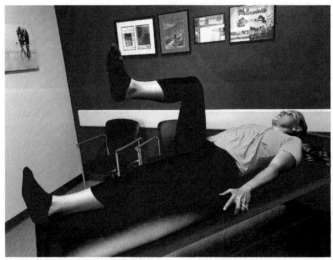

FIG. 11.10 Bicycle test. Patient laying supine, cycles their legs as if riding a bicycle with the hips alternating from flexion to extension bilaterally and the ipsilateral knee of the flexed hip also flexed to 90 degrees.

iliopsoas tendon anteriorly and pain with resisted hip flexion are signs of iliopsoas tendonitis/bursitis related to internal snapping hip syndrome.[46]

While imaging is not always required to diagnose internal snapping hip, it is helpful in determining the likely location of iliopsoas contact with the anterior pelvic structures and can aid in management.[14,15] Additionally, imaging can identify concomitant pathology such as FAI and the sources of intra-articular snapping hip, such as chondromatosis and loose bodies.[15,43] Snapping psoas is commonly associated with hip dysplasia and ligamentous laxity. A standing anteroposterior radiograph of the pelvis and false profile view of the affected hip are the primary radiographic imaging views preferred by the senior author, as they allow for identification of bony abnormalities, such as exostoses or osteophytes, causing the symptomatic contact with the iliopsoas tendon, sites of impingement (including FAI), or evidence of dysplasia.

MRI has been thought of as a limited study in the past owing to the dynamic nature of the internal coxa saltans and the static nature of the imaging modality,[15] but more recent studies describe the consistent ability of MRI to diagnose abnormalities associated with the iliopsoas tendon, anterior capsule, bursa, and the surrounding musculature that correspond to the patient's complaints.[45] Inflammation of the iliopsoas muscle and/or tendon can give indirect evidence of internal snapping hip syndrome.[47] The key to utilize MRI is to compare the patient's symptoms and examination findings, as some large abnormalities in the iliopsoas

tendon and/or surrounding structures may be present in a patient without symptoms.[45] Therefore MRI can be a useful adjunct to physical examination and ultrasound, but it should not be used in isolation.

Dynamic ultrasound is the most valuable imaging modality used in diagnosing internal snapping hip syndrome, especially because it is a dynamic phenomenon.[44,45] Winston et al.[44] reviewed snapping hips in ballet dancers and found snapping in 29 of 46 hips (63%) utilizing ultrasound, with 27 being from the iliopsoas and 2 of 29 from the ITB. Pelsser et al.[48] studied 40 hips in 20 patients with unilateral or bilateral symptoms and visualized snapping on ultrasound in 26 of 40 (65%) hips, with 2 of 26 being from ITB external snapping and the rest from the iliopsoas. An additional benefit of ultrasound is that it is noninvasive and of relatively low cost but does require a skilled ultrasonographer.[47]

Treatment

The large majority of patients with internal coxa saltans require nonoperative treatment alone.[15,45–47] Since internal snapping hip syndrome is usually from overuse, the mainstay of treatment is nonsurgical intervention focusing on activity modifications, including a significant rest period, ice, pain control with antiinflammatory agents, and physical therapy.[15,45,46] Physical therapy targets muscle imbalances, especially anterior musculature tightness, through active and passive stretching regimens.[47,49] Stretching and conservative treatment should start making improvements within

2—4 weeks.[45] If no improvement is noted after that time, rapid return to play and training remains an ultimate priority, or an athlete is unable or unwilling to avoid the exacerbating activity, therapeutic injections of local anesthetic and corticosteroid have shown clinical improvements.[45] These improvements are maximized when combined with continued rest, avoidance of aggravating activities (e.g., hip flexion >90 degrees), stretching, use of modalities (e.g., cryotherapy, electric stimulation), and use of nonsteroidal antiinflammatory drugs (NSAIDs).[45] Wahl et al.[45] report their tendon sheath cocktail of choice as including 40 mg of triamcinolone acetonide (Kenalog), 0.5 mL of 1% lidocaine, and 0.5 mL of 0.5% bupivacaine. They report utilizing this injection with stretching, NSAIDs, and temporary avoidance of training and drills and have found athletes able to return to sport in as little as 1 week.[45]

Consistent conservative treatment may take 6—12 months to regain normal hip function without evidence of snapping or pain. Despite this duration, continued postural and movement patterns and stretching activities are encouraged to prevent recurrence.[47] Several authors agree that conservative treatment should continue for at least 3—4 months before considering surgical intervention.[43,45,47] However, after that time, surgical treatment can be pursued especially if an athlete needs to return to sport and all other diagnoses have been excluded.

Surgical intervention is focused on functionally lengthening the iliopsoas tendon by either transection or fractional lengthening. Additionally, the location of lengthening has also varied in the literature but tends to be one of the following zones: central compartment (at the level of the femoral head and hip capsule and pelvic brim), peripheral compartment (at the level of the inferior hip capsule and superior to the lesser trochanter), and at the lesser trochanter.[43] A level I randomized trial and a level IV comparative study found that the location of release at either the lesser trochanter or the central compartment yielded nonsignificant differences between the two and favorable results for both.[1,43,50]

Outcomes

Surgical intervention has been approached both open and arthroscopically, although arthroscopic treatments currently show less morbidity and improved results compared with an open approach.[43,51] A systematic review of open versus arthroscopic treatments of internal snapping hip syndrome found that an arthroscopic approach was associated with a decreased failure rate, lower complication rate, and decreased postoperative pain.[51]

While overall outcomes seem to be good, the largest complication with open or arthroscopic approaches seems to be transient iliopsoas muscle weakness.[43] This weakness seems to resolve by 3—6 months postoperatively, with no difference regarding the level of tendon release.[43] Return to sports can be expected around 9 months postoperatively.[52]

ILIOTIBIAL BAND TIGHTNESS AND EXTERNAL SNAPPING HIP SYNDROME

External snapping hip syndrome, or external coxa saltans, is due to the posterior aspect of the ITB or the anterior aspect of the gluteus maximus muscle snapping across the greater trochanter at the lateral aspect of the hip. It is usually a visible, dynamic phenomenon and one that patients describe as catching, "giving way," or even the sensation of hip dislocation.[47] External snapping hip is more common than its internal counterpart, but is diagnosed and treated similarly.

The iliotibial tract is formed proximally from two muscles: the tensor fascia lata (TFL) anteriorly and the gluteus maximus posteriorly.[15] The TFL originates along the lateral iliac crest between the anterior superior iliac spine and the tubercle of the iliac crest. It then inserts on to the ITB or iliotibial tract, which continues down the lateral thigh and inserts at Gerdy's tubercle on the anterolateral aspect of the proximal tibia.[42] The gluteus maximus, which can also attribute to external coxa saltans, also originates on the iliac crest, but only crosses the hip joint inserting on the posterior aspect of the ITB and the linea aspera distal to the greater trochanter via the gluteal sling.[15,42] Functionally, the ITB crosses both the hip and knee joints and acts to help stabilize the pelvis in one-legged stance with abduction of the TFL and helps stabilize the knee in extension. The ITB lies posterior to the greater trochanter in extension and mechanistically glides anteriorly over the greater trochanter when the hip moves to flexion.[15,47]

Clinical Symptoms, Examination, Radiology, and Diagnosis

Due to the often visible nature of external snapping hip syndrome, coxa saltans externa is typically easier to diagnose than coxa saltans interna. Patients tend to locate pain and symptoms at the lateral aspect of the hip and may complain of dislocating their hip, snapping, catching, or giving way.[15,46,47] The patient will frequently offer to demonstrate the snapping.[15]

On physical examination, having the patient lie on his/her side with the affected hip up will allow for evaluation with the Ober test, bicycle test, and direct palpation. To perform the Ober test, the patient will first flex

(A)   **(B)**

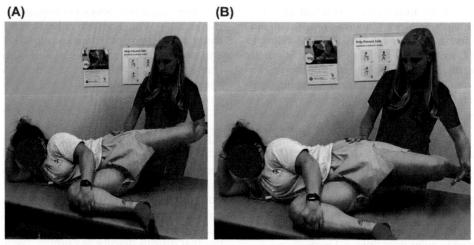

FIG. 11.11 The Ober test for detecting external snapping hip syndrome and iliotibial band (ITB) contracture. The examiner stands behind the patient who is lying on the unaffected side. With both hips and knees flexed, the examiner passively abducts the affected leg past neutral and passively extends the hip, with the other hand palpating the greater trochanter for a snap **(A,B)**. Then the examiner slowly lets go of the leg allowing to enter adduction while still maintaining extension of the affected hip. If the patient's leg remains abducted, it is a positive test result and the patient has an ITB contracture. If the patient's leg is able to adduct past neutral, the test result is negative.

the unaffected and affected hips, and the affected hip will be extended and adducted by the examiner. If a snap is palpated as the hip is extended, this is positive for external snapping. If the affected leg cannot adduct past neutral, this test is positive for ITB tightness (Fig. 11.11). The bicycle test is performed with the patient lying on the unaffected side and cycling the affected hip as if peddling a bicycle. The examiners hand rests on the greater trochanter to feel the snap.

Imaging is similar to the methods used in internal snapping hip syndrome, where dynamic ultrasound is usually the most valuable modality. Usually a thickened ITB and/or focal thickening of the anterior gluteus maximus is visualized snapping over the greater trochanter.[47]

Treatment

Similar to internal snapping hip, the treatment of choice for external snapping hip syndrome is conservative therapy.[15,47] Activity modification, rest, cryotherapy, antiinflammatory agents, and focused physical therapy are critical to symptomatic resolution. Commonly, an imbalance between gluteus maximus and TFL activation contributes to the pathology and can be an area of focus with biofeedback and neuromuscular retraining.[47]

If conservative measures are not offering improvement for the athlete, and rapid return to sport remains

a priority, then consideration of an ITB bursa injection with local anesthestic and corticosteroid is warranted.[53]

Recalcitrant painful snapping after conservative treatments for 3—4 months is rare but can be escalated to surgical intervention.[43,45,47] Goals of surgery for external snapping hip syndrome is to minimize the forces and tension the ITB undergoes when gliding across the greater trochanter.[46,47] This is usually achieved by lengthening the ITB and various methods have been visited in the literature, including a formal Z-lengthening,[53] a Z-shaped release,[54] a cross-shaped release,[47,53] and a release of the gluteus maximus tendon insertion to the femur.[55] A formal Z-lengthening was originally described by Brignall and Stainsby[56] where a 10-cm incision is made over the greater trochanter laterally, with two-thirds of the incision below the greater trochanter.[53] An 8-cm longitudinal incision is made in the fascia lata and the proximal limb is made posterocaudally and the distal limb is made anteroproximally at 45 degrees to the longitudinal incision.[53] The flaps are reoriented to gain more length to the ITB and sutured in place. Intraoperative Ober test and range of motion ensure no snapping of the ITB is visualized or palpated.[53] Variations of the shape of ITB incision have been described.[54,57] Polesello et al.[55] describe a newer technique of releasing the gluteus maximus insertion instead of the ITB in hopes of creating a more physiologic approach to decrease ITB tension. Many options exist, with no randomized controlled trials comparing the various methods. While participant numbers are low in most studies, overall outcomes appear good with the majority of patients returning to preinjury levels and painful snapping resolving.

TROCHANTERIC BURSITIS

Greater trochanteric bursitis is an inflammatory condition part of a larger entity called greater trochanteric pain syndrome (GTPS). GTPS also includes gluteus medius and minimus tendinopathy (see more details in the section Gluteal Tendonitis and Tears) and external coxa saltans (see the section Iliotibial Band Tightness and External Snapping Hip Syndrome).[58] Several authors agree that greater trochanteric bursitis is largely a sequela of another inciting pathology that should be addressed to obtain full resolution of the greater trochanteric pain.[58,59]

The peritrochanteric bursae have been described as three fluid-filled sacs to protect and decrease friction of the gluteal tendons, the ITB, and the TFL, with some anatomic variations having four in total. Each bursal sac is named with respect to the location under which tendon it resides: the subgluteus maximus bursa (aka trochanteric bursa), the subgluteus medius bursa, and the subgluteus maximus bursa. The first one is the largest and most commonly indicated in GTPS.[58]

Clinical Symptoms, Examination, Radiology, and Diagnosis

Being aware of the associated hip diagnosis in the setting of greater trochanteric bursitis is critical in fully diagnosing and therefore appropriately treating the patient. Concomitant diagnoses including external coxa saltans, gluteus medius or minimus tendinopathy, and recalcitrant greater trochanteric bursitis are important to delineate when examining the patient.[54,58]

Direct palpation over the greater trochanter can help discern the location of pathology and the associated cause. With the patient lying on the contralateral leg in a lateral position, tenderness to palpation over the anterior superior greater trochanter likely indicated gluteus minimus pathology, as this is the location of insertion on the greater trochanter. The gluteus medius inserts along the posterosuperior aspect of the greater trochanter, indicating tenderness along this region is more likely associated with the gluteus medius tendon. Tenderness to palpation along the central and distal portions of the greater trochanter aligns with the pathology focused at the trochanteric bursa, also known as the subgluteus maximus bursa. A tight ITB can also

cause or worsen trochanteric bursal pain, so there will be indications of a tight ITB on examination, such as during the Ober test (described in further detail in the Section Iliotibial Band Tightness and External Snapping Hip Syndrome).

Treatment

Treatment for greater trochanteric bursitis and GTPS is largely nonoperative with focus on rest, cryotherapy, stretching the ITB and gluteal musculature, and antiinflammatory agents.[47,58] Corticosteroid injections are commonly initiated once other more conservative measures fail.

Once extensive nonoperative modalities have been exhausted for 6−12 months, and the athlete is unable to return to training or competition, surgical intervention may be discussed. Surgical options include, open versus endoscopic bursectomy, proximal or distal Z-plasty of the ITB, longitudinal release of the ITB, trochanteric reduction osteotomy, and repair of gluteus medius and/or minimus tears.[59]

GLUTEAL TENDONITIS AND TEARS

Commonly described as "rotator cuff" disease of the hip, the spectrum of gluteal tendinitis, tendinopathy, and tears is an important cause of lateral greater trochanteric hip pain, particularly in female patients.[60] Although the precise prevalence of gluteal tendinopathy in the overall population is unknown, increasing awareness of this diagnosis has led to the thought that the majority of lateral greater trochanteric pain is attributable not to bursitis, but to gluteal tendinopathy.[61] Radiologic studies of patients with symptomatic greater trochanter pain have demonstrated that bursitis is rarely the primary underlying cause of pain, with one study demonstrating a rate of only 20% of trochanteric bursitis in 877 patients with lateral greater trochanteric hip pain. In addition, 49% of these patients were found to have abnormalities of the gluteus medius, gluteus minimus, or both.[62]

Although gluteal tears and tendinosis are typically seen in patients in the fourth through sixth decades of life, recognition of this pathology will become increasingly important in the management of female athletes. The average age of road race participants was 40 years in the United States in 2011, and with both the overall aging population and the increased participation of females in triathlons and long-distance running, the incidence of symptomatic gluteal tears and tendinosis will likely increase.[63,64]

The abductor complex of the hip includes the gluteus minimus, gluteus medius, and TFL. These muscles all originate on different portions of the iliac crest and have different sites of tendinous insertion. The TFL becomes contiguous with the ITB and inserts on Gerdy's tubercle on the lateral condyle of tibia, whereas the gluteus medius and minimus tendons insert onto different portions of the greater trochanter. An anatomic cadaver study of the insertion site of the gluteus medius demonstrated that the posterior portion of the gluteus medius tendon was thicker and inserts on the superoposterior facet of the greater trochanter in a straight line, whereas the anterolateral tendon was thinner in substance and inserted on the lateral facet of the greater trochanter via a posteroinferior direction.[65] This may have important implications in the surgical treatment of gluteus medius tears as well as provide some explanation for why tears of the anterior fibers are generally reported to be of greater frequency than those of posterior fibers.[65] The gluteus minimus additionally has dual insertion at both the lateral facet of the greater trochanter as well as the hip capsule itself.

The posterior portion of the gluteus medius tendon as well as the gluteus minimus have been shown to be important dynamic femoral head stabilizers.[66,67] Although traditionally gluteus medius was thought to be the main hip abductor for single-leg stance and pelvic balance during walking, it is likely the force vector of the TFL that generates the most hip abduction power and contributes the greatest force to these activities.[67]

The main function of gluteus medius and minimus is as pelvic and hip joint stabilizers. Weakness of the hip abductor complex can lead to overuse injuries, strains of the hip adductors, patellofemoral pain, and the Trendelenburg gait.[68] Tears of the gluteus medius and minimus are usually degenerative akin to rotator cuff tendinopathy, but traumatic tears of the gluteus tendons have also been rarely reported.[69]

Clinical Symptoms, Examination, Radiology, and Diagnosis

Typically, patients with gluteal tendinopathy present with an insidious onset of greater trochanteric hip pain and tenderness. Pain is often worse at night, exacerbated by direct pressure on the lateral aspect of their hip, and may be worse with activities such as walking or climbing stairs. Some patients will have a limp to varying degrees and will exhibit the Trendelenburg gait.[70,71] Rarely, a patient will give a history of an acute inciting injury just prior to the onset of symptoms.[69]

Clinical examination of a patient presenting with GTPS will help aid in the diagnosis of the underlying condition. Assessing for other coexisting or unrelated pathology should be performed, including a thorough lumbar spine examination for spondylolisthesis, lysis, and lumbar stenosis.

Both active and passive hip range of motion should be evaluated to assess for underlying OA or, as can be particularly relevant in the case of female athletes, an occult stress fracture of the proximal femur.[72] Superior gluteal nerve disease is generally rare but can be seen in conditions of diabetes mellitus. The provider should maintain a higher level suspicion of iatrogenic gluteal neuropathy in patients presenting with abduction weakness and muscle wasting in the setting of previous hip surgery.[73]

Assessing for tenderness, examining for atrophy of peritrochanteric musculature, and testing muscle strength should all be performed. Physical examination should include the assessment of gait, specifically watching for any antalgic limping or the Trendelenburg sign. Single-leg stance can also be performed to identify abductor weakness. Pain within 30 s of a single-leg stance can be very predictive (98%) of gluteal tendinosis when combined with MRI abnormalities.[74] Hip abduction strength should be tested in a side-lying position and has shown to be the most valid and reliable assessment of unilateral abduction strength.[68] A single-leg squat is another test that may be utilized in athletes to assess for gluteal weakness.[75] Patients with dysfunction of their hip abductors or weakness have been found to have both difficulty in performing a single-leg squat and delayed onset of gluteus medius activation during single-leg squat based on electromyographic findings.[75]

Trochanteric bursitis can be present in the setting of gluteal tendinosis, or less commonly, in isolation.[62] Many of the symptoms of gluteal tendinosis and trochanteric bursitis can be overlapping, but continued pain and residual abduction weakness after a corticosteroid injection into the bursa has been performed can be suggestive of gluteal tendon pathology.

Ultrasound is one imaging modality that can be utilized to further diagnose GTPS. Tendinosis is demonstrated on ultrasound by decreased echogenicity within the tendon. Partial- and full-thickness tears can also be seen on ultrasound as an anechoic defect disrupting the continuity of the tendon.[76] One study correlated ultrasound and intraoperative findings and found that in 17 of 19 patients with gluteal tendinopathy, ultrasound correctly diagnosed the underlying condition. However, ultrasound demonstrated poor specificity when identifying gluteal tendinosis in five of the six patients with normal gluteal tendon anatomy.[77] Another study with a small series of patients, published in 2010, demonstrated a positive predictive value of 1.0

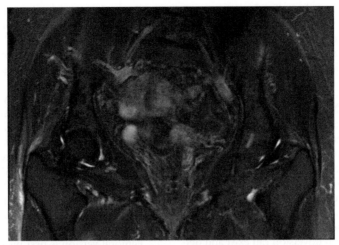

FIG. 11.12 Magnetic resonance image showing gluteus medius tearing at the insertion on the superior and lateral facet of the greater trochanter on the right hip.

for diagnosing gluteal tendon tears with ultrasound findings as described earlier.[78]

Plain radiographs are useful in the setting of lateral trochanteric hip pain to evaluate for any underlying or concomitant hip OA. Specific radiographic findings of gluteal tendinosis can be seen on plain radiographs and can include sclerosis or osteophytes of the greater trochanter.[60]

MRI has aided significantly in the diagnosis of gluteal tendinosis and tears (Fig. 11.12). Previous MRI studies of this pathology have identified that gluteus medius tears are far more common than gluteus minimus tears.[79] The diagnostic accuracy has been reported in a wide range with most studies showing good sensitivity and specificity for the identification of gluteal tendon tears.[80,81] MRI can also be utilized to quantify the percentage of fatty infiltration of the gluteus medius and minimus, which has been shown to influence outcomes following repair.[82]

Treatment

Nonoperative management remains the first line of treatment for patients with symptomatic tears or tendinopathy. This can involve modalities including physical therapy, activity and functional modifications, injections, and oral medications such as NSAIDs. There is little conclusive evidence on the efficacy of these therapies (as well as a paucity of high-quality research by which to draw conclusions).[83]

Both cortisone and platelet-rich plasma (PRP) injections have been used in the treatment of gluteal tendinosis. A randomized controlled trial published in 2018 showed that patients who took PRP injection achieved better clinical improvement compared with those treated with corticosteroid at 12 weeks.[84]

Typically, after 3 months of conservative management fails, including combinations of the abovementioned modalities, operative intervention can be considered. Surgical intervention for both partial and complete gluteal tears has been increasing in frequency over the past decade. There are a number of different techniques utilized, including open and arthroscopic repair and augmentation of the repair with synthetic or allograft materials.

Open techniques have been described using bone tunnels and suture anchors.[85,86] Good to excellent results are generally reported with improvement in pain, ambulation without assistive devices, and subjective outcomes scores.[85,86] As expected, the poorest results occurred in patients with the largest tears.[86] For larger tears that cannot be repaired with suture anchors alone, other surgical procedures have been described, including partial transfer of the gluteus maximus or TFL, or advancement of the vastus lateralis.[87–89] These techniques have been reported only in small case series, with variable results of patient satisfaction and complication rates up to 27%. An alternative technique that has been described is the use of allograft or synthetic augmentation for open or arthroscopic repair.[89] Results were directly impacted by the rate of fatty degeneration of the muscle, as patients with less than 75% fatty degeneration had better functional outcomes postoperatively.

Endoscopic repair of the gluteus tendons has also increased in popularity as techniques improve.[90] A systematic review of open versus endoscopic abductor tendon repairs demonstrated similar functional outcomes between groups, with a higher rate of complications in patients who underwent open repair.[91] Notably, no re-tears or surgical-site infections were reported in the endoscopic group.[91]

FEMORAL TORSIONAL ABNORMALITIES

Femoral torsion, or version, is used to describe the position of the femoral head and neck relative to the rest of the femur. At birth, average femoral anteversion is approximately 40 degrees, which decreases to 16 degrees at skeletal maturity.[92] There is a wide range of "normal" anteversion in adults with no uniform agreement, but the average adult femoral anteversion is reported between 10 and 20 degrees.[92–100] Excessive femoral anteversion and retroversion can exist and definitions of this vary. Femoral retroversion is typically defined as less than 5 degrees of femoral anteversion and femoral anteversion as >20 degrees. Definitions based on rotational examination also exist, with femoral anteversion defined as >80 degrees internal rotation in the setting of <20 degrees external rotation.[96] There are accepted gender-based differences in normal of femoral version, with females having an average greater femoral version than males.[100,101]

Clinical Symptoms, Examination, Radiology, and Diagnosis

On its most basic level, excessive femoral anteversion or retroversion can result in an in-toeing or out-toeing gait, respectively. Both in-toeing and out-toeing exist in the normal adult population based on foot progression angles without any known pathologic significance. Extremes in femoral version can exist in isolation or can be seen in combination with tibial torsion or acetabular version abnormalities.

Excessive femoral anteversion can cause hip instability, damage to the articular cartilage or labrum, and potentially contribute to the development of OA, although this last statement is controversial.[96,102,103] Excessive femoral anteversion can cause rotational abnormalities at the level of the knee and have been shown to increase the risk of anterior knee pain, patellofemoral maltracking, and potentially increased rates of anterior cruciate ligament rupture.[103–105] One study examining femoral anteversion in young adults with hip pain found that females were more likely to have increased femoral anteversion compared with males and also had smaller alpha angles, and they were subsequently more likely to have subtle cam lesions, which could still be symptomatic.[100]

Femoral retroversion is associated with hip impingement secondary to the position of the femoral neck in relation to the acetabulum.[95] This hip impingement can lead to damage to the labrum and articular cartilage. Femoral retroversion has been shown to potentially increase the risk of a slipped capital femoral epiphysis (SCFE) in skeletally immature individuals, as well as a higher risk for posterior hip dislocation in contact athletes.[106] From an arthroscopic standpoint, residual femoral retroversion is seen in a higher proportion of patients who have poorer outcomes after arthroscopic decompression for FAI compared with those with normal femoral version.[107] However, arthroscopic decompression in patients with femoral retroversion can still achieve satisfactory results with regard to pain and function.[102]

Femoral version is best measured on axial CT scans of the proximal portion of the femur in relation to the femoral condyles distally (Fig. 11.13). There are many different methods of measuring the proximal femur morphology described in the literature.[94] A study published in CORR in 2019 compared the five most common methods and found that femoral version of the same specimen changed depending on the method of measuring the proximal femur.[94] The variation in calculated femoral torsion based on measurements tended to increase in patients with excessive version, whereas in patients with less version, all methods tended to be more precise with regard to one another. They concluded that it is important to identify which method is being utilized to calculate femoral version, as measurements of anteversion can differ up to 17 degrees depending on which method of calculation is used.[94]

Treatment

Treatment for symptomatic femoral torsion can begin with a course of rest from aggravating activities and physical therapy aimed at gait and functional movement retraining of periarticular muscles. However, therapy cannot correct bony deformities, and so if activity modification and therapy cannot overcome the bony abnormality, surgical intervention may be indicated.

Surgery to address rotational deformities of the femur is well described. The surgeries can be performed in isolation or with other surgical procedures as needed to address the patient's specific underlying pathology. Osteotomies can be performed at the level of the intertrochanteric region, subtrochanteric region, or distally.[108] Both open plating and intramedullary nails have been used and reported. Buly et al.[95] described performing a subtrochanteric osteotomy with derotation over an intramedullary nail in 43 patients and

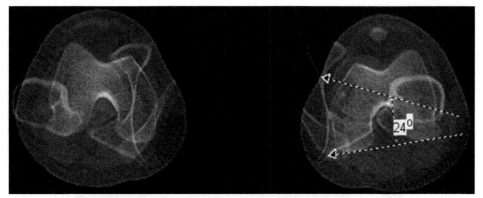

FIG. 11.13 Axial computed tomographic scan with femoral torsion measured as the angle between a line bisecting the greater trochanter and middle of the femoral head and a line connecting the posterior femoral condyles.

reported a 93% success rate. The advantages of using an intramedullary device with this type of osteotomy are the limited dissection necessary when compared to proximal femoral plating as well as immediate weight-bearing. Compared to an intertrochanteric or metaphyseal osteotomy, the location of this osteotomy means that complete bony healing does take longer to complete. Additionally, the authors noted that 70% of patients required a secondary surgery for nail removal.[95] Failures of surgery in this study were in patients with underlying connective tissue disorders. There is no literature to currently support one osteotomy location or fixation option over another.[109]

HIP OSTEOARTHRITIS IN FEMALE ATHLETES

There is a large body of evidence suggesting that OA of the hip is caused by underlying structural abnormalities of the hip joint and is not just a consequence of aging.[1,28,29,50,110-112] FAI including cam and pincer deformities, developmental dysplasia of the hip, Perthes disease, and SCFE type deformities are all known to lead to articular degeneration and eventual OA of the hip.[28,110] These conditions cause mechanical dysfunction including concentric or eccentric overloading, dynamic instability, impingement, or some combination of these features, which in turn leads to articular damage and the progression of OA. Over 90% of patients with hip OA show radiographic evidence of structural abnormalities, mostly common acetabular dysplasia or "pistol-grip" deformity.[28]

With regard to athletes, there has long been the thought that elite athletic activity predisposes individuals to develop OA of the hip and knee.[111,113,114]

A review of collegiate Division I female athletes found that they are less likely than male athletes to have femoroacetabular impingement but were more likely to have acetabular dysplasia than the general population.[114] In this study, 48% of female athletes had signs of FAI, whereas 21% had an LCEA less than 20 degrees indicating acetabular dysplasia, and 46% had borderline dysplasia with LCEA between 20 and 25 degrees. One meta-analysis compared the incidence of hip OA in competitive and recreational runners, as well as the general population, and found that recreational runners had a decreased incidence of hip OA compared with the general population, whereas competitive (professional) runners had an increased incidence of hip OA compared with recreational runners as well as the general sedentary population.[113]

Clinical Symptoms, Examination, Radiology, and Diagnosis

The differential diagnosis of hip OA in the athletic, younger patient includes many of the conditions previously mentioned, including developmental dysplasia of the hip, FAI, osteonecrosis, GTPS, and femoral neck stress fractures. Typically, patients with OA complain of groin or anterior thigh pain. Range of motion will become limited over time, usually characterized by limited internal rotation and abduction preceding other physical examination findings. An antalgic gait can be present. Radiographic assessment typically begins with plain radiographs as in other conditions discussed in this chapter. Plain radiographs may show sclerosis of the acetabulum or femoral head, joint space narrowing, osteophyte formation, or cystic changes (Fig. 11.14). Advanced imaging, such as MRI, can be helpful when the plain film assessment is borderline or when more

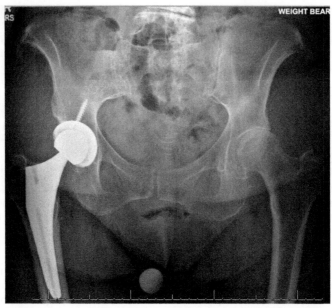

FIG. 11.14 Anteroposterior pelvis radiograph of a patient who has undergone total hip replacement for osteoarthritis on the right hip and has symptomatic osteoarthritis with joint space narrowing and sclerosis of the acetabular roof on the left side.

detail of soft tissue structures is needed. These images can help the provider diagnose the underlying structural abnormalities, diagnose the extent of OA, and guide further treatment regarding the ability to perform joint preservation surgery versus the need for replacement.

Treatment

First-line treatment for symptom management of OA includes the use of NSAIDs and is given a "strong" recommendation level by the American Academy of Orthopaedic Surgeons (AAOS) Appropriate Use Criteria.[115] Other medical treatment options include intra-articular injections including hyaluronic acid (HA), PRP, and corticosteroid injections. The benefit to the use of any or all these injections is controversial. The AAOS appropriate use guidelines give a "strong" recommendation to the use of intra-articular corticosteroid injections for short-term pain relief of hip OA, but concluded there was not enough evidence to support the use of HA for pain relief.[115] One randomized controlled trial investigating the use of PRP, PRP + HA, and HA alone demonstrated that PRP alone had the greatest impact on WOMAC scores up to 6 months (but not at 12 months) and the lowest VAS scores at all time points up to 1 year.[116] Unfortunately, the results of this study are limited secondary to the lack

of blinding of patients and providers, as well as the lack of a true control "sham" injection.[116]

The operative management of the young adult with hip OA consists of joint preservation or hip replacement surgery. Joint preservation surgery, when possible, is preferable in younger patients because of concerns of longevity of the implants as well as the increased rates of wear and aseptic loosening in younger, active patients compared with their older counterparts. The goals of hip preservation surgery include optimizing the hip joint mechanics in order to help prevent or prolong the development of OA requiring replacement. The ideal candidate for joint preservation is one who is young, is active, and has minimal degeneration of the joint. The use of hip arthroscopy in patients with early OA of the hip is controversial, and several studies have shown limited improvement of symptoms after arthroscopy for the treatment of OA.[110]

Periacetabular osteotomy has been shown to be very effective in young adults with hip dysplasia and minimal underlying OA in prolonging the need for a hip replacement surgery, with a 60% survival rate of the native hip joint at 19 years.[117] More advanced grades of OA and older age at time of surgery were associated with poorer outcomes.[117]

Resurfacing arthroplasty of the hip is another procedure that can be considered in young patients with hip OA. However, it must be mentioned that there are numerous complications associated with metal-on-metal resurfacing arthroplasty, including elevated levels of metallic ions and much higher rates of failure in females than in males, which is thought to be due to the smaller size of implants necessarily used in female hips compared with those used in males.[118,119]

Total hip arthroplasty is an option for young patients with end-stage OA that is not amenable to joint preservation procedures. Although this is an excellent option for pain relief, the concern in younger patients includes higher rates of aseptic loosening and the need for potentially multiple revisions throughout a younger person's lifetime.[120]

When reviewing the results of modern uncemented total hip arthroplasties in patients younger than 50 years, failure rates ranged from 2.9% to 49%, although all but one study had low failure rates.[120] High-quality evidence regarding return to sport for athletes after total hip arthroplasty, particularly in young patients, is sparse. One study showed a 91% return to sporting activity within 6 months of total hip arthroplasty.[121] The study population was stratified into <60, 60−70, and >70 years of age, and the youngest group of patients were more likely to return to sporting activities than older patients. However, participation in high-impact sporting activities decreased after total hip arthroplasty, whereas participation in most low-impact activities did not significantly decrease.[121] A systematic review published in 2018 examining rates of return to work and sporting activities after total hip replacement included 37 studies and found a mean return to sports level of 104% compared to presurgery level (meaning that more patients were involved in sporting activities than prior to surgery) and a 82% level compared to their presymptomatic sporting level.[122] Although this data can be used to help counsel older and recreational female athletes as to return to low-impact activities, evidence supporting the return to athletics by elite-level athletes is lacking in the literature.

REFERENCES

1. Ganz R, Parvizi J, Beck M, Leunig M, Nötzli H, Siebenrock KA. Femoroacetabular impingement: a cause for osteoarthritis of the hip. *Clin Orthop Relat Res.* 2003; (417):112−120. https://doi.org/10.1097/01.blo.00000 96804.78689.c2.
2. Beck M, Kalhor M, Leunig M, Ganz R. Hip morphology influences the pattern of damage to the acetabular cartilage: femoroacetabular impingement as a cause of early osteoarthritis of the hip. *J Bone Joint Surg Br.* 2005; 87-B(7):1012−1018. https://doi.org/10.1302/0301-620X.87B7.15203.
3. Griffin DR, Dickenson EJ, O'Donnell J, et al. The Warwick Agreement on femoroacetabular impingement syndrome (FAI syndrome): an international consensus statement. *Br J Sports Med.* 2016;50(19):1169−1176. https://doi.org/10.1136/bjsports-2016-096743.
4. Larson CM, Pierce BR, Giveans MR. Treatment of athletes with symptomatic intra-articular hip pathology and athletic pubalgia/sports hernia: a case series. *Arthrosc J Arthrosc Relat Surg.* 2011;27(6):768−775. https://doi.org/10.1016/j.arthro.2011.01.018.
5. Nawabi DH, Bedi A, Tibor LM, Magennis E, Kelly BT. The demographic characteristics of high-level and recreational athletes undergoing hip arthroscopy for femoroacetabular impingement: a sports-specific analysis. *Arthrosc J Arthrosc Relat Surg.* 2014;30(3):398−405. https://doi.org/10.1016/j.arthro.2013.12.010.
6. Byrd JWT. Femoroacetabular impingement in athletes: current concepts. *Am J Sports Med.* 2014;42(3): 737−751. https://doi.org/10.1177/0363546513499136.
7. Griffin DR, Dickenson EJ, Wall PDH, et al. Hip arthroscopy versus best conservative care for the treatment of femoroacetabular impingement syndrome (UK FASHIoN): a multicentre randomised controlled trial. *Lancet.* 2018;391(10136):2225−2235. https://doi.org/10.1016/S0140-6736(18)31202-9.
8. Kelly BT, Maak TG, Larson CM, Bedi A, Zaltz I. Sports hip injuries: assessment and management. *Instr Course Lect.* 2013;62:515−531.
9. Lynch TS, Bedi A, Larson CM. Athletic hip injuries. *J Am Acad Orthop Surg.* 2017;25(4):269−279. https://doi.org/10.5435/JAAOS-D-16-00171.
10. Nepple JJ, Prather H, Trousdale RT, et al. Diagnostic imaging of femoroacetabular impingement. *J Am Acad Orthop Surg.* 2013;21(Suppl.):S20−S26. https://doi.org/10.5435/JAAOS-21-07-S20.
11. Tannast M, Siebenrock KA, Anderson SE. Femoroacetabular impingement: radiographic diagnosis—what the radiologist should know. *Am J Roentgenol.* 2007;188(6): 1540−1552. https://doi.org/10.2214/AJR.06.0921.
12. Tannast M, Hanke MS, Zheng G, Steppacher SD, Siebenrock KA. What are the radiographic reference values for acetabular under- and overcoverage? *Clin Orthop Relat Res.* 2015;473(4):1234−1246. https://doi.org/10.1007/s11999-014-4038-3.
13. Hapa O, Bedi A, Gursan O, et al. Anatomic footprint of the direct head of the rectus femoris origin: cadaveric study and clinical series of hips after arthroscopic anterior inferior iliac spine/subspine decompression. *Arthrosc J Arthrosc Relat Surg.* 2013;29(12):1932−1940. https://doi.org/10.1016/j.arthro.2013.08.023.
14. Philippon MJ, Devitt BM, Campbell KJ, et al. Anatomic variance of the iliopsoas tendon. *Am J Sports Med.* 2014; 42(4). https://doi.org/10.1177/0363546513518414.

15. Allen WC, Cope R. Coxa saltans: the snapping hip revisited. *J Am Acad Orthop Surg*. 1995;3(5):303−308. https://doi.org/10.5435/00124635-199509000-00006.

16. Byrd JWT, Bardowski EA, Civils AN, Parker SE. The safety of hip arthroscopy within 3 months of an intra-articular injection. *J Bone Joint Surg*. 2019;101(16):1467−1469. https://doi.org/10.2106/JBJS.19.00147.

17. Beck EC, Kunze KN, Friel NA, et al. Is there a correlation between outcomes after hip arthroscopy for femoroacetabular impingement syndrome and patient cortical bone thickness? *J Hip Preserv Surg*. 2019;6(1):16−24. https://doi.org/10.1093/jhps/hnz010.

18. Kuhns BD, Hannon CP, Makhni EC, et al. A comparison of clinical outcomes after unilateral or bilateral hip arthroscopic surgery: age- and sex-matched cohort study. *Am J Sports Med*. 2017;45(13):3044−3051. https://doi.org/10.1177/0363546517719020.

19. Stone AV, Mehta N, Beck EC, et al. Comparable patient-reported outcomes in females with or without joint hypermobility after hip arthroscopy and capsular plication for femoroacetabular impingement syndrome. *J Hip Preserv Surg*. 2019;6(1):33−40. https://doi.org/10.1093/jhps/hnz004.

20. Poehling-Monaghan KL, Krych AJ, Levy BA, Trousdale RT, Sierra RJ. Female sex is a risk factor for failure of hip arthroscopy performed for acetabular retroversion. *Orthop J Sports Med*. 2017;5(11). https://doi.org/10.1177/2325967117737479.

21. Wolfson TS, Ryan MK, Begly JP, Youm T. Outcome trends after hip arthroscopy for femoroacetabular impingement: when do patients improve? *Arthrosc J Arthrosc Relat Surg*. 2019;35(12):3261−3270. https://doi.org/10.1016/j.arthro.2019.06.020.

22. Bryan AJ, Krych AJ, Pareek A, Reardon PJ, Berardelli R, Levy BA. Are short-term outcomes of hip arthroscopy in patients 55 years and older inferior to those in younger patients? *Am J Sports Med*. 2016;44(10):2526−2530. https://doi.org/10.1177/0363546516652114.

23. Frank RM, Lee S, Bush-Joseph CA, Salata MJ, Mather RC, Nho SJ. Outcomes for hip arthroscopy according to sex and age: a comparative matched-group analysis. *J Bone Joint Surg*. 2016;98(10):797−804. https://doi.org/10.2106/JBJS.15.00445.

24. Gala L, Clohisy JC, Beaulé PE. Hip dysplasia in the young adult. *J Bone Joint Surg*. 2016;98(1):63−73. https://doi.org/10.2106/JBJS.O.00109.

25. Weinstein SL, Mubarak SJ, Wenger DR. Developmental hip dysplasia and dislocation: part II. *Instr Course Lect*. 2004;53:531−542.

26. Clohisy JC, Beaulé PE, O'Malley A, Safran MR, Schoenecker P. Hip disease in the young adult: current concepts of etiology and surgical treatment. *J Bone Jt Surg Am*. 2008;90(10):2267−2281. https://doi.org/10.2106/JBJS.G.01267.

27. Klaue K, Durnin CW, Ganz R. The acetabular rim syndrome. A clinical presentation of dysplasia of the hip. *J Bone Joint Surg Br*. 1991;73(3):423−429.

28. Ganz R, Leunig M, Leunig-Ganz K, Harris WH. The etiology of osteoarthritis of the hip: an integrated mechanical concept. *Clin Orthop Relat Res*. 2008;466(2):264−272. https://doi.org/10.1007/s11999-007-0060-z.

29. Wyles CC, Heidenreich MJ, Jeng J, Larson DR, Trousdale RT, Sierra RJ. The John Charnley award: redefining the natural history of osteoarthritis in patients with hip dysplasia and impingement. *Clin Orthop Relat Res*. 2017;475(2):336−350. https://doi.org/10.1007/s11999-016-4815-2.

30. Sankar WN, Duncan ST, Baca GR, et al. Descriptive epidemiology of acetabular dysplasia: the academic network of conservational hip outcomes research (ANCHOR) periacetabular osteotomy. *J Am Acad Orthop Surg*. 2017;25(2):150−159. https://doi.org/10.5435/JAAOS-D-16-00075.

31. Nepple JJ, Wells J, Ross JR, Bedi A, Schoenecker PL, Clohisy JC. Three patterns of acetabular deficiency are common in young adult patients with acetabular dysplasia. *Clin Orthop Relat Res*. 2017;475(4):1037−1044. https://doi.org/10.1007/s11999-016-5150-3.

32. Schmitz MR, Murtha AS, Clohisy JC. Developmental dysplasia of the hip in adolescents and young adults. *J Am Acad Orthop Surg*. 2020;28(3):91−101. https://doi.org/10.5435/JAAOS-D-18-00533.

33. Jacobsen JS, Bolvig L, Hölmich P, et al. Muscle−tendon-related abnormalities detected by ultrasonography are common in symptomatic hip dysplasia. *Arch Orthop Trauma Surg*. 2018;138(8):1059−1067. https://doi.org/10.1007/s00402-018-2947-4.

34. Philippon MJ, Zehms CT, Briggs KK, Manchester DJ, Kuppersmith DA. Hip instability in the athlete. *Operat Tech Sports Med*. 2007;15(4):189−194. https://doi.org/10.1053/j.otsm.2007.10.004.

35. Kalisvaart MM, Safran MR. Hip instability treated with arthroscopic capsular plication. *Knee Surg Sports Traumatol Arthrosc*. 2017;25(1):24−30. https://doi.org/10.1007/s00167-016-4377-6.

36. Beighton P. Hypermobility scoring. *Rheumatology*. 1988;27(2):163. https://doi.org/10.1093/rheumatology/27.2.163.

37. Leunig M, Podeszwa D, Beck M, Werlen S, Ganz R. Magnetic resonance arthrography of labral disorders in hips with dysplasia and impingement. *Clin Orthop Relat Res*. 2004;418:74−80. https://doi.org/10.1097/00003086-200401000-00013.

38. Sankar WN, Beaulé PE, Clohisy JC, et al. Labral morphologic characteristics in patients with symptomatic acetabular dysplasia. *Am J Sports Med*. 2015;43(9):2152−2156. https://doi.org/10.1177/0363546515591262.

39. Larson CM, Moreau-Gaudry A, Kelly BT, et al. Are normal hips being labeled as pathologic? A CT-based method for defining normal acetabular coverage. *Clin Orthop Relat Res*. 2015;473(4):1247−1254. https://doi.org/10.1007/s11999-014-4055-2.

40. Ganz R, Klaue K, Vinh TS, Mast JW. A new periacetabular osteotomy for the treatment of hip dysplasias. Technique and preliminary results. *Clin Orthop Relat Res*. 1988;232:26−36.

41. Wells J, Schoenecker P, Duncan S, Goss CW, Thomason K, Clohisy JC. Intermediate-term hip survivorship and patient-reported outcomes of periacetabular osteotomy: the Washington University experience. *J Bone Joint Surg.* 2018;100(3):218–225. https://doi.org/10.2106/JBJS.17.00337.

42. Drake RL, Vogl W, Mitchell AWM, Gray H. Lower limb. In: Gray H, ed. *Gray's Anatomy for Students.* Vol. 1. Elsevier/Churchill Livingstone; 2005:519.

43. Anderson CN. Iliopsoas: pathology, diagnosis, and treatment. *Clin Sports Med.* 2016;35(3):419–433. https://doi.org/10.1016/j.csm.2016.02.009.

44. Winston P, Awan R, Cassidy JD, Bleakney RK. Clinical examination and ultrasound of self-reported snapping hip syndrome in elite ballet dancers. *Am J Sports Med.* 2007;35(1):118–126. https://doi.org/10.1177/0363546506293703.

45. Wahl CJ, Warren RF, Adler RS, Hannafin JA, Hansen B. Internal coxa saltans (snapping hip) as a result of overtraining: a report of 3 cases in professional athletes with a review of causes and the role of ultrasound in early diagnosis and management. *Am J Sports Med.* 2004;32(5):1302–1309. https://doi.org/10.1177/0336354650325877.

46. Telhan R, Kelly BT, Moley P. Hip and pelvis overuse syndromes. In: Miller MD, Thompson SR, eds. *DeLee & Drez's Orthopaedic Sports Medicine: Principles and Practice.* Vol. 4. Philadelphia, PA: Elsevier; 2015:991–995.

47. Yen YM, Lewis CL, Kim YJ. Understanding and treating the snapping hip. *Sports Med Arthrosc Rev.* 2015;23(4):194–199. https://doi.org/10.1097/JSA.0000000000000095.

48. Pelsser V, Cardinal É, Hobden R, Aubin B, Lafortune M. Extraarticular snapping hip: sonographic findings. *Am J Roentgenol.* 2001;176(1):67–73. https://doi.org/10.2214/ajr.176.1.1760067.

49. Stopka C, Morley K, Siders R, Schuette J, Houck A, Gilmet Y. Stretching techniques to improve flexibility in special olympics athletes and their coaches. *J Sport Rehabil.* 2002;11(1):22–34. https://doi.org/10.1123/jsr.11.1.22.

50. Gosvig KK, Jacobsen S, Sonne-Holm S, Palm H, Troelsen A. Prevalence of malformations of the hip joint and their relationship to sex, groin pain, and risk of osteoarthritis: a population-based survey. *J Bone Joint Surg Am.* 2010;92(5):1162–1169. https://doi.org/10.2106/JBJS.H.01674.

51. Khan M, Adamich J, Simunovic N, Philippon MJ, Bhandari M, Ayeni OR. Surgical management of internal snapping hip syndrome: a systematic review evaluating open and arthroscopic approaches. *Arthrosc J Arthrosc Relat Surg.* 2013;29(5):942–948. https://doi.org/10.1016/j.arthro.2013.01.016.

52. Anderson SA, Keene JS. Results of arthroscopic iliopsoas tendon release in competitive and recreational athletes. *Am J Sports Med.* 2008;36(12):2363–2371. https://doi.org/10.1177/0363546508322130.

53. Provencher MT, Hofmeister EP, Muldoon MP. The surgical treatment of external coxa saltans (the snapping hip) by Z-plasty of the iliotibial band. *Am J Sports Med.* 2004;32(2):470–476. https://doi.org/10.1177/0363546503261713.

54. Voos JE, Rudzki JR, Shindle MK, Martin H, Kelly BT. Arthroscopic anatomy and surgical techniques for peritrochanteric space disorders in the hip. *Arthrosc J Arthrosc Relat Surg.* 2007;23(11):1246.e1–1246.e5. https://doi.org/10.1016/j.arthro.2006.12.014.

55. Polesello GC, Queiroz MC, Domb BG, Ono NK, Honda EK. Surgical technique: endoscopic gluteus maximus tendon release for external snapping hip syndrome. *Clin Orthop Relat Res.* 2013;471(8):2471–2476. https://doi.org/10.1007/s11999-012-2636-5.

56. Brignall CG, Stainsby GD. The snapping hip. Treatment by Z-plasty. *J Bone Joint Surg Br.* 1991;73(2):253–254.

57. White RA, Hughes MS, Burd T, Hamann J, Allen WC. A new operative approach in the correction of external coxa saltans: the snapping hip. *Am J Sports Med.* 2004;32(6):1504–1508. https://doi.org/10.1177/0363546503262189.

58. Redmond JM, Chen AW, Domb BG. Greater trochanteric pain syndrome. *J Am Acad Orthop Surg.* 2016;24(4):231–240. https://doi.org/10.5435/JAAOS-D-14-00406.

59. Lustenberger DP, Ng VY, Best TM, Ellis TJ. Efficacy of treatment of trochanteric bursitis: a systematic review. *Clin J Sport Med.* 2011;21(5):447–453. https://doi.org/10.1097/JSM.0b013e318221299c.

60. Bird PA, Oakley SP, Shnier R, Kirkham BW. Prospective evaluation of magnetic resonance imaging and physical examination findings in patients with greater trochanteric pain syndrome. *Arthritis Rheum.* 2001;44(9):2138–2145. https://doi.org/10.1002/1529-0131(200109)44:9<2138::AID-ART367>3.0.CO;2-M.

61. Grimaldi A, Fearon A. Gluteal tendinopathy: integrating pathomechanics and clinical features in its management. *J Orthop Sports Phys Ther.* 2015;45(11):910–922. https://doi.org/10.2519/jospt.2015.5829.

62. Long SS, Surrey DE, Nazarian LN. Sonography of greater trochanteric pain syndrome and the rarity of primary bursitis. *Am J Roentgenol.* 2013;201(5):1083–1086. https://doi.org/10.2214/AJR.12.10038.

63. Grimaldi A, Mellor R, Hodges P, Bennell K, Wajswelner H, Vicenzino B. Gluteal tendinopathy: a review of mechanisms, assessment and management. *Sports Med.* 2015;45(8):1107–1119. https://doi.org/10.1007/s40279-015-0336-5.

64. Fields KB. Running injuries - changing trends and demographics. *Curr Sports Med Rep.* 2011;10(5):299–303. https://doi.org/10.1249/JSR.0b013e31822d403f.

65. Tsutsumi M, Nimura A, Akita K. The gluteus medius tendon and its insertion sites: an anatomical study with possible implications for gluteus medius tears. *J Bone Joint Surg.* 2019;101(2):177–184. https://doi.org/10.2106/JBJS.18.00602.

66. Semciw AI, Green RA, Murley GS, Pizzari T. Gluteus minimus: an intramuscular EMG investigation of anterior and posterior segments during gait. *Gait Posture.* 2014;

39(2):822–826. https://doi.org/10.1016/j.gaitpost.2013. 11.008.

67. Gottschalk F, Kourosh S, Leveau B. The functional anatomy of tensor fasciae latae and gluteus medius and minimus. *J Anat.* 1989;166:179–189.

68. Widler KS, Glatthorn JF, Bizzini M, et al. Assessment of hip abductor muscle strength. A validity and reliability study. *J Bone Joint Surg.* 2009;91(11):2666–2672. https://doi.org/10.2106/JBJS.H.01119.

69. Godshaw B, Wong M, Ojard C, Williams G, Suri M, Jones D. Acute traumatic tear of the gluteus medius and gluteus minimus in a marathon runner. *Ochsner J.* 2019;19(4):405–409. https://doi.org/10.31486/toj.18. 0090.

70. Allison K, Salomoni SE, Bennell KL, et al. Hip abductor muscle activity during walking in individuals with gluteal tendinopathy. *Scand J Med Sci Sports.* 2018;28(2): 686–695. https://doi.org/10.1111/sms.12942.

71. Pierce TP, Issa K, Kurowicki J, Festa A, McInerney VK, Scillia AJ. Abductor tendon tears of the hip. *JBJS Rev.* 2018;6(3):e6. https://doi.org/10.2106/JBJS.RVW.17. 00076.

72. Teitz CC, Hu SS, Arendt EA. The female athlete: evaluation and treatment of sports-related problems. *J Am Acad Orthop Surg.* 1997;5(2):87–96. https://doi.org/ 10.5435/00124635-199703000-00004.

73. Lachiewicz PF. Abductor tendon tears of the hip: evaluation and management. *J Am Acad Orthop Surg.* 2011; 19(7):385–391. https://doi.org/10.5435/00124635-201 107000-00001.

74. Grimaldi A, Mellor R, Nicolson P, Hodges P, Bennell K, Vicenzino B. Utility of clinical tests to diagnose MRI-confirmed gluteal tendinopathy in patients presenting with lateral hip pain. *Br J Sports Med.* 2017;51(6): 519–524. https://doi.org/10.1136/bjsports-2016-096175.

75. Crossley KM, Zhang W-J, Schache AG, Bryant A, Cowan SM. Performance on the single-leg squat task indicates hip abductor muscle function. *Am J Sports Med.* 2011;39(4):866–873. https://doi.org/10.1177/0363546 510395456.

76. Kong A, Van der Vliet A, Zadow S. MRI and US of gluteal tendinopathy in greater trochanteric pain syndrome. *Eur Radiol.* 2007;17(7):1772–1783. https://doi.org/10.1007/ s00330-006-0485-x.

77. Docking SI, Cook J, Chen S, et al. Identification and differentiation of gluteus medius tendon pathology using ultrasound and magnetic resonance imaging. *Musculoskelet Sci Pract.* 2019;41:1–5. https://doi.org/10.1016/ j.msksp.2019.01.011.

78. Fearon AM, Scarvell JM, Cook JL, Smith PN. Does ultrasound correlate with surgical or histologic findings in greater trochanteric pain syndrome? A pilot study. *Clin Orthop Relat Res.* 2010;468(7):1838–1844. https:// doi.org/10.1007/s11999-009-1174-2.

79. Kingzett-Taylor A, Tirman PF, Feller J, et al. Tendinosis and tears of gluteus medius and minimus muscles as a cause of hip pain: MR imaging findings. *Am J Roentgenol.*

1999;173(4):1123–1126. https://doi.org/10.2214/ajr. 173.4.10511191.

80. Cvitanic O, Henzie G, Skezas N, Lyons J, Minter J. MRI diagnosis of tears of the hip abductor tendons (gluteus medius and gluteus minimus). *Am J Roentgenol.* 2004; 182(1):137–143. https://doi.org/10.2214/ajr.182.1. 1820137.

81. Westacott DJ, Minns JI, Foguet P. The diagnostic accuracy of magnetic resonance imaging and ultrasonography in gluteal tendon tears - a systematic review. *HIP.* 2011; 21(6):637–645. https://doi.org/10.5301/HIP.2011.8759.

82. Ebert JR, Smith A, Breidahl W, Fallon M, Janes GC. Association of preoperative gluteal muscle fatty infiltration with patient outcomes in women after hip abductor tendon repair augmented with LARS. *Am J Sports Med.* 2019;47(13):3148–3157. https://doi.org/10.1177/0363 546519873672.

83. Barratt PA, Brookes N, Newson A. Conservative treatments for greater trochanteric pain syndrome: a systematic review. *Br J Sports Med.* 2017;51(2):97–104. https://doi.org/10.1136/bjsports-2015-095858.

84. Fitzpatrick J, Bulsara MK, O'Donnell J, McCrory PR, Zheng MH. The effectiveness of platelet-rich plasma injections in gluteal tendinopathy: a randomized, double-blind controlled trial comparing a single platelet-rich plasma injection with a single corticosteroid injection. *Am J Sports Med.* 2018;46(4):933–939. https://doi.org/ 10.1177/0363546517745525.

85. Walsh MJ, Walton JR, Walsh NA. Surgical repair of the gluteal tendons. *J Arthroplasty.* 2011;26(8):1514–1519. https://doi.org/10.1016/j.arth.2011.03.004.

86. Davies JF, Stiehl JB, Davies JA, Geiger PB. Surgical treatment of hip abductor tendon tears. *J Bone Jt Surg Am.* 2013;95(15):1420–1425. https://doi.org/10.2106/JBJS. L.00709.

87. Whiteside LA. Surgical technique: gluteus maximus and tensor fascia lata transfer for primary deficiency of the abductors of the hip. *Clin Orthop Relat Res.* 2014;472(2): 645–653. https://doi.org/10.1007/s11999-013-3161-x.

88. Whiteside LA. Surgical technique: transfer of the anterior portion of the gluteus maximus muscle for abductor deficiency of the hip. *Clin Orthop Relat Res.* 2012;470(2): 503–510. https://doi.org/10.1007/s11999-011-1975-y.

89. Beck M, Leunig M, Ellis T, Ganz R. Advancement of the vastus lateralis muscle for the treatment of hip abductor discontinuity. *J Arthroplasty.* 2004;19(4):476–480. https://doi.org/10.1016/j.arth.2003.11.014.

90. Okoroha KR, Beck EC, Nwachukwu BU, Kunze KN, Nho SJ. Defining minimal clinically important difference and patient acceptable symptom state after isolated endoscopic gluteus medius repair. *Am J Sports Med.* 2019;47(13):3141–3147. https://doi.org/10.1177/0363 546519877179.

91. Chandrasekaran S, Lodhia P, Gui C, Vemula SP, Martin TJ, Domb BG. Outcomes of open versus endoscopic repair of abductor muscle tears of the hip: a systematic review. *Arthrosc J Arthrosc Relat Surg.* 2015;

31(10):2057–2067.e2. https://doi.org/10.1016/j.arthro.2015.03.042.

92. Fabry G, MacEwen GD, Shands AR. Torsion of the femur. A follow-up study in normal and abnormal conditions. *J Bone Joint Surg Am.* 1973;55(8):1726–1738.

93. Tönnis D, Heinecke A. Current concepts review - acetabular and femoral anteversion: relationship with osteoarthritis of the hip*. *J Bone Joint Surg.* 1999;81(12):1747–1770. https://doi.org/10.2106/00004623-199912000-00014.

94. Schmaranzer F, Lerch TD, Siebenrock KA, Tannast M, Steppacher SD. Differences in femoral torsion among various measurement methods increase in hips with excessive femoral torsion. *Clin Orthop Relat Res.* 2019;477(5):1073–1083. https://doi.org/10.1097/CORR.0000000000000610.

95. Buly RL, Sosa BR, Poultsides LA, Caldwell E, Rozbruch SR. Femoral derotation osteotomy in adults for version abnormalities. *J Am Acad Orthop Surg.* 2018;26(19):e416–e425. https://doi.org/10.5435/JAAOS-D-17-00623.

96. Weinberg DS, Park PJ, Morris WZ, Liu RW. Femoral version and tibial torsion are not associated with hip or knee arthritis in a large osteological collection. *J Pediatr Orthop.* 2017;37(2):e120–e128. https://doi.org/10.1097/BPO.0000000000000604.

97. Maruyama M, Feinberg JR, Capello WN, D'Antonio JA. The Frank Stinchfield Award: morphologic features of the acetabulum and femur: anteversion angle and implant positioning. *Clin Orthop Relat Res.* 2001;393:52–65.

98. Litrenta JM, Domb BG. Normative data on femoral version. *J Hip Preserv Surg.* 2018;5(4):410–424. https://doi.org/10.1093/jhps/hny048.

99. Tanzer M, Noiseux N. Osseous abnormalities and early osteoarthritis: the role of hip impingement. *Clin Orthop Relat Res.* 2004;429:170–177.

100. Hetsroni I, Dela Torre K, Duke G, Lyman S, Kelly BT. Sex differences of hip morphology in young adults with hip pain and labral tears. *Arthrosc J Arthrosc Relat Surg.* 2013;29(1):54–63. https://doi.org/10.1016/j.arthro.2012.07.008.

101. Bråten M, Terjesen T, Rossvoll I. Femoral anteversion in normal adults: ultrasound measurements in 50 men and 50 women. *Acta Orthop Scand.* 1992;63(1):29–32. https://doi.org/10.3109/17453679209154844.

102. Hartigan DE, Perets I, Walsh JP, Chaharbakhshi EO, Yuen LC, Domb BG. Clinical outcomes of hip arthroscopic surgery in patients with femoral retroversion: a matched study to patients with normal femoral anteversion. *Orthop J Sports Med.* 2017;5(10). https://doi.org/10.1177/2325967117732726.

103. Eckhoff DG, Montgomery WK, Kilcoyne RF, Stamm ER. Femoral morphometry and anterior knee pain. *Clin Orthop Relat Res.* 1994;302:64–68.

104. Zhang Z, Zhang H, Song G, Zheng T, Ni Q, Feng H. Increased femoral anteversion is associated with inferior clinical outcomes after MPFL reconstruction and combined tibial tubercle osteotomy for the treatment of recurrent patellar instability. *Knee Surg Sports Traumatol Arthrosc.* 2020;28(7):2261–2269. https://doi.org/10.1007/s00167-019-05818-3.

105. Alpay Y, Ezici A, Kurk MB, Ozyalvac ON, Akpinar E, Bayhan AI. Increased femoral anteversion related to infratrochanteric femoral torsion is associated with ACL rupture. *Knee Surg Sports Traumatol Arthrosc.* https://doi.org/10.1007/s00167-020-05874-0. Published online February 6, 2020.

106. Canham CD, Yen Y-M, Giordano BD. Does femoroacetabular impingement cause hip instability? A systematic review. *Arthrosc J Arthrosc Relat Surg.* 2016;32(1):203–208. https://doi.org/10.1016/j.arthro.2015.07.021.

107. Fabricant PD, Fields KG, Taylor SA, Magennis E, Bedi A, Kelly BT. The effect of femoral and acetabular version on clinical outcomes after arthroscopic femoroacetabular impingement surgery. *J Bone Jt Surg Am.* 2015;97(7):537–543. https://doi.org/10.2106/JBJS.N.00266.

108. Pailhé R, Bedes L, Sales de Gauzy J, Tran R, Cavaignac E, Accadbled F. Derotational femoral osteotomy technique with locking nail fixation for adolescent femoral antetorsion: surgical technique and preliminary study. *J Pediatr Orthop B.* 2014;23(6):523–528. https://doi.org/10.1097/BPB.0000000000000087.

109. Nelitz M. Femoral derotational osteotomies. *Curr Rev Musculoskelet Med.* 2018;11(2):272–279. https://doi.org/10.1007/s12178-018-9483-2.

110. Parvizi J, Campfield A, Clohisy JC, Rothman RH, Mont MA. Management of arthritis of the hip in the young adult. *J Bone Joint Surg Br.* 2006;88-B(10):1279–1285. https://doi.org/10.1302/0301-620X.88B10.17859.

111. Spector TD, Harris PA, Hart DJ, et al. Risk of osteoarthritis associated with long-term weight-bearing sports: a radiologic survey of the hips and knees in female ex-athletes and population controls. *Arthritis Rheum.* 1996;39(6):988–995. https://doi.org/10.1002/art.1780390616.

112. Hartofilakidis G, Karachalios T. Idiopathic osteoarthritis of the hip: incidence, classification, and natural history of 272 cases. *Orthopedics.* 2003;26(2):161–166.

113. Alentorn-Geli E, Samuelsson K, Musahl V, Green CL, Bhandari M, Karlsson J. The association of recreational and competitive running with hip and knee osteoarthritis: a systematic review and meta-analysis. *J Orthop Sports Phys Ther.* 2017;47(6):373–390. https://doi.org/10.2519/jospt.2017.7137.

114. Kapron AL, Peters CL, Aoki SK, et al. The prevalence of radiographic findings of structural hip deformities in female collegiate athletes. *Am J Sports Med.* 2015;43(6):1324–1330. https://doi.org/10.1177/0363546515576908.

115. AAOS. *Appropriate Use Criteria for the Management of Osteoarthritis of the Hip.* 2017.

116. Dallari D, Stagni C, Rani N, et al. Ultrasound-guided injection of platelet-rich plasma and hyaluronic acid, separately and in combination, for hip osteoarthritis: a randomized controlled study. *Am J Sports Med.* 2016;

44(3):664–671. https://doi.org/10.1177/03635465156 20383.

117. Steppacher SD, Tannast M, Ganz R, Siebenrock KA. Mean 20-year followup of bernese periacetabular osteotomy. *Clin Orthop Relat Res.* 2008;466(7):1633–1644. https://doi.org/10.1007/s11999-008-0242-3.

118. McGrory B, Barrack R, Lachiewicz PF, et al. Modern metal-on-metal hip resurfacing. *Am Acad Orthop Surg.* 2010;18(5):306–314. https://doi.org/10.5435/001246 35-201005000-00007.

119. Sands D, Schemitsch EH. The role of metal-on-metal bearings in total hip arthroplasty and hip resurfacing: review article. *HSS J.* 2017;13(1):2–6. https://doi.org/10.1007/s11420-016-9521-9.

120. Polkowski GG, Callaghan JJ, Mont MA, Clohisy JC. Total hip arthroplasty in the very young patient. *J Am Acad Orthop Surg.* 2012;20(8):487–497. https://doi.org/10.5435/JAAOS-20-08-487.

121. Schmidutz F, Grote S, Pietschmann M, et al. Sports activity after short-stem hip arthroplasty. *Am J Sports Med.* 2012;40(2):425–432. https://doi.org/10.1177/0363546 511424386.

122. Hoorntje A, Janssen KY, Bolder SBT, et al. The effect of total hip arthroplasty on sports and work participation: a systematic review and meta-analysis. *Sports Med.* 2018; 48(7):1695–1726. https://doi.org/10.1007/s40279-018-0924-2.

CHAPTER 12

Ankle Anatomy and Biomechanics

JOHN W. YUREK, DO • ARIANNA L. GIANAKOS, DO • MARY K. MULCAHEY, MD

INTRODUCTION

The ankle joint is composed of bones, ligaments, and tendons that provide an inherent balance between structure and function. Ligamentous structures connect the bones of the ankle to create a strong foundation for transmission of forces during weight-bearing activities. Traversing tendons work synergistically to create motion and generate power during ankle movement. Nerves and blood vessels provide sensation, proprioceptive feedback, and oxygen to all structures of the ankle. Each of these vital components work together biomechanically and play a critical role in the gait cycle. Understanding anatomy and biomechanics is important when evaluating and treating athletic injuries involving the ankle joint. In addition, gender-related differences including structure, kinematics, laxity, and neuromuscular control should also be addressed when managing injuries in the female athlete. This chapter will review the ankle bony, soft tissue, and neurovascular anatomy; the biomechanics underlying the gait cycle; and gender-related differences within the ankle joint.

BONY ANATOMY

The distal tibia, distal fibula, and talus articulate to form the bony structure of the ankle joint. The distal tibial articular surface, also known as the tibial plafond, is a quadrilateral surface that is wider anteriorly.[1-4] This surface is concave in the sagittal plane and slightly convex in the transverse plane.[1-4] This allows smooth articulation with the dorsal surface of the talus, also called the trochlea, which is convex in the sagittal plane and approximately 4 mm wider anteriorly.[5,6] The distal end of the tibia has an inferomedial projection, the medial malleolus, which articulates with the medial articular surface of the talus during ankle motion.[1-4] The distal aspect of the medial malleolus has two rounded projections, the anterior colliculus and the posterior colliculus. The anterior colliculus projects more distally. The distal, lateral tibia contains a notch

for the fibula, also known as the incisura fibularis, and is surrounded by strong ligaments that make up the ankle syndesmosis, which will be discussed later. The distal aspect of the fibula projects past the tibial plafond and is referred to as the lateral malleolus. The medial aspect of the lateral malleolus articulates with the lateral surface of the talus. The tibial plafond, medial malleolus, and lateral malleolus together are known as the ankle mortise. With an intact syndesmosis, the ankle mortise acts to contain the talus and prevent its medial and lateral translation. The concavity of the tibial plafond in the sagittal plane creates a posterior, distal protrusion known as the posterior malleolus. This structure differs from the medial and lateral malleoli by not providing a vertical bony wall to prevent talar translation.[1-4]

SOFT TISSUE ANATOMY

The lateral ankle joint is stabilized by the lateral ligamentous complex, which is composed of the anterior talofibular ligament (ATFL), the calcaneofibular ligament (CFL), and the posterior talofibular ligament (PTFL).[1-4] The ATFL extends from the anterior tip of the lateral malleolus proximally to the anterolateral surface of the talus distally (Fig. 12.1). The CFL runs from the middle aspect of the tip of the lateral malleolus, courses deep to the peroneal tendons, and attaches to the lateral surface of the calcaneus. The PTFL courses from the posterior part of the lateral malleolus to the posterolateral talar surface.[1-4]

The medial ankle joint is stabilized by the medial ligamentous complex, also referred to as the deltoid ligamentous complex, which connects the medial malleolus to the navicular, talus, and calcaneus.[7] The deltoid ligamentous complex functions to limit lateral, anterior, and posterior talar translation and prevents talar abduction. It is composed of a superficial layer containing four ligaments and a deep layer containing two ligaments (Fig. 12.2). The superficial and deep layers are separated by a thin layer of adipose tissue

The Female Athlete. https://doi.org/10.1016/B978-0-323-75985-4.00019-2

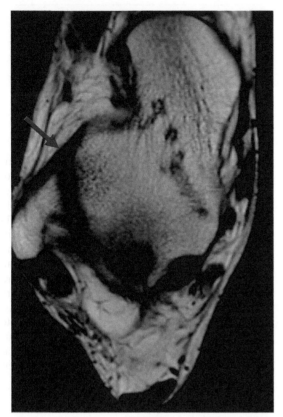

FIG. 12.1 Normal anterior talofibular ligament on axial T2 magnetic resonance imaging. Arrow indicates intact ATFL. (Courtesy of Brian Everist, MD and Bryan Vopat, MD, University of Kansas Medical Center.)

and all six ligaments are named for their attachment sites. The four ligaments that compose the superficial layer include the tibionavicular ligament, the tibiocalcaneal ligament, the superficial posterior tibiotalar ligament, and the tibiospring ligament. The deep layer consists of the deep anterior tibiotalar ligament and the deep posterior tibiotalar ligament. The entire deltoid ligamentous complex sits deep to the tendons and neurovascular structures that traverse the medial ankle.[7]

The distal articulation between the tibia and fibula is stabilized by the syndesmotic ligament complex and is composed of three main parts: the anteroinferior tibiofibular ligament (AITFL), the posteroinferior tibiofibular ligament (PITFL), and the interosseous tibiofibular ligament (IOTFL).[8-10] The AITFL originates on the anterior tubercle of the distal tibia approximately 5 mm proximal to the articular surface and runs in a lateral and distal orientation to its attachment site on the

anterior margin of the lateral malleolus (Fig. 12.3). Often the AITFL can appear to be divided into fascicles by perforating branches of the peroneal artery. The PITFL is composed of superficial and deep layers. The superficial layer originates from the posterior tibial tubercle and runs distally and laterally to attach to the posterior margin of the lateral malleolus. This layer is homologous to the AITFL. The deep layer of the PITFL, also known as the transverse ligament, originates on the posterior edge of the distal tibia as far medial as the medial malleolus and projects laterally to attach to the proximal aspect of the lateral malleolar fossa. The transverse ligament is cone shaped owing to its broad attachment to the posterior tibia and can aid in ankle joint stability by acting as a labrum preventing posterior talar translation. The IOTFL is a dense network of short fibers spanning directly between the distal tibia and fibula. It is the distal continuation of the interosseous membrane at the level of the syndesmosis and helps provide stability to the syndesmotic ligamentous complex.[8-10]

The tendinous portions of muscles that cross the ankle joint act in synchronicity to provide movement.[11] Anteriorly, from medial to lateral, the tibialis anterior, extensor hallucis longus, extensor digitorum longus, and peroneus tertius tendons cross over the ankle joint. They all work to dorsiflex the ankle joint and have varying functions distally within the foot. Posteromedially, from medial to lateral, the tibialis posterior, flexor digitorum longus, and flexor hallucis longus tendons cross the ankle and aid in plantar flexion of the ankle, with varying functions distally within the foot. Directly posterior, the Achilles tendon crosses the ankle and provides the majority of plantar flexion strength. Posterolaterally, the peroneus brevis and peroneus longus tendons cross the ankle just posterior to the lateral malleolus. The peroneus brevis runs anterior to the peroneus longus and together they assist in plantar flexion of the ankle.[11]

NEUROVASCULAR ANATOMY

Neurologic structures provide sensation to the skin overlying the ankle and innervate muscles that create motion at the ankle joint. Sensation about the ankle, as in all parts of the body, can be described in either dermatomal or peripheral nerve distributions. The anterior ankle dermatomes are supplied by the L4 nerve root medially and L5 laterally.[11] The posterior ankle is supplied by S1 laterally and S2 medially. L5 supplies an area of skin between S1 and S2 over the posterior ankle. Sensation to the ankle can also be described by the individual peripheral nerves

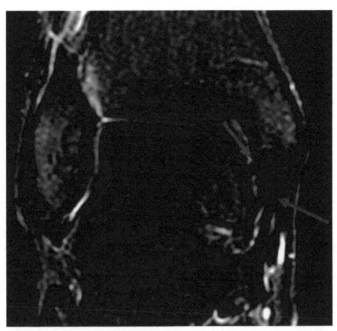

FIG. 12.2 Coronal T2FS magnetic resonance imaging with normal deep deltoid and superficial deltoid (tibiospring component). Small arrow indicates intact deep deltoid ligament. Long arrow indicates intactd superficial deltoid ligament. (Courtesy of Brian Everist, MD and Bryan Vopat, MD, University of Kansas Medical Center.)

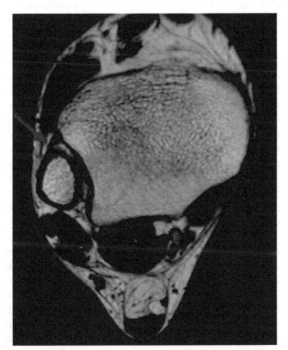

FIG. 12.3 Anteroinferior tibiofibular ligament on axial T2 magnetic resonance imaging. Arrow indicated intact AITFL. (Courtesy of Brian Everist, MD and Bryan Vopat, MD, University of Kansas Medical Center.)

supplying skin branches. The superficial peroneal nerve provides sensation to the anterior ankle, the saphenous nerve supplies the medial and posteromedial ankle, and the sural nerve supplies the lateral and posterolateral ankle. The distal tibiofibular joint receives innervation from the deep peroneal, tibial, and saphenous nerves. The ankle joint is innervated by the deep peroneal and tibial nerves. The muscles that cross the ankle are innervated by three peripheral nerves that are supplied by the L4-S2 nerve roots. The anterior compartment muscles are all innervated by the deep peroneal nerve, the peroneal muscles are innervated by the superficial peroneal nerve, and all three posteromedial muscles are innervated by the tibial nerve.[11]

Blood supply to the ankle is provided by three main arteries: the anterior tibial artery, posterior tibial artery, and peroneal artery.[11,12] Around the ankle, the anterior tibial artery runs from proximal to distal just lateral to the tibialis anterior tendon and deep to the extensor hallucis longus, which crosses superficially from lateral to medial. This main artery provides the anterior medial and anterior lateral malleolar branches, which course perpendicularly toward those structures they are named for. The anterior tibial artery continues distally into the foot as the dorsalis pedis artery. The peroneal artery courses longitudinally along the posterolateral ankle.

It provides a branch named the peroneal perforating artery that pierces the distal tibiofibular syndesmosis 5 cm proximal to the tip of the lateral malleolus to anastomose with the anterior lateral malleolar artery. The peroneal artery also gives off a posterior lateral malleolar artery, which courses perpendicularly, deep to the peroneal tendons, to anastomose with the anterior lateral malleolar artery and perforating artery to create a vascular network around the lateral malleolus. A communicating branch arises from the peroneal artery 6 cm proximal to the tip of the lateral malleolus to anastomose with the posterior tibial artery. Lastly, the peroneal artery branches into the lateral calcaneal artery, which supplies the heel pad and calcaneus distally. The posterior tibial artery crosses the ankle joint between the flexor digitorum longus tendon medially and flexor hallucis longus tendon laterally and courses next to the tibial nerve. This artery gives rise to the posterior medial malleolar artery, which courses perpendicularly, deep to the posterior tibialis and flexor digitorum longus tendons, to anastomose with the anterior medial malleolar artery and create a vascular network in this area. Distally, the posterior tibial artery provides a branch named the medial calcaneal artery, which anastomoses with the lateral calcaneal artery over the posterior calcaneus.[11,12]

BIOMECHANICS OF THE ANKLE-GAIT CYCLE

The anatomic structures of the ankle discussed earlier work together to power ankle motion, which plays an important role throughout the gait cycle. The gait cycle is a series of pelvis and lower extremity motions that allow humans to walk or run. One cycle of gait is described as occurring between the initial ground contact of one foot and continues until that same foot contacts the ground again.[13,14] This cycle can be divided into a stance phase and a swing phase. The stance phase is a continuum from the initial heel strike, the foot lying flat on the floor with the body passing over, the heel rising from the floor, and to the eventual toe rise. After toe rise, that foot goes through the swing phase. With slower speed gait cycles, such as during walking, there are periods where both feet are in contact with the ground and there is always one foot in contact with the ground throughout all time points of the cycle. As the speed of the gait cycle increases, such as during running, a float phase will start to be incorporated where neither foot is touching the ground. Also, with increasing speeds, the duration and percentage of the stance phase in the gait cycle decreases and the float phase increases.[13,14]

The various muscles that cross the ankle joint work together during the gait cycle to create a smooth transition between dorsiflexion and plantar flexion through both concentric and eccentric contractions.[13,14] The posterior (deep and superficial) and lateral lower leg compartment muscles provide plantar flexion force, whereas the anterior compartment lower leg muscles drive ankle dorsiflexion. During gait, the anterior compartment concentrically contracts at the end of toe-off phase to bring the ankle from plantar flexion to dorsiflexion. Dorsiflexion is maintained throughout the swing phase with continued anterior compartment muscle contraction. This contraction continues during heel strike and the concentric contraction then stops and eccentric contraction begins to control the rapid plantar flexion that occurs during the transition to foot-flat phase. At this point, the anterior compartment becomes dormant until the end of toe-off phase. The posterior compartment musculature first becomes active with eccentric contraction during the foot-flat phase to control the forward movement of the tibia over the foot. Then concentric contraction occurs to drive ankle plantar flexion during the heel-off and toe-off phases. This contraction ceases before full plantar flexion once the opposite limb begins weight-bearing and the terminal portion of plantar flexion occurs passively through gravity without muscle contraction.[13,14]

During walking, the vertical ground reaction force is 1.0–1.5 times the body weight, and during running, it is 2.0–2.9 times the body weight.[15] These forces can be even greater during sports that require push-off, acceleration, or jumping. During walking, the ankle joint experiences a force of approximately five times the body weight and is the highest during the flat foot portion of the stance phase.[16] With running, the force transmitted across the ankle joint can increase to 13 times the body weight.[16] Approximately 83% of the total force is transmitted across the tibiotalar joint, whereas 17% is transmitted through the fibula.[17] The load-bearing area of the tibiotalar joint is relatively large, approximately 12 cm^2, which aids in distribution of the high amount of force seen by this joint.[18] Because of the major forces experienced by the ankle joint, the bony architecture and ligaments are pivotal in providing adequate stability to transmit forces, while being supple enough to help absorb the large forces experienced during impact.

The majority of plantar flexion and dorsiflexion of the ankle is thought to occur at the tibiotalar joint, with only a few degrees of motion occurring through the subtalar joint.[19] Inversion and eversion have been shown to be distributed between the tibiotalar joint and the subtalar joint.[17] The sagittal plane range of motion of the ankle joint during the gait cycle encompasses a 70-degree arc with 20 degrees of dorsiflexion to 50 degrees of plantar flexion.[20,21] This range of motion occurs twice during the normal gait cycle. Just before heel strike, the ankle is dorsiflexed, and at heel strike, rapid plantar flexion occurs. During flat foot, as the body moves over the foot, the ankle goes from plantar flexion to dorsiflexion. Then plantar flexion occurs again during heel rise and toe-off phase.

GENDER-RELATED DIFFERENCES IN ANKLE ANATOMY AND BIOMECHANICS

Previous studies have demonstrated various gender-related differences in ankle anatomy and biomechanics that may attribute to the variability in the development of injuries about the foot and ankle (Table 12.1).

TABLE 12.1 Ankle Anatomy and Biomechanics Differences in Females Compared With Males.	
	Females (Compared With Males)
Proportional foot length	↓
Forefoot width	↑
Arch of foot length	↓
Metatarsal length	↓
Trochlear breadth of talus	↓
Ligamentous laxity	↑
Ankle dorsiflexion	↑
Ankle plantar flexion	↑
Talocrural dorsiflexion	↑
Talocrural plantar flexion	↑
Subtalar inversion	↑
Subtalar eversion	↑
Subtalar internal/external rotation	↑
Neuromuscular control	↓
Syndesmosis laxity	↑
Mobility during gait	↑
Cadence	↑
Stride length	↓

Arrow up indicates female value greater than male value. Arrow down indicates female value less than male value.

Females typically have proportionately shorter foot and arch lengths, wider forefoot widths, and shorter metatarsal lengths when compared with males.[22,23] Nozaki et al.[24] conducted a study evaluating the morphologic differences in talar anatomy between males and females. The authors found that the female talus had a longer neck; a narrower head width, which was more twisted and elongated in the dorsoplantar direction; and a more lateral superiorly tilted trochlea. These factors can potentially alter the subtalar and talonavicular joint kinematics during gait.[24]

Variability in ankle ligamentous laxity between males and females has also been established within the literature. Studies have demonstrated that females have an increase in ligamentous laxity, resulting in increased mobility about the ankle joint.[25,26] Fukano et al.[25] evaluated fluoroscopic images to determine three-dimensional bone orientation and reported that females had a statistically significant larger range of motion in talocrural dorsiflexion/plantar flexion, subtalar eversion/inversion, and subtalar external/internal rotation while walking when compared with males. Several studies have evaluated ankle ligamentous laxity during the anterior drawer and talar tilt test under stress radiography using the Telos device and reported greater ankle laxity in females than in males.[27,28] In addition, previous studies have demonstrated gender-related differences in the viscoelastic properties of tendon structures around the ankle joint. Males typically have greater passive ankle joint stiffness and higher hysteresis of tendons when compared with females.[29]

There have been several biomechanical studies that have also demonstrated differences in walking and running between males and females. Takabayashi et al.[30] investigated three-dimensional rearfoot, midfoot, and forefoot kinematics, as well as spatiotemporal parameters, during running. The authors found that females had significantly increased range of motion in the sagittal plane of the rearfoot and midfoot, with larger peak plantar flexion angles of the rearfoot and larger peak dorsiflexion angles of the midfoot, when compared with their male counterparts.[30] In addition, studies have demonstrated that females typically have weaker gross motor strength of ankle plantar flexion and dorsiflexion, as well as less arch stiffness, than males.[31,32] Fukano et al.[25] demonstrated an increase in talocrural dorsiflexion, inversion, and subtalar internal rotation in the early stance phase in females compared with males. Chiu et al.[33] reported that females have a more inverted position at the talocrural joint during the early stance phase of gait. Kinematic differences between males and females tend to be greatest at the early phase of stance into toe-off during the gait cycle. Therefore males and females may have differing adaptation patterns when ambulating on different surfaces and at different speeds. In addition, during running, females typically require an increase in plantar flexion strength as a result of proportionately shorter foot lengths in order to maintain kinematics at other joints.[22,34] Lastly, Ko et al. conducted a gait analysis study utilizing reflective markers, three-dimensional motion capture cameras, and ground reaction forces to determine differences between males and females. The authors found that females walked with a higher cadence and shorter stride length and had less hip range of motion, greater ankle range of motion in the sagittal plane, and greater hip range of motion in the frontal plane.[35] These findings demonstrate that males and females rely on different hip and ankle kinematics, leading to variable energy expenditure, during gait.

SUMMARY

The bony and soft tissue anatomy of the ankle joint functions biomechanically to allow for efficient gait. Understanding the function of the various tendons, ligaments, and bones is important in order to better assess and manage the pathology of athletic injuries involving the ankle joint. Gender-related differences should also be considered when managing injuries. Female and male athletes may have different presentations of symptoms as well as different functional outcomes with both conservative and/or surgical treatment.

REFERENCES

1. Standring S. *Gray's Anatomy: The Anatomical Basis of Clinical Practice*. 41st ed. Elsevier; 2015.
2. Moore KL, Dalley AF. *Clinically Oriented Anatomy*. 5th ed. LWW; 2005.
3. Kelikian AS, Sarrafian SK. *Sarrafian's Anatomy of the Foot and Ankle: Descriptive, Topographic, Functional*. 3rd ed. LWW; 2011.
4. Bozkurt M, Doral MN. Anatomic factors and biomechanics in ankle instability. *Foot Ankle Clin*. 2006;11(3):451–463.
5. Romanes GJ. *Cunningham's Textbook of Anatomy*. 10th ed. Oxford University Press; 1964.
6. Inman VT. *The Joints of the Ankle*. Williams & Wilkins; 1976.
7. Campbell KJ, Michalski MP, Wilson KJ, et al. The ligament anatomy of the deltoid complex of the ankle: a qualitative and quantitative anatomical study. *J Bone Joint Surg Am*. 2014;96(8):e62.
8. Lin CF, Gross MT, Weinhold P. Ankle syndesmosis injuries: anatomy, biomechanics, mechanism of injury, and clinical guidelines for diagnosis and intervention. *J Orthop Sports Phys Ther*. 2006;36(6):372–384.
9. Golanó P, Vega J, de Leeuw PAJ, et al. Anatomy of the ankle ligaments: a pictorial essay. *Knee Surg Sports Traumatol Arthrosc*. 2010;18(5):557–569.
10. Van den Bekerom MPJ, Raven EEJ. The distal fascicle of the anterior inferior tibiofibular ligament as a cause of tibiotalar impingement syndrome: a current concepts review. *Knee Surg Sports Traumatol Arthrosc*. 2007;15(4):465–471.
11. Riegger CL. Anatomy of the ankle and foot. *Phys Ther*. 1988;68(12):1802–1814.
12. Attinger C, Cooper P, Blume P. Vascular anatomy of the foot and ankle. *Operat Tech Plast Reconstr Surg*. 1997;4(4):183–198.
13. Brockett CL, Chapman GJ. Biomechanics of the ankle. *Orthop Trauma*. 2016;30(3):232–238.
14. Miller M, Thompson S. *DeLee, Drez and Miller's Orthopaedic Sports Medicine: 2-Volume Set*. 5th ed. Elsevier; 2019.
15. Nilsson J, Thorstensson A, Halbertsma J. Changes in leg movements and muscle activity with speed of locomotion and mode of progression in humans. *Acta Physiol Scand*. 1985;123(4):457–475.
16. Burdett RG. Forces predicted at the ankle during running. *Med Sci Sports Exerc*. 1982;14(4):308–316.
17. Calhoun JH, Li F, Ledbetter BR, Viegas SF. A comprehensive study of pressure distribution in the ankle joint with inversion and eversion. *Foot Ankle Int*. 1994;15(3):125–133.
18. Nordin M, Frankel V. *Basic Biomechanics of the Musculoskeletal System*. Fourth, North American edition. LWW; 2012.
19. Valderrabano V, Hintermann B, Horisberger M, Fung TS. Ligamentous posttraumatic ankle osteoarthritis. *Am J Sports Med*. 2006;34(4):612–620.
20. Stauffer RN, Chao EY, Brewster RC. Force and motion analysis of the normal, diseased, and prosthetic ankle joint. *Clin Orthop Relat Res*. 1977;127:189–196.
21. Grimston SK, Nigg BM, Hanley DA, Engsberg JR. Differences in ankle joint complex range of motion as a function of age. *Foot Ankle*. 1993;14(4):215–222.
22. Bruening DA, Frimenko RE, Goodyear CD, Bowden DR, Fullenkamp AM. Sex differences in whole body gait kinematics at preferred speeds. *Gait Posture*. 2015;41(2):540–545.
23. Wunderlich RE, Cavanagh PR. Gender differences in adult foot shape: implications for shoe design. *Med Sci Sports Exerc*. 2001;33(4):605–611.
24. Nozaki S, Watanabe K, Kamiya T, Katayose M, Ogihara N. Morphological variations of the human talus investigated using three-dimensional geometric morphometrics. *Clin Anat*. Published online March 20, 2020.
25. Fukano M, Fukubayashi T, Banks SA. Sex differences in three-dimensional talocrural and subtalar joint kinematics during stance phase in healthy young adults. *Hum Mov Sci*. 2018;61:117–125.
26. Kinney RC, Schwartz Z, Week K, Lotz MK, Boyan BD. Human articular chondrocytes exhibit sexual dimorphism in their responses to 17 beta-estradiol. *Osteoarthritis Cartilage*. 2005;13(4):330–337.

27. Beynnon BD, Bernstein IM, Belisle A, et al. The effect of estradiol and progesterone on knee and ankle joint laxity. *Am J Sports Med.* 2005;33(9):1298–1304.

28. Wilkerson RD, Mason MA. Differences in men's and women's mean ankle ligamentous laxity. *Iowa Orthop J.* 2000;20:46–48.

29. Kubo K, Kanehisa H, Fukunaga T. Gender differences in the viscoelastic properties of tendon structures. *Eur J Appl Physiol.* 2003;88(6):520–526.

30. Takabayashi T, Edama M, Nakamura M, Nakamura E, Inai T, Kubo M. Gender differences associated with rearfoot, midfoot, and forefoot kinematics during running. *Eur J Sport Sci.* 2017;17(10):1289–1296.

31. Holmbäck AM, Porter MM, Downham D, Andersen JL, Lexell J. Structure and function of the ankle dorsiflexor muscles in young and moderately active men and women. *J Appl Physiol.* 2003;95(6):2416–2424.

32. Buchanan PA, Vardaxis VG. Lower-extremity strength profiles and gender-based classification of basketball players ages 9-22 years. *J Strength Cond Res.* 2009;23(2):406–419.

33. Chiu M-C, Wu H-C, Chang L-Y. Gait speed and gender effects on center of pressure progression during normal walking. *Gait Posture.* 2013;37(1):43–48.

34. Gianakos AL, George N, Merklein M, et al. Foot and ankle related sex-specific analysis within high-impact journals. *Foot Ankle Int.* 2020;41(3):356–363.

35. Ko S, Tolea MI, Hausdorff JM, Ferrucci L. Sex-specific differences in gait patterns of healthy older adults: results from the Baltimore Longitudinal Study of Aging. *J Biomech.* 2011;44(10):1974–1979.

CHAPTER 13

Ankle Instability

ARIANNA L. GIANAKOS, DO • MARY K. MULCAHEY, MD

INTRODUCTION

Ankle sprains are common injuries accounting for up to 40% of all athletic injuries.[1] It has been estimated that 75% of ankle sprains involve the lateral ligamentous complex.[2] More than 23,000 ankle sprains occur per day in the United States affecting both males and females at approximately the same rates.[3] Previous studies demonstrate that ankle sprains account for up to 53% of basketball injuries and 29% of soccer injuries.[4] Most injuries respond well to conservative treatment with physical therapy emphasizing proprioceptive training, restoration of motion, and strengthening of the supporting musculature. Unfortunately, up to 34% of patients will resprain their ankle and up to 33% of ankle sprains will develop mechanical instability (MI) or functional instability (FI) that may ultimately lead to chronic ankle instability.[5] Previous studies have demonstrated associated intra-articular pathology in upward 93% of patients with ankle instability, with up to 78% of patients developing posttraumatic arthritis.[6,7] Therefore proper diagnosis and management is critical in order to prevent long-term sequelae of ankle instability.

ANATOMY/BIOMECHANICS

The lateral ligament complex of the ankle is composed of the anterior talofibular ligament (ATFL), the calcaneofibular ligament (CFL), and the posterior talofibular ligament (PTFL) (Fig. 13.1).

The ATFL, which is the weakest of the three ligaments, originates 10 mm proximal to the tip of the fibula and inserts onto the lateral talar neck just distal to the articular surface.[1] The CFL is an extra-articular ligament originating on the distal tip of the fibula and inserting onto the calcaneus 13 mm distal to the subtalar joint.[1] The CFL forms the floor of the peroneal tendon sheath.[2] The PTFL is the strongest of the lateral ligaments and extends from the posterior border of the distal fibula to the posterolateral tubercle of the talus.

The ATFL functions as the primary restraint to inversion in plantar flexion and resists anterolateral translation of the talus.[1] It is the most commonly injured ligament in lateral ankle sprains. The CFL is the primary restraint to subtalar inversion in neutral and dorsiflexed positions. Although the PTFL limits posterior talar displacement, it does not play an integral role in ankle stability when both the ATFL and CFL are intact.[1]

The most common mechanism of injury to the lateral ankle ligament complex involves excessive supination of the rearfoot about an externally rotated lower leg after contact with the ground.[8] Plantar flexion during injury increases the likelihood of injury. The ATFL is typically the first ligament injured during an ankle sprain. Attarian et al.[8] conducted a biomechanical study evaluating 20 human cadaver ankles and performed cyclic loading of each isolated bone-ligament-bone preparation, constant velocity load-deflection tests at varying deflection rates, and extremely rapid load to failure tests. The authors demonstrated that maximum load to failure for the CFL was 2−3.5 times greater than that for the ATFL, further supporting the increased rate of injury to the ATFL when compared with the CFL.[8] The CFL is involved in 50%−75% of ankle sprains, whereas the PTFL is involved in less than 10% of all ankle sprains.[9]

RISK FACTORS

Several studies have examined the relationship between intrinsic and extrinsic risk factors for ankle sprains. Extrinsic risk factors include training errors, type of sport, type of equipment, level of competition, and environmental conditions.[10] Intrinsic risk factors include age, gender, weight, aerobic fitness, alignment, strength, range of motion, proprioception, joint laxity, and foot morphology.[11] McKay et al.[12] conducted a study evaluating the risk of ankle sprain in elite and recreational male and female basketball players and demonstrated an increased risk in patients who had a history of ankle

The Female Athlete. https://doi.org/10.1016/B978-0-323-75985-4.00025-8

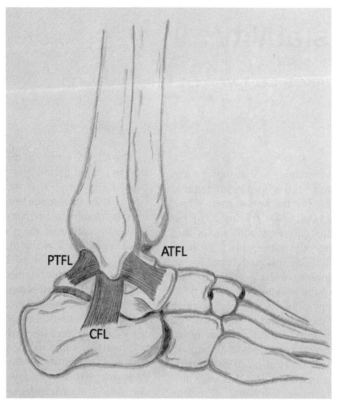

FIG. 13.1 **Lateral Ankle Ligament Complex.** *ATFL*, anterior talofibular ligament; *CFL*, calcaneofibular ligament; *PTFL*, posterior talofibular ligament.

injury and in patients who failed to stretch before games. Insufficient rehabilitation and earlier perceived healing of the injury may contribute to this increased risk.[11] Baumhauer et al.[10] demonstrated that individuals with a muscle strength imbalance and a smaller dorsiflexion-to-plantar flexion ratio had a higher incidence of ankle sprain. Willems et al. performed a prospective study evaluating risk factors for inversion ankle sprains in collegiate physical education female students aged 17—26 years. The authors identified several risk factors including less accurate passive joint inversion position sense, less postural control, and higher extension range of motion at the first metatarsophalangeal joint.[13] Sport activities that involve running, jumping, and cutting movements place athletes at an increased risk for inversion sprains.[11] Previous studies have demonstrated that ankle sprains most commonly occur in basketball, football, and soccer.[14]

CLINICAL PRESENTATION

Patients with acute ankle ligament injuries typically present with lateral ankle pain and swelling, and they often describe a sensation of "rolling over" his or her ankle. Patients may be unable to bear weight on the affected extremity during the initial presentation. In cases of chronic instability, patients report experiencing recurrent ankle sprains and describe a sensation of the ankle "giving way."

PHYSICAL EXAMINATION

Physical examination may demonstrate localized tenderness directly over the ligament origin/insertion points. The anterior drawer test performed in 10—15 degrees of plantar flexion is considered positive for an ATFL tear when there is greater than 8 mm of forward translation on the lateral radiograph.[2] The talar tilt test assesses for CFL integrity. The angle formed by the tibial plafond and talar dome is measured as inversion force is applied to the hindfoot.[2] Angles greater than 5 degrees indicate CFL disruption. These test results should always be compared to those of the contralateral ankle. In addition to the standard tests, patients should also be evaluated for peroneal tendon pathology, deformity, and neurovascular compromise.

IMAGING

Standard radiographic assessment, including weight-bearing anteroposterior, lateral, and mortise views, is initially performed after acute ankle injury in order to rule out ankle fracture. The Ottawa Ankle Rules were described to determine which patients presenting with lateral ankle sprain symptoms warranted proper radiographic workup. The three rules include (1) bony tenderness at the base of the fifth metatarsal, (2) inability to bear weight, and (3) bony tenderness at the tip of the malleolus.[15] Ultrasound can also be used to assess for ligamentous injury. Computed tomography and magnetic resonance imaging (MRI) are typically utilized only when associated injuries are suspected, including fracture, tendon pathology, osteochondral lesions or fractures, and other ligamentous injuries.[2]

GRADING OF LATERAL ANKLE SPRAINS

Ankle sprains are typically graded as I (no tear), II (partial tear), or III (complete rupture).[1] Lateral ankle ligament injury can also be classified by ligament involvement, including grade I (ATFL stretched), grade II (ATFL torn ± CFL tear), and grade III (ATFL, CFL torn ± capsular tear ± PTFL tear). Clinical grading is subjective and may be inaccurate depending on the amount of pain and swelling of the ankle, especially following an acute injury.

CONCOMITANT INJURIES

Lateral ankle sprains may be associated with concomitant intra-articular and extra-articular ankle injuries. Previous studies have demonstrated associated pathology including osteochondral defects, peroneal tendon injuries, deltoid ligament injury, intra-articular loose bodies, and fractures.[16] The most common fractures include those of the fifth metatarsal base, anterior process of the calcaneus, and lateral/posterior process of the talus. Previous studies have reported high prevalence of peroneal weakness in individuals following lateral ankle sprain, with 66% of patients presenting with residual peroneal related symptoms.[17]

NONOPERATIVE TREATMENT

Early functional rehabilitation is the standard of care for acute lateral ankle sprains. Management typically includes rest, ice, compressions, and elevation (RICE); early range of motion; progressive weight-bearing; and physical therapy.[18] Previous studies have recommended that therapy includes proprioception, range of motion, inversion/eversion strengthening, and peroneal strengthening and that exercises be continued for up to 12 weeks.[16] Kerkhoffs et al.[19] performed a meta-analysis of 2184 adult male and female patients evaluating immobilization versus early functional rehabilitation for the treatment of acute lateral ankle sprains. Early functional rehabilitation was defined as functional treatment with tape, bandages, or wraps that only supported the ankle joint.[19] The authors reported higher return to sports/work, fewer symptoms, better range of motion, and higher patient satisfaction in patients treated with early functional rehabilitation.[19] Surgical intervention is typically reserved for patients who present with persistent lateral ankle instability and pain after nonoperative interventions have failed.

CHRONIC ANKLE INSTABILITY

It has been estimated that up to 20%−30% of patients with acute lateral ankle ligament rupture will develop chronic ankle instability.[20,21] Patients presenting with recurrent ankle sprains may have persistent ankle instability and pain due to MI or FI. MI results from anatomic changes leading to increased risk of ankle sprain. These include pathologic laxity, impaired kinematics, synovial changes, and osteoarthritis.[3] FI is the presence of symptoms of "giving way," which is typically attributed to impaired proprioception and sensation, postural control, and strength deficits.[3] MRI can be helpful in these cases to evaluate for other causes of ankle pain, including tendon tears, chondral defects, and ligamentous injuries.

OPERATIVE TREATMENT

Patients who have failed conservative treatment typically require surgical intervention. Numerous surgical techniques for the treatment of chronic lateral ankle ligament instability have been described, along with various modifications of each procedure. Categories of techniques include nonanatomic tenodesis reconstruction, anatomic repair, and anatomic reconstruction.[22,23]

Repair of mid-substance tears of the ATFL was first described by Brostrom (Fig. 13.2) and was later modified to include repair of the CFL and incorporation of the inferior extensor retinaculum and lateral talocalcaneal ligament by Gould.[24]

These procedures typically involve shortening the ATFL and/or CFL and reattaching the ligaments through drill holes in their anatomic position.[25] Previous studies demonstrate excellent outcomes following early and late anatomic repair of the lateral ligament

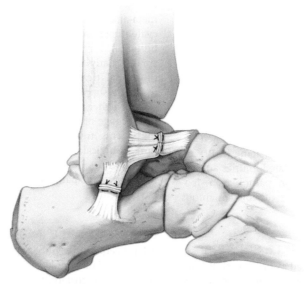

FIG. 13.2 **Brostrom Anterior Talofibular Ligament Repair. (**Yasui Y, Shimozono Y, Kennedy JG. Surgical procedures for chronic lateral ankle instability. *J Am Acad Orthop Surg* 2018;26(7):223–230.)

complex, with over 85% of patients reporting good postoperative outcomes, including patient satisfaction, return to daily activity, and range of motion.[26,27] Karlsson et al.[28] demonstrated improved results following imbrication of the damaged ATFL and CFL through bone tunnels in the fibula (Fig. 13.3).

A subset of patients with poor tissue quality, long-standing instability, history of previous repair, generalized ligamentous laxity, and cavovarus foot deformity may require augmentation in order to enhance the repair and improve outcomes.[1,2] Kennedy et al. described a hybrid anatomic lateral ligament reconstruction technique using peroneus longus autograft to substitute for the native ATFL and demonstrated improved functional outcomes and mechanical stability (Fig. 13.4).[29]

Several additional techniques include reconstruction with a local periosteal flap from the fibula as well as allograft tendon reconstruction utilizing semitendinosis, fascia lata, gracilis, palmaris longus, and plantaris allografts. Pagenstert et al.[30] reported excellent results utilizing a plantaris graft and Coughlin et al.[31] demonstrated good functional outcomes with ATFL augmentation using the gracilis tendon in the treatment of chronic lateral ligament instability. Notably, allografts have been associated with a higher rate of infection, immune response, and cost compared with autografts.[25]

Several examples of nonanatomic tenodesis stabilization of the lateral ankle ligamentous complex have been described in the literature. The Watson-Jones technique involves weaving the peroneus brevis tendon through the calcaneus and talus to reconstruct the ATFL.[32] Evans modified this technique by rerouting the tendon through drill holes in the distal fibula.[33] Chrisman and Snook[34] described a technique for lateral ankle stabilization in which the peroneus brevis was split and transferred to the base of the fifth metatarsal in order to augment the repair. Although patient outcomes have been reported as good to excellent, several studies have demonstrated higher complication rates, peroneal muscle fatigue, persistent instability, and decreased range of motion with nonanatomic tenodesis techniques.[35,36]

Lastly, arthroscopic ligament repair utilizing outside-in and inside-out suture passing techniques has also gained increased popularity. Previous studies have demonstrated no significant difference in outcomes when comparing arthroscopic with open lateral ligament repair/reconstruction.[37] Contraindications to arthroscopic repair include severely frayed ligaments, prior failed reconstruction, hyperlaxity syndromes, isolated subtalar instability, morbid obesity, and high-demand athletes.[38]

Ferkel [7] demonstrated that up to 93% of patients with chronic lateral ankle instability have an associated

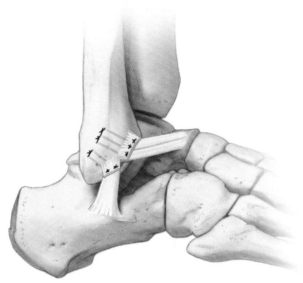

FIG. 13.3 **Imbrication of the Anterior Talofibular Ligament and the Calcaneofibular Ligament Through Fibular Bone Tunnels.** (Yasui Y, Shimozono Y, Kennedy JG. Surgical procedures for chronic lateral ankle instability. *J Am Acad Orthop Surg* 2018;26(7):223–230.)

intra-articular lesion. The most common intra-articular abnormalities include loose bodies, synovitis, osteochondral lesions of the talus, ossicles, osteophytes, adhesions, and chondromalacia.[7] Taga et al.[39] reported chondral lesions in 95% of chronic injuries and 89% of acute injuries, with lesions predominantly located on the medial aspect of the tibial plafond. Therefore arthroscopic assessment prior to (or at the time of) repair/reconstruction is often recommended in order to adequately identify and treat concomitant pathology.[7]

REHABILITATION
Postoperative rehabilitation following lateral ligament repair/reconstruction typically consists of 4–8 weeks of immobilization and protected weight-bearing, followed by 6 weeks of physical therapy.[21] Mattacola et al. demonstrated the importance of early functional rehabilitation with range of motion exercises initiated 72 h after surgery. Once normal range of motion is achieved and swelling resolves, isometric and isotonic strength-training exercises can be started.[40] Postoperatively, early rehabilitation goals should consist of decreasing inflammation and pain and should progress to increasing range of motion, muscular strength,

power, and endurance.[40] In addition, improving both balance and proprioception to prevent future ankle injuries should be a primary focus. Full athletic activity is permitted at 3–6 months, pending the type of surgery performed and the degree of damage found at the time of surgery.[1]

GENDER-RELATED DIFFERENCES
Increased ligamentous laxity in female athletes may alter injury patterns leading to ankle sprains and may ultimately affect the risk of both acute and chronic instability. Previous studies have demonstrated that females have increased inversion-eversion laxity and talocrural laxity when compared with males.[41,42] Females typically sustain lateral ankle sprains, while males more often sustain medial ankle sprains (relative to females); however, overall lateral ankle sprains remain the most common injury pattern encountered in both males and females. Waterman et al. reported on a military cohort of patients and found that overall, ankle sprains were more common in females than in males. In this specific subset of patients, males were three times more likely to sustain a medial ankle sprain, as well as a syndesmotic injury, than their female counterparts.[43] Although the literature is limited on this topic,

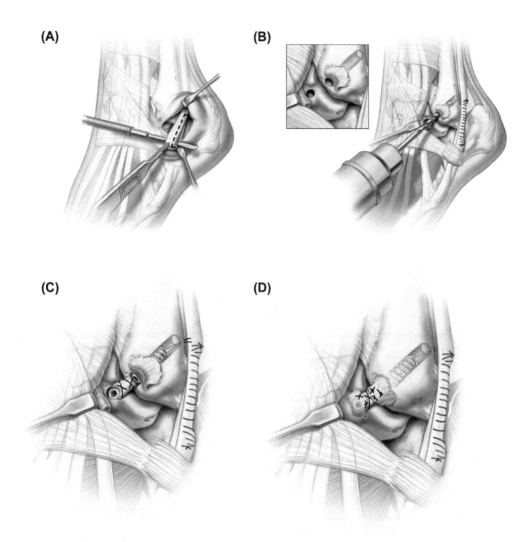

FIG. 13.4 Anterior Talofibular Ligament Reconstruction Utilizing the Hybrid Technique. *Inlet,* Image of position of bone tunnels. (Kennedy JG, Smyth NA, Fansa AM, et al. Anatomic lateral ligament reconstruction in the ankle: a hybrid technique in the athletic population. *J Am Acad Orthop Surg* 2012;40(10):2309–2317.)

understanding these anatomic differences is important when determining injury patterns and management strategies.

SUMMARY

Ankle sprains are common athletic injuries, and up to 30% of acute ankle sprains can develop a FI or an MI resulting in chronic ankle instability. Although most acute ankle sprains can be managed conservatively with good functional outcomes, patients with underlying instability and unsuccessful nonsurgical treatment may require operative intervention. Up to 90% of patients may have concomitant intra-articular pathology; therefore the authors suggest arthroscopic evaluation at the time of surgical intervention. High success rates have been reported with both anatomic and nonanatomic repair/reconstruction. Functional rehabilitation focusing on range of motion, stretching, strengthening, balance, and proprioception is critical to manage athletes and improve their ability to safely return to high-level sports participation.

REFERENCES

1. DiGiovanni CW, Brodsky A. Current concepts: lateral ankle instability. *Foot Ankle Int.* 2006;27(10):854–866.
2. Chan KW, Ding BC, Mroczek KJ. Acute and chronic lateral ankle instability in the athlete. *Bull NYU Hosp Jt Dis.* 2011; 68(1):17–26.
3. Hertel J. Functional anatomy, pathomechanics, and pathophysiology of lateral ankle instability. *J Athl Train.* 2002;37(4):364–375.
4. Garrick JG. The frequency of injury, mechanism of injury, and epidemiology of ankle sprains. *Am J Sports Med.* 1977; 5:241–242.
5. van Rijn RM, van Os AG, Bernsen RM, et al. What is the clinical course of acute ankle sprains? A systematic literature review. *Am J Sports Med.* April 2008;121(4): 324–331.e326.
6. Harrington KD. Degenerative arthritis of the ankle secondary to long-standing lateral ligament instability. *J Bone Joint Surg Am.* April 1979;61(3):354–361.
7. Komenda GA, Ferkel RD. Arthroscopic findings associated with the unstable ankle. *Foot Ankle Int.* November 1999; 20(11):708–713.
8. Attarian DE, McCrackin HJ, DeVito DP, et al. Biomechanical characteristics of human ankle ligaments. *Foot Ankle Int.* October 1985;6(2):54–58.
9. Ferran NA, Maffulli N. Epidemiology of sprains of the lateral ankle ligament complex. *Foot Ankle Clin.* 2006;11: 659–662.
10. Baumhauer JF, Alosa DM, Renstrom AF, et al. A prospective study of ankle injury risk factors. *Am J Sports Med.* 1995;23(5):564–570.
11. McCriskin BJ, Cameron KL, Orr JD, et al. Management and prevention of acute and chronic lateral ankle instability in athletic patient populations. *World J Orthop.* March 18, 2015;6(2):161–171.
12. McKay G, Goldie P, Payne W, et al. Ankle injuries in basketball: injury rate and risk factors. *Br J Sports Med.* 2001;35:103–108.
13. Willems TM, Witvrouw E, Delbaere K, et al. Intrinsic risk factors for inversion ankle sprains in females – a prospective study. *Scan J Med Sci Sports.* October 2005;15(5): 336–345.
14. Waterman BR, Owens BD, Davey S, et al. The epidemiology of ankle sprains in the United States. *J Bone Joint Surg Am.* 2010;92:2279–2284.
15. Steill I. Ottawa ankle rules. *Can Fam Physician.* March 1996;42:478–480.
16. Digiovanni BF, Fraga CJ, Cohen BE, et al. Associated injuries found in chronic lateral ankle instability. *Foot Ankle Int.* October 2000;21(10):809–815.
17. Bosien WR, Staples OS, Russel SW. Residual disability following acute ankle sprains. *J Bone Joint Surg Am.* 1955; 37:1237–1243.
18. Frey C. Ankle sprains. *Instr Course Lect.* 2001;50:515–520.
19. Kerkhoffs GM, Rowe BH, Assendelft WJ, et al. Immobilisation and functional treatment for acute lateral ankle ligament injuries in adults. *Cochrane Database Syst Rev.* 2002;3:CD003762.
20. Krips R, de Vries J, van Dijk CN. Ankle instability. *Foot Ankle Clin.* 2006;11:311–329.
21. Shakked RJ, Sheskier S. Acute and chronic lateral ankle instability – diagnosis, management, and new concepts. *Bull NYU Hosp Jt Dis.* 2017;75(1):71–80.
22. Ferran NA, Oliva F, Maffulli N. Ankle instability. *Sports Med Arthrosc Rev.* 2009;17:139–145.
23. Watson-Jones R. Recurrent forward dislocation of the ankle joint. *J Bone Joint Surg Br.* 1952;134:519.
24. Gould N. Repair of lateral ligament of ankle. *Foot Ankle.* 1987;8.
25. Mafulli N, Del Buono A, Mafulli GD, et al. Isolated anterior talofibular ligament Brostrom repair for chronic lateral ankle instability: 9-year follow-up. *Am J Sports Med.* April 2013;41(4):858–864.
26. Bell SJ, Mologne TS, Sitler DF, et al. Twenty-six-year results after Brostrom procedure for chronic lateral ankle instability. *Am J Sports Med.* June 2006;34(6):975–978.
27. Hamilton WG, Thompson FM, Snow SW. The modified Brostrom procedure for lateral ankle instability. *Foot Ankle.* January 1993;14(1):1–7.
28. Karlsson J, Bergsten T, Lansinger O, et al. Reconstruction of the lateral ligaments of the ankle for chronic lateral instability. *J Bone Joint Surg Am.* April 1988;70(4): 581–588.
29. Kennedy JG, Smyth NA, Fansa AM, et al. Anatomic lateral ligament reconstruction in the ankle – a hybrid technique in the athletic population. *J Am Acad Orthop Surg.* 2012; 40(10):2309–2317.
30. Pagenstert GI, Hintermann B, Knupp M. Operative management of chronic ankle instability: plantaris graft. *Foot Ankel Clin.* 2006;11(3):567–583.
31. Coughlin MU, Schenck RC, Grebing BR, et al. Comprehensive reconstruction of the lateral ankle for chronic instability using a free gracilis graft. *Foot Ankle Int.* 2004;25: 231–241.
32. Watson-Jones R. Recurrent forward dislocation of the ankle joint. *J Bone Joint Surg.* 1952;34-B:519.
33. Evans DL. Recurrent instability of the ankle-a method of surgical treatment. *Proc R Soc Med.* 1953;46:343–344.
34. Chrisman OD, Snook GA. Reconstruction of lateral ligament tears of the ankle: an experimental study and clinical evaluation of seven patients treated by a new modification of the Elmslie procedure. *J Bone Joint Surg.* 1969;51-A: 904–912.
35. van der Rijt AJ, Evans GA. The long-term results of Watson-Jones tenodesis. *J Bone Joint Surg Br.* May 1984;66(3): 371–375.
36. Karlsson J, Bergsten T, Lansinger O, Peterson L. Lateral instability of the ankle treated by the Evans procedure. A long-term clinical and radiological follow-up. *J Bone Joint Surg Br.* May 1988;70(3):476–480.
37. Drakos MC, Behrens SB, Paller D, et al. Biomechanical comparison of an open vs arthroscopic approach for

lateral ankle instability. *Foot Ankle Int.* August 2014;25(8): 809–815.

38. Acevedo JI, Mangone PG. Arthroscopic lateral ankle ligament reconstruction. *Tech Foot Ankle Surg.* 2011;10: 111–116.

39. Taga I, Shino K, Inoue M, et al. Articular cartilage lesions in ankles with lateral ligament injury: an arthroscopic study. *Am J Sports Med.* 1993;21:120–127.

40. Mattacola C, Dwyer MK. Rehabilitation of the ankle after acute sprain or chronic instability. *J Athl Train.* October– December 2002;37(4):413–429.

41. Ericksen H, Gribble PA. Sex differences, hormone fluctuations, ankle stability, and dynamic postural control. *J Athl Train.* March–April 2012;47(2):143–148.

42. Beynnon B, Murphy DF, Alosa DM. Predictive factors for lateral ankle sprains: a literature review. *J Athl Train.* October–December 2002;37(4):376–380.

43. Waterman BR, Belmont PJ, Cameron KL, et al. Epidemiology of ankle sprain at the United States Military Academy. *Am J Sports Med.* April 2020;38(4):797–803.

CHAPTER 14

Shoulder Anatomy and Biomechanics

LJILJANA BOGUNOVIC, MD • MEGAN LISSET JIMENEZ, DO • JODY LAW, BA

OSTEOLOGY

A variety of bony structures including the scapula, humerus, clavicle, and sternum are connected via soft tissue throughout the shoulder complex. The scapula is a flat, triangular bone that forms the posterior aspect of the pectoral girdle. Numerous muscles originate at and insert on the scapula. The four rotator cuff muscles (supraspinatus, infraspinatus, teres minor, and subscapularis), teres major, triceps, deltoid, and several other muscles all originate from the scapula (Fig. 14.1A and B).[1]

The scapula has three borders named by their location: the superior border, medial border, and lateral (axillary) border. The superior border is the shortest and extends from the superior angle of the scapula to the suprascapular notch at the base of the coracoid.[2] The medial border is the longest of the three and runs parallel to the spinous processes of the thoracic vertebrae. It extends from the superior angle to the inferior angle of the scapula and serves as the insertion site of the levator scapulae, serratus anterior, and rhomboid muscles.[3] The lateral border is thick and runs obliquely downward from the lateral angle to the inferior angle of the scapula. It is the attachment site for the teres minor, teres major, subscapularis, and long head of the triceps brachii.[2] The borders of the scapula meet at three distinct angles: superior, lateral, and inferior. The superior angle serves as the insertion site for the levator scapulae and serratus anterior.[1] The inferior angle is located at the junction of the lateral and medial borders. It serves as the origin of the teres major and latissimus dorsi muscles and the insertion of the serratus anterior. The superior and lateral borders form the lateral angle, which gives rise to one of the scapula's most important structures, the glenoid.[1]

The glenoid is a shallow, pyriform recess, which is wider inferiorly. Overall, females have smaller glenoids than males. The mean glenoid height ranges from 31.7 to 39 mm, with females having, on average, 2.9–3.18 mm smaller glenoid heights than males.[1,2,4,5] The mean glenoid anteroposterior width ranges from 23 to 29 mm, with females having 3.4 mm smaller glenoid widths than males.[1,2,4–6] Additionally, males tend to have slightly more retroverted glenoids than females.[2,5] The glenoid has, on average, 1–3 degrees of retroversion, but can vary from 14 degrees of anteversion to 12 degrees of retroversion.[1] It has been reported that males have between 1 and 8.4 degrees more glenoid retroversion than females.[2,5] Glenoid retroversion can theoretically help prevent anterior translation of the humeral head.[7]

The scapula has three processes: the spine, the acromion, and the coracoid. The spinous process is a prominent, horizontal ridge that divides the dorsal scapula into the supraspinatus and infraspinatus fossae. The spine of the scapula suspends the acromion and functions as a lever arm to aid in deltoid motion.[2] The acromion is a lateral and anterior continuation of the spine that forms the summit of the shoulder. Three acromion types have been described: flat (Type I), curved (Type II), and hooked (Type III).[3] Types II and III acromions are associated with subacromial impingement, whereas Type I has the lowest risk for impingement[2] (Fig. 14.2). The lateral border of the acromion provides an origin for the deltoid muscle, while the medial border acts as an insertion point for the trapezius muscle.[1] Additionally, the acromion articulates with the distal end of the clavicle at the acromioclavicular (AC) joint (ACJ). The apex, located at the anteroinferior aspect of the acromion, serves as the attachment site for the coracoacromial ligament, which extends between the acromion and the coracoid process of the scapula and helps provide stability to the glenohumeral joint (GHJ).[1] The coracoid process is a bony projection that arises from the superior border of the scapula. It projects superiorly and anteriorly above the glenoid fossa.[1] The coracoid process works to stabilize the scapula and provides the attachment for the coracoclavicular (CC) ligament, the short head of the biceps brachii, the coracobrachialis the pectoralis minor, the coracoacromial ligament, and the coracohumeral ligament (CHL).[2] The coracoid

(A)

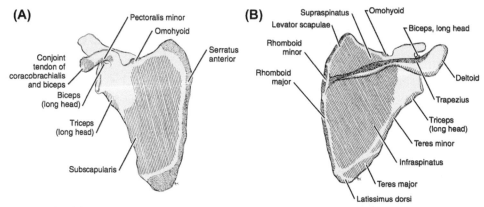

FIG. 14.1 **(A,B)** Scapula muscle origins and attachments. ((A) Rockwood CA, Matsen FA, Wirth MA, Lippitt SB, Fehringer EV, Sperling JW. *Rockwood and Matsen's the Shoulder*. 5th ed; 2017:41. Figure 2.10; **(B)** Rockwood CA, Matsen FA, Wirth MA, Lippitt SB, Fehringer EV, Sperling JW. *Rockwood and Matsen's the Shoulder*. 5th ed; 2017:41. Figure 2.11.)

measures approximately 15.9 mm in width and 10.4 mm in thickness.[1] The CC ligament varies in length from 22 to 28 mm measuring from the tip of the coracoid, and the normal CC distance is approximately 11−13 mm.[1,8]

The proximal humerus consists of the humeral head, which articulates with the glenoid fossa; the greater and lesser tuberosities, which serve as attachment sites for the rotator cuff muscles; and the humeral shaft.[1] The humeral head is covered by hyaline cartilage. The thickness of the cartilage on the humeral head ranges from 0.2 to 2.0 mm, with the thickest portion located at the center of the head.[1,9] The humeral head articular surface has a radius of curvature ranging from 22 to 55 mm.[1,3] The most superior aspect of the humeral head lies 8 mm superior to the greater tuberosity.[1] The narrow groove separating the articular cartilage of the humeral head and the tuberosities is referred to as the anatomic neck of the humerus.[2] The greater tuberosity provides the insertion site for the supraspinatus, infraspinatus, and teres minor. The lesser tuberosity serves as the insertion site for the subscapularis tendon. Below the level of the tuberosities, the humerus narrows into the surgical neck of the humerus where the shaft begins (Fig. 14.3).[2] The average angle of the humeral head and neck ranges from 130 to 150 degrees, and the shaft is retroverted about 20−30 degrees.[2,3]

The clavicle is an S-shaped bone that consists of an anteriorly convex greater medial curve and a posteriorly convex lesser lateral curve.[2] The medial end of the clavicle connects to the sternum, the first rib, and its costal cartilage via the sternoclavicular (SC) joint.[2,3] The lateral end of the clavicle articulates with the acromion at the ACJ.[1] The clavicle acts as a site of muscle attachment and plays an important role in maintaining the

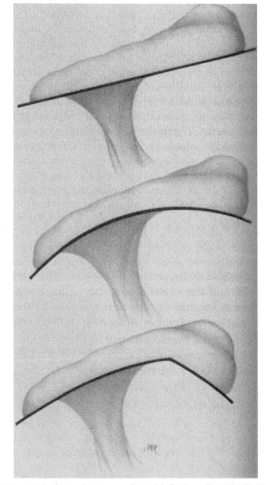

FIG. 14.2 Acromion types. (Peat M, Culham E, Wilk KE. *The Athlete's Shoulder*. 2nd ed. Elsevier; 2009:7. Figure 1.6.)

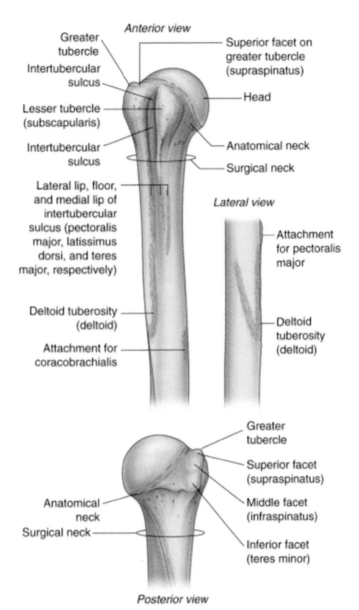

FIG. 14.3 Anterior and posterior proximal humerus anatomy. (Drake RL, Vogl W, Mitchell AWM, Gray H. *Gray's Anatomy for Students*. 4th ed. Elsevier; 2019. Figure 7.22.)

positioning and kinematics of the scapula.[1] Muscles that originate from the clavicle include the deltoid, pectoralis major, sternocleidomastoid, and sternohyoid, while the trapezius and the subclavius insert on the clavicle (Fig. 14.4A and B).[2]

ARTHROLOGY

The shoulder complex is composed of four different articulations: glenohumeral (GH), acromioclavicular (AC), strenoclavicular (SC), and scapulothoracic. The GH jointt is the most complex articulation in the body. Together, the four articulations allow the shoulder to function normally in space.

The GH joint is a multiaxial spheroidal joint, which has minimal inherent stability.[9] It allows for the largest range of motion in the human body, with multiple degrees of freedom including flexion/extension, abduction/adduction, translation, and internal/external rotation (Fig. 14.5).[1,9,10] The humerus is

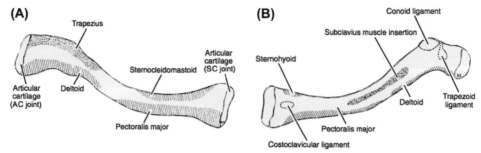

FIG. 14.4 **(A)** Superior clavicle muscle attachment sites. **(B)** Inferior clavicle muscle attachment sites. *AC*, acromioclavicular; *SC*, sternoclavicular. (**(A)** Rockwood CA, Matsen FA, Wirth MA, Lippitt SB, Fehringer EV, Sperling JW. *Rockwood and Matsen's the Shoulder*. 5th ed; 2017:41. Figure 2.6; **(B)** Rockwood CA, Matsen FA, Wirth MA, Lippitt SB, Fehringer EV, Sperling JW. *Rockwood and Matsen's the Shoulder*. 5th ed; 2017:41. Figure 2.7.)

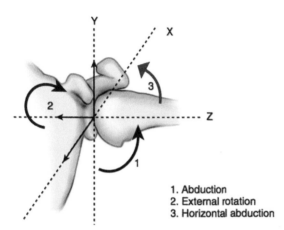

1. Abduction
2. External rotation
3. Horizontal abduction

FIG. 14.5 Shoulder motions. (Mologne TS. *DeLee, Drez, and Miller's Orthopedics Sport's Medicine*. 5th ed; 2019: 395. Figure 36.5.)

stabilized in the concave glenoid fossa by dynamic and static stabilizers. As noted earlier, the radius of curvature of the humeral head ranges from 22 to 55 mm.[1,3] The radius of curvature of the glenoid is slightly larger than that of the humeral head, which allows the humeral head to be compressed into the glenoid.[11] The glenoid only covers 25%–30% of the humeral head in any given position, which further demonstrates the importance of the static and dynamic stabilizers for shoulder stability.[12,13]

The AC joint is an articulation between the convex, lateral end of the clavicle and the concave acromion process of the scapula.[3] Additionally, it is a synovial joint that consists of an intra-articular disk and a joint capsule, which is thickest superiorly and posteriorly.[1] The AC joint is supported by two sets of ligaments: the AC ligaments and the CC ligaments. The CC

ligaments consist of the conoid and the trapezoid. The conoid attaches approximately 45 mm from the distal clavicle, whereas the trapezoid attaches approximately 25 mm from the distal clavicle (Fig. 14.6).[14]

The SC joint consists of the proximal end of the clavicle and the upper sternum and is the only joint connecting the shoulder complex to the axial skeleton.[2] The clavicular articular surface is covered by fibrocartilage, and the joint is divided by an articular disk.[9] The articular surface of the sternum is small and lacks congruency with the irregular surface of the clavicle.[1] Consequently, the SC joint has minimal bony stability.[2] Several ligamentous structures, including the SC ligaments, the interclavicular ligament, and the costoclavicular ligaments, provide stability to the joint (Fig. 14.7).[1] The SC ligaments connect the clavicle and sternum and stabilize the joint against anteroposterior movement of the clavicle.[3] The interclavicular ligament runs across the sternum and connects the medial aspects of the bilateral clavicles, providing joint stabilization against superior translation.[3] The costoclavicular ligaments, which are attached to the inferior surface of the clavicle and the first rib, resist medial and lateral displacement of the clavicle relative to the thorax.[2] The SC joint allows elevation, depression, retraction, and rotation of the clavicle.

The scapulothoracic articulation is a collective unit composed of the AC joint, the SC joint, and the fascial spaces between the anterior surface of the scapula and the thorax.[2] It serves as an important insertion site for several stabilizing muscles and contributes largely to scapular motion.[1] The scapulothoracic articulation allows for elevation by the trapezius and levator scapulae, depression by the serratus anterior and pectoralis minor, protraction by the serratus anterior and pectoralis minor, retraction by the trapezius and rhomboids,

Acromioclavicular joint

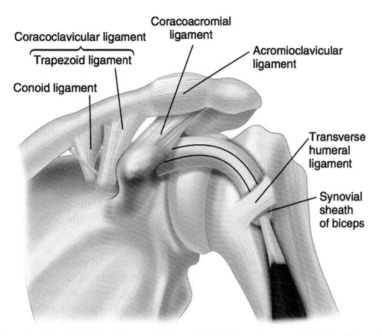

FIG. 14.6 Acromioclavicular joint anatomy. (Mologne TS. *DeLee, Drez, and Miller's Orthopedics Sport's Medicine*. 5th ed; 2019:394. Figure 36.3.)

Sternoclavicular joint

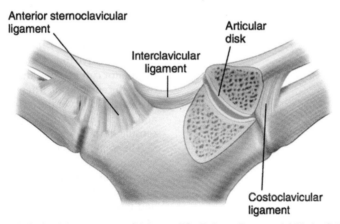

FIG. 14.7 Sternoclavicular joint anatomy. (Mologne TS. *DeLee, Drez, and Miller's Orthopedics Sport's Medicine*. 5th ed; 2019:397. Figure 36.7.)

lateral rotation by the trapezius and serratus anterior, and medial rotation by the levator scapulae and rhomboids.[15] Smooth movement at this articulation is crucial for proper shoulder mechanics.[1]

STATIC STABILIZERS

There are three main static stabilizers of the GH joint: the labrum, the glenohumeral ligaments, and the capsule. The labrum is a fibrocartilaginous extension of the glenoid, which increases the depth of the glenoid by 50%.[16] The labrum resists translation forces of the humeral head on the glenoid and serves as an attachment for the glenohumeral ligaments.[3] The inferior labrum is attached more firmly to the glenoid, whereas the anterosuperior labrum is more loosely attached.[1] The glenohumeral ligaments are thickened areas of the capsule and consist of the superior glenohumeral ligament (SGHL), the middle glenohumeral ligament (MGHL), the inferior glenohumeral ligament (IGHL), and the CHL (Fig. 14.8).[3] These ligaments are important for protecting against instability during extremes of joint motion as well as during midranges of motion.[17] Furthermore, the capsule, the SGHL, and the CHL make up the rotator interval. The size of the rotator

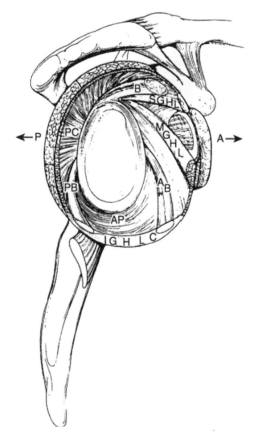

FIG. 14.8 Glenohumeral capsular ligamentous anatomy. *AB,* anterior band; *AP,* axillary pouch; *IGHLC,* inferior glenohumeral ligament complex; *MGCHL,* middle glenohumeral ligament; *PB,* posterior band; *SGHL,* superior glenohumeral ligament. (Peat M, Culham E, Wilk KE. *The Athlete's Shoulder.* 2nd ed. Elsevier; 2009:8. Figure 1.9.)

interval varies, and the larger the interval, the greater the potential for inferior and posterior instability.[18] The SGHL arises from the anterosuperior labrum and inserts onto the lesser tuberosity.[19] It is located in the rotator interval, which is the area between the superior border of the subscapularis and the anterior margin of the supraspinatus.[17] The MGHL has been described as having the most variation in size of all the glenohumeral ligaments, and it may be absent in up to 40% of individuals.[3,13] It has a wide attachment and extends from the SGHL along the anterior margin of the glenoid fossa to the anatomic neck of the humerus.[3] The IGHL is the thickest and runs from the anterior, inferior, and posterior glenoid margins to the humeral metaphysis.[3] It is composed of three distinct portions: the anterior band (AIGHL), the posterior band (PIGHL), and the axillary pouch.[20] The AIGHL and axillary pouch act as anterior stabilizers, while the PIGHL acts as a posterior stabilizer.[21] The CHL originates from the base and lateral border of the coracoid process, and it makes up the rotator interval, along with the SGHL. As it descends obliquely, it separates into two bands that insert onto the lesser and greater tuberosities.[3] The capsule surrounds the GHJ and is loose, allowing for a large range of humeral motion.[17] It is attached medially to the glenoid fossa and laterally to the circumference of the anatomic neck.[3] The capsule is relatively thin, varying anywhere between 1.3 and 4.5 mm, with the thickest portion in the anteroinferior quadrant and the thinnest in the rotator interval and posterior quadrant.[13,22]

DYNAMIC STABILIZERS

The primary dynamic stabilizers of the shoulder include the rotator cuff muscles, the deltoid, and the long head of the biceps brachii. These muscles contribute to the dynamic stability of the GH joint via joint compression and tightening of the glenohumeral ligamentous capsule during muscle contraction.[17]

The rotator cuff consists of the supraspinatus, infraspinatus, teres minor, and subscapularis muscles. The supraspinatus, which is located on the superior portion of the scapula, originates from the supraspinatus fossa and inserts into the greater tuberosity.[1] It acts as a primary abductor of the humerus and contributes to glenohumeral compression during active shoulder motion.[13] The infraspinatus originates from the infraspinatus fossa and inserts into the greater tuberosity, along with the supraspinatus. It is a main external rotator of the humerus, accounting for 60%–70% of external rotation force.[1,2] It also depresses the humeral head and stabilizes the shoulder against posterior subluxation during internal rotation.[2] The teres minor is another main external rotator that originates on the posterior aspect of the scapula and inserts on the posterior aspect of the greater tuberosity.[13] Compared with the infraspinatus, it provides greater external rotation force at increased levels of abduction and elevation.[1] It is also important for stabilizing the GH joint in the anterior direction.[23] The subscapularis originates along the costal surface of the scapula and inserts onto the lesser tuberosity of the humerus. It is the largest and most powerful rotator cuff muscle, occupying nearly the entire anterior scapular surface.[13] Functions of the subscapularis include internal rotation and adduction of the humerus. The muscle also stabilizes the shoulder from 0 to 45 degrees of abduction.[24]

The deltoid is another important primary dynamic stabilizer of the shoulder. It consists of three portions (anterior, middle, and posterior) that originate from the clavicle, acromion, and scapular spine and insert on the deltoid tubercle of the humerus.[2] The anterior and middle portions of the deltoid contribute to arm abduction, the anterior portion aids in arm flexion, and the posterior portion assists in arm adduction and extension.[1]

The long head of the biceps brachii is thought to contribute to dynamic stabilization of the shoulder when the static stabilizers or rotator cuff muscles are overwhelmed, but its true function remains debated.[13] It attaches to the superior aspect of the labrum and exits the GH joint in the rotator interval before passing distally in the bicipital groove.[1] The biceps tendon is stabilized within the groove by a pulley composed of fibers from the CHL and SGHL, with reinforcement from the subscapularis tendon.[1,2]

NERVES

The shoulder complex is innervated by the brachial plexus and its branches, which include the spinal accessory nerve (CN XI) and the supraclavicular nerves.[2] The brachial plexus is a network made up of the anterior rami of C5, C6, C7, and T1. It is divided into roots, trunks, divisions, cords, and branches. They give rise to five terminal branches: the musculocutaneous nerve, axillary nerve, median nerve, radial nerve, and ulnar nerve. The brachial plexus also gives off several minor branches including the dorsal scapular nerve, long thoracic nerve, small nerve to the subclavius, suprascapular nerve, lateral pectoral nerve, medial pectoral nerve, upper and lower subscapular nerves, thoracodorsal nerve, medial brachial cutaneous nerve, and medial antebrachial cutaneous nerve (Fig. 14.9). The nerves of particular importance to shoulder anatomy and function are the axillary, suprascapular, subscapular, and musculocutaneous nerves.[3] The axillary nerve (C5 and C6) arises from the posterior cord. It is accompanied by the posterior circumflex humeral artery as it passes through a quadrangular

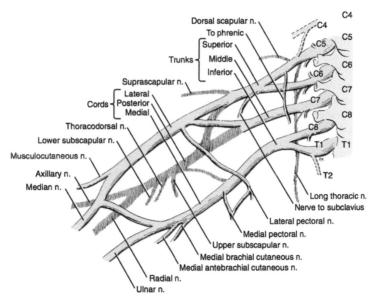

FIG. 14.9 The brachial plexus. (Rockwood CA, Matsen FA, Wirth MA, Lippitt SB, Fehringer EV, Sperling JW. *Rockwood and Matsen's the Shoulder.* 5th ed; 2017:66. Figure 2.39.)

space bounded by the subscapularis, teres minor, teres major, long head of the triceps, and surgical neck of the humerus.[15] The axillary nerve divides into an anterior branch that supplies motor innervation to the anterior two-thirds of the deltoid and a posterior branch that provides motor innervation to the teres minor and the posterior third of the deltoid. It gives off the lateral brachial cutaneous nerve, which supplies sensory information from the skin overlying the inferior region of the deltoid muscle.[25] The axillary nerve also supplies sensory innervation to the articular structures on the anterior portion of the GHJ.[3]

The suprascapular nerve (C5 and C6) originates from the upper trunk and supplies motor innervation to the supraspinatus before curving around the lateral border of the spine of the scapula, with the suprascapular artery supplying the infraspinatus via two branches.[15] The suprascapular nerve also provides two articular branches: one to the AC joint and superior GH joint and one to the posterosuperior GH joint.[2] The subscapular nerves consist of the upper and lower subscapular nerves (C5 and C6), both arising from the posterior cord. The upper subscapular nerve innervates the upper two-thirds of the subscapularis muscle, while the lower subscapular nerve innervates the lower portion of the subscapularis muscle and the teres major.[2]

The musculocutaneous nerve (C5−C7) branches off from the lateral cord and pierces the brachioradialis muscle distal to the coracoid process.[2] After supplying a motor nerve branch to the brachioradialis muscle, it branches further to supply the biceps brachii and brachialis as it descends down the lateral side of the arm. Below these branches, the musculocutaneous nerve continues as the lateral antebrachial cutaneous nerve and provides sensation to the lateral forearm.[15]

The spinal accessory nerve (CN XI) originates from the medulla and upper spinal cord and supplies the sternocleidomastoid and trapezius muscles. Owing to its superficial location in the posterior cervical triangle, it is especially susceptible to injury, and damage can result in lateral scapular winging.[25] The supraclavicular nerves (C3 and C4) provide sensation to the superior and upper posterior aspects of the shoulder region.[3] The medial supraclavicular nerve supplies the medial clavicular skin, including the skin over the SC joint. The middle supraclavicular nerve innervates the skin over the clavicle and anterior chest, including the anterior axillary fold. The lateral supraclavicular nerve supplies the skin over the lateral clavicle, acromion, and deltoid.[15]

ARTERIES

The shoulder is supplied by a rich plexus of arteries that anastomose around the scapula and associated muscles (Fig. 14.10). The vascular supply of the shoulder begins with the subclavian artery. This vessel can be divided into three parts in relation to the anterior scalene muscle. Branching off of the first part are the vertebral artery, the internal thoracic artery, and the thyrocervical trunk.[2] The suprascapular artery, a branch of the thyrocervical trunk, is of particular importance because it supplies the supraspinatus and infraspinatus and contributes to the scapular anastomosis found in the posterior scapular region.[26] Other vessels involved in this anastomosis are the dorsal scapular artery, the subscapular artery, and the circumflex scapular artery.[27] The internal costocervical trunk arises from the second section. The dorsal scapular artery arises from the third section; however, variations have been reported in which the dorsal scapular artery comes off of the thyrocervical trunk.[15] After reaching the lateral border of the first rib, the subclavian artery continues as the axillary artery. Similar to the subclavian artery, the axillary artery is separated into three sections by its relation to the pectoralis minor.[2]

The superior thoracic artery arises from the first section of the axillary artery and supplies the thoracic wall and parts of pectoralis major and minor.[17,18] The second section has two branches: the thoracoacromial artery and the lateral thoracic artery. The thoracoacromial artery gives off four branches, which supply the deltoid, acromion, clavicle, and both pectoralis muscles.[19] The lateral thoracic artery supplies the pectoralis minor, serratus anterior, and intercostal spaces 3 to 5. It also participates in an anastomosis with intercostal arteries 2 to 5, the pectoral artery, and the thoracodorsal artery.[17] The branches of the third section are the subscapular artery, the anterior humeral circumflex artery, and the posterior humeral circumflex artery. The suprascapular artery is the largest branch of the axillary artery and divides into the circumflex scapular artery and the thoracodorsal artery.[25] The circumflex scapular artery anastomoses with the suprascapular and dorsal scapular arteries, thus contributing greatly to shoulder girdle circulation.[3,13] The thoracodorsal artery runs with the thoracodorsal nerve and supplies the intercostal muscles, teres major, latissimus dorsi, and serratus anterior.[3] The anterior humeral circumflex artery supplies the deltoid, teres major and minor, the head of the humerus, and the GH joint.[17] It anastomoses with the posterior humeral circumflex artery, which curves around the surgical neck of the humerus. The posterior humeral circumflex artery supplies the deltoid, teres major and

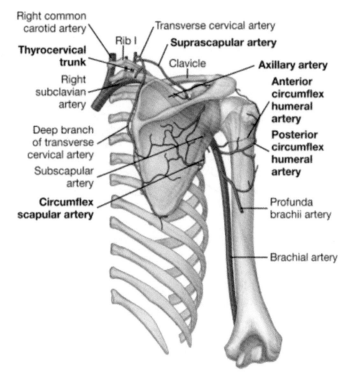

FIG. 14.10 Arterial anastomosis of the shoulder. (Drake R, Vogl W, Mitchell A. *Gray's Basic Anatomy*. 2nd ed. Elsevier; 2017. Figure 7.27.)

minor, the GH joint, and the long and lateral heads of triceps.[3]

BIOMECHANICS

The shoulder is among the most complex joints in the body with several planes of motion and multiple articulations. Given the limited osseous constraints of the GH joint, the surrounding soft tissue structures play a significant role in maintaining shoulder stability.[28,29]

Scapula Biomechanics

The scapulothoracic joint is an important contributor to shoulder motion, as most activities are performed in the plane of the scapula.[28,30] The scapula floats on the posterior aspect of the thoracic spine and ribs and is angled about 30–45 degrees anteriorly (Fig. 14.11). The scapulothoracic joint is complex and provides enhanced stability for the glenohumeral articulation. The scapula moves along three axes of rotation as well as in translation (Fig. 14.12). The motions include elevation/depression, adduction/abduction, posterior/anterior

tilt, internal/external rotation, and medial/lateral rotation. Several muscles contribute to scapular motion, including the upper and lower trapezius, rhomboids, levator scapulae, and serratus anterior.[31] Elevation and depression are predominantly powered by the upper trapezius, the levator scapulae, and the rhomboids.[28,32] The serratus anterior and pectoralis major abduct the arm, while the rhomboids, middle trapezius, and lower trapezius adduct the arm.[28] Downward rotation is powered by the rhomboids, levator scapulae, and pectoralis minor.[28]

The glenoid and humerus are extremely congruent, with a difference in their radii of curvature of 0.99 ± 0.05, which aids in glenohumeral stability by promoting rotation rather than translation.[33] Glenohumeral abduction/flexion and scapulothoracic rotation occurs at a 2:1 ratio. The scapula moves laterally during the first 30–50 degrees of glenohumeral abduction, then rotates about 65 degrees as the upper extremity reaches a maximum abduction of about 120 degrees.[34–36] Finally, passive scapular motion is far different than active motion. During passive motion, the muscles

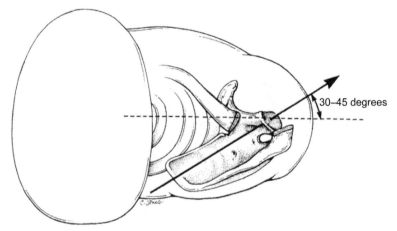

FIG. 14.11 The scapular plane.

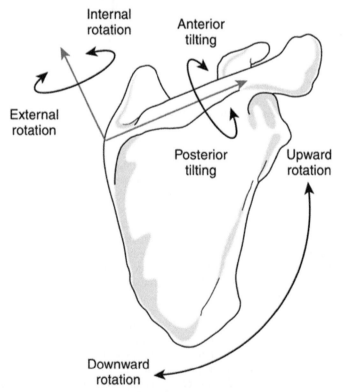

FIG. 14.12 Scapular motion.

surrounding the scapula are inactive. Therefore scapula motion typically begins around 70–90 degrees of glenohumeral forward elevation or abduction.[36]

The AC joint connects the scapula to the distal clavicle. The average size of this joint is 9 mm in the superior-posterior direction by 19 mm in the anteroposterior direction.[37] This joint moves in three planes of motion including vertical, horizontal, and translation.[37] The AC ligaments provide anteroposterior stability, while the CC ligaments control vertical stability of the AC joint.[2] The trapezoid provides 75% of the constraint against axial compression.[38] The conoid provides 60% of the restraint against superior translation and 70% of the restraint against anterior translation.[38] While relatively little motion occurs at this joint, it plays an important role in total arm movement and transmission of forces between the clavicle and acromion, which can occur in a frontal, vertical, or sagittal axis.[3] The main movements at this joint include clavicular rotation during abduction and adduction of the shoulder, as well as joint translation during overhead motion.[1] Finally, this joint undergoes 10 degrees of rotation during the first 30 degrees of shoulder flexion and abduction, followed by another 10 degrees of rotation throughout the final 45 degrees of shoulder motion.[35]

Rotator Cuff Biomechanics

The rotator cuff muscles provide stability to the GH joint both at the beginning of shoulder motion and throughout a full arc of motion.[39] Lippitt et al.[40] found that the rotator cuff provides compression of the humerus into the glenoid cavity at midrange of motion when the capsuloligamentous structures are lax (Fig. 14.13). The rotator cuff has multiple other functions as well, including dynamic stabilization, humeral head depression, humeral head rotation, and humeral head abduction.[13] The muscles of the rotator cuff generate far less force than the larger surrounding muscles (i.e., deltoid, pectoralis major, latissimus dorsi, and trapezius) mainly because of the shorter lever arm and their proximity to the center of rotation.[13]

Force couples play an important role in glenohumeral kinematics. There are essentially two muscle groups that contract in opposing directions to generate a symmetric movement. The deltoid brings the humeral head superiorly, while the subscapularis, infraspinatus, and teres minor work in opposition to bring the humeral head inferiorly.[35] Burkhart[41] examined the importance of balanced forces in both the coronal and transverse planes with regard to glenohumeral kinematics. Furthermore, it is critical that the anterior and posterior portions of the cuff are maintained for normal shoulder range of motion (Fig. 14.14).[41]

The rotator cuff also assists in preventing dislocations (in addition to the labrum and capsule, as noted in the subsequent section). The subscapularis works in conjunction with the capsule to prevent anterior translation of the humerus.[28] If the capsuloligamentous structures become incompetent (i.e., with subsequent dislocations), then the subscapularis becomes the primary restraint to anterior translation. In addition, the posterior cuff helps pull the humeral head posteriorly, thus preventing anterior shear.[23]

LABRUM, BICEPS, GLENOHUMERAL LIGAMENTS, AND CAPSULE

The labrum is a fibrocartilaginous ring, which encircles the glenoid.[28] The main function of the labrum is to deepen the glenoid by 50%.[16] Although many authors believe that the labrum acts as a buttress, or physical block, against humeral head translation, other authors argue that the labrum is more important in linking the capsule to the glenoid.[42,43]

The superior labrum, along with the supraglenoid tubercle, provides an attachment site for the long head of the biceps. The superior labrum resists external rotation with the arm abducted and internally rotated.[44] As noted previously, the function of the long head of the biceps is controversial, but it is thought to function as a humeral head depressor (in concordance with the rotator cuff), an anterior stabilizer, and a posterior stabilizer.[45] The long head of the biceps functions specifically as an anterior stabilizer when

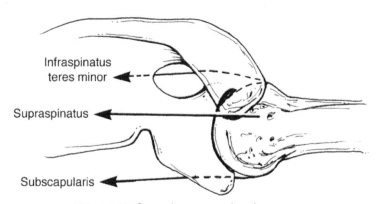

FIG. 14.13 Concavity-compression phenomenon.

Infraspinatus teres minor

Supraspinatus

Subscapularis

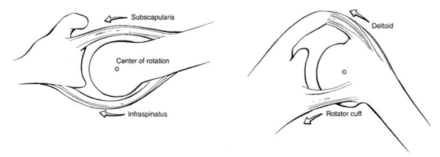

FIG. 14.14 Rotator cuff force couples.

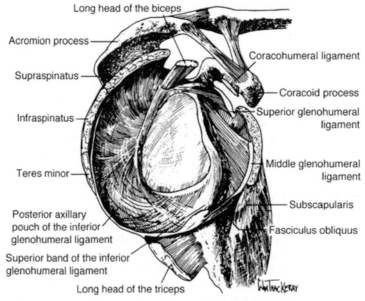

FIG. 14.15 Cross-sectional image of the capsuloligamentous structures.

the upper extremity is abducted to 90 degrees and maximally externally rotated.[28] The anteroinferior labrum is described to be weaker than the posterior labrum, especially in younger athletes under the age of 30 years.[46] This is especially true when incremental, constant loads are applied to the anterior labrum and capsule.

The GH joint capsule is a complex structure that consists of many different thickenings that form ligaments, each contributing to glenohumeral stability. They predominantly prevent against translation and aid in articular compression when they are taut.[28] By itself, the capsule contributes little to the stability of the joint. However, with reinforcement from the glenohumeral ligaments and muscle tendons, the capsule contributes greatly in maintaining the intra-articular vacuum that stabilizes the joint.[13]

The rotator interval, which consists of the SGHL and the CHL, prevents inferior and posterior translation of the adducted shoulder (Fig. 14.15).[28] The SGHL assists in preventing inferior humeral subluxation in 0 degree of abduction; it also acts against anterior and posterior stress at 0 degree of abduction.[13] The MGHL is important for anterior stability of the joint and limits anterior translation within the lower to middle ranges of shoulder abduction, specifically at 0 and 45 degrees.[13] The IGHL is one of the most important stabilizing structures during overhead motion in which the shoulder is abducted and externally rotated.[13] The posterior band of the IGHL and the axillary pouch restrict posterior subluxation/dislocation with the arm internally rotated at 90 degrees of abduction.[20] Key functions of the CHL include limitation of external rotation of the adducted arm and stabilization against inferior translation.[13] Finally, the posterior capsule functions to limit internal rotation, flexion, and abduction (Fig. 14.15).[28]

SUMMARY

Shoulder anatomy and biomechanics are extremely complex. Although there are differences in shoulder anatomy between females and males, they appear to be less significant with regard to injury patterns compared to the knee. The coordination of four articulations, namely, the GH joint, the AC joint, the SC joint, and the scapulothoracic articulation, allows the shoulder to move in multiple planes. In addition to bony stability, the shoulder requires a significant amount of soft tissue support to function properly and aid in keeping the humeral head centered in the glenoid cavity. Shoulder dysfunction and pain can result from injury or overuse.

REFERENCES

1. Mologne TS. Shoulder anatomy and biomechanics. In: *DeLee Drez & Miller's Orthopaedic Sports Medicine*. 5th ed. 2019.
2. Hsu JE, Lippitt SB, Matsen III FA. Rockwood and Matsen's the shoulder. In: *Rockwood and Matsen's the Shoulder*. 5th ed. 2016.
3. Peat M, Culham E, Wilk KE. Functional anatomy of the shoulder complex. In: *The Athlete's Shoulder*. 2009.
4. Merrill A, Guzman K, Miller SL. Gender differences in glenoid anatomy: an anatomic study. *Surg Radiol Anat*. 2009; 31(3):183–189.
5. Piponov HI, et al. Glenoid version and size: does gender, ethnicity, or body size play a role? *Int Orthop*. 2016; 40(11):2347–2353.
6. Bueno RS, et al. Correlation of coracoid thickness and glenoid width: an anatomic morphometric analysis. *Am J Sports Med*. 2012;40(7):1664–1667.
7. Saha AK. Mechanism of shoulder movements and a plea for the recognition of "zero position" of glenohumeral joint. *Indian J Surg*. 1950;12(2):153–165.
8. Alyas F, et al. MR imaging appearances of acromioclavicular joint dislocation. *Radiographics*. 2008;28:463–479.
9. Standring S. *Gray's Anatomy*. 41st ed. Elsevier; 2016.
10. Andrews J, Wilk K, Reinold M. *The Athlete's Shoulder*. 2009.
11. Iannotti JP, Schneck L, Gabriel P. The normal glenohumeral relationships: an anatomical study of 140 shoulders. *J Bone Joint Surg*. 1992;74(4):491–500.
12. Saha AK. Dynamic stability of the glenohumeral joint. *Acta Orthop*. 1971;42(6):491–505.
13. Cole BJ, et al. Anatomy, biomechanics, and pathophysiology of glenohumeral instability. In: *Disorders of the Shoulder: Diagnosis and Management*. 2007.
14. Rios CG, Arciero RA, Mazzocca AD. Anatomy of the clavicle and coracoid process for reconstruction of the coracoclavicular ligaments. *Am J Sports Med*. 2007;35(5):811–817.
15. Stranding S. Gray's anatomy. 42nd edition. *Emerg Med J*. 2020.
16. Howell SM, Galinat BJ. The glenoid-labral socket: a constrained articular surface. *Clin Orthop Relat Res*. 1989;243: 122–125.
17. Wilk KE, Arrigo CA, Andrews JR. Current concepts: the stabilizing structures of the glenohumeral joint. *J Orthop Sports Phys Ther*. 1997;25(6):364–379.
18. Harryman DT, et al. The role of the rotator interval capsule in passive motion and stability of the shoulder. *J Bone Joint Surg*. 1992;74:53–66.
19. Kask K, et al. Anatomy of the superior glenohumeral ligament. *J Shoulder Elbow Surg*. 2010;19(6):908–916.
20. O'Brien SJ, et al. The anatomy and histology of the inferior glenohumeral ligament complex of the shoulder. *Am J Sports Med*. 1990;18(5):449–456.
21. Urayama M, et al. Function of the 3 portions of the inferior glenohumeral ligament: a cadaveric study. *J Shoulder Elbow Surg*. 2001;10(6):589–594.
22. Ciccone WJ, et al. Multiquadrant digital analysis of shoulder capsular thickness. *Arthroscopy*. 2000;16(5):457–461.
23. Cain PR, et al. Anterior stability of the glenohumeral joint: a dynamic model. *Am J Sports Med*. 1987;15(2):144–148.
24. Turkel SJ, et al. Stabilizing mechanisms preventing anterior dislocation of the glenohumeral joint. *J Bone Joint Surg*. 1981;63(8):1208–1217.
25. Slavin KV. Peripheral nerve. In: *Essential Neuromodulation*. 13th ed. Elsevier; 2011.
26. Drake RL, et al. *Gray's Basic Anatomy*. 2012.
27. Moore KL, Dalley AF, Agur AM. *Clinically Oriented Anatomy*. 7th ed. Lippincott Williams & Wilkins; 2014.
28. Eckenrode BJ, Kelley MJ. Clinical biomechanics of the shoulder complex. In: *The Athlete's Shoulder*. 2nd ed. 2009.
29. Hsu JE, et al. Restoration of anterior-posterior rotator cuff force balance improves shoulder function in a rat model of chronic massive tears. *J Orthop Res*. 2011;29(7): 1028–1033.
30. Forthomme B, Crielaard JM, Croisier JL. Scapular positioning in athlete's shoulder: particularities, clinical measurements and implications. *Sports Med*. 2008;38(5): 369–386.
31. DiGiovine NM, et al. An electromyographic analysis of the upper extremity in pitching. *J Shoulder Elbow Surg*. 1992; 1(1):15–25.
32. Oatis CA. *Kinesiology. The Mechanics and Pathomechanics of Human Movement*. Kinesiology. 2nd ed. 2013.
33. Soslowsky LJ, et al. Articular geometry of the glenohumeral joint. *Clin Orthop Relat Res*. 1992;285:181–190.
34. Poppen NK, Walker PS. Normal and abnormal motion of the shoulder. *J Bone Joint Surg*. 1976;58(2):195–201.
35. Inman VT, Saunders JB, Abbott LC. Observations of the function of the shoulder joint. *Clin Orthop Relat Res*. 1996;330:3–12.
36. Kibler WB. The role of the scapula in athletic shoulder function. *Am J Sports Med*. 1998;26(2):325–337.
37. Bosworth BM. Complete acromioclavicular dislocation. *N Engl J Med*. 1949;241:221–225.

38. Fukuda K, et al. Biomechanical study of the ligamentous system of the acromioclavicular joint. *J Bone Joint Surg.* 1986;68(3):434–440.

39. Yamamoto N, Itoi E. A review of biomechanics of the shoulder and biomechanical concepts of rotator cuff repair. *Asia-Pac J Sports Med Arthrosc Rehab Technol.* 2015; 2(1):27–30.

40. Lippitt SB, et al. Glenohumeral stability from concavity-compression: a quantitative analysis. *J Shoulder Elbow Surg.* 1993;2(1):27–35.

41. Burkhart SS. Fluoroscopic comparison of kinematic patterns in massive rotator cuff tears: a suspension bridge model. *Clin Orthop Relat Res.* 1992;284:144–152.

42. Bankart ASB. The pathology and treatment of recurrent dislocation of the shoulder-join. *Br J Surg.* 1938;26: 23–29.

43. Rowe CR, Patel D, Southmayd WW. The Bankart procedure. A long-term end-result study. *J Bone Joint Surg.* 1978; 60(1):1–16.

44. Rodosky MW, Harner CD, Fu FH. The role of the long head of the biceps muscle and superior glenoid labrum in anterior stability of the shoulder. *Am J Sports Med.* 1994;22(1): 121–130.

45. Nho SJ, et al. Long head of the biceps tendinopathy: diagnosis and management. *J Am Acad Orthop Surg.* 2010; 18(111):645–656.

46. Hara H, Ito N, Iwasaki K. Strength of the glenoid labrum and adjacent shoulder capsule. *J Shoulder Elbow Surg.* 1996;5(4):263–268.

CHAPTER 15

Shoulder Instability in the Female Athlete

LESLIE B. VIDAL, MD

INTRODUCTION

The shoulder is notable for being the most mobile joint in the body. Optimal function requires a delicate balance of stability and flexibility. This balance is achieved by contributions from both static and dynamic stabilizers. It is important to understand that some athletes, such as swimmers and dancers, inherently require greater amounts of flexibility, while others, such as overhead athletes, depend more on stability. Shoulder instability is a pathologic spectrum in which the motion of the humeral head exceeds the containment of the glenoid labral complex resulting in pain and dysfunction. Instability of the shoulder can occur in the anterior, posterior, or inferior direction, or in a combination of these directions.[1]

Shoulder instability is a common problem in the young athletic population.[2,3] Interestingly, studies have reported that young males are 2.7 times more likely to present with shoulder instability than young females.[2,4] Therefore male participants comprise the majority of patients in research cohorts related to shoulder instability.[5] However, when comparing shoulder instability rates between young males and females in gender-comparable sports (e.g., soccer, basketball, and rugby), the rates of shoulder instability are nearly equal.[2,6]

FUNCTIONAL ANATOMY

Stability of the shoulder is conferred by both static and dynamic restraints. The static stabilizers of the glenohumeral joint include the bony anatomy (i.e., the humeral head and glenoid), as well as the glenoid labrum, capsule, and glenohumeral ligaments. The dynamic stabilizers of the shoulder include the surrounding muscles, specifically the rotator cuff (i.e., supraspinatus, infraspinatus, subscapularis, and teres minor) and scapular stabilizers.[7]

The proximal humerus consists of the humeral head and articular surface; the greater and lesser tuberosities, which are the attachment sites for the rotator cuff muscles; and the humeral shaft. The scapula is a relatively flat, triangular bone that sits on the posterior lateral aspect of the chest wall at the level of the second to the seventh rib. The superolateral corner of the scapula gives rise to the glenoid fossa, which is angled slightly posterior and inferior relative to the body (Fig. 15.1).

The glenoid labrum is a fibrocartilaginous ring that is located circumferentially around the rim of the

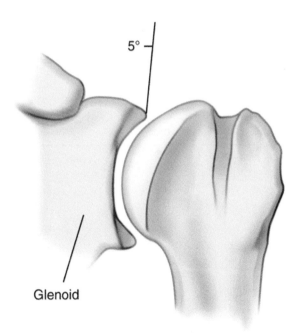

FIG. 15.1 Relative to the plane of the scapula, the fossa is angled slightly inferior and posterior, offering little bony support to inferior instability with the arm at the side.

The Female Athlete. https://doi.org/10.1016/B978-0-323-75985-4.00026-X

glenoid and is continuous with the articular surface of the glenoid face. It has a bumper effect, limiting abnormal translation of the humeral head on the shallow glenoid bone (Fig. 15.2). On cross section, the labrum is wedge shaped and functionally increases the depth of the glenoid cavity by up to 50%.[8] The glenohumeral joint capsule encapsulates the articular portion of the humeral head and glenoid. Three main thickenings in the capsule, the superior glenohumeral ligament (SGHL), the middle glenohumeral ligament (MGHL), and both the anterior and posterior bands of the inferior glenohumeral ligament (IGHL), also provide restraint against glenohumeral translation. The IGHL is a hammocklike structure, as its anterior and posterior bands extend along the inferior aspect of the glenohumeral joint. The IGHL predominantly stabilizes the arm in the abducted, externally rotated position.[9-11] The MGHL can demonstrate variable anatomy,[12] and in general, it originates from the anterior superior labrum or glenoid rim and inserts on the anatomic neck of the humerus, providing stability against anterior translation when the arm is in 45 degrees of abduction.[13] Finally, the SGHL arises from the anterosuperior glenoid, runs parallel to the biceps tendon in the rotator interval, and inserts on the lesser tuberosity.[14] In some studies, it is thought to be the most important stabilizer against inferior translation,[15] while other studies have shown it is the coracohumeral ligament (CHL)[16] and/or the IGHL[17] that resist inferior translation[18] (Fig. 15.3).

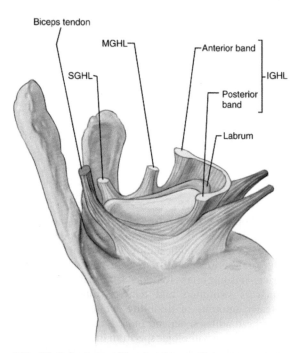

FIG. 15.3 Anatomy of the glenohumeral ligaments: superior glenohumeral ligament (SGHL), middle glenohumeral ligament (MGHL), and inferior glenohumeral ligament (IGHL). The view is from the posterior aspect, as traditionally seen in lateral-position arthroscopy.

The glenohumeral joint is the most mobile joint in the body and allows range of motion with 6 degrees of freedom. Additionally, the humeral head can translate as much as 8–14 mm anteriorly, posteriorly, or inferiorly on the glenoid fossa. Given the significant mobility and wide range of motion inherent to the glenohumeral joint, it is not surprising that the shoulder is not only the most mobile joint in the body but also the most unstable. While shoulder joint stability is predominantly achieved through a combination of the static and dynamic stabilizers, there is also inherent negative intra-articular pressure due to the glenoid concavity "plunger" effect on the humeral head. The glenohumeral joint capsule is important in maintaining this intra-articular vacuum effect.[19]

PATHOANATOMY OF ANTERIOR INSTABILITY

When the humeral head dislocates from the glenoid, the resulting pathoanatomy can be capsulolabral, osseous, or both. In anterior shoulder instability, the "essential lesion" involves an injury to the anteroinferior glenoid labrum and the anterior band of the

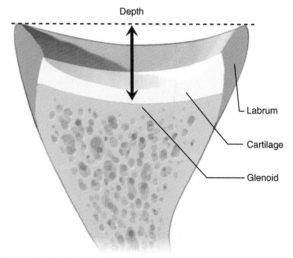

FIG. 15.2 Glenoid concavity is deepened by both the articular cartilage and labrum.

IGHL. This is often referred to as the "Bankart lesion," which is seen in 97% of cases of acute, first-time, traumatic, anterior dislocations.[20] When there is an osseous component (i.e., an associated fracture of the anteroinferior glenoid rim), it is referred to as a "bony Bankart lesion." Recurrent anterior instability can lead to anterior glenoid bone loss due to medial displacement of a bony fracture or erosion of the anterior glenoid.[21]

Concomitant osseous injury to the posterosuperior humeral head (i.e., Hill-Sachs lesion) can occur via a compression fracture as the softer humeral head impacts the anterior glenoid rim during anterior shoulder subluxation or dislocation.[22,23] Hill-Sachs lesions are seen in approximately 40% of patients with recurrent subluxation, in 70%–90% of patients with a single dislocation, and in almost 100% of patients with recurrent shoulder dislocations.[20,24–26] The majority of Hill-Sachs lesions are small and are likely clinically insignificant. However, they can be large and clinically significant.[27] Additional intra-articular and extra-articular pathology that needs to be identified include tears of the superior labrum anterior to posterior (SLAP tears), circumferential labral lesions, humeral avulsion of the glenohumeral ligament (HAGL) lesions, anterior labral periosteal sleeve avulsion (ALPSA) lesions, glenoid labrum articular disruption (GLAD) lesions, and rotator cuff injuries.[28] These lesions may alter surgical management as well as rehabilitation for the patient.

As males are more commonly afflicted with shoulder instability, females are underrepresented in the majority of studies describing the pathoanatomy. In an attempt to better understand the unique pathology associated with shoulder instability in collegiate female athletes, Patzkowski et al.[3] performed a retrospective analysis of a consecutive series of female students at a National Collegiate Athletic Association (NCAA) Division I military service academy, who were treated operatively for shoulder instability. The authors described the pathoanatomy seen at the time of arthroscopy in 36 female student athletes with an average age of 20 years. They reported that shoulder instability in female athletes presents commonly as multiple subluxation events. Soft tissue Bankart lesions were found with a frequency similar to those published in previous mixed-gender studies; however, bony Bankart lesions were much less common in females. Additionally, the presence of combined anterior and posterior labral tears and HAGL lesions in females was noted to be much more common in this group than previously reported.[3]

PATHOANATOMY OF POSTERIOR INSTABILITY

Posterior shoulder instability can be thought of as a spectrum of pathology. The posterior labrum, capsule, and posterior band of the IGHL are the primary stabilizers to posterior translation of the humeral head when the arm is between 45 and 90 degrees of abduction.[10] A frank posterior dislocation may occur in the setting of a traumatic posteriorly directed blow to an adducted, internally rotated, and forward-flexed upper extremity (e.g., fall on an outstretched arm), which can result in an acute posterior capsulolabral detachment (i.e., a reverse Bankart tear). On the other end of the spectrum, because the posterior capsule is the thinnest segment of the shoulder capsule and does not contain any supporting ligamentous structures like that seen anteriorly and inferiorly, it is more susceptible to attenuation from repetitive stress.[29] Therefore in overhead athletes (e.g., throwers and swimmers), in whom there is repetitive direct stress on the posterior capsular labral complex, athletes can develop recurrent posterior shoulder subluxation in the absence of frank dislocation. It is thought that the progressive laxity of the posterior capsule and fatigue of both static and dynamic stabilizers lead to attenuation and deformation of the posterior capsule, resulting in a patulous posterior inferior capsular pouch and labral tearing. This can be seen on both magnetic resonance arthrography (MRA) and arthroscopy.[30]

PATHOANATOMY OF MULTIDIRECTIONAL INSTABILITY

Multidirectional instability (MDI) of the shoulder refers to anterior and posterior instability associated with involuntary inferior subluxation or dislocation. While glenohumeral stability results from a complex interplay of static and dynamic stabilizers, anatomically it has been noted that the depth of the glenoid cavity in patients with MDI is more shallow than that of age-matched control subjects.[31–33] However, the characteristic pathologic entity in patients with MDI is increased capsular redundancy.[34–36] The redundancy may be congenital and associated with a connective tissue disorder (e.g., Ehlers-Danlos syndrome, Marfan syndrome, benign joint hypermobility syndrome, and osteogenesis imperfecta). Alternatively, it can be acquired from repetitive microtrauma and/or repetitive overuse during activities that result in stretching of the capsuloligamentous restraints. The most significant restraint to inferior subluxation of the humeral head is the rotator interval complex, which is made up of the SGHL, the CHL, and the superior joint capsule. Incompetence of the rotator interval is often seen in patients with MDI.[37,38]

EVALUATION OF THE FEMALE ATHLETE WITH SHOULDER INSTABILITY

History

The importance of taking a good history is both to establish the diagnosis of shoulder instability and to obtain information that will help direct treatment. Unidirectional, anterior shoulder instability most often results from a discrete traumatic event, and joint manipulation is often required to obtain reduction. If the athlete has had a true dislocation event, it is helpful to determine the mechanism of injury, use radiographs to determine the direction of the dislocation, establish if there was a need for manual reduction versus if the patient experienced a spontaneous reduction, and determine if there is any associated disability resulting from the dislocation (e.g., paresthesias or weakness in the involved extremity). If the patient has had numerous dislocations, it is important to ascertain if the mechanism of injury has changed; for example, if the instability events are becoming more frequent and occurring with less traumatic force. Additionally, it is important to document the age at the time of the first dislocation and at the time of the subsequent dislocations, as age is a significant prognostic indicator for recurrence.[27]

Symptoms of shoulder subluxation without dislocation tend to be more vague and difficult to evaluate. Patients may report an insidious onset of symptoms and a feeling of looseness and achiness in the shoulder. Occasionally, these complaints can occur with concomitant transient neurologic symptoms. The precipitating factors may be unpredictable and symptoms may occur with activities of daily living or even during sleep.[1]

To distinguish between anterior instability, posterior instability, and MDI, it is helpful to determine the arm position that makes the patient feel uncomfortable. Most patients with anterior instability will be apprehensive with the arm in an abducted and externally rotated position. Patients with posterior instability will report pain with the arm in the forward-flexed, internally rotated, and adducted positions (i.e., reaching forward to open a door). Patients with MDI may report pain with the arm in several different positions; however, by definition, they should have symptoms, with inferior translation among their constellation of complaints.[27]

In addition to understanding the direction and frequency of the instability events as well as concomitant symptoms, it is important to understand the demands the patient puts on the affected shoulder. This includes inquiring about which sports they participate in; if they throw, hit, or swing with the affected extremity; and about their occupation and if it is affected by their symptoms. Understanding their social history as well as their instability history will help guide treatment for the patient.[27]

Physical Examination

A general physical examination of the cervical spine and scapula is performed followed by a thorough examination of the shoulder. Once inspection, palpation, range of motion, and strength testing are carefully performed, specific provocative maneuvers can be done to elicit symptoms suggestive of the different instability patterns. Ligamentous laxity should be evaluated in all patients presenting with complaints of shoulder instability. Beighton scoring is the most common way to quantify generalized hypermobility. The patient is awarded one point for each positive test result for a possible total of 0–9. The higher the score, the more generalized joint hypermobility the patient has. The components of this test include passive dorsiflexion of the small fingers beyond 90 degrees, passive apposition of the thumbs to the volar forearm, hyperextension of the elbows greater than 10 degrees, hyperextension of the knees beyond 10 degrees, and touching the floor with the palms of the hands while flexing forward with the trunk and keeping the knees extended.[39–41] Female athletes have been noted to have more signs of generalized joint hyperlaxity than male athletes as measured by the Beighton criteria.[42]

Provocative Tests for Anterior, Posterior, and Multidirectional Shoulder Instability

Anterior apprehension test

With the patient in the supine position and the scapula stabilized on the examination table, the shoulder is passively brought into 90 degrees of abduction and then into maximal external rotation, while slight anterior pressure is applied to the posterior aspect of the humeral head (Fig. 15.4). A positive test result is signified by a sense of impending anterior shoulder dislocation.[43]

Jobe relocation test

In this test, a posteriorly directed manual force is applied to the humeral head with the arm in 90 degrees of abduction and maximal external rotation. A positive relocation test result is signified by relief of the patient's sense of impending shoulder dislocation[43] (Fig. 15.5).

Anterior and posterior drawer test

The anterior drawer test is performed with the patient in the supine position on an examination table. The scapula is again stabilized on the table and the examiner brings the arm to 80–120 degrees of abduction, slight forward flexion, and slight external rotation. The arm is then translated anteriorly.[44] The movement can be graded by the modified Hawkins scale,[45] with type 1 being translation to the glenoid rim, type 2 as translation over the glenoid rim, and type 3 as translation over the glenoid rim that does not spontaneously reduce. Any apprehension noted during the anterior drawer test should be considered positive for anterior shoulder instability. Translation should also be compared to the contralateral shoulder to determine what is normal for the patient.

The posterior drawer test is also performed with the patient in the supine position. In this case, the examiner holds the patient's proximal forearm and flexes the elbow

to 120 degrees. The arm is brought into 80–120 degrees of abduction and 20–30 degrees of forward flexion. With the contralateral hand, the examiner stabilizes the scapula. The arm is then internally rotated and flexed to 60–80 degrees, and the examiner's thumb is used to subluxate the humeral head posteriorly. Any apprehension is considered a positive test result for posterior instability.[44]

Load and shift test

The patient can be positioned in the seated position, with the examiner standing behind the patient. The scapula and shoulder girdle are stabilized with one hand, and the humeral head is then loaded and shifted anteriorly and posteriorly with the other hand. The amount of translation is noted and graded with the same modified Hawkins scale of translation.[46] Alternatively, the patient can be placed in the supine position and the arm brought into 20 degrees of abduction and 20 degrees of forward flexion so that it is centered on the glenoid fossa. The examiner then applies an anterior and posterior force to assess the translation of the humeral head relative to the glenoid room[46] (Fig. 15.6). The affected shoulder should always be compared to the contralateral shoulder to establish the pathologic translation relative to the patient's physiologic laxity.[41]

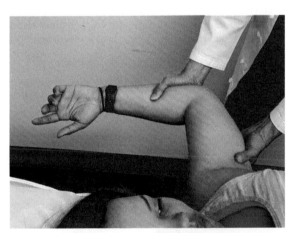

FIG. 15.4 Anterior Apprehension Test.

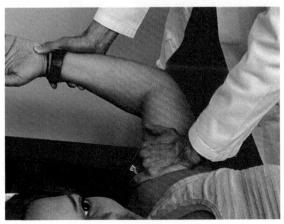

FIG. 15.5 Jobe Relocation Test.

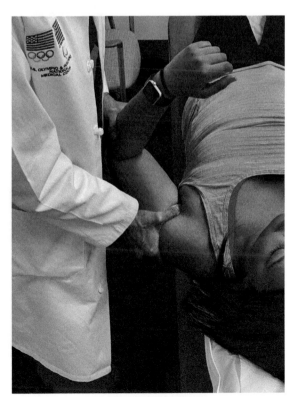

FIG. 15.6 Load and Shift Test.

Jerk test

The jerk test is used to evaluate for posterior instability. With the patient in the sitting position, the examiner stabilizes the patient's scapula with one hand while the arm is abducted to 90 degrees and internally rotated to 90 degrees. The examiner's other hand then axially loads the patient's arm at the elbow and applies a horizontal adduction force. A positive test result is defined by the presence of a sharp pain with or without a clunk in the posterior aspect of the shoulder.[41,47]

Kim test

The Kim test is another test for posterior shoulder instability. It is performed with the patient in the sitting position and the arm in 90 degrees of abduction. The examiner holds the patient's elbow and lateral upper arm and applies an axial force and 45 degrees of upward diagonal elevation, while also pushing inferiorly and posteriorly on the upper arm. Posterior shoulder pain with or without a clunk is considered a positive test result for posterior labral pathology[41,47] (Fig. 15.7).

Sulcus test

When evaluating for inferior instability or MDI, it is important to evaluate for a sulcus sign. With the patient in the upright position and the arm relaxed by the side, downward traction is applied to the patient's upper arm (Fig. 15.8). A positive sulcus sign is when this reproduces pain or instability and a depression is created between the lateral edge of the acromion and the humeral head. The depression can be measured and reported in centimeters. Type I is less than 1 cm of depression, type II is 1−2 cm of depression, and type III is greater than 2 cm of depression.[45] Additionally, a positive sulcus sign noted with the arm at 30 degrees of external rotation can suggest pathologic laxity of the rotator interval[45] (Fig. 15.9).

Gagey test

An additional test evaluating glenohumeral laxity is the Gagey test. The examiner's forearm pushes down firmly on the shoulder girdle. The examiner then lifts the relaxed upper limb of the patient with the elbow flexed to 90 degrees into abduction with his/her other hand. Excessive   abduction   (i.e.,   >105   degrees)   or

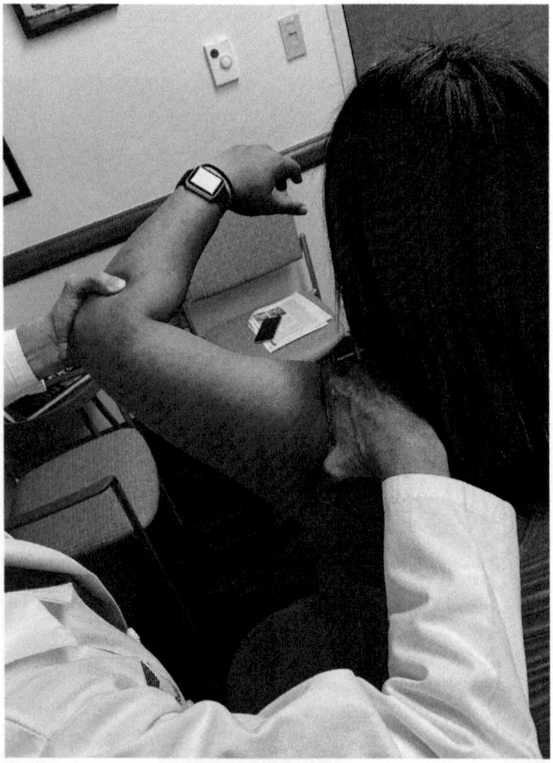

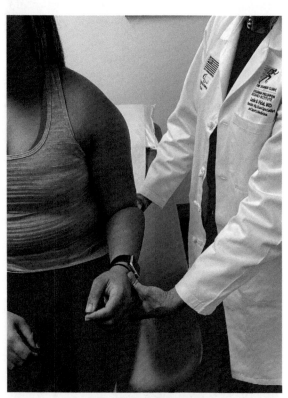

FIG. 15.7 Kim Test

FIG. 15.8 Sulcus Test.

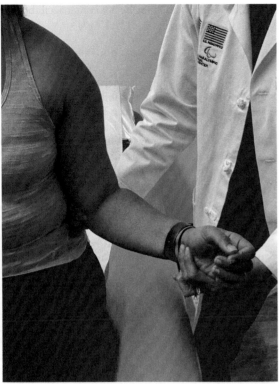

FIG. 15.9 Sulcus in External Rotation.

apprehension limiting passive abduction is a positive finding for laxity of the IGHL.[48]

Imaging

Initial workup of any patient presenting with shoulder instability should include obtaining plain radiographs (true anteroposterior, scapular Y, axillary lateral). Variations of the axillary lateral include the Velpeau view as well as the West Point view. The scapular Y view is more easily obtained in the setting of pain or acute trauma. It is obtained with the arm at the side and the patient seated upright or in the prone position and rotated 30—45 degrees toward the cassette. The projection that results is the Y-shaped intersection of the scapular body, coracoid process, and scapular spine, with the humeral head superimposed on top of the glenoid fossa. This view can also be used to visualize anterior or posterior shoulder dislocations.[49]

Advanced imaging with magnetic resonance imaging (MRI) or MRA is often warranted to evaluate for labral or other soft tissue pathology. MRI also allows for the evaluation of bony impactions, fractures, and osseous edema, which may be present in the setting of shoulder instability (Fig. 15.10). Computed tomography may be

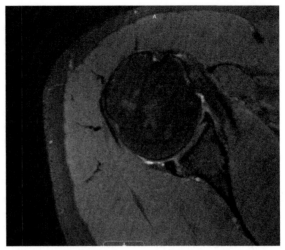

FIG. 15.10 MRI Axial Fat Suppressed Proton Density Posterior Labral Tear.

warranted to obtain more detailed evaluation of bony anatomy, especially in the setting of trauma or significant glenoid bone loss.[49]

MANAGEMENT OF ANTERIOR SHOULDER INSTABILITY

Nearly half of all anterior shoulder dislocations occur in patients 15—29 years old. The incidence of true dislocations is nearly three times higher in males than in females.[50] When evaluating the mechanism of injury between young male and female athletes, it has been reported that females are more than twice as likely to experience an episode of shoulder instability after contact with an object or the ground, whereas male athletes are more likely to experience instability after collision with another player.[2]

Understanding the natural history and consequences of recurrent anterior shoulder instability is important to help determine the indications for nonoperative versus operative intervention.

As described earlier, detachment of the anterior inferior glenoid labrum is considered the essential injury required to allow anterior instability. In some cases, this isolated Bankart lesion alone may not be sufficient to produce anterior glenohumeral instability. It is thought that concomitant elongation of the anterior capsule and associated ligaments is required to allow for anterior instability. It is important to recognize not only injury to the anterior glenohumeral ligament complex but also normal anatomic variants. Many female athletes will demonstrate a variant known as a sublabral foramen, which is a nonpathologic area where the anterior superior labrum may not be fully attached to the anterior superior glenoid. Additionally, patients may demonstrate the "Buford complex," which is an absence of the anterior superior labrum in the presence of a cordlike MGHL.[51]

Nonsurgical Management

The overall recurrence rate following nonsurgical management of traumatic anterior shoulder instability ranges from 33% to 67%.[52] The recurrence rate increases in higher risk individuals. Risk factors for recurrent instability have been identified as young age, athletic activity, male gender, and the presence of a bony Bankart lesion.[53,54] Nonsurgical management continues to be the initial treatment of choice for first-time dislocation in many cases.[55] However, there is increasing acceptance for operating on patients following a first-time traumatic anterior dislocation in the high-risk population. Nonsurgical management consists of a period of sling immobilization followed by supervised physical therapy exercises focusing on scapular stabilization, progressive range of motion, and subsequent strengthening.

Surgical Management

Decision-making regarding surgery and timing is challenging. Many studies demonstrate that the risk of recurrent instability is significantly lower following surgical treatment in high-risk patients. However, most surgeons continue to recommend a period of rehabilitation and return to normal activities and sports and consider surgery only in case of recurrence. Management of the in-season athlete following a first-time shoulder dislocation can be particularly challenging. Many authors will initially recommend nonsurgical treatment, rehabilitation, and possibly the use of a brace, with the goal of letting the athletes finish their season, and then consider surgical stabilization at the end of the season.[56,57]

Arthroscopic Shoulder Stabilization

Surgical stabilization can be performed open or arthroscopically. Advantages of an arthroscopic approach include the opportunity to thoroughly evaluate the glenohumeral joint and identify any coexistent shoulder pathology. Arthroscopic stabilization is associated with less postoperative pain, fewer risks for iatrogenic nerve injury, lower morbidity, and improved cosmesis.[58] Additionally, because arthroscopic stabilization does not violate the subscapularis tendon, there is a very low risk of subscapularis insufficiency or scarring. While labral repair and capsular plication techniques can be reliably performed arthroscopically, some coexistent pathology (e.g., HAGL lesion) can be more

difficult to address and may be better managed through an open approach (Figs. 15.11–15.13).

Results of Arthroscopic Shoulder Stabilization

While early studies showed inferior results of arthroscopic versus open shoulder stabilization, arthroscopic surgical techniques and implants have improved significantly. In a meta-analysis, it was shown that modern arthroscopic techniques with suture anchor fixation have redislocation rates similar to open surgery.[58] Recurrent instability occurred in approximately 7% of

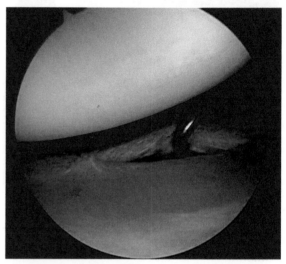

FIG. 15.11 Arthroscopic Image of Bankart Tear.

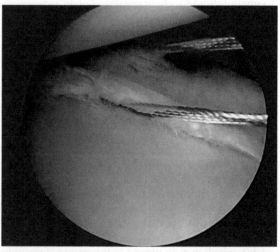

FIG. 15.12 Arthroscopic Image of Suture Passage for Bankart Repair.

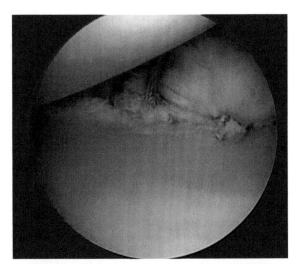

FIG. 15.13 Arthroscopic Image of Bankart Repair.

TABLE 15.1	
Instability Severity Index Score Based on a Preoperative Questionnaire, Clinical Examination, and Radiographs.	
Prognostic Factors	**Points**
AGE AT SURGERY (YEARS)	
≤20	2
>20	0
DEGREE OF PREOPERATIVE SPORTS PARTICIPATION	
Competitive	2
Recreational or none	0
TYPE OF PREOPERATIVE SPORTS PARTICIPATION	
Contact or forced overhead	1
Other	0
SHOULDER HYPERLAXITY	
Shoulder hyperlaxity (anterior or inferior)	1
Normal laxity	0
HILL-SACHS ON AP RADIOGRAPH	
Visible in external rotation	2
Not visible in external rotation	0
GLENOID LOSS OF CONTOUR ON AP RADIOGRAPH	
Loss of contour	2
No lesion	0
Total points possible	**10**

AP, anteroposterior.

patients, and 90% of patients returned to their preinjury level of sports. Reported risk factors for recurrent instability following arthroscopic stabilization are ligamentous laxity, anterior glenoid bone deficiency of 20% −30%, a large Hill-Sachs lesion, and an engaging Hill-Sachs lesion during physiologic range of motion.[59,60] These findings have been corroborated in other studies, in addition to brief postoperative immobilization of less than 4 weeks and glenoid bone loss of more than 15%.[53,61,62] To help surgeons determine preoperatively who will do well with an arthroscopic procedure and who will likely require an open stabilization, Balg and Boileau developed the Instability Severity Index Score (ISIS), which attempts to quantify a patient's risk for failure following an arthroscopic stabilization. It is based on a preoperative questionnaire, clinical examination, and radiographs that are scaled on a 0- to 10-point system (Table 15.1). The risk for recurrence following arthroscopic stabilization was found to be 3% for patients with a score ≤3, 10% for those with a score ≤6, and 70% for those with a score ≥7. This group concluded that patients with an elevated ISIS are likely better managed with an open surgical stabilization as opposed to an arthroscopic procedure.

Open Shoulder Stabilization

Open surgery is often recommended for the management of failed previous arthroscopic stabilizations, significant glenoid or humeral bone loss, HAGL lesions, associated subscapularis tears, and patients who have a high ISIS.[63] However, some surgeons still prefer to address anterior shoulder instability through an open approach as their primary treatment for anterior

shoulder instability. Many open procedures have been described. Historically, some led to significant scarring, subscapularis insufficiency, stiffness, and postoperative arthritis due to overconstraining the glenohumeral joint.[64] Modern open techniques for capsulolabral repair have been successful in protecting the subscapularis, repairing the labrum, imbricating the capsule, and augmenting or bone grafting areas of significant bone loss on the glenoid or humeral head.

Results of Open Surgical Stabilization

Many authors have reported long-term outcomes of open Bankart repair. Most studies report a low recurrence rate of 3%−5% with a high patient satisfaction rate. However, full range of motion is less predictably achieved, and degenerative joint disease can be seen postoperatively.[65−67] Therefore although the recurrence rates after open Bankart repair are favorable, long-term studies have shown patients to be at risk of developing osteoarthritis.[29]

Rehabilitation Following Anterior Shoulder Stabilization

The goals of postoperative rehabilitation following anterior glenohumeral stabilization are to protect the soft tissues as they heal and restore range of motion, strength, proprioception, and function. Most postoperative protocols recommend a period of relative sling immobilization for approximately 4 weeks, during which time passive range of motion and scapular stabilization exercises are encouraged. Range of motion is then progressed from active assisted to active range of motion. Full range of motion is expected by 12 weeks. Progressive strengthening and sports-specific activities are initiated, and return to sport can be expected sometime between 5 and 6 months following surgery.

MANAGEMENT OF POSTERIOR SHOULDER INSTABILITY

Nonsurgical Management

Similar to anterior shoulder instability, the goals of treating posterior glenohumeral instability should focus on reducing pain, improving function, and preventing recurrence.[68] The natural history of an acute traumatic posterior instability event as well as that of a recurrent posterior instability is more poorly understood than that of anterior shoulder instability. That being said, it is felt that a patient sustaining a single traumatic posterior instability event is more likely to experience recurrent instability if surgical stabilization is not performed.[69] It is not clear which anatomic features such as bone loss, bone morphology, and hyperlaxity or which demographic factors such as age, gender, and type of sports participation are most associated with recurrence.[68] Nonsurgical management of posterior shoulder instability incorporates activity modification in order to avoid activities that aggravate the symptoms, physical therapy focusing on regaining range of motion, scapulothoracic and subscapularis strengthening, and proprioception. This approach has shown encouraging results in both patients with generalized laxity and patients with a traumatic cause of symptoms.[70,71]

Surgical Management

Surgical stabilization for posterior shoulder instability is recommended for patients who remain symptomatic despite nonsurgical treatment as well as in patients with an acute traumatic cause and identifiable soft tissue or osseous pathology.[68] Posterior instability can often be treated successfully with an arthroscopic repair. This allows for a thorough evaluation of the entire glenohumeral joint and the opportunity to address concomitant intra-articular and extra-articular pathology, including SLAP tears, circumferential labral tears, rotator cuff tears, and less common pathologies such as ALPSA lesions, GLAD lesions, and reverse HAGL lesions. If not identified and addressed, these concomitant injuries can lead to suboptimal surgical outcomes. Identification may alter surgical management as well as the rehabilitation protocol for the patient.[28]

Open approaches for posterior shoulder stabilization are less frequently performed. Because of the challenging dissection necessary to obtain adequate visualization for open posterior capsulolabral stabilization, arthroscopic procedures result in less surgical site morbidity and improved surgeon familiarity with the anatomy.[72,73] Open posterior shoulder stabilization may need to be considered in some cases of failed arthroscopic repairs, particularly in the setting of posterior glenoid bone loss or significant glenoid retroversion. Bone augmentation techniques include glenoid osteotomy, rotational osteotomy of the proximal humerus, and bone block augmentation of the posterior glenoid with autograft or allograft.[74,75] Recent data suggests that posterior glenoid augmentation with iliac crest autograft and distal tibia allograft results in similar biomechanical properties. Therefore the use of distal tibial allograft when compared with the use of autograft may be advantageous because of the lack of donor-site morbidity and the osteoarticular nature of the distal tibial allograft graft.[76] Additional research on the clinical and radiographic outcomes of posterior glenoid bone augmentation with this technique is needed.

Results of Posterior Shoulder Stabilization

The outcomes of both arthroscopic and open posterior shoulder stabilization are good. A large meta-analysis concluded that patients undergoing arthroscopic stabilization had superior outcomes with lower recurrence rates and higher return-to-play rates than patients undergoing open stabilization procedures.[77,78] However, it is difficult to draw conclusions given the significant heterogeneity of the studies included. Each patient should have an individualized clinical decision made based on their specific history, physical examination, and pathoanatomy.

Rehabilitation Following Posterior Shoulder Stabilization

Rehabilitation following posterior shoulder stabilization is similar to that for anterior shoulder stabilization.

The arm is immobilized in a sling with an abduction pillow for 4–6 weeks. Passive range of motion and scapular stabilization are initiated early. Active assisted and active range of motion are then progressed. Gentle progressive strengthening and proprioception are initiated. Return to sport is typically permitted between 4 and 6 months postoperatively.

MULTIDIRECTIONAL INSTABILITY OF THE SHOULDER

Nonsurgical Management

Symptomatic MDI occurs when both static and dynamic restraints are insufficient to maintain healthy glenohumeral stability. The goal of management is to rehabilitate or reconstruct deficient structures to restore stability and alleviate symptoms.[31] Many, if not most, patients with MDI can be managed nonoperatively. Treatment of scapulothoracic dyskinesia is the primary focus of physical therapy. The resultant improvement of the dynamic positioning of the scapula in combination with proprioceptive exercises can improve the efficiency of dynamic glenohumeral stabilizers. Additionally, strengthening of the rotator cuff can improve the dynamic concavity compression effect, which also enhances shoulder stability.[31] Studies suggest that rehabilitation results in substantially increased rotator cuff activation, which functionally reduces instability. Motivated patients typically do well with the rehabilitative protocol and report diminished pain and improved stability.[79] Historical data from Burkhead and Rockwood[71] demonstrated good or excellent results in 35 of 39 patients with MDI treated with a directed rehabilitation program. More recently, less encouraging long-term results were reported in a cohort of young athletic patients with MDI treated with rehabilitation. Among 36 patients, 19 experienced poor results, and only 8 were free of pain and instability at a mean of 8-year follow-up. Athletic patients with MDI may have a less favorable response to rehabilitation.[80]

Surgical Management

Surgical treatment for MDI should be considered for patients who continue to have debilitating symptoms despite an extensive course of nonoperative treatment. Common surgical procedures include open inferior capsular shift and arthroscopic capsular plication. The humeral open inferior capsular shift, as described by Neer and Foster in 1980,[34] has been considered the gold standard for surgical treatment of MDI. A T-shaped incision is made between the MGHL and IGHL. Capsular flaps are elevated from the neck of the humerus and advanced to reduce posterior capsular redundancy and to reduce the volume of the inferior capsular pouch. The subscapularis is then repaired superficial to the reconstructed capsule. Additional open capsular shift procedures have been popularized and include subscapularis sparing and glenoid-based techniques.[81,82]

Arthroscopic capsular plication is a less invasive treatment option for patients who require soft tissue repair, and it has become more common, as advanced techniques have made arthroscopic management of MDI more viable. Like arthroscopic treatment for other instability patterns, the advantages of arthroscopic techniques for MDI include decreased morbidity, visual confirmation of decreased capsule laxity, and avoidance of subscapularis detachment.[31] The direction and magnitude of instability should be established preoperatively and confirmed with an examination under anesthesia. Diagnostic arthroscopy may demonstrate a patulous capsule and labral abnormalities. Following capsular abrasion to promote healing, the capsule can then be imbricated or plicated sequentially with or without the use of anchor fixation to decrease capsular volume. It has been shown in a cadaver model that multiple pleated anterior, inferior, and posterior capsular plications can result in a significantly larger decrease in capsular volume compared with open inferior capsular shift.[83] A question remains as to the necessity or indications to perform a concomitant closure of the rotator interval. Biomechanical data suggests that rotator interval closure should be considered in patients with MDI when capsular laxity is not sufficiently addressed, despite adequate capsular plication.[84,85] However, there is no consensus on when concomitant rotator interval closure should be performed. Clinically, satisfactory results have been obtained both with and without routine interval closure.[86,87]

Rehabilitation Following Multidirectional Instability Shoulder Stabilization

Postoperative rehabilitation should be individualized and based on the direction and severity of primary instability as well as the robustness of the repair. In general, the shoulder is immobilized in an abduction sling in neutral rotation for 4–6 weeks. Gentle progressive range of motion and strengthening is then initiated. Anticipated return to sport is approximately 4–6 months postoperatively if patients have regained full range of motion and strength and successfully completed an appropriate sports-specific training program.

CONCLUSION

The diagnosis and management of shoulder instability requires a thoughtful history, thorough physical examination, and careful review of appropriate imaging. Treatment options vary widely and interventions should be tailored to each patient, particularly the female athlete, based on the patient's individual symptoms, pathology, and activity level.

REFERENCES

1. Carlisle RM, Tokish JM. Multidirectional instability of the shoulder. In: Miller MD, Thompson SR, eds. *DeLee, Drez & Miller's Orthopaedic Sports Medicine Principles and Practice*. Philadelphia, PA: Elsevier; 2020:476–488.
2. Owens BD, Agel J, Mountcastle SB, Cameron KL, Nelson BJ. Incidence of glenohumeral instability in collegiate athletics. *Am J Sports Med*. 2009;37(9):1750–1754.
3. Patzkowski JC, Dickens JF, Cameron KL, Bokshan SL, Garcia EJ, Owens BD. Pathoanatomy of shoulder instability in collegiate female athletes. *Am J Sports Med*. 2019;47(8):1909–1914.
4. Owens BD, Dawson L, Burks R, Cameron KL. Incidence of shoulder dislocation in the United States military: demographic considerations from a high-risk population. *J Bone Jt Surg Am*. 2009;91(4):791–796.
5. Blomquist J, Solheim E, Liavaag S, Schroder CP, Espehaug B, Havelin L. Shoulder instability surgery in Norway: the first report from a multicenter register, with 1-year follow-up. *Acta Orthop*. 2012;83(2):165–170.
6. Peck KY, Johnston DA, Owens BD, Cameron KL. The incidence of injury among male and female intercollegiate rugby players. *Sport Health*. 2013;5:327–333.
7. Wuelker N, Korell M, Thren K. Dynamic glenohumeral joint stability. *J Shoulder Elbow Surg*. 1998;7(1):43–52.
8. Howell SM, Galinat BJ. The glenoid-labral socket. A constrained articular surface. *Clin Orthop Relat Res*. 1989; (243):122–125.
9. O'Brien SJ, Neves MC, Arnoczky SP, et al. The anatomy and histology of the inferior glenohumeral ligament complex of the shoulder. *Am J Sports Med*. 1990;18(5):449–456.
10. O'Brien SJ, Schwartz RS, Warren RF, Torzilli PA. Capsular restraints to anterior-posterior motion of the abducted shoulder: a biomechanical study. *J Shoulder Elbow Surg*. 1995;4(4):298–308.
11. Urayama M, Itoi E, Hatakeyama Y, Pradhan RL, Sato K. Function of the 3 portions of the inferior glenohumeral ligament: a cadaveric study. *J Shoulder Elbow Surg*. 2001; 10(6):589–594.
12. Ide J, Maeda S, Takagi K. Normal variations of the glenohumeral ligament complex: an anatomic study for arthroscopic Bankart repair. *Arthroscopy*. 2004;20(2):164–168.
13. Turkel SJ, Panio MW, Marshall JL, Girgis FG. Stabilizing mechanisms preventing anterior dislocation of the glenohumeral joint. *J Bone Jt Surg Am*. 1981;63(8):1208–1217.
14. Kask K, Põldoja E, Lont T, et al. Anatomy of the superior glenohumeral ligament. *J Shoulder Elbow Surg*. 2010; 19(6):908–916.
15. Warner JJ, Deng XH, Warren RF, Torzilli PA. Static capsuloligamentous restraints to superior-inferior translation of the glenohumeral joint. *Am J Sports Med*. 1992;20(6): 675–685.
16. Boardman ND, Debski RE, Warner JJ, et al. Tensile properties of the superior glenohumeral and coracohumeral ligaments. *J Shoulder Elbow Surg*. 1996;5(4):249–254.
17. Soslowsky LJ, Malicky DM, Blasier RB. Active and passive factors in inferior glenohumeral stabilization: a biomechanical model. *J Shoulder Elbow Surg*. 1997;6(4): 371–379.
18. Mologne TS. Shoulder anatomy and biomechanics. In: Miller MD, Thompson SR, eds. *DeLee, Drez, & Miller's Orthopedic Sports Medicine Principles and Practice*. Philadelphia, PA: Elsevier; 2020:393–401.
19. Mologne TS. Shoulder anatomy and biomechanics. In: Miller MD, Thompson SR, eds. *DeLee, Drez, & Miller's Orthopedic Sports Medicine Principles and Practice*. Philadelphia, PA: Elsevier; 2020:9.
20. Taylor DC, Arciero RA. Pathologic changes associated with shoulder dislocations. Arthroscopic and physical examination findings in first-time, traumatic anterior dislocations. *Am J Sports Med*. 1997;25(3):306–311.
21. Griffith JF, Antonio GE, Yung PSH, et al. Prevalence, pattern, and spectrum of glenoid bone loss in anterior shoulder dislocation: CT analysis of 218 patients. *Am J Roentgenol*. 2008;190(5):1247–1254.
22. Hill HA, Sachs MD. The grooved defect of the humeral head. *Radiology*. 1940;35:11.
23. Reider B. Conquering the Hill-Sachs. *Am J Sports Med*. 2016;44(11):2767–2770.
24. Rowe CR, Zarins B. Recurrent transient subluxation of the shoulder. *J Bone Jt Surg Am*. 1981;63(6):863–872.
25. Nakagawa S, Ozaki R, Take Y, Iuchi R, Mae T. Relationship between glenoid defects and Hill-Sachs lesions in shoulders with traumatic anterior instability. *Am J Sports Med*. 2015;43(11):2763–2773.
26. Calandra JJ, Baker CL, Uribe J. The incidence of Hill-Sachs lesions in initial anterior shoulder dislocations. *Arthroscopy*. 1989;5(4):254–257.
27. Thompson SR, Menzer H, Brockmeier SF. Anterior shoulder instability. In: MD M, SR T, eds. *DeLee, Drez & Miller Orthopaedic Sports Medicine Principles and Practice*. Philadelphia, PA: Elsevier; 2020:440–462.
28. Forsythe B, Frank RM, Ahmed M, et al. Identification and treatment of existing copathology in anterior shoulder instability repair. *Arthroscopy*. 2015;31(1):154–166.
29. Pagnani MJ, Warren RF. Stabilizers of the glenohumeral joint. *J Shoulder Elbow Surg*. 1994;3(3):173–190.
30. Bradley JP, Tjoumakaris FP. Posterior shoulder instability. In: MD M, SR T, eds. *DeLee, Drez & Miller's Orthopaedic Sports Medicine Principles and Practice*. Philadelphia, PA: Elsevier; 2020:463–475.

31. Gaskill TR, Taylor DC, Millett PJ. Management of multidirectional instability of the shoulder. *J Am Acad Orthop Surg.* 2011;19(12):10.

32. von Eisenhart-Rothe R, Mayr HO, Hinterwimmer S, Graichen H. Simultaneous 3D assessment of glenohumeral shape, humeral head centering, and scapular positioning in atraumatic shoulder instability: a magnetic resonance-based in vivo analysis. *Am J Sports Med.* 2010;38(2):375−382.

33. Kim SH, Noh KC, Park JS, Ryu BD, Oh I. Loss of chondrolabral containment of the glenohumeral joint in atraumatic posteroinferior multidirectional instability. *J Bone Jt Surg Am.* 2005;87(1):92−98.

34. Neer CS, Foster CR. Inferior capsular shift for involuntary inferior and multidirectional instability of the shoulder. A preliminary report. *J Bone Jt Surg Am.* 1980;62(6):897−908.

35. Shafer BL, Mihata T, McGarry MH, Tibone JE, Lee TQ. Effects of capsular plication and rotator interval closure in simulated multidirectional shoulder instability. *J Bone Jt Surg Am.* 2008;90(1):136−144.

36. Mallon WJ, Speer KP. Multidirectional instability: current concepts. *J Shoulder Elbow Surg.* 1995;4(1 Pt 1):54−64.

37. Jost B, Koch PP, Gerber C. Anatomy and functional aspects of the rotator interval. *J Shoulder Elbow Surg.* 2000;9(4):336−341.

38. Ovesen J, Nielsen S. Experimental distal subluxation in the glenohumeral joint. *Arch Orthop Trauma Surg.* 1985;104(2):78−81.

39. Beighton P, Solomon L, Soskolne CL. Articular mobility in an African population. *Ann Rheum Dis.* 1973;32(5):413−418.

40. Juul-Kristensen B, Røgind H, Jensen DV, Remvig L. Inter-examiner reproducibility of tests and criteria for generalized joint hypermobility and benign joint hypermobility syndrome. *Rheumatology.* 2007;46(12):1835−1841.

41. Hippensteel KJ, Brophy R, Smith MV, Wright RW. Comprehensive review of provocative and instability physical examination tests of the shoulder. *J Am Acad Orthop Surg.* 2019;27(11):10.

42. Cameron KL, Duffey ML, DeBerardino TM, Stoneman PD, Jones CJ, Owens BD. Association of generalized joint hypermobility with a history of glenohumeral joint instability. *J Athl Train.* 2010;45(3):253−258.

43. van Kampen DA, van den Berg T, van der Woude HJ, Castelein, RM, Terwee, CB, Willems WJ. Diagnostic value of patient characteristics, history, and six clinical tests for traumatic anterior shoulder instability. *J Shoulder Elbow Surg.* 2013;22(10):1310−1319.

44. Gerber C, Ganz R. Clinical assessment of instability of the shoulder. With special reference to anterior and posterior drawer tests. *J Bone Jt Surg Br.* 1984;66(4):551−556.

45. McFarland EG, Kim TK, Park HB, Neira CA, Gutierrez MI. The effect of variation in definition on the diagnosis of multidirectional instability of the shoulder. *J Bone Jt Surg Am.* 2003;85(11):2138−2144.

46. Tennent TD, Beach WR, Meyers JF. A review of the special tests associated with shoulder examination. Part II: laxity, instability, and superior labral anterior and posterior (SLAP) lesions. *Am J Sports Med.* 2003;31(2):301−307.

47. Kim SH, Park JS, Jeong WK, Shin SK. The Kim test: a novel test for posteroinferior labral lesion of the shoulder—a comparison to the jerk test. *Am J Sports Med.* 2005;33(8):1188−1192.

48. Gagey OJ, Gagey N. The hyperabduction test. *J Bone Jt Surg Br.* 2001;83(1):69−74.

49. Burge AJ, Konin GP. Glenohumeral joint imaging. In: Miller MD, Thompson SR, eds. *DeLee, Drez & Miller's Orthopaedic Sports Medicine Principles and Practice.* Philadelphia, PA: Elsevier; 2020:408−432.

50. Zacchilli MA, Owens BD. Epidemiology of shoulder dislocations presenting to emergency departments in the United States. *J Bone Jt Surg Am.* 2010;92(3):542−549.

51. Williams MM, Snyder SJ, Buford D. The Buford complex—the "cord-like" middle glenohumeral ligament and absent anterosuperior labrum complex: a normal anatomic capsulolabral variant. *Arthroscopy.* 1994;10(3):241−247.

52. Rhee YG, Cho NS, Cho SH. Traumatic anterior dislocation of the shoulder: factors affecting the progress of the traumatic anterior dislocation. *Clin Orthop Surg.* 2009;1(4):188−193.

53. Boileau P, Villalba M, Héry, JY, Balg F, Ahrens P, Neyton L. Risk factors for recurrence of shoulder instability after arthroscopic Bankart repair. *J Bone Jt Surg Am.* 2006;88(8):1755−1763.

54. Calvo E, Granizo JJ, Fernández-Yruegas D. Criteria for arthroscopic treatment of anterior instability of the shoulder: a prospective study. *J Bone Jt Surg Br.* 2005;87(5):677−683.

55. Paterson WH, Throckmorton TW, Koester M, Azar FM, Kuhn JE. Position and duration of immobilization after primary anterior shoulder dislocation: a systematic review and meta-analysis of the literature. *J Bone Jt Surg Am.* 2010;92(18):2924−2933.

56. Buss DD, Lynch GP, Meyer CP, Huber M S, Freehill MQ. Nonoperative management for in-season athletes with anterior shoulder instability. *Am J Sports Med.* 2004;32(6):1430−1433.

57. Owens BD, Dickens JF, Kilcoyne KG, Rue JP. Management of mid-season traumatic anterior shoulder instability in athletes. *J Am Acad Orthop Surg.* 2012;20(8):518−526.

58. Brophy RH, Marx RG. The treatment of traumatic anterior instability of the shoulder: nonoperative and surgical treatment. *Arthroscopy.* 2009;25(3):298−304.

59. Voos JE, Livermore RW, Feeley BT, et al. Prospective evaluation of arthroscopic bankart repairs for anterior instability. *Am J Sports Med.* 2010;38(2):302−307.

60. Streubel PN, Krych AJ, Simone JP, et al. Anterior glenohumeral instability: A pathology-based surgical treatment strategy. *J Am Acad Orthop Surg.* 2014;22(5):12.

61. Sisto DJ. Revision of failed arthroscopic bankart repairs. *Am J Sports Med.* 2007;35(4):537−541.

62. Porcellini G, Campi F, Pegreffi F, Castagna A, Paladini P. Predisposing factors for recurrent shoulder dislocation after arthroscopic treatment. *J Bone Jt Surg Am.* 2009;91(11):2537−2542.

63. Balg F, Boileau P. The instability severity index score. A simple pre-operative score to select patients for arthroscopic or open shoulder stabilisation. *J Bone Jt Surg Br.* 2007;89(11):1470–1477.

64. Kiss J, Mersich I, Perlaky, GY, Szollas L. The results of the Putti-Platt operation with particular reference to arthritis, pain, and limitation of external rotation. *J Shoulder Elbow Surg.* 1998;7(5):495–500.

65. Cheung EV, Sperling JW, Hattrup SJ, Cofield RH. Long-term outcome of anterior stabilization of the shoulder. *J Shoulder Elbow Surg.* 2008;17(2):265–270.

66. Rowe CR, Zarins B, Ciullo JV. Recurrent anterior dislocation of the shoulder after surgical repair. Apparent causes of failure and treatment. *J Bone Jt Surg Am.* 1984;66(2):159–168.

67. Pagnani MJ. Open capsular repair without bone block for recurrent anterior shoulder instability in patients with and without bony defects of the glenoid and/or humeral head. *Am J Sports Med.* 2008;36(9):1805–1812.

68. RM F, AA R, MT P. Posterior glenohumeral instability: evidence-based treatment. *J Am Acad Orthop Surg.* 2017;25(9):14.

69. Provencher MT, Bell SJ, Menzel KA, Mologne TS. Arthroscopic treatment of posterior shoulder instability: results in 33 patients. *Am J Sports Med.* 2005;33(10):1463–1471.

70. Fronek J, Warren RF, Bowen M. Posterior subluxation of the glenohumeral joint. *J Bone Jt Surg Am.* 1989;71(2):12.

71. Burkhead J WZ, Rockwood J CA. Treatment of instability of the shoulder with an exercise program. *J Bone Jt Surg Am.* 1992;74(6):7.

72. Wolf EM, Eakin CL. Arthroscopic capsular plication for posterior shoulder instability. *Arthroscopy.* 1998;14(2):153–163.

73. Hawkins RJ, Janda DH. Posterior instability of the glenohumeral joint. A technique of repair. *Am J Sports Med.* 1996;24(3):275–278.

74. Servien E, Walch G, Cortes ZE, Edwards TB, O'Connor DP. Posterior bone block procedure for posterior shoulder instability. *Knee Surg Sports Traumatol Arthrosc.* 2007;15(9):1130–1136.

75. Gupta AK, Chalmers PN, Klosterman E, Harris JD, Provencher MT, Romeo AA. Arthroscopic distal tibial allograft augmentation for posterior shoulder instability with glenoid bone loss. *Arthrosc Tech.* 2013;2(4):e405–e411.

76. Frank RM, Shin J, Saccomanno MF, et al. Comparison of glenohumeral contact pressures and contact areas after posterior glenoid reconstruction with an iliac crest bone graft or distal tibial osteochondral allograft. *Am J Sports Med.* 2014;42(11):2574–2582.

77. DeLong JM, Jiang K, Bradley JP. Posterior instability of the shoulder: a systematic review and meta-analysis of clinical outcomes. *Am J Sports Med.* 2015;43(7):1805–1817.

78. Bradley JP, McClincy MP, Arner JW, Tejwani SG. Arthroscopic capsulolabral reconstruction for posterior instability of the shoulder: a prospective study of 200 shoulders. *Am J Sports Med.* 2013;41(9):2005–2014.

79. Illyés A, Kiss J, Kiss RM. Electromyographic analysis during pull, forward punch, elevation and overhead throw after conservative treatment or capsular shift at patient with multidirectional shoulder joint instability. *J Electromyogr Kinesiol.* 2009;19(6):e438–e447.

80. Misamore GW, Sallay PI, Didelot W. A longitudinal study of patients with multidirectional instability of the shoulder with seven- to ten-year follow-up. *J Shoulder Elbow Surg.* 2005;14(5):466–470.

81. Bak K, Spring BJ, Henderson JP. Inferior capsular shift procedure in athletes with multidirectional instability based on isolated capsular and ligamentous redundancy. *Am J Sports Med.* 2000;28(4):466–471.

82. Altchek DW, Warren RF, Skyhar MJ, Ortiz G. T-plasty modification of the Bankart procedure for multidirectional instability of the anterior and inferior types. *J Bone Jt Surg Am.* 1991;73(1):105–112.

83. Sekiya JK, Willobee JA, Miller MD, Hickman AJ, Willobee A. Arthroscopic multi-pleated capsular plication compared with open inferior capsular shift for reduction of shoulder volume in a cadaveric model. *Arthroscopy.* 2007;23(11):1145–1151.

84. Provencher MT, Mologne TS, Hongo M, Zhao K, Tasto JP, An KN. Arthroscopic versus open rotator interval closure: biomechanical evaluation of stability and motion. *Arthroscopy.* 2007;23(6):583–592.

85. Mologne TS, Hongo M, Romeo AA, An KN, Provencher MT. The addition of rotator interval closure after arthroscopic repair of either anterior or posterior shoulder instability: effect on glenohumeral translation and range of motion. *Am J Sports Med.* 2008;36(6):1123–1131.

86. Kim SH, Ha KI, Yoo JC, Noh KC. Kim's lesion: an incomplete and concealed avulsion of the posteroinferior labrum in posterior or multidirectional posteroinferior instability of the shoulder. *Arthroscopy.* 2004;20(7):712–720.

87. Gartsman GM, Roddey TS, Hammerman SM. Arthroscopic treatment of multidirectional glenohumeral instability: 2- to 5-year follow-up. *Arthroscopy.* 2001;17(3):236–243.

CHAPTER 16

Rotator Cuff Function and Injury in the Female Athlete

SHEILA M. ALGAN, MD • KATHERINE SPROUSE, MD

INTRODUCTION

Shoulder problems in the female athlete occur most commonly in sports that require repetitive or forceful use of the upper extremity. While there is extensive research in male overhead athletes, most notably baseball players and in particular pitchers, there is much less research involving female athletes. There is some research in sports where both male and female athletes compete in the same events or under the same set of rules, but research often includes only males.[1-3] Injury to the rotator cuff or chronic overuse of rotator cuff musculature is often not clearly defined in observational injury prevalence studies, making it difficult to ascertain the true extent of rotator cuff problems.[4,5] Overuse problems may not be reported by the athlete who may fear loss of a position on the team or by the athletic training staff if the injury does not involve time lost from participation. Club sports often do not have access to athletic training staff to track or report injuries. For these reasons, it is difficult to know the actual incidence or prevalence of rotator cuff problems in the female athlete for most sports, outside of "captured" athlete populations, such as the National Collegiate Athletic Association (NCAA).

There are clear similarities between the movement patterns of various men's and women's overhead sports, but differences in muscle firing patterns may only be observed with electromyographic (EMG) studies correlated with kinetic and kinematic information for the specific sport.[6,7] This chapter will discuss rotator cuff injury patterns for various women's sports and the activity of the rotator cuff musculature in female athletes participating in overhead sports and will incorporate information related to injury prevention programs.

SOFTBALL

The typical softball is 12 inches in circumference with a weight between 6¼ and 7 oz. A baseball has a circumference of 9¼ inch and a weight of 5¼ oz.[8] Softball pitchers frequently throw far more innings and pitches over the course of a week in season than baseball pitchers. Werner et al.[9] reviewed the number of pitches for a typical softball tournament weekend. The authors found that a pitcher may pitch as many as 10 games, with 7 innings per game, and a total of 1500−2000 pitches thrown over a 3-day period. There are no mandated pitch counts for fast pitch junior or senior division softball as there are for Little League Baseball. Little League Baseball mandates no more than 95 pitches per day for its oldest age group (13−16 years), with required rest periods depending on the number of pitches thrown.[10] College and professional baseball and softball do not require pitch counts.

There is extensive literature detailing the overhead baseball pitch. EMG studies have described the muscle activation patterns (Fig. 16.1).[11] The rotator cuff acts to decelerate the arm and compress the glenohumeral joint in overhead throwing sports. The windmill pitch technique used in fast pitch softball is less studied, but the throwing cycle is well-described.[12] The phases of the windmill pitch (Fig. 16.2)[12] include (1) windup, first ball movement to 6 o'clock; (2) 6 o'clock to 3 o'clock (ends with shoulder flexed 90 degrees); (3) 3 o'clock to 12 o'clock (shoulder flexed/abducted near 180 degrees); (4) 12 o'clock to 9 o'clock (shoulder abducted to 90 degrees); (5) 9 o'clock to ball release; and (6) ball release to completion of throw (followthrough). The total arc of movement during the windmill pitch is 450−500 degrees.[11,13]

Werner et al.[9] have described the kinematics and kinetics of the elite windmill (rising) softball pitch by evaluating 24 elite female Olympic pitchers by using high-speed cameras during the 1996 Olympic Games. The authors found that shoulder distraction forces averaged 80% body weight, and they postulated that these distraction forces, which are similar to those in

The Female Athlete. https://doi.org/10.1016/B978-0-323-75985-4.00002-7

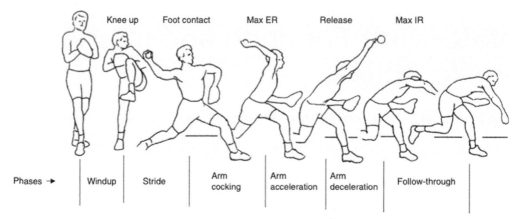

FIG. 16.1 Pitching phases and key events (adapted from Fleisig et al.[6] with permission). *ER*, external rotation; *IR*, internal rotation; *max*, maximum. (From Escamilla RF, Andrews JR. Shoulder muscle recruitment patterns and related biomechanics during upper extremity sports. *Sports Med*. 2009;39(7):572. www.littleleague.org/playing-rules/pitch-count. Accessed May 2020.)

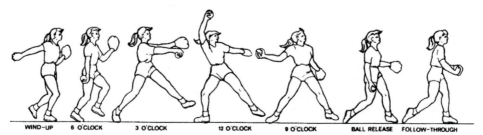

FIG. 16.2 Six phases of the windmill pitch. (From Maffet MW, Jobe FW, Pink MM, Brault J, Mathiyakom W. Shoulder muscle firing patterns during the windmill softball pitch. *Am J Sports Med*. 1997;25(3):370.)

overhead throwers, place windmill pitchers at risk for overuse injuries. Injury data was not reported in this study.

Barrentine et al.[13] also examined the kinematics and kinetics of the windmill fastball pitch in eight healthy female collegiate or previous collegiate pitchers. The authors found that peak forces resisting shoulder distraction occurred during the acceleration phase, as opposed to overhead pitching where the peak resistance to distraction is during deceleration.[13] The supraspinatus and infraspinatus muscles had their highest EMG activity during phase 2. The distractive force at the shoulder was approximately 20%–40% body weight during the upward swing of the arm, resisted by the supraspinatus and infraspinatus. During phase 3, teres minor and infraspinatus reached peak activity, facilitating external rotation and resisting the approximately 50% body weight distractive force. Rapid downward acceleration and internal rotation (2000–3000 degrees/second) occur in phase 4, with the subscapularis muscle

showing increased activity and peaking during phase 5. Subscapularis activity resists the distractive force, which peaks to full body weight distractive force, meaning a distractive force equal to the athlete's body weight that the subscapularis must resist. Shoulder internal rotation also peaks at 4600 degrees/second.[13]

Maffet et al.[12] studied collegiate softball pitchers whose release included contact of the arm with the lateral thigh at ball release, decreasing the need for shoulder muscles to decelerate the arm (Table 16.1). The study included EMG and high-speed cinematography motion analysis. The authors found that the supraspinatus was most active between 6 o'clock and 3 o'clock during arm elevation. The posterior cuff and infraspinatus were most active from 3 o'clock to 12 o'clock, and the pectoralis accelerated the arm from 12 o'clock to ball release. Activity in all muscles decreased during follow-through, due to arm contact with the body, which slowed the forward momentum of the arm, decreasing the need for muscles to

TABLE 16.1
Differences and Similarities Between the Baseball and Softball Pitch.

Vol. 25, No. 3, 1997   *Shoulder Muscle Firing During the Windmill Pitch* **373**

The 12 to 9 o'clock Phase

Activity of the posterior deltoid and teres minor muscles diminished but remained at a moderate level. Infraspinatus muscle activity dropped compared with previous phases. These muscles are perhaps controlling the arm as it is accelerated through this and the following phase.

    The EMG activity increased significantly in the pectoralis major, subscapularis, and serratus anterior muscles.

major, serratus anterior, and subscapularis muscles continue their high levels of activity as the arm is further adducted across the body until the arm contacts the lateral thigh, beginning the follow-through phase of the pitch. The pectoralis major muscle performs the powerful adduction and internal rotation of the humerus and the serratus anterior muscle acts simultaneously to stabilize the scapula and maintain glenohumeral congruency. The subscapularis muscle most likely is contributing to the

From Maffet, MW, Jobe, FW, Pink, MM, Brault, J, Mathiyakom, W. Shoulder muscle firing patterns during the windmill softball pitch. *Am J Sports Med*, 1997;25(3):373.

decelerate the arm. Escamilla and Andrews[11] reviewed EMG studies of several overhead sports and made a distinction between the overhead throw, which involves high forces and torques during the follow-through after ball release when muscles are decelerating the arm, and the windmill pitch, which has the highest forces and torques during the acceleration phase. This is an important difference to note between the overhead pitch and the windmill pitch, in which the rotator cuff muscles are not firing to decelerate the arm during the windmill pitch compared to the overhead throw, where the rotator cuff is active in decelerating the arm.

Lear and Patel[8] reviewed the literature on softball injury risk in youth and collegiate softball players, noting overuse injuries to be generally more common than acute injuries and shoulder injuries to be more common than injuries to other joints, especially in pitchers. Many of the studies they reviewed focused on injuries sustained by pitchers. There was no consensus as to whether there are more reinjuries versus acute injuries or whether serious injuries (i.e., those that involve time loss from participation) are more common than nonserious injuries.[8]

In 1992, Loosli et al.[14] surveyed athletic trainers regarding injuries to pitchers from 8 of the top 15 NCAA collegiate softball teams that season, noting a significant number of minor to severe rotator cuff injuries among pitchers. All were reported as a strain or tendinitis/overuse injuries. No full-thickness or partial thickness rotator cuff tears were reported, likely, at least in part, because this study predated the widespread use of magnetic resonance imaging (MRI).[14]

An interesting study by Chu et al.[15] made a comparison of female versus male overhead baseball pitchers. Although females predominantly play softball, there is growing interest in baseball for females. The authors studied 11 female overhead baseball pitchers, noting a few significant differences compared with male pitchers including a shorter more open stride, lower ball velocity, and lower maximal proximal forces at the shoulder and elbow. Females also took longer to progress through the pitching cycle.[15]

VOLLEYBALL

While ankle injuries are the most common injury in volleyball, shoulder injuries account for approximately 8%–10% of all injuries in high-school and collegiate volleyball players. Studies often do not distinguish between rotator cuff and other shoulder injuries.[16] In female collegiate volleyball players, the shoulder accounted for 10% of non-time-loss injuries versus only 4% of time loss injuries.[17]

The volleyball serve and spike involve overhead use of the arm, but unlike the throwing motion, the ball is only in contact with the hand for a brief period at the point of ball impact. In the United States, competitive volleyball is a sport played most commonly by female athletes. Rokito et al.[18] studied glenohumeral muscle firing patterns in the volleyball serve and spike. Each skill is divided into five phases: (1) windup, consisting of shoulder abduction and extension; (2) cocking, initiation to maximum external rotation; (3) acceleration, which begins at maximum external rotation and transitions into internal rotation to ball impact; (4) deceleration, ball impact to arm perpendicular to trunk; and (5) follow-through, arm perpendicular to the end of arm movement (Figs. 16.3 and 16.4).[18]

Rokito et al.[18] described peak supraspinatus EMG activity at deceleration (45% manual muscle test [MMT]) during the serve (Table 16.2). Activity was much higher for the supraspinatus during the windup for the spike (71% MMT). EMG activity for the infraspinatus muscle

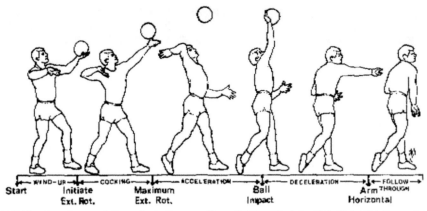

FIG. 16.3 The five phases of the volleyball serve. (From Rokito AS, Jobe FW, Pink MM, Perry J, Brault J. Electromyographic analysis of shoulder function during the volleyball serve and spike. *J Shoulder Elbow Surg.* 1998;7(3):257.)

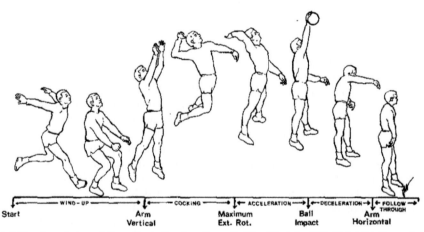

FIG. 16.4 The five phases of the volleyball spike. (From Rokito AS, Jobe FW, Pink MM, Perry J, Brault J. Electromyographic analysis of shoulder function during the volleyball serve and spike. *J Shoulder Elbow Surg.* 1998;7(3):257.)

was lower during windup for the serve but higher during windup for the spike. Teres minor had the lowest activity during windup for the serve (7% MMT) and increased to 54% MMT at acceleration during the serve. Teres minor had higher activity during windup for the spike at 39% MMT, with peak activity during cocking and acceleration at 51% MMT. Windup for the serve was associated with minimal activity in the subscapularis (8% MMT). Peak activity for subscapularis (56% MMT) for the serve occurred during acceleration. EMG activity in the subscapularis muscle during windup for the spike was relatively higher (46% MMT), dropping during cocking then rising to maximal activity (65% MMT) during acceleration.[18]

Muscle activity during windup and follow-through was low for the volleyball serve.[18] In contrast, supraspinatus and infraspinatus had peak activity during windup of the spike. Infraspinatus and teres minor had high activity during cocking to produce external rotation. The rotator cuff is also necessary for joint compression to resist the shoulder distraction force generated by these motions. An important difference in muscle firing occurs during the acceleratory phase between spike and serve. The acceleratory muscles (subscapularis, teres major, latissimus dorsi, and pectoralis major) are much more active in the spike than the serve, as velocity is the primary goal for a spike, whereas a more parabolic trajectory is used for the serve. During

TABLE 16.2
Mean and Standard Deviations (Percent Manual Muscle Test) for Each Muscle Tested for the Volleyball Serve and Spike.

Muscle	Windup	Cocking	Acceleration	Deceleration	Follow-Through
ANTERIOR DELTOID					
Serve	21 ± 11	31 ± 13	27 ± 22	42 ± 17	16 ± 16
Spike	58 ± 26	49 ± 19	23 ± 17	27 ± 10	15 ± 7
SUPRASPINATUS					
Serve	25 ± 10	32 ± 18	37 ± 25	45 ± 13	24 ± 16
Spike	71 ± 31	40 ± 17	21 + 27	37 + 23	27 ± 15
INFRASPINATUS					
Serve	17 ± 10	36 ± 16	32 ± 22	39 ± 21	13 ± 11
Spike	60 ± 17	49 ± 16	27 ± 18	38 ± 19	22 ± 11
TERES MINOR					
Serve	7 ± 8	44 ± 20	54 ± 26	30 ± 23	8 ± 9
Spike	39 ± 20	51 ± 17	51 ± 24	34 ± 13	17 ± 7
SUBSCAPULARIS					
Serve	8 ± 8	27 ± 25	56 ± 18	27 ± 15	13 ± 11
Spike	46 ± 16	38 ± 21	65 ± 25	23 ± 11	16 ± 15
TERES MAJOR					
Serve	1 ± 1	11 ± 7	47 ± 24	7 ± 8	3 ± 3
Spike	28 ± 14	20 ± 11	65 ± 31	21 ± 18	15 ± 16
LATISSIMUS DORSI					
Serve	1 ± 2	9 ± 18	37 ± 39	6 ± 9	3 ± 3
Spike	20 ± 13	16 ± 17	59 ± 28	20 ± 21	15 ± 10
PECTORALIS MAJOR					
Serve	3 ± 6	31 ± 14	36 ± 14	7 ± 11	7 ± 6
Spike	35 ± 17	46 + 17	59 ± 24	20 ± 16	21 ± 12

From Rokito AS, Jobe FW, Pink MM, Perry J, Brault J. Electromyographic analysis of shoulder function during the volleyball serve and spike. *J Shoulder Elbow Surg.* 1998;7(3):259.

deceleration, infraspinatus and supraspinatus activity was greatest during the serve rather than the spike.[11] During the spike, the ball is struck and the ball in turn imparts an opposing force on the arm. This may help decelerate the arm, thereby requiring less activation from the rotator cuff muscles to control arm deceleration, which differentiates this action from throwing, where muscles must decelerate the arm.[18]

Lajtai et al.[19] studied 84 professional beach volleyball players (54 males and 30 females) using a questionnaire, physical examination, and ultrasound, as well as MRI, in 29 male athletes to assess typical clinical and imaging findings in the hitting shoulder of this population. The mean age of athletes was 28 years (range, 20–39 years). About 63% (50 of 80) of players reported shoulder pain in the hitting shoulder. Infraspinatus muscle atrophy was noted in 25 of 84 (30%) athletes without evidence of suprascapular nerve compression. Male and female athletes were not significantly different in this measure (31% vs. 27%, respectively). External rotation strength was significantly decreased in the hitting shoulder for both male and female athletes. Five of the male (9%) and four of the female (13%) players had undergone previous shoulder surgery. Among the 84 players, 12 (14%) had a partial rotator cuff tear as documented by ultrasound. One explanation for external rotation weakness and infraspinatus atrophy in the absence of a compressive structure, such as thickened spinoglenoid or transverse scapular ligament or ganglion cyst, is a stretch neuropathy of the suprascapular nerve.[19]

Notarnicola et al.[20] evaluated perfusion of the supraspinatus tendon at its insertion to the tuberosity of male and female elite volleyball players using oximetry to study microcirculation, based on the theory that relative hypoxia caused by functional overload of the tendon can lead to a neovascularization response within the tissue. Only athletes with no complaints or physical findings of shoulder pain or problems were included in the study. The authors found no difference between male and female athletes, but they did note a difference between athletes playing different positions. Rotator cuff oximetric percentages increased by position, with the middle hitter having the lowest percentage and the outside hitter having the highest in the dominant arm.[20]

TENNIS

Tennis, similar to softball and baseball, involves considerable overhead use of the dominant arm for the serve and volley. There is limited research on EMG activity in the rotator cuff musculature of tennis players. Ryu and Kibler have conducted EMG studies in male tennis players.[3,21] The authors found that the subscapularis was most active in the overhead serve and the forehand stroke, while supraspinatus and infraspinatus were more active in the backhand stroke.[21] Serratus anterior was active for all three strokes. Kibler et al.[3] focused more on the timing of muscle firing patterns, noting that the scapular positioning muscles were active prior to the shoulder elevators and cuff musculature that serve as a force couple to center the humeral head. In addition, Kibler et al.[3] found infraspinatus to be relatively inactive in the overhead serve. No EMG studies were found specific to the muscle firing patterns of the rotator cuff of female tennis players.

Lynall et al.[22] reported on injury rates in men's and women's collegiate tennis players using the NCAA Injury Surveillance Program (ISP), which included data from 19 men's varsity programs and 25 women's varsity programs between the 2009/10 and 2014/15 seasons. Injury rates were similar between males and females, with the majority of injuries occurring to the lower extremities. About 14% injuries in males and 11.9% in females were to the shoulder/clavicle area, with an injury rate of 0.7 and 0.58 per 1000 athlete-exposures (AEs), respectively.[22]

Dakic et al.[23] evaluated injuries in 52 women's professional tennis circuit players competing in the 2015 Australian Open. The authors found that 9.3% of injuries reported by players were to the shoulder/clavicle area for a rate of 8.2 injuries per 1000 match-hours. Lower extremity injuries were much more common, comprising 51% of injuries and an injury rate of 42.2 per 1000 match-hours by comparison. They did not report rotator cuff injuries separate from shoulder injuries, in general.[23]

In 2012, Abrams et al.[24] conducted a literature review of tennis injuries and found that shoulder injuries composed 4%—17% of all injuries. The study did not detail information on female players specifically. The authors noted that younger athletes tended to have more instability issues, while older athletes tended to have more rotator cuff issues. The authors cited scapular dyskinesis as well as glenohumeral internal rotation deficit as frequent contributing factors for shoulder injury in tennis players.[24]

SWIMMING

Competitive swimming often begins at a young age with intense training hours. There are two main phases to the stroke cycle: (1) pull-through, where speed is generated, and (2) recovery, where the arm is out of the water and includes body roll for some strokes. The repetitive stroke cycle leads to overuse of the shoulder joint; in particular, the shoulder adductors and internal rotators become hypertrophied.[25] About 40%—91% of competitive swimmers have reported shoulder pain, making it the most common musculoskeletal injury in this population.[26] As with many sports where female athletes compete similar to male athletes, many studies are conducted using only male swimmers. This results in an unfortunate deficiency in our understanding of the female swimmer. It may not be safe to assume that the muscle firing patterns and response to various interventions will be the same for female swimmers as for male swimmers.

"Swimmer's shoulder" is a common injury cited in the literature, with presenting symptoms of anterior shoulder pain due to repetitive impingement on the rotator cuff tendons. Both intrinsic and extrinsic factors contribute to the development of "swimmer's shoulder." Intrinsic factors include joint hypermobility, core instability, thoracic kyphosis, scapular dyskinesis, rotator cuff imbalance, and lack of flexibility (Tables 16.3 and 16.4).[26,27] Extrinsic factors include increase in training hours, lack of dry-land shoulder strengthening, and use of resistance devices such as hand paddles.[27] The supraspinatus

TABLE 16.3
Etiology of Swimmer's Shoulder.

EXTRINSIC FACTORS

Training volume—absolute and sudden increases
Technical errors
Hand paddles

INTRINSIC FACTORS

Excessive laxity/general joint hypermobility
Isolated joint hyperlaxity
Posture, core stability, and increased thoracic
    kyphosis
Scapular dyskinesis
Glenohumeral internal rotation deficit
Rotator cuff imbalance
Lack of flexibility/stiffness (posterior capsule, anterior
    capsule, anterior cuff, and pectoralis minor)

From Bak K. Practical management of Swimmer's painful shoulder: etiology, diagnosis and treatment. *Clin J Sports Med*. 2010;20(5):387.

TABLE 16.4
Tissues Under Risk During Swimming.

RECOVERY

Subacromial bursa
Supraspinatus tendon
Posterior-superior labrum

EARLY PULL-THROUGH

Anterior capsulolabral complex
Posterior-superior labrum

LATE PULL-THROUGH

Supraspinatus tendon

From Bak K. Practical management of swimmer's painful shoulder: etiology, diagnosis and treatment. *Clin J Sports Med*, 2010;20(5):387

tendon is most commonly involved because of subacromial impingement causing repetitive trauma to a relatively avascular region of the tendon.[28] Supraspinatus tendinopathy was reported in up to 91% of elite swimmers and is associated with a positive impingement sign.[26] Specifically, the supraspinatus tendon is put under stress during the recovery phase and the late pull-through phase of the swimmer's stroke cycle.[27]

Sein et al.[29] reported on 80 youth elite swimmers (mean age, 15.9 years), noting that 91% reported shoulder pain. Most of the swimmers (84%) had a positive impingement sign, which correlated strongly with supraspinatus tendinopathy demonstrated on MRI. Increased tendon thickness also correlated with tendinopathy. Training hours per week and weekly mileage

correlated significantly with supraspinatus tendinopathy, but preferred stroke did not. Shoulder laxity had only weak correlation to shoulder impingement pain. Female swimmers had significantly more laxity than male swimmers (1.72 vs. 1.28 mm); however, it is unclear if this is clinically significant.[29]

Wolf et al.[30] reported on a single men's and women's Division I collegiate swimming and diving team for the period of 2002–07. The shoulder and arm were the most commonly reported injury sites, accounting for 36% of injuries in males and 50% of injuries in females during practice. Freshmen sustained the most frequent injuries. There was no noted difference between male and female swimmers.[30] Kerr et al.[31] reported on injury rates in NCAA collegiate male and female swimmers and divers between 2009/10 and 2013/14, using the NCAA ISP, which included data from 9 men's and 13 women's programs. Female divers had a higher injury rate than female swimmers (2.49/1000 AE vs. 1.63/1000 AE), whereas there was no significant difference between male divers and swimmers (1.94 vs. 1.48/1000 AE). Overuse injury rate was higher for female than male swimmers (1.04 vs. 0.66/1000 AE). Shoulder strain and overuse were the most common injuries reported in this population.[31]

EMG studies have been conducted to determine shoulder muscle activity for various swim strokes. Pink et al.[32] studied normal muscle activity of shoulder musculature during the butterfly stroke, which involves both arms entering and exiting the water simultaneously. The study included male and female collegiate- and masters-level swimmers with a mean age of 39 years. The supraspinatus was active at the start of the stroke (hand entry), increased through the first half of early pull-through phase, dropped off at the middle of early pull-through, and increased throughout late pull-through, peaked at the end of late pull-through (hand exit) into early recovery, and then gradually decreased during late recovery. The infraspinatus had lower activity amplitude throughout the swim stroke cycle, although it mirrored that of the supraspinatus with about half the amplitude. The teres minor had a lesser peak in activity just after hand entry and its greatest activity at mid-pull-through. The subscapularis remained active throughout with a slightly higher plateau at mid-pull-through.[32]

Pink et al. also studied the painful shoulder during the butterfly stroke, noting increased activity in the posterior deltoid during hand entry and decreased activity in the upper trapezius and the serratus anterior.[33] Hand entry occurred with a wider position in the painful shoulder, a compensatory movement pattern that decreases impingement and avoids the painful arc.

The supraspinatus showed decreased activity, as did the teres minor and the serratus anterior throughout pulling. The decrease in activity was attributed to fatigue. The subscapularis demonstrated increased activity in the painful shoulder, especially just before mid-pull-through, and infraspinatus demonstrated increased activity as the hand left the water in the painful shoulder compared with the pain-free shoulder. Both muscles acted to depress the humeral head.[33]

Pink et al.[34] also studied EMG muscle firing patterns in the normal and painful shoulders in freestyle swimmers (Fig. 16.5). Many of the muscle firing patterns and function in the normal shoulder are similar to those described for the butterfly stroke. The supraspinatus mirrored the firing pattern of the deltoid: midrange at hand entry, dropping to 6% MMT at mid-pull-through, and eventually peaking at the end of pull-through to early recovery (74% MMT). Infraspinatus reached its peak activity at mid-pull-through. The teres minor reached peak activity (57% MMT) at mid-pull-through, staying relatively low otherwise. The subscapularis stayed active throughout, ranging from 26% at early pull-through to 64% and 71% at late pull-through and early recovery, respectively. Likewise, the serratus anterior remained active throughout the stroke cycle.[34]

Scovazzo et al.[35] compared the results in the normal shoulder to EMG activity in the painful shoulder in 14 collegiate- and masters-level swimmers (9 males, 5 females). With respect to the rotator cuff, the infraspinatus was significantly more active at terminal pull-through in the painful shoulder compared with the normal shoulder. Additionally, the subscapularis was significantly less active at mid-recovery compared with the normal shoulder. The supraspinatus and the teres minor did not demonstrate significant differences between the normal and the painful shoulder. The scapular stabilizers also were significantly different, with the rhomboids and upper trapezius in the painful shoulder being less active at hand entry than the normal shoulders. The painful shoulder at mid-pull-through showed increased activity in the rhomboid and decreased activity in the serratus anterior. The serratus anterior was also less active shortly after hand entry in the painful versus the normal shoulder. It was noted that the hand entered the water further from the midline with the humerus lower to the water (dropped elbow).[35]

Two portions of the freestyle stroke are more apt to produce shoulder pain: early pull-through to mid-pull-through and mid-recovery (Fig. 16.6).[36] During the freestyle stroke, 70% of shoulder pain occurred during early pull-through, while 18% occurred during early

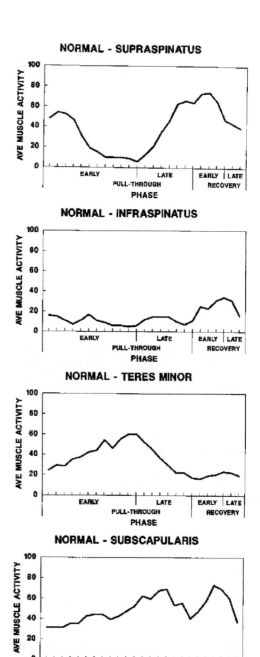

FIG. 16.5 Muscle activity firing patterns in the rotator cuff muscles. (From Pink M, Perry J, Browne A, Scovazzo ML, Kerrigan J. The normal shoulder during freestyle swimming. *Am J Sports Med.* 1991;19(6):572.)

recovery. Swimmers tended to report an increase in intensity and distance of workout sessions as common factors contributing to aggravated shoulder pain.[36]

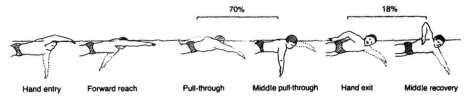

FIG. 16.6   (From Pink MM, Tibone JE. The painful shoulder in the swimming athlete. *Orthop Clin N Am.* 2000;31(2):248.)

Pink and Tibone[36] note that muscle firing patterns remain essentially similar for freestyle in the normal versus the painful shoulder for the primary muscles of propulsion (pectoralis major, latissimus dorsi, posterior deltoid) and for teres minor (force couple with pectoralis major). The supraspinatus firing pattern remains unchanged, compressing the humeral head on the glenoid. The serratus anterior is active throughout the normal swim cycle (stable scapula platform); however, there is decreased activity in the painful shoulder, along with the subscapularis. The decreased activity is thought to be related to fatigue. A pathologic movement pattern noted in swimmers with a painful shoulder is to drop the elbow in recovery. This compensatory movement pattern allows the athlete to avoid painful humeral internal rotation. This is consistent with EMG studies showing increased activity in infraspinatus, with a wider hand entry into the water. Other changes that may be noted include difficulty staying centered in the lane, decreasing pull on the nonpainful side, altered kick, early hand exit, and excessive body roll. The scapula moves in an asynchronous pattern, with an apparent, but not real, overactivity of the upper trapezius in comparison to its force couple, the serratus anterior, which demonstrates decreased activity. This causes early excessive scapular elevation and upward rotation. Pink and Tibone[36] point out that the "normal" strength ratio for internal to external rotators is approximately 3:2, rather than 1:1.

It is interesting to note that both swimmers and overhead throwers demonstrate a compensatory movement pattern described as a "dropped elbow" or "dropped arm." The EMG data explains the change in muscle firing patterns that correspond to the compensatory movement pattern. It also explains why coaches' instructions to athletes to "stop dropping your elbow" are unlikely to be successful without addressing the kinesthetic reasons behind the compensatory movement patterns.

Ciullo and Stevens[28] describe a three-phase approach to rotator cuff impingement syndrome in the swimmer. Phase 1 is described as edema and hemorrhage presenting with symptoms of aching at rest and limited range of motion. At this stage, the rotator cuff may be irritated; however, the cross-striations between the superior and inferior walls of the subacromial bursa are not injured. Conservative management with nonsteroidal antiinflammatory drugs and ice promotes full recovery at this phase. Phase 2 is promoted by repeated inflammation leading to recurrent tendonitis. Pain occurs with activity in this phase and continues until the shoulder is at complete rest. Phase 3 consists of rotator cuff tears, bony changes, and biceps rupture. Pain is constant, is located deep in the shoulder, and may prevent the athlete from sleeping. Treatment at this phase consists of surgical repair to the damaged structures. Rotator cuff tears are uncommon in the female swimmer.[28]

INJURY PREVENTION PROGRAMS

Injury prevention programs for lower extremity injuries are well-described and include the F-MARC 11+ (FIFA [Federation Internationale de Football Association] Medical Assessment and Research Center), the PEP (Prevent Injury and Enhance Performance) program, and the Sportsmetrics program.[37,38] All three programs have been extensively studied and shown to have some success in decreasing the rate of lower extremity injury. However, there is a paucity of information available on injury prevention programs for the shoulder.

One concern in the throwing athlete is that the posterior (external rotators) rotator cuff musculature is utilized in an eccentric firing pattern to decelerate the arm late in the throwing cycle. Neiderbracht et al.[39] attempted to address this deficiency by studying female tennis players in a nonisokinetic dynamometer-based strength training program (six athletes) versus control tennis players (six athletes). Exercises included external rotation at 90 degrees, seated row, scaption, chest press, and external shoulder rotation (rubber tubing). They found significant gains in eccentric external rotation total work versus the control group. The 3 athletes in the experimental group with an eccentric external/concentric internal total work ratio of <1.0 before training all converted to a ratio >1 after training. Two control athletes with a ratio less than one before training remained <1 after training. Injury rates over the course of the season were not studied.[39]

Management of "swimmer's shoulder" begins with a complete evaluation for diagnosis and contributing factors.[26] A dry-land program for strengthening the scapular stabilizers and rotator cuff as well as a core and flexibility program are considered standard management, in addition to avoidance of pain generating training, elimination of hand paddles, more kicking, and proper warm-up (Table 16.5).[26]

Repetitive swimming motion leads to an increase in the strength of the internal rotational torque muscles compared with the external rotation torque muscles.[40] As a result, the antagonist-agonist muscle pairs become imbalanced leading to suboptimal shoulder mechanics

---

TABLE 16.5
"Swimmer's Shoulder" Treatment and Prevention Strategies.

DRY-LAND TREATMENT

Strengthening
Scapular stabilizers—serratus anterior, scapular retractors (lower trapezius, rhomboids), subscapularis
Rotator cuff (especially external rotators, goal = ER/IR ratio of ≥65%)

Stretching
Posterior rotator cuff
Scapular stabilizers
Posterior capsule
Pectoralis major
Pectoralis minor

Note: Generally do not need to stretch the anterior shoulder

IN-THE-POOL TREATMENT

Avoid strokes and training that exacerbate pain

Eliminate hand paddles

More kicking sets emphasizing lower extremities

Proper warm-up

Stroke corrections
Increase body roll
Widen hand entry (butterfly)
Reduce internal rotation of upper extremity at hand entry (freestyle)
Breathe bilaterally (freestyle)
Shorten follow-through (freestyle and butterfly)

From Nichols AW. Medical care of the aquatics athlete. *Curr Sports Med Rep.* 2015;14(5):392. doi:10.1249/JSR.0000000000000194.

---

and overuse injuries.[26] Hence the prevention of "swimmer's shoulder" aims to decrease antagonist-agonist imbalance with a dry-land strength training program, with the goal of external rotation torque to internal rotation torque of 65%.[26] In addition, treatment aims at strengthening of the scapular stabilizers to prevent scapular dyskinesias as well as stretching of the posterior rotator cuff, scapular stabilizers, posterior capsule, pectoralis major, and pectoralis minor (Table 16.5).[26] Lastly, stretching of the anterior shoulder should be avoided.

Lynch et al.[41] evaluated the efficacy of an exercise program designed to improve swimmer posture in 28 Division I NCAA collegiate swimmers. Training load predisposes swimmers to a head forward, rounded shoulder (thoracic kyphosis/lumbar lordosis) posture. The 8-week exercise program included flexibility and scapular stabilization exercises. The authors noted an improvement in posture as measured by cervical angle. Shoulder function, as measured by the American Shoulder and Elbow Surgeons (ASES) scores, was not significantly different following intervention; however, 79% of athletes had improved or had no pain following intervention, while 50% of controls had increased pain over the same period.[41]

Pink and Tibone[36] recommended a series of exercises for swimmers, starting with elevation in the scapular plane and progressing to frontal and coronal planes. The swimmers then progress to a modified military press, standing four-count horizontal row, and push-ups, plus endurance exercises, such as arm bike and swim bench. The authors recommended using an isokinetic device for subscapularis endurance work. They emphasized the importance of maintaining proper scapular position and control throughout the exercise program. The authors did not report data on the use of the program for injury prevention; however, it seems reasonable to assume that implementing these exercises would be helpful in preventing chronic injuries.[36]

Muniz-Pardos et al.[42] conducted a systematic review of land-based resistance training and water-based swimming power training on swimming performance. The authors did not assess the ability of the programs to prevent injury. Land-based programs included exercises performed on land with movements similar to those used during swimming. The water-based programs included tethered swimming, active drag swimming, and velocity through perturbation. A total of 25 studies met their inclusion criteria. The authors concluded that the water-based inertial programs seemed most effective. Female swimmers were included in at least some studies, but the authors did not comment specifically on female swimmers.[42]

Batalha et al.[25] studied the effect of a 16-week land-based shoulder exercise program in 40 (83%) male youth swimmers. The experimental group did a land-based strengthening program in addition to water training followed by a "detraining" period. The control group did water training only throughout the season. The exercise group did see gains in external rotation strength and external rotation to internal rotation ratios that returned to baseline once the program stopped (detraining), after the 16 weeks while still in-season, indicating the importance of a sustained land-based exercise program, in addition to the water-based training. Female athletes were not included in the study, so it is unknown whether these results are applicable to the female swimmer.[25]

SHOULDER SURGERY IN THE FEMALE ATHLETE

There are very few reports in the literature of surgical management of rotator cuff tears in high-level athletes, particularly in female athletes. Tibone et al.[43] reported their results on open rotator cuff repair in 45 athletes, including 6 female patients who participated in dance, javelin, tennis, volleyball, bowling, and skiing preoperatively. Half (three of six) of the female patients had a good result, whereas the other half had a fair result, compared to 56% good results in the overall population. Three of five (60%) patients who participated in overhead sports reported problems with overhead activity after surgery. One of the six (17%) patients was able to go back to a higher level of play, two were unchanged (33%), and three (50%) had decreased level of participation. Five of 6 females (83%) reported participating in a different sport after surgery, but two went back to sports that involve overhead use of the arm.[43]

Shaffer et al.[44] reviewed the literature regarding rotator cuff surgery in the throwing athlete. The current recommendation is initial nonoperative management with rehabilitation, especially for asymptomatic tears. For partial thickness tears up to 75% of the tendon thickness, where nonoperative management has failed, debridement is recommended. Repair of the tear is generally indicated for tears approaching or exceeding 75% of tendon thickness. Care must be taken not to overconstrain the repaired tendon. Patients should be advised of the significant risk of failure to return to the same level of competition for high-level overhead athletes.[44]

Little is known regarding return to play following shoulder surgery in the female tennis player. Young et al.[45] reported on return to play of eight WTA (Women's Tennis Association) female professional tennis players following shoulder surgery. Procedures included rotator cuff debridement (n = 3) or repair (n = 2), labral repair for instability (n = 3), superior labrum anterior-posterior (SLAP) repair (n = 1), neurolysis of the suprascapular nerve (n = 2), and subacromial decompression (n = 3). Seven of eight (88%) players returned to professional play, but only two of eight (25%) returned to preinjury ranking by 18 months.[45] Owing to the small number of patients and the need to preserve patient privacy, the authors could not comment on which patients had rotator cuff surgery relative to their return to play.

Brushoj et al.[46] examined arthroscopic management of painful shoulder in 18 (8 females, 10 males) competitive swimmers. The most common finding was labral pathology (61%) followed by subacromial impingement (28%). There were no rotator cuff tears. Of the 18 patients, 11 (61%) underwent debridement, with 4 (22%) undergoing bursectomy and 4 (22%) undergoing partial release of the coracoacromial ligament. Only 9 of the 18 (56%) patients were able to return to the same level of competition by 4 months, including 2 (12%) patients with pain and 7 (44%) patients without pain. Among the 16 patients, 7 (44%) never returned to competitive swim, and among the 7 patients, 6 (86%) did not return because of shoulder pain. Results were not reported separately for female and male athletes. At final follow-up, 2 of the 18 athletes could not be reached.[46]

SUMMARY

While there is documentation of muscle activation patterns about the shoulder in the female athlete for many overhead sports (e.g., softball, volleyball, swim), there is a paucity of information related to rotator cuff injuries in the female overhead athlete. Future studies should attempt to better define common shoulder injury patterns in this patient population. Additionally, more research is needed to better understand and develop clear, sport-specific injury prevention programs for the female overhead athlete.

REFERENCES

1. Jost B, Zumstein M, Pfirrmann CWA, Zanetti M, Gerber C. MRI findings in throwing shoulders. Abnormalities in professional handball players. *Clin Orthop Relat Res.* 2005;434: 130−137.
2. Reynolds SB, Dugas JR, Cain EL, McMichael CS, Andrews JR. Debridement of small partial-thickness rotator cuff tears in elite overhead throwers. *Clin Orthop Relat Res.* 2008;466:614−621.

3. Kibler WB, Chandler TJ, Shapiro R, Conuel M. Muscle activation in coupled scapulohumeral motions in the high performance tennis serve. *Br J Sports Med.* 2007;41: 745−749.

4. Nelson CE, Rayan GM, Judd DI, Ding K, Stoner JS. Survey of hand and upper extremity injuries among rock climbers. *Hand.* 2017;12(4):389−394.

5. Baugh CM, Kerr ZY. High school rowing injuries: athletic treatment, injury, and outcomes network (NATION). *J Athl Train.* 2016;51(4):317−320.

6. Fleisig GS, Barrentine SW, Escamilla RF, Andrews JR. Biomechanics of overhand throwing. *Sports Med.* 1996; 21(6):421−437.

7. Atwater AE. Biomechanics of overarm throwing movements and of throwing injuries. *Exerc Sport Sci Rev.* 1979; 7:43−85.

8. Lear AL, Patel N. Softball pitching and injury. *Curr Sports Med Rep.* 2016;15(5):336−341.

9. Werner SL, Jones DG, Guido JA, Brunet ME. Kinematics and kinetics of elite windmill softball pitching. *Am J Sports Med.* 2006;34(4):597−603.

10. www.littleleague.org/playing-rules/pitch-count, Accessed May, 2020.

11. Escamilla RF, Andrews JR. Shoulder muscle recruitment patterns and related biomechanics during upper extremity sports. *Sports Med.* 2009;39(7):569−590.

12. Maffet MW, Jobe FW, Pink MM, Brault J, Mathiyakom W. Shoulder muscle firing patterns during the windmill softball pitch. *Am J Sports Med.* 1997;25(3):369−374.

13. Barrentine SW, Fleisig GS, Whiteside JA, Escamilla RF, Andrews JR. Biomechanics of windmill softball pitching with implications about injury mechanisms at the shoulder and elbow. *JOSPT.* 1998;28(6):405−414.

14. Loosli AR, Requa RK, Garrick JG, Hanley E. Injuries to pitchers in women's collegiate fast-pitch softball. *Am J Sports Med.* 1992;20(1):35−37.

15. Chu Y, Fleisig GS, Simpson KJ, Andrews JR. Biomechanical comparison between elite female and male baseball pitchers. *J Appl Biomech.* 2009;25:22−31.

16. Kerr ZY, Gregory AJ, Wosmek J, et al. The first decade of web-based sports injury surveillance: descriptive epidemiology of injuries in US high school girls' volleyball (2005−2006 through 2013−2014) and National Collegiate Athletic Association women's volleyball (2004−2005 through 2013−2014). *J Athl Train.* 2018; 53(10):926−937.

17. Baugh CM, Weintraub GS, Gregory AJ, Djoko A, Dompier TP, Kerr ZY. Descriptive epidemiology of injuries sustained in national collegiate athletic association men's and women's volleyball, 2013−2014 to 2014−2015. *Sport Health.* 2018;10(1):60−69.

18. Rokito AS, Jobe FW, Pink MM, Perry J, Brault J. Electromyographic analysis of shoulder function during the volleyball serve and spike. *J Shoulder Elbow Surg.* 1998; 7(3):256−263.

19. Lajtai G, Pfirrmann CWA, Aitzetmuller G, Pirkl C, Gerber C, Jost B. The shoulders of professional beach volleyball players. High prevalence of infraspinatus muscle atrophy. *Am J Sports Med.* 2009;37(7):1375−1383.

20. Notarnicola A, Fischetti F, Gallone D, et al. Overload and neovascularization of shoulder tendons in volleyball players. *BMC Res Notes.* 2012;5:397.

21. Ryu RK, McCormick J, Jobe FW, Moynes DR, Antonelli DJ. An electromyographic analysis of shoulder function in tennis players. *Am J Sports Med.* 1988;16(5):481−485.

22. Lynall RC, Kerr ZY, Djoko A, Pluim BM, Hainline B, Dompier TP. Epidemiology of national collegiate athletic association men's and women's tennis injuries, 2009/2010−2014/2015. *Br J Sports Med.* 2016;50:1211−1216.

23. Dakic JG, Smith B, Gosling CM, Perraton LG. Musculoskeletal injury profiles in professional women's tennis association players. *Br J Sports Med.* 2018;52:723−729.

24. Abrams GD, Renstrom PA, Safran MR. Epidemiology of musculoskeletal injury in the tennis player. *Br J Sports Med.* 2012;46:492−498.

25. Batalha NM, Raimundo AM, Tomas-Carus P, Marques MAC, Silva AJ. Does an in-season detraining period affect the shoulder rotator cuff strength and balance of young swimmers? *J Strength Condit Res.* 2014;28(7): 2054−2062.

26. Nichols AW. Medical care of the aquatics athlete. *Curr Sports Med Rep.* 2015;14(5):389−396.

27. Bak K. The practical management of swimmer's painful shoulder: Etiology, diagnosis, and treatment. *Clin J Sport Med.* 2010;20(5):386−390.

28. Ciullo JV, Stevens GG. The prevention and treatment of injuries to the shoulder in swimming. *Sports Med.* 1989;7(3): 182−204.

29. Sein ML, Walton J, Linklater J, et al. Shoulder pain in elite swimmers: primarily due to swim-volume-induced supraspinatus tendinopathy. *Br J Sports Med.* 2010;44:105−113.

30. Wolf BR, Ebinger AE, Lawler MP, Britton CL. Injury patterns in division I collegiate swimming. *Am J Sports Med.* 2009;37(10):2037−2042.

31. Kerr ZY, Baugh CM, Hibberd EE, Snook EM, Hayden R, Dompier TP. Epidemiology of National Collegiate Athletic Association men's and women's swimming and diving injuries from 2009/2010 to 2013/2014. *Br J Sports Med.* 2015;49:465−471.

32. Pink M, Jobe FW, Perry J, Kerrigan J, Browne A, Scovazzo ML. The normal shoulder during the butterfly swim stroke. An electromyographic and cinematographic analysis of twelve muscles. *Clin Orthop Relat Res.* 1993; 288:48−59.

33. Pink M, Jobe FW, Perry J, Browne A, Scovazzo ML, Kerrigan J. The painful shoulder during the butterfly stroke. An electromyographic and cinematographic analysis of twelve muscles. *Clin Orthop Relat Res.* 1993;288: 60−72.

34. Pink M, Perry J, Browne A, Scovazzo ML, Kerrigan J. The normal shoulder during freestyle swimming. *Am J Sports Med.* 1991;19(6):569−576.

35. Scovazzo ML, Browne A, Pink M, Jobe FW, Kerrigan J. The painful shoulder during freestyle swimming: and

electromyographic cinematographic analysis of twelve muscles. *Am J Sports Med.* 1991;19(6):577–582.

36. Pink MM, Tibone JE. The painful shoulder in the swimming athlete. *Orthop Clin N Am.* 2000;31(2):247–261.

37. Herman K, Barton C, Malliaras P, Morrissey D. The effectiveness of neuromuscular warm up strategies that require no additional equipment for preventing lower limb injuries in sports participation: a systematic review. *BMC Med.* 2012;10:75.

38. Noyes FR, Barber-Westin SD. Neuromuscular retraining intervention programs: do they reduce noncontact anterior cruciate ligament injury rates in adolescent female athletes? *J Arthroscopy Relat Surg.* 2014;30(2):245–255.

39. Niederbracht Y, Shim AL, Sloniger MA, Paternostra-Bayles M, Short TH. Effects of a shoulder injury prevention strength training program on eccentric external rotator muscle strength and glenohumeral joint imbalance in female overhead activity athletes. *J Strength Condit Res.* 2008;22(1):140–145.

40. Batalha NM, Raimundo AM, Tomas-Carus P, Barbosa TM, Silva AJ. Shoulder rotator cuff balance, strength, and endurance in young swimmers during a competitive season. *J Strength Condit Res.* 2013;27(9):2562–2568.

41. Lynch SS, Thigpen CA, Mihalik JP, Prentice WE, Padua D. The effects of an exercise intervention on forward head and rounded shoulder postures in elite swimmers. *Br J Sports Med.* 2010;44:376–381.

42. Muniz-Pardos B, Gomez-Bruton A, Matute-Llorente A, et al. Swim-specific resistance training: a systematic review. *J Strength Condit Res.* 2019;33(10):2875–2881.

43. Tibone JE, Elrod B, Jobe FW, et al. Surgical treatment of tears of the rotator cuff in athletes. *JBJS.* 1986;68-A(6):887–891.

44. Shaffer B, Huntman D. Rotator cuff tears in the throwing athlete. *Sports Med Arthrosc Rev.* 2014;22(2):101–109.

45. Young SW, Dakic JD, Stroia K, Nguyen ML, Safran MR. Arthroscopic shoulder surgery in female professional tennis players: ability and timing to return to play. *Clin J Sport Med.* 2017;27:357–360.

46. Brushoj C, Bak K, Johannsen HV, Fauno P. Swimmers' painful shoulder arthroscopic findings and return rate to sports. *Scand J Med Sci Sports.* 2007;17:373–377.

CHAPTER 17

Elbow Anatomy and Biomechanics

TIFFANY LIU, MD • SARA EDWARDS, MD

INTRODUCTION

The elbow consists of three joints: the ulnohumeral joint, radiocapitellar joint, and proximal radioulnar joint (PRUJ). Together, these three joints enable the elbow to flex and extend as a hinge joint as well as rotate about a longitudinal axis for pronation-supination. As such, the elbow is classified as a trochoginglymoid joint.

The distal humerus has a 30-degree anterior tilt relative to the humeral shaft; therefore the anterior cortex of the humeral shaft should intersect the capitellum between the anterior and middle thirds of the capitellum. The trochlea is shaped like a spool of thread; the medial ridge of the trochlea is more prominent than the lateral ridge, and the trochlea extends more distal and posterior than the capitellum. As a result, the joint line is in about 6 degrees of valgus and 5 degrees of internal rotation.[1,2] This also contributes to the valgus carrying angle of the elbow, which is defined as the angle between the long axis of the humerus and the long axis of the ulna, and ranges between 10 and 15 degrees in males and 15−20 degrees in females.[3] The distal humerus consists of two articulations: medially, the trochlea articulates with the greater sigmoid notch of the proximal ulna and laterally, the capitellum articulates with the radial head.

The ulnohumeral joint acts as a hinge joint. Anteriorly, the proximal aspect of the ulna is known as the coronoid process, which plays a critical role in elbow stability. It provides a highly congruent articulation, and several key soft tissue structures such as the medial collateral ligament (MCL), anterior capsule, and brachialis insert on the coronoid process. Posteriorly, the olecranon limits the extension of the elbow.

The radiocapitellar joint not only acts in flexion and extension but also allows for rotation. Here, the radial head articulates with the capitellum. The concave radial head provides stability at this joint through a concavity-compression method.[4] Rotation occurs via the PRUJ.

The PRUJ consists of the articulation between the radial head and the lesser sigmoid notch of the ulna. Approximately 240−280 degrees of the circumference of the radial head are covered with cartilage to allow for pronation and supination.[1,2,5,6]

In the skeletally immature elbow, the ossification centers of the elbow appear in a predictable manner. The mnemonic "CRITOE," or some variation, is often used to describe the pattern of ossification. The capitellum appears first, followed by the radial head, medial ("internal") epicondyle, trochlea, olecranon, and lateral ("external") epicondyle. On imaging, it is particularly important to examine the relationships between the anterior humeral line and capitellum and the radial head and capitellum to ensure appropriate reduction.

MUSCULAR ANATOMY

The elbow flexors consist of the biceps, brachialis, and brachioradialis. The biceps tendon attaches to the radial tuberosity, while the brachialis attaches 11 mm distal to the tip of the coronoid.

The triceps attaches to the olecranon and acts to extend the elbow. While the anconeus also contributes to elbow extension, it functions more as a restraint to varus and posterolateral rotatory instability (PLRI).

The forearm flexor-pronator group originates from the medial epicondyle of the elbow and consists of the flexor carpi radialis, palmaris longus, pronator teres, flexor digitorum superficialis (FDS), and flexor carpi ulnaris (FCU). The forearm extensors arise from a common origin of the lateral epicondyle and include the brachioradialis, extensor carpi radialis longus, extensor carpi radialis brevis, extensor carpi ulnaris, extensor digiti minimi, and extensor digitorum communis. The supinator also has one head that arises from the lateral epicondyle, while the other originates from the proximal ulna.

The Female Athlete. https://doi.org/10.1016/B978-0-323-75985-4.00028-3

NEUROVASCULAR ANATOMY

The median nerve arises from the medial and lateral cords of the brachial plexus. It crosses the elbow anteriorly, medial to the brachial artery, and at the level of the elbow joint, it lies deep to the bicipital aponeurosis and superficial to the brachialis. Distally, it continues deep to the pronator teres and then between the two heads of the FDS.

The musculocutaneous nerve arises from the lateral cord of the brachial plexus, travels between the biceps and the brachialis, and becomes the lateral antebrachial cutaneous nerve.

The radial nerve originates from the posterior cord of the brachial plexus, travels along the spiral groove of the humerus, and pierces the lateral intermuscular septum 7.5 cm above the trochlea. It crosses the elbow anteriorly, between the brachialis and brachioradialis. At the level of the joint, it divides into the posterior interosseus nerve, which enters the forearm between the two heads of the supinator, and the superficial radial nerve, which courses deep to the brachioradialis.

The ulnar nerve arises from the medial cord of the brachial plexus. In the arm, it travels medial to the brachial artery and pierces the medial intermuscular septum at the arcade of Struthers to pass into the posterior compartment. It then runs along the back of the medial epicondyle; dives between the two heads of the FCU, giving off the first motor branch to the FCU; and then runs along the anterior surface of the FDP.

The brachial artery also travels in the cubital fossa lateral to the median nerve and divides into the radial and ulnar arteries in the cubital fossa. The radial artery then passes medial to the biceps tendon and runs anterior to the supinator. The ulnar artery passes deep to the deep head of the pronator teres.

ELBOW BIOMECHANICS

While full elbow range of motion is from 0 degrees (some individuals may be capable of up to 15 degrees of hyperextension) to 140 degrees of flexion with a 180-degree arc of pronation/supination, the functional arc of motion of the elbow is from 30 to 130 degrees of flexion, as well as 50 degrees of pronation and 50 degrees of supination.[7] The ulnohumeral joint bears roughly 40% of the axial load across the elbow, while the radiocapitellar joint bears the other 60%.[8] However, this distribution can vary depending on the degree of flexion. Forces across the radiocapitellar joint are greatest in 0–30 degrees of flexion and in pronation.[9] During activities of daily living, joint reaction forces vary from a maximum of 350 N with activities, such as

eating and dressing, to 2000 N with maximal isometric flexion.[10] During push-ups, the elbow bears 45% of body weight.[11]

The stabilizers of the elbow can be divided into (1) primary and secondary static stabilizers and (2) dynamic stabilizers. Primary stabilizers are those that lead to laxity when they are released. Injury or release of a secondary stabilizer alone does not lead to instability, but increased laxity occurs when a secondary stabilizer is damaged in addition to a compromised primary stabilizer.

Primary Stabilizers

Primary static stabilizers of the elbow include the bony anatomy (i.e., ulnohumeral joint), the MCL, and the lateral collateral ligament (LCL) complex. The articular anatomy provides 50% or more of the stability to valgus and varus stress, most notably at the extremes of flexion and extension when the coronoid and olecranon engage into the coronoid and olecranon fossae, respectively.[2,4,6,12] At mid-flexion, stabilization from ligamentous structures predominates.[13] Prior studies have shown that with a loss of 50% of coronoid height, the elbow develops posterior instability, which is greater in positions of flexion, as well as varus laxity, particularly at lower flexion angles, because of the loss of soft tissue attachments.[14–16]

The elbow MCL, or ulnar collateral ligament, originates from the medial epicondyle posterior to the axis of rotation and acts as a restraint against valgus stress and posteromedial rotatory instability.[17] The elbow MCL consists of an anterior bundle, a posterior bundle, and oblique or transverse fibers between the two. The anterior bundle inserts on the sublime tubercle of the coronoid process and can be further divided into anterior, central, and posterior bands. While there is no true isometric point for the MCL, the central band originates closest to the axis of rotation of the ulnohumeral joint, and so it is nearly isometric throughout the elbow's arc of motion.[18–20] The anterior band acts as the primary restraint to valgus stress in flexion up to 90 degrees; at 120 degrees, the anterior and posterior bands of the anterior bundle act as coprimary restraints.[21] The anterior band also resists internal rotation.[22] Overall, the effect of anterior bundle deficiency is greatest in 70–90 degrees of flexion.[21,23] The posterior bundle of the MCL inserts on the medial olecranon and provides restraint to valgus stress when the elbow is in greater than 90 degrees of flexion.[20,24] The posterior bundle also forms the floor of the cubital tunnel.

The LCL complex protects against PLRI and contributes about 10% of overall restraint to varus instability.[5]

It consists of the radial collateral ligament (RCL), lateral ulnar collateral ligament (LUCL), accessory collateral ligament, and annular ligament. The LUCL and RCL originate from the lateral epicondyle at the isometric point.[5] The LUCL inserts on the supinator crest of the ulna and is the primary ligamentous stabilizer to varus stress throughout the elbow's arc of motion. The annular ligament encircles the radial head and attaches at the lesser sigmoid notch, and the RCL attaches to the annular ligament to stabilize the radial head.[1] Studies have suggested that if the annular ligament is intact, stability is maintained even if the LUCL and RCL are transected.[25]

Secondary Stabilizers

Secondary static stabilizers include the radiocapitellar joint, joint capsule, and flexor and extensor origins. The radial head is the second most important restraint to valgus stress following the anterior bundle of the MCL. This is most notable from 0 to 30 degrees of flexion. While some studies have shown that the radial head provides approximately 30% of valgus stability,[26] Morrey et al.[17] demonstrated that as long as the MCL is intact, loss of the radial head does not lead to clinical instability.

The capsule provides its greatest contribution to stability at maximum extension.[5] It can be maximally distended at about 70–80 degrees of flexion, and intra-articular volumes up to 25–35 mL can be achieved.[27,28]

Dynamic Stabilizers

The dynamic stabilizers of the elbow include the muscles that cross the joint, such as the biceps, brachialis, triceps, and anconeus. These muscles provide stability through compressive forces. In general, the flexor mass resists valgus forces and the extensors resist varus forces. In particular, the anconeus provides restraint against varus and PLRI.[2] In fact, muscle tension after release of the MCL can restore near-normal patterns of motion.[17]

SUMMARY

The elbow is a complex joint involving multiple different articulations with a variety of osseous and soft tissue support structures. A fundamental knowledge of elbow anatomy and biomechanics is critical to understand how sports-related injuries impact the structure and function of the elbow joint.

REFERENCES

1. Smith JM, Bell J-E. Anatomy of the elbow. In: Tashjian RZ, ed. *The Unstable Elbow: An Evidence-Based Approach to Evaluation and Management.* Springer International Publishing; 2017:3–11. https://doi.org/10.1007/978-3-319-46019-2_1.
2. Bryce CD, Armstrong AD. Anatomy and biomechanics of the elbow. *Orthop Clin North Am.* 2008;39(2):141–154. https://doi.org/10.1016/j.ocl.2007.12.001.
3. Chalmers PN, Chamberlain AM. Biomechanics of the elbow. In: Tashjian RZ, ed. *The Unstable Elbow: An Evidence-Based Approach to Evaluation and Management.* Springer International Publishing; 2017:13–26. https://doi.org/10.1007/978-3-319-46019-2_2.
4. Wolfe SW, Pederson WC, Hotchkiss RN, Kozin SH, Cohen MS. *Green's Operative Hand Surgery: Expert Consult: Online and Print.* Elsevier Health Sciences; 2010.
5. Karbach LE, Elfar J. Elbow instability: anatomy, biomechanics, diagnostic maneuvers, and testing. *J Hand Surg.* 2017;42(2):118–126. https://doi.org/10.1016/j.jhsa.2016.11.025.
6. Rooker JC, Smith JRA, Amirfeyz R. Anatomy, surgical approaches and biomechanics of the elbow. *Orthop Trauma.* 2016;30(4):283–290. https://doi.org/10.1016/j.mporth.2016.05.008.
7. Morrey BF, Askew LJ, Chao EY. A biomechanical study of normal functional elbow motion. *J Bone Joint Surg Am.* 1981;63(6):872–877.
8. Halls AA, Travill A. Transmission of pressures across the elbow joint. *Anat Rec.* 1964;150(3):243–247. https://doi.org/10.1002/ar.1091500305.
9. Morrey BF, An KN, Stormont TJ. Force transmission through the radial head. *J Bone Joint Surg Am.* 1988;70(2):250–256.
10. Kincaid BL, An K-N. Elbow joint biomechanics for preclinical evaluation of total elbow prostheses. *J Biomech.* 2013;46(14):2331–2341. https://doi.org/10.1016/j.jbiomech.2013.07.027.
11. An KN, Chao EY, Morrey BF, Donkers MJ. Intersegmental elbow joint load during pushup. *Biomed Sci Instrum.* 1992;28:69–74.
12. Morrey BF, An K-N. Articular and ligamentous contributions to the stability of the elbow joint. *Am J Sports Med.* 1983;11(5):315–319. https://doi.org/10.1177/036354658301100506.
13. Wilps T, Kaufmann RA, Yamakawa S, Fowler JR. Elbow biomechanics: bony and dynamic stabilizers. *J Hand Surg.* 2020;45(6):528–535. https://doi.org/10.1016/j.jhsa.2020.01.016.
14. Closkey RF, Goode JR, Kirschenbaum D, Cody RP. The role of the coronoid process in elbow stability. A biomechanical analysis of axial loading. *J Bone Joint Surg Am.* 2000; 82(12):1749–1753. https://doi.org/10.2106/00004623-200012000-00009.

15. Beingessner DM, Dunning CE, Stacpoole RA, Johnson JA, King GJW. The effect of coronoid fractures on elbow kinematics and stability. *Clin Biomech.* 2007;22(2):183–190. https://doi.org/10.1016/j.clinbiomech.2006.09.007.

16. Hull JR, Owen JR, Fern SE, Wayne JS, Boardman ND. Role of the coronoid process in varus osteoarticular stability of the elbow. *J Shoulder Elbow Surg.* 2005;14(4):441–446. https://doi.org/10.1016/j.jse.2004.11.005.

17. Morrey BF, Tanaka S, An K-N. Valgus stability of the elbow: a definition of primary and secondary constraints. *Clin Orthop Relat Res.* 1991;265:187–195.

18. Ochi N, Ogura T, Hashizume H, Shigeyama Y, Senda M, Inoue H. Anatomic relation between the medial collateral ligament of the elbow and the humero-ulnar joint axis. *J Shoulder Elbow Surg.* 1999;8(1):6–10. https://doi.org/10.1016/S1058-2746(99)90046-0.

19. Armstrong AD, Ferreira LM, Dunning CE, Johnson JA, King GJW. The medial collateral ligament of the elbow is not isometric: an in vitro biomechanical study. *Am J Sports Med.* 2004;32(1):85–90. https://doi.org/10.1177/0363546503258886.

20. Fuss FK. The ulnar collateral ligament of the human elbow joint. Anatomy, function and biomechanics. *J Anat.* 1991; 175:203–212.

21. Callaway GH, Field LD, Deng XH, et al. Biomechanical evaluation of the medial collateral ligament of the

elbow. *J Bone Joint Surg Am.* 1997;79(8):1223–1231. https://doi.org/10.2106/00004623-199708000-00015.

22. Kaufmann RA, Wilps T, Musahl V, Debski RE. Elbow biomechanics: soft tissue stabilizers. *J Hand Surg.* 2020; 45(2):140–147. https://doi.org/10.1016/j.jhsa.2019.10.034.

23. Floris S, Olsen BS, Dalstra M, Søjbjerg JO, Sneppen O. The medial collateral ligament of the elbow joint: anatomy and kinematics. *J Shoulder Elbow Surg.* 1998;7(4):345–351. https://doi.org/10.1016/S1058-2746(98)90021-0.

24. Regan WD, Korinek SL, Morrey BF, An KN. Biomechanical study of ligaments around the elbow joint. *Clin Orthop.* 1991;(271):170–179.

25. Dunning CE, Zarzour ZD, Patterson SD, Johnson JA, King GJ. Ligamentous stabilizers against posterolateral rotatory instability of the elbow. *J Bone Joint Surg Am.* 2001;83(12):1823–1828. https://doi.org/10.2106/00004623-200112000-00009.

26. Hotchkiss RN, Weiland AJ. Valgus stability of the elbow. *J Orthop Res.* 1987;5(3):372–377. https://doi.org/10.1002/jor.1100050309.

27. O'Driscoll SW, Morrey BF, An KN. Intraarticular pressure and capacity of the elbow. *Arthroscopy.* 1990;6(2): 100–103. https://doi.org/10.1016/0749-8063(90)90007-z.

28. Van Den Broek M, Van Riet R. Intra-articular capacity of the elbow joint. *Clin Anat.* 2017;30(6):795–798. https://doi.org/10.1002/ca.22915.

CHAPTER 18

Elbow Ulnar Collateral Ligament Injuries in the Female Athlete

JENNIFER J. BECK, MD, FAAOS • KELLY E. CLINE, MD • PAMELA J. LANG, MD

INTRODUCTION

While there is abundant literature on ulnar collateral ligament (UCL) injuries in male athletes, predominantly professional baseball players, research remains sparse on the pathoanatomy, epidemiology, treatment, and outcomes of UCL injuries in female athletes. A literature review by Gardner and Bedi[1] demonstrated that only 79 of 1902 (4.15%) patients within UCL studies are female. The majority of elbow UCL studies consist of either small case reports or limited case series or otherwise involve larger studies where a predominant cohort of the athletes are male. A small subset of these larger studies includes female athletes; however, many of the studies do not separate out the female athlete when specifically discussing outcomes.

Several recent studies have highlighted gender-related differences in orthopedic conditions; however, there remains a paucity of literature on outcomes following the treatment of UCL injuries in female athletes. The majority of studies on elbow UCL injuries focus on professional baseball pitchers. Baseball is a sport dominated by male athletes, whereas softball is dominated by female athletes. Softball pitchers have a significantly different throwing pattern (underhand/windmill) than baseball pitchers (overhand), which may protect them from UCL injuries.

Electromyographic study of the windmill pitch demonstrates that the highest level of biceps eccentric contraction occurs at the 9 o'clock position, just prior to ball release when the shoulder is experiencing maximum distraction stress and the elbow is experiencing maximum extension torque.[2] Peak biceps motor activation was significantly higher than that during an overhand throwing motion where the biceps is responsible for providing elbow flexion torque.[2] Alteration of peak forces with the elbow flexed (overhand) versus extended (underhand/windmill) may be related to the incidence of UCL injury. When standard overhand throwing kinematics and kinetics are compared between genders, females were found to have lower ball velocity, lower elbow extension angular velocity, lower proximal forces on the elbow and shoulder joints, lower pelvis and upper torso rotation, and shorter stride length.[3] Notably, in this study, these reductions were not compared to the overall athlete stature or body muscle composition, but rather were compared as absolute values.

Gymnastics represents a more female-dominated sport (compared with male athlete participation). Elbow UCL injuries tend to occur from the overhead, weight-bearing/compression, and the rotational forces on the upper extremity caused by the unique movements of the sport. Therefore gymnasts represent a large proportion of female athletes with UCL injuries. Floor exercises followed by balance beam have been shown to have the highest rates of acute injuries, with bars and vault having lower injury rates.[4] Large lateral compression and valgus forces have been noted during the double-arm support phase of a backhand spring (a maneuver performed on both floor and balance beam), which may explain the pathogenesis of lateral capitellar osteochondritis dissecans (OCD) and UCL injuries during this maneuver.[5]

NONOPERATIVE MANAGEMENT OF ULNAR COLLATERAL LIGAMENT INJURIES IN FEMALE ATHLETES

Nonoperative management of UCL injuries consists of a combination of rest, use of nonsteroidal antiinflammatory medications, immobilization with casting or bracing, and rehabilitation exercises.[6–9] Rehabilitation programs progress through phases with the initial goal of reducing pain and maintaining or restoring full range of motion.[6,7] Athletes then focus on periscapular and rotator cuff strengthening with the goal of regaining

The Female Athlete. https://doi.org/10.1016/B978-0-323-75985-4.00016-7

strength at or above baseline. An interval throwing program can then be initiated, provided athletes are pain-free.[6,7] Throwing athletes generate increased forces at the elbow when utilizing an effort-based return to the throwing program; therefore a relative velocity return to the throwing approach may be more successful.[10] Modalities that may be used in conjunction with therapy include soft tissue mobilization, electric stimulation, ultrasound, and laser therapy.[6] In some cases, injections with platelet-rich plasma (PRP) can be performed.[11–13]

Nonoperative treatment of UCL insufficiency has been most commonly evaluated among throwing athletes, with return to play being the primary outcome variable. Ford et al.[6] reported 84% return to the same level of play in 31 professional baseball players with partial UCL injury diagnosed by magnetic resonance imaging (MRI), with 3 athletes failing rehabilitation and going on to have surgery. The authors concluded that rehabilitation was a viable option for treating partial UCL injuries, even among professional baseball players.[6] Conversely, in a series of baseball players with an average age of 18 years, only 42% of the athletes were able to return to their previous level of participation following a minimum of 3 months of rest along with rehabilitation exercises.[7] Diagnosis of UCL insufficiency or tear was made by physical examination findings of tenderness over the anterior band of the UCL and pain with both the milking maneuver and valgus stress in all patients. All patients had radiographs taken of the affected elbow; some had stress radiographs comparing the involved side to the asymptomatic elbow and some had MRI to confirm the diagnosis.[7] Athletes who were able to return to the same level of play following nonoperative treatment did so about 6 months following diagnosis, and no factors could be identified to predict the success of nonoperative treatment.[7]

The efficacy of nonoperative treatment of UCL injuries among female athletes is not well understood. Nicolette and Gravlee[14] presented a series of five Division I collegiate gymnasts who sustained acute UCL injuries from a valgus load to the elbow. Among the five athletes, four (80%) were able to return to basic gymnastic skills between 1.5 and 12 weeks following a structured rehabilitation program.[14] In gymnastics, athletes can return to one, some, or all events, which may speed up recovery time by selecting an event that least precipitates symptoms. Although this is a series of only five athletes, it does suggest that for an acute injury in a nonthrowing athlete, nonoperative treatment can be successful.

More recently, PRP has been used as an adjunct to rest and rehabilitation in the nonoperative treatment of UCL injuries.[12,13] Podesta et al. utilized PRP injection as a supplement to rehabilitation for the treatment of MRI-confirmed partial UCL tears in a cohort of 35 athletes (28 males and 6 females consisting of 27 baseball players, 3 softball players, 2 tennis players, and 2 volleyball players; mean age of 18 years).[11] Following a single PRP injection, 88% of athletes had successfully returned to play at an average of 12 weeks.[11] The PRP injections were administered for continued symptoms following a minimum of 2 months of rehabilitation.[11] Deal et al.[12] treated 25 adolescent and young adult throwing athletes with MRI-diagnosed partial UCL injuries using a combination of a varus loading hinged elbow brace, rehabilitation, and two sequential ultrasound-guided PRP injections spaced 2 weeks apart. Only two of these athletes were female, both of whom played softball.[12] Following the two PRP injections, 96% of the athletes with a primary injury were able to return to play at the same level or a higher level and had stable elbows on ultrasound evaluation.[12] In the athletes who were able to return to their sport, all but two showed healing of the UCL on posttreatment MRI.[12] The only complication reported among athletes receiving PRP injections was localized swelling that resolved over 24 h.[12]

With studies showing mixed results for nonoperative treatment of UCL injuries, some authors have tried to identify factors that may predict an individual's response to conservative management.[6,15] Among the professional baseball pitchers who failed nonoperative management, 82% had a distal UCL tear on MRI, whereas among those who were able to return to pitching following rehabilitation alone, 81% had proximal tears.[15] Currently, no study has evaluated UCL tear location in female athletes or nonprofessional athletes as a predictor of successful nonoperative management.

Not only the location of the UCL injury but also the extent of injury seem to be important in predicting the need for surgery. MRI staging (or grading) has been proposed, with four injury grades: grade I injuries involve an intact ligament with or without edema, grade IIA includes partial injuries, grade IIB represents chronic healed injuries as indicated by ligament thickening without tearing, and grade III injuries involve a complete tear of the UCL.[6,16] A study of professional baseball pitchers treated nonoperatively showed that the rate of return to play was 100%, 83%, and 94% for grade I, grade IIA, and grade IIB injuries, respectively.[6] Using a different MRI grading scale, Kim et al.[17] similarly reported intact continuity of the ligament and low-grade partial tears more commonly in baseball players who were managed with rehabilitation alone, whereas high-grade partial tears and complete ruptures were more common in those requiring surgical intervention. So far, no study has evaluated the UCL tear grade in female athletes or nonprofessional athletes as a predictor of successful nonoperative management.

OPERATIVE MANAGEMENT OF ULNAR COLLATERAL LIGAMENT INJURIES IN FEMALE ATHLETES

There is currently limited data on the operative management of UCL injuries in female athletes.[9,14,18] While specific indications for acute repair or reconstruction are unclear, failure of sufficient nonoperative management is an indication for surgical intervention.

Case series, including those evaluating outcomes following operative management of UCL injuries in female gymnasts, have limited follow-up and lack detailed outcome measures. Nicolette et al. reported on five female Division I collegiate gymnasts with UCL injuries; however, only one patient underwent surgery: a 19-year-old female gymnast who sustained a valgus load to the elbow resulting in a distal UCL tear with "complete tear at the insertion of the anterior band of the UCL off the sublime tubercle," as demonstrated on magnetic resonance arthrogram of the elbow.[14] After a thorough nonoperative rehabilitation program, the patient underwent UCL reconstruction because continued pain and instability limited her participation in gymnastics. Postoperatively, she began light tumbling at 5 months and was cleared for full participation 6 months after surgery. Grumet et al.[19] published an isolated case report on a 16-year-old female high-school gymnast who was found to have a bony avulsion of her sublime tubercle, which contained the anterior band of her UCL. The patient underwent open repair of her bony avulsion using two suture anchors because of persistent elbow instability with valgus stress. Postoperatively, the injury was splinted for 2 weeks that was then converted to a hinged elbow brace set 30−105 degrees. At 2 month after repair, a strengthening program was initiated. At her final postoperative follow-up (6 months), the patient had full elbow range of motion, no tenderness to palpation, and her elbow was stable to valgus stress. The patient noted pain (1/10) with "heavy lifting or repeated elbow movements," yet had returned to full competition at her preinjury level. Final radiographs at 1 year did not show any degenerative joint changes.[19]

A large cohort study by Cain Jr et al.[18] was performed to evaluate the results of UCL reconstruction at a minimum of 2-year follow-up in an athletic population. This population of athletes primarily involved baseball players (95%); however, it also included football, javelin, softball, tennis, wrestling, soccer, gymnastics, cheerleading, and pole vaulting athletes. This study highlights the rarity of UCL surgery in female athletes: only 28 of 1281 (2.2%) patients were female.[18] A majority of the patients in this study underwent reconstruction (1266 patients, 98.8%) versus repair (15 patients, 1.2%). Indications for UCL reconstruction included failure to progress through a rehabilitation program after 3 months. Reconstruction involved the use of autograft palmaris longus, gracilis, or plantaris, along with concomitant subcutaneous ulnar nerve transposition using a modification of the original Jobe technique.[18] Although 2-year outcomes were reported, they were not separated by gender. About 83% of athletes with reconstructions and 70% of those with UCL repair returned to the same or higher level of sport. The average time from surgery to throwing was 4.4 months, and the average time for return to full competition was 11.6 months. Complications with operative treatment were reported in 20% of cases, with the most common being a minor postoperative ulnar nerve neuropraxia, which involved only sensory changes and was resolved by 6 weeks. A total of 55 patients underwent subsequent elbow surgery between 6 and 7 months after the initial reconstruction (1% required revision UCL reconstruction).[18] Without gender as an independent variable, it is difficult to make any gender-specific conclusions about UCL reconstruction or repair from this study.

Only two available studies report on young athletes with UCL injuries. Savoie et al.[20] reported on primary repairs of the UCL in elbows of young athletes with age ranging from 14.8 to 22 years (mean, 17.2 years) and 13 of 60 (21.67%) athletes included were female. Nonoperative treatment was attempted for an average of 4.1 months before proceeding with repair. This study found that 56 of 60 (93%) athletes were able to return to sports within 6 months with good to excellent functional results. In this study, four patients had failures according to the functional results and the Andrews-Carson rating scale. None of the four patients were female athletes.[20]

Jones et al.[21] reported on the docking technique of UCL reconstruction in adolescent athletes and 4 of 55 (7.27%) athletes included were female. While they did not give the specific breakdown by sport, three gymnasts and five javelin throwers were included in addition to the majority cohort of baseball players (n = 47). Overall, 87% of athletes reported excellent

TABLE 18.1
The Conway Scale.[22]

LEVEL OF COMPETITION	
Excellent	Able to compete at same or higher level for >12 months
Good	Able to compete at lower level for >12 months
Fair	Able to play regularly at recreational level
Poor	Unable to participate in sports

results using the Conway scale (Table 18.1).[22] However, two of three (66%) female gymnasts (average age, 15 years) had poor outcomes according to the Conway scale. Both of these female athletes had OCD lesions of the capitellum, in addition to their UCL injuries, complicating interpretation of the results. Additionally, two gymnasts and two javelin throwers had postoperative complications of a transient ulnar neuritis after UCL reconstruction; however, the gender of these patients is unknown.[21]

One of the largest studies specifically addressing the operative treatment of UCL insufficiency of the elbow in female athletes was a retrospective cohort by Argo and colleagues.[9] A total of 19 female athletes (average age, 22 years; range, 15.1–37.2 years) were included, with an average follow-up of 38.8 months (range, 12.4–68.6 months). Among them, 42% ($n = 8$) were softball players, 21% ($n = 4$) were gymnasts, and 10.5% ($n = 2$) were tennis players. Operative intervention followed failure of nonoperative treatment (mean duration of 5.1 months). The decision to reconstruct or repair the ligament was made intraoperatively, with 18 of 19 (94.7%) patients undergoing repair of the UCL.[9] Repair techniques varied based on ligament injury pattern.[9] This strongly contrasts reports regarding male athletes in general and baseball players specifically, in whom surgical intervention often involves UCL reconstruction. Postoperatively, the patients were initially on splint and then placed into a hinged brace initially set at 30 degrees to full flexion. The brace use was discontinued after 12 weeks in the repair group and 16 weeks for the patient who underwent reconstruction.[9] The athletes started sport-specific rehabilitation while remaining in a brace by 6 weeks postoperatively, with 94.4% returning to play at a mean of 2.5 months (range, 2.0–3.5 months), which was one of the remarkable reported outcomes. Based on the Andrews-Carson scoring

system, the overall postoperative outcome was excellent in 16 patients and good in 3 patients.[9] There were no reported postoperative failures in this time range. The rapid return to play may be due to a muscle splitting approach used in 79% of patients, a less invasive repair versus reconstruction technique, or an improved postoperative rehabilitation.

While the majority of female athletes in this study underwent repair, there is no current literature comparing UCL repair to reconstruction specifically regarding the female athlete. Conway et al.[22] compared repair to reconstruction in throwing athletes, where 14 patients (all male) underwent direct UCL repair and 56 (55 males and 1 female) underwent UCL reconstruction using a free tendon graft. A total of 10 of 14 (71.4%) patients in the repair group had an excellent or a good result, while 45 of 56 (80.4%) patients in the reconstruction group had good or excellent results. However, in this study, only 7 of 14 (50%) patients who underwent repair returned to their previous level of sports participation compared to 38 of 56 (68%) athletes in the reconstruction group.

CONCLUSION

Elbow UCL injuries are rarely reported in female athletes. Larger cohort studies do not define results based on gender. Treatment algorithms, indications for repair versus reconstruction, and the method of reconstruction have not been well-defined within the female athlete population. Despite this, successful outcomes of nonoperative and operative management have been reported.

REFERENCES

1. Gardner E, Bedi A. Ulnar collateral ligament injury in female athletes. In: Dines J, Altchek D, eds. *Elbow Ulnar Collateral Ligament Injury*. Boston: Springer; 2015: 205–212. https://doi.org/10.1007/978-1-4899-7540-9_24.
2. Rojas IL, Provencher MT, Bhatia S, Foucher KC, Bach Jr BR, Romeo AA, et al. Biceps activity during windmill softball pitching: injury implications and comparison with overhand throwing. *Am J Sports Med*. 2009;37(3):558–565.
3. Chu Y, Simpson K, Andrews J. Biomechanical comparison between elite female and male baseball pitchers. *J Appl Biomech*. 2009;25:22–31.
4. Caine D, Cochrane B, Caine C, Zemper E. An epidemiologic investigation of injuries affecting young, competitive female gymnasts. *Am J Sports Med*. 1989;17(6):811–820.
5. Koh T, Grabiner MD, Weiker G. Technique and ground reaction forces in the back handspring. *Am J Sports Med*. 1992;20(1):61–66.

6. Ford GM, Genuario J, Kinkartz J, Githens T, Noonan T. Return-to-Play outcomes in professional baseball players after medial ulnar collateral ligament injuries: comparison of operative versus nonoperative treatment based on magnetic resonance imaging findings. *Am J Sports Med.* 2016; 44(3):723–728. https://doi.org/10.1177/036354651562 1756.

7. Rettig AC, Sherrill C, Snead DS, Mendler JC, Mieling P. Nonoperative treatment of ulnar collateral ligament injuries in throwing athletes. *Am J Sports Med.* 2001;29(1): 15–17. https://doi.org/10.1177/03635465010290010601.

8. Biz C, Crimi A, Belluzzi E, et al. Conservative versus surgical management of elbow medial ulnar collateral ligament injury: a systematic review. *Orthop Surg.* 2019;11(6): 974–984. https://doi.org/10.1111/os.12571.

9. Argo D, Trenhaile SW, Savoie 3rd FH, Field LD. Operative treatment of ulnar collateral ligament insufficiency of the elbow in female athletes. *Am J Sports Med.* 2006;34(3): 431–437. https://doi.org/10.1177/0363546505281240.

10. Lizzio VA, Smith DG, Jildeh TR, et al. Importance of radar gun inclusion during return-to-throwing rehabilitation following ulnar collateral ligament reconstruction in baseball pitchers: a simulation study. *J Shoulder Elbow Surg.* 2019. https://doi.org/10.1016/j.jse.2019.08.014.

11. Podesta L, Crow SA, Volkmer D, Bert T, Yocum LA. Treatment of partial ulnar collateral ligament tears in the elbow with platelet-rich plasma. *Am J Sports Med.* 2013;41(7): 1689–1694. https://doi.org/10.1177/0363546513487979.

12. Deal JB, Smith E, Heard W, O'Brien MJ, Savoie 3rd FH. Platelet-rich plasma for primary treatment of partial ulnar collateral ligament tears: MRI correlation with results. *Orthop J Sports Med.* 2017;5(11). https://doi.org/10.1177/2325967117738238.

13. McCrum CL, Costello J, Onishi K, Stewart C, Vyas D. Return to play after PRP and rehabilitation of 3 elite ice hockey players with ulnar collateral ligament injuries of the elbow. *Orthop J Sports Med.* 2018;6(8).

14. Nicolette GW, Gravlee JR. Ulnar collateral ligament injuries of the elbow in female division I collegiate gymnasts: a report of five cases. *Open Access J Sports Med.* 2018;9: 183–189. https://doi.org/10.2147/OAJSM.S159624.

15. Frangiamore SJ, Lynch TS, Vaughn MD, et al. Magnetic resonance imaging predictors of failure in the nonoperative management of ulnar collateral ligament injuries in professional baseball pitchers. *Am J Sports Med.* 2017; 45(8):1783–1789. https://doi.org/10.1177/0363546517 699832.

16. Ramos N, Limpisvasti O. UCL injury in the non-throwing athlete. *Curr Rev Musculoskelet Med.* 2019. https://doi.org/10.1007/s12178-019-09590-2.

17. Kim NR, Moon SG, Ko SM, Moon W-J, Choi JW, Park J-Y. MR imaging of ulnar collateral ligament injury in baseball players: value for predicting rehabilitation outcome. *Eur J Radiol.* 2011;80(3):e422–e426. https://doi.org/10.1016/j.ejrad.2010.12.041.

18. Cain ELJ, Andrews JR, Dugas JR, et al. Outcome of ulnar collateral ligament reconstruction of the elbow in 1281 athletes: results in 743 athletes with minimum 2-year follow-up. *Am J Sports Med.* 2010;38(12):2426–2434. https://doi.org/10.1177/0363546510378100.

19. Grumet RC, Friel NA, Cole BJ. Bony avulsion of the medial ulnar collateral ligament in a gymnast: a case report. *J Shoulder Elbow Surg.* 2010;19(7):e1–e6. https://doi.org/10.1016/j.jse.2010.04.007.

20. Savoie 3rd FH, Trenhaile SW, Roberts J, Field LD, Ramsey JR. Primary repair of ulnar collateral ligament injuries of the elbow in young athletes: a case series of injuries to the proximal and distal ends of the ligament. *Am J Sports Med.* 2008;36(6):1066–1072. https://doi.org/10.1177/0363546508315201.

21. Jones KJ, Dines JS, Rebolledo BJ, et al. Operative management of ulnar collateral ligament insufficiency in adolescent athletes. *Am J Sports Med.* 2014;42(1):117–121. https://doi.org/10.1177/0363546513507695.

22. Conway JE, Jobe FW, Glousman RE, Pink M. Medial instability of the elbow in throwing athletes. Treatment by repair or reconstruction of the ulnar collateral ligament. *J Bone Jt Surg Am.* 1992;74(1):67–83.

CHAPTER 19

Osteochondritis Dissecans of the Elbow

LAURA MOORE, MD • SARA EDWARDS, MD

INTRODUCTION AND EPIDEMIOLOGY

Osteochondritis dissecans (OCD) was first described by König in 1887 as a possible explanation for the presence of loose bodies within a joint.[1] Initially, he postulated that inflammation led to the atraumatic formation of loose bodies, hence the designation of "osteochondritis." Although the exact cause of OCD remains elusive, we recognize it to be acquired, focal lesions of subchondral bone with varying degrees of osseous resorption, fragmentation, and sclerosis that risk possible disruption of superficial articular cartilage.[2–5]

OCD lesions remain a disease of maturing joints. The overall incidence of OCD across all joints declines to 2.52 (female) and 4.41 (male) per 100,000 person-years in patients aged 20–45 years.[6] Several authors have noted an increasing incidence of OCD in the elbow with time and decreasing age at presentation[7,8] and suggest that it may correlate with the increasing popularity of competitive sports among young athletes.

Of all the OCD lesions diagnosed in adolescent athletes, the elbow represents only 12% of lesions.[9] The reported incidence of elbow OCD lesions in patients aged 6–19 years is 2.2 per 100,000, with 3.8 per 100,000 in males and 0.6 per 100,000 in females.[10] This represents a 6.8 times greater odds ratio in males than females. Additionally, the same study found that the odds ratio was 21.7 times higher in patients aged 12–19 years when compared with those aged 6–11 years. The vast majority of elbow OCD lesions (97.5%) are found in the capitellum, with rare lesions seen on the trochlea (2.5%) and radial head[10,11] (Fig. 19.1).

Capitellar OCD lesions are typically seen in adolescent athletes engaging in repetitive overhead activities such as baseball, gymnastics, football, javelin, or overhead weight lifting.[3–5] Kida et al.[12] describe a prevalence of 3.4% among adolescent baseball players (14.5 ± 1.5 years), as detected by ultrasound. The authors also found that players with elbow OCD had played for longer periods, started playing at an earlier age, and experienced more elbow pain. Furthermore, patients who had continued to pitch despite having elbow pain demonstrated more advanced lesions. This was additionally confirmed by Matsuura et al.[13] who found a prevalence of 3.2% among baseball players aged 10–12 years using ultrasound.

Although no large-scale studies have been undertaken with female athletes, several reports note an elevated risk of capitellar OCD in female gymnasts.[14–16]

(A) **(B)**

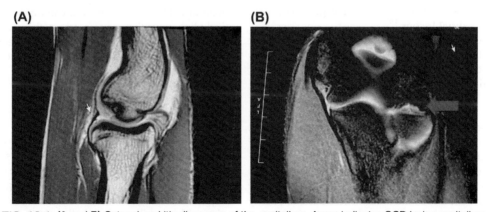

FIG. 19.1 **(A** and **B)** Osteochondritis dissecans of the capitellum. Arrow indicates OCD lesion capitellum.

The Female Athlete. https://doi.org/10.1016/B978-0-323-75985-4.00003-9

Although Kessler et al.[10] noted a 6.8 times greater odds ratio of having elbow OCD in adolescent males as opposed to females, these findings are likely biased by sport popularity in Southern California. A similar, but much smaller, cohort out of Boston noted similar rates of OCD among male and female athletes.[17] Interestingly, in the cohort out of Boston, female gymnasts were noted to be more likely to present at a younger physical and skeletal age and to have an injury to their nondominant arm compared to the group of largely male baseball players.

MECHANISM OF INJURY

Although the initial description by König in 1887 suggested a central role for inflammation in the formation of osteochondral fragments, this has since been disproven by multiple histologic studies.[2] Currently, the most widely accepted cause for OCD formation across joints is repetitive microtrauma. Within the elbow, this theory is supported by the relatively high prevalence of capitellar OCD in adolescent baseball players and gymnasts, where the elbow is subjected to repetitive valgus loading.[12–15] For baseball players, the elbow is subjected to high valgus stress during the late cocking and early acceleration phases of throwing, which generates both compressive and shear forces across the radiocapitellar joint.[18] In contrast, the stress experienced during gymnastics appears to be an axial load, 60% of which is born by the radiocapitellar joint.[19,20] Interestingly, female gymnasts' events result in increased axial loading and adduction moment, potentially placing them at higher risk of elbow injury than their male counterparts.[21,22] The variation in loading pattern between baseball and gymnastics translates into different locations for capitellar OCD between baseball players, who have more anterior lesions, and gymnasts, who have more distal lesions.[19]

However, repetitive microtrauma may only be part of the elbow OCD story. The European Pediatric Orthopedic Society conducted a large multicenter study, which demonstrated that only 55% of patients with knee OCD regularly participated in sports or strenuous physical activity.[23] Importantly, OCD may also result from obesity or anatomic variations. Kessler et al. found that extreme childhood obesity, as defined by body mass index >35 kg/m^2 or weight 1.2× the 95th percentile, increases the risk of OCD formation across all joints by 86%.[24] Interestingly, the highest risk joints in this study were the elbow and ankle, where extreme obesity conferred 3.1 and 3.0 times increased risk of OCD formation, respectively.

Lower extremity alignment plays a significant role in the development of OCD in the knee, with varus knees tending to develop medial femoral condyle OCD lesions and valgus knees tending to develop lateral femoral condyle OCD lesions.[25] Anatomic considerations appear to be critical to elbow OCD development as well. First, the converse pattern appears to be true for the elbow, where patients with capitellar OCD are more likely to have a varus carrying angle than matched controls.[26] Second, Schenck et al.[27] demonstrated in cadaveric studies that a stiffness mismatch is present in the radiocapitellar joint, which may lead the lateral capitellum to experience a higher strain environment during valgus load. Third, healing after injury may be compromised by limited vascular supply to the distal/anterior capitellum. The immature capitellum lacks a substantial metaphyseal blood supply and instead relies on branches from the radial recurrent and interosseous recurrent arteries.[5,28] This leaves the capitellum vulnerable to ischemia, particularly in the setting of repetitive injury.

One potentially unifying theory involves disordered ossification of a portion of the epiphysis.[29,30] According to this theory, there is an unspecified insult (single or repetitive) to the epiphysis that leads to either temporary or permanent cessation of ossification in one region. The remainder of the epiphysis continues to grow and undergo endochondral ossification, leading to the development of a growing defect. Here, a complete cessation in ossification would generate a completely cartilaginous OCD, whereas a temporary stop would generate a partially ossified fragment. Although Barrie[29,30] did not provide any direct evidence to support this mechanism, unpublished MRI data out of the Research in Osteochondritis of the Knee (ROCK) group suggest it may be visible on MRI.[2] Regardless, capitellar OCD formation is likely the result of a combination of factors including repetitive stresses across the radiocapitellar joint, tenuous vascular supply to the capitellum, and a mismatch in stiffness between the radial head and lateral capitellum.

TREATMENT AND OUTCOMES
Nonoperative Management

The initial approach to the management of capitellar OCD is generally dictated by the lesion's stability. Of note, because of the near-complete absence of outcome data for noncapitellar OCD, the following discussion on treatment and outcomes will focus on capitellar lesions. The stability of capitellar OCD is affected by several factors including patient age, elbow motion, and radiographic and MRI findings (Fig. 19.1A and B). Nonoperative treatment, consisting of elbow rest for 6 months, has been found to be successful in managing early capitellar OCD in multiple studies.[31–33] Matsuura et al.[31] reported radiographic healing in 91% of early capitellar lesions, as defined by capitellar radiolucency only, with conservative treatment. These results were confirmed by Mihara et al.[32] who reported an 88% radiographic healing rate with conservative treatment for patients presenting with radiolucency or capitellar flattening. Takahara et al.[33] also investigated the impact of presenting symptoms and the status of the capitellar growth plate on nonoperative treatment. They reported successful nonoperative treatment of patients with an open capitellar growth plate, localized flattening or radiolucency of the subchondral bone on radiograph, and good elbow motion at presentation. All three studies noted that patients who continued to stress their elbows after activity restrictions had been prescribed were more likely to have lesion progression and to fail conservative treatment.[31–33]

Although Takahara et al. used plain radiographs in their study, more recent studies have moved toward using MRI owing to the lack of sensitivity of radiography in detecting OCD.[34,35] Pill et al.[36] demonstrated that MRI could be utilized to assist in predicting the success of nonoperative treatment of OCD in the knee. Although multiple studies have verified that preoperative MRI is consistently able to identify stable versus unstable lesions of the capitellum as confirmed via arthroscopy,[34,37–40] these studies do not provide any correlation with the outcome of operative or nonoperative treatment. Niu et al.[41] studied 89 patients (45% female, average age 13 years) with 93 OCD lesions in an effort to identify predictors of successful nonoperative management. The authors found that patients with lower Helfi grade, smaller lesion size, and the absence of cystlike lesions on MRI were more likely to go on to clinical and radiographic healing. Interestingly, age, gender, handedness, sport, and physeal status were not significant predictors of outcome. Of note, Niu et al. also reported healing rates of 64% for Helfi grade I lesions, which is much lower than the findings reported by Takahara, Matsuura, and Mihara, suggesting that there may be a difference in the prognostic value of radiographic and MRI findings that should be investigated further.

Operative Management

Multiple surgical procedures have been described for the management of capitellar OCD lesions that have failed conservative management or have radiographic

indicators of instability. Surgical treatment options include fragment removal with or without curettage or drilling,[33,42–44] direct fragment fixation,[45–49] reconstruction with autograft,[50–53] reconstruction with allograft or autologous chondrocytes,[54–56] and closing wedge osteotomy of the distal humerus.[57] Early surgical treatments consisted of open fragment removal with or without drilling or curettage of the donor site.[33,42–44] Although there were short-term improvements in elbow symptoms after surgical treatment, all four studies noted residual symptoms in 42%–65% of patients at long-term follow-up.

An alternative surgical treatment is arthroscopic removal of loose bodies, debridement, and chondroplasty[45–49] (Figs. 19.2 and 19.3). All studies describing this technique demonstrate improvements in pain postoperatively, with return to preinjury levels of sport ranging from 40% to 92%. When combined in a meta-analysis, the overall return to any level of sport rate was 87%, with 71% returning to their previous level of activity at a mean time of 4 ± 1.5 months after arthroscopy with or without microfracture.[58] These results are supported by the long-term case series in adolescent baseball players by Matsuura et al., which showed an 87% return-to-sport rate and durable symptom relief at a minimum of 10-year follow-up.[59] Importantly, this study notes that although their return to sport rate was high overall, it was much lower for pitchers, where only one of five patients returned to pitching. Of note, poorer results from arthroscopy were seen in patients with lesions that extended to the lateral border of the capitellum, as such lesions may compromise elbow biomechanics.[46,47]

Microfracture has also been described as an option for full-thickness osteochondral lesions of the capitellum. A retrospective review of 23 patients (25 elbows) demonstrated that 77.3% of patients were able to return to sport. In female gymnasts, however, only 50% were able to return to sport. The authors concluded that use of osteochondral allograft should be the preferred treatment for a large osteochondral defect in a gymnast, whereas other sports such as swimming and water polo had greater success with microfracture[60] (Fig. 19.4A and B).

Multiple studies have also evaluated the utility of OCD fixation using wires, Herbert screws, or dynamic stapling.[61–66] All methods of fixation provide good short-term improvements in symptoms, with variable return-to-sport rates ranging from 66% to 100%. However, when the data was combined in a meta-analysis completed by Westermann et al.,[58] patients who underwent fixation of capitellar OCD lesions had a

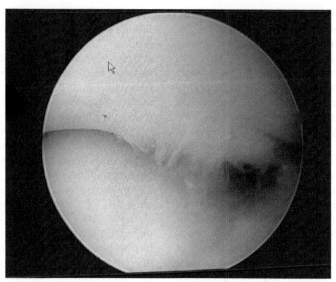

FIG. 19.2 Osteochondritis dissecans lesion of the capitellum, uncontained lesion. Arrow indicates OCD lesion capitellum.

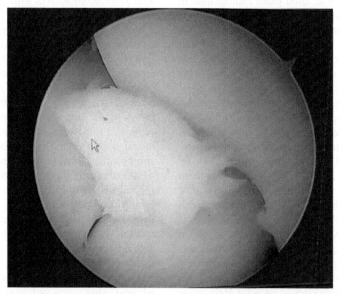

FIG. 19.3 Large loose body in the posterior compartment of the elbow. Arrow indicates OCD lesion capitellum.

return-to-sport rate of only 64%. This data is strongly influenced by the studies from Nobuta et al.[61] and Hennrikus et al.[65] which had much lower return-to-sport rates than the other studies included in the analysis. In the level II study completed by Takahara et al.,[33] the authors found similar outcomes for fragment fixation and removal with smaller unstable lesions (<50% capitellar articular width). However,

with unstable lesions larger than 50% of the capitellar width, the authors reported superior outcomes with either fragment fixation or reconstruction as compared with removal alone.

Another surgical option for large, advanced or irreparable capitellar OCD lesions is osteochondral autograft transfer (OATS), which has been described using autografts from both the rib and the knee.[32,50,51,53,67]

(A)   **(B)**

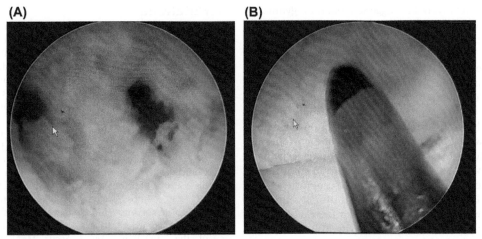

FIG. 19.4 **(A)** Microfracture of osteochondritis dissecans (OCD) defect after debridement. **(B)** OCD lesion after microfracture. Arrow indicates OCD lesion capitellum.

In the previously mentioned meta-analysis by Westermann et al.,[58] the authors found a 95% return to any level of sport rate and 94% return to previous level of sport rate at a mean of 5.9 ± 0.9 months following OATS for capitellar OCD. Notably, the authors reported that OATS provided superior return-to-sport rates when compared with debridement and marrow stimulation (71%) and fragment fixation (64%).

Similar to the knee, there are a number of other cartilage restoration and offloading procedures that are currently being investigated in the literature. One technique of interest is autologous chondrocyte implantation, which has long been studied in the knee.[68,69] Although there are no outcome studies in the elbow published at present, Patzer et al.[56] published a technique paper describing the procedure for arthroscopic autologous chondrocyte implantation for the capitellum. Additionally, Dunn et al.[54] reported on one case with the associated technique for particulated juvenile cartilage transfer. Finally, Mirzayan et al. reported good outcomes and near 100% pain relief with fresh osteochondral allograft transplantation in nine adolescent baseball players.[55]

Another technique of interest is distal humeral osteotomy, originally reported by Yoshizu and colleagues.[70] Similar to the concepts of high tibial osteotomy and distal femoral osteotomy of the knee, the closing wedge distal humeral osteotomy seeks to offload the radiocapitellar joint to allow for OCD healing. Since then, there have been multiple small case series evaluating the utility of the procedure. Kiyoshige et al.[70] reported on the treatment of seven adolescent baseball players, with six of seven players returning to

their prior level of sport. Ueki et al.[57] reported on a series of 17 patients treated with distal humeral osteotomy for capitellar OCD with a minimum follow-up of 2 years. The authors reported poor healing in 2 of 17 lesions, and although all patients returned to sport, only 11 of 17 returned to their preinjury sport of choice. Although promising, the reported outcomes are inferior to other cartilage restoration procedures, suggesting that distal humeral osteotomy alone may find utility as an adjunct or salvage procedure.

OUTCOMES IN FEMALE ATHLETES

Perhaps because of the popularity of baseball in both the United States and Japan, the vast majority of studies on outcomes of OCD treatment have focused on male athletes. Early studies of OCD in female athletes, predominantly gymnasts, suggest that they may have inferior outcomes than their male counterparts.[15,71] Maffulli et al.[71] looked at a series of 12 gymnasts, 6 males and 6 females, and found that only 1 of 12 athletes was able to continue competing at a high level at skeletal maturity. Jackson et al.[15] reported similarly poor results in a series of seven female gymnasts treated with arthroscopic removal of loose bodies, curettage of loose articular margins, and drilling, with only one of seven athletes continuing to compete at follow-up. These findings are in contrast to the earlier series from Singer and Roy,[14] where they found four of five female gymnasts were able to return to sport. The variability of these studies is unquestionably due to the small sizes of these case series and lack of data on lesion grading.

More recent work has suggested that both gymnasts and female athletes have similar outcomes with both conservative and surgical management of elbow OCD. Niu et al.[41] found that gender and sport had no impact on the healing of stable OCD lesions with conservative management. Jones et al.[72] evaluated outcomes of patients after arthroscopic debridement and loose body removal with or without drilling and bone grafting. This study included return-to-sport data on their subgroups, with 8 of 10 baseball players and 4 of 5 gymnasts returning to their preinjury sporting activities. Brownlow et al.[48] also included return-to-sport information for their subgroups after arthroscopic treatment of capitellar OCD. They reported an overall return-to-sport rate of 85%, with six of seven female gymnasts returning to their prior level of activity. This data is supported by the larger case series presented by Yehyawi et al.[73] at the American Society for Hand Surgery in 2018. The authors evaluated 80 OCD lesions in 64 gymnasts that were managed surgically and reported a return to sport rate of 81%. Unfortunately, they did not specify whether the study patients were male or female. However, overall, the data indicates that lesion stability has a much stronger impact on outcomes than gender or sport.

SUMMARY

OCD is a well-recognized cause of elbow pain and disability in adolescent athletes, both male and female. OCD lesions are most commonly seen in athletes who participate in sports that subject the elbow to high valgus and/or axial loads, such as baseball and gymnastics. Female gymnasts may be at particular risk for capitellar injury than their male counterparts. Although the exact mechanism for OCD formation in the elbow has yet to be determined, it likely involves single or repetitive microtrauma to the capitellar epiphysis, which is vulnerable to disordered ossification and necrosis due to a tenuous blood supply. Good treatment outcomes have been seen in early or stable capitellar OCD managed conservatively, regardless of patient gender or sport. Surgical management of advanced or unstable lesions may consist of removal of loose bodies via an open or arthroscopic technique, fragment fixation, or articular surface reconstruction. Good outcomes have been seen with arthroscopic management of smaller (<50% of capitellar width) lesions, regardless of sport or gender. However, larger, unstable lesions may benefit from articular surface reconstruction with OATS or other reconstructive procedures.

REFERENCES

1. Nagura S. The so-called osteochondritis dissecans of König. *Clin Orthop Relat Res.* 1960:18. Available from: https://journals.lww.com/clinorthop/Fulltext/1960/00180/.
2. Edmonds EW, Polousky J. A review of knowledge in osteochondritis dissecans: 123 years of minimal evolution from könig to the ROCK study group general. *Clin Orthop Relat Res.* 2013:1118−1126. Available from: pmc/articles/PMC3586043/reportabstract.
3. Nissen CW. Osteochondritis dissecans of the elbow. *Clin Sports Med.* 2014:251−265. PMID: 24698041. Available from: https://pubmed.ncbi.nlm.nih.gov/24698041/.
4. Churchill RW, Munoz J, Ahmad CS. Osteochondritis dissecans of the elbow. *Curr Rev Musculoskel Med.* 2016:232−239. https://doi.org/10.1007/s12178-016-9342-y. Available from: https://link.springer.com/article/.
5. Baker CL, Romeo AA, Baker CL. Osteochondritis dissecans of the capitellum. *Am J Sports Med.* 2010;38(9):1917−1928. Available from: https://pubmed.ncbi.nlm.nih.gov/20097927/.
6. Weiss JM, Shea KG, Jacobs JC, et al. Incidence of osteochondritis dissecans in adults. *Am J Sports Med.* 2018;46(7):1592−1595. Available from: https://pubmed.ncbi.nlm.nih.gov/29613834/.
7. Lindén B. The incidence of osteochondritis dissecans in the condyles of the femur. *Acta Orthop.* 1976;47(6):664−667. https://doi.org/10.3109/17453677608988756. Available from: https://www-tandfonline-com.ucsf.idm.oclc.org/.
8. Cahill BR. Osteochondritis dissecans of the knee: treatment of juvenile and adult forms. *J Am Acad Orthop Surg.* 1995;3(4):237−247. PMID: 10795030. Available from: https://pubmed.ncbi.nlm.nih.gov/10795030/.
9. Weiss JM, Nikizad H, Shea KG, et al. The incidence of surgery in osteochondritis dissecans in children and adolescents. *Orthop J Sport Med.* 2016;4(3). Available from: pmc/articles/PMC4797230/.
10. Kessler JI, Jacobs JC, Cannamela PC, Weiss JM, Shea KG. Demographics and epidemiology of osteochondritis dissecans of the elbow among children and adolescents. *Orthop J Sport Med.* 2018;6(12). Available from: pmc/articles/PMC6302285.
11. Patel DN, ElAttrache NS, Banffy MB. Osteochondritis dissecans lesion of the radial head. *Am J Orthop.* 2018;47(8). Available from: https://pubmed.ncbi.nlm.nih.gov/30180223/.
12. Kida Y, Morihara T, Kotoura Y, et al. Prevalence and clinical characteristics of osteochondritis dissecans of the humeral capitellum among adolescent baseball players. *Am J Sports Med.* 2014;42(8):1963−1971. Available from: https://pubmed.ncbi.nlm.nih.gov/24944293/.
13. Matsuura T, Suzue N, Iwame T, Nishio S, Sairyo K. Prevalence of osteochondritis dissecans of the capitellum in young baseball players: results based on ultrasonographic findings. *Orthop J Sport Med.* 2014;2(8):1−5. Available from: pmc/articles/PMC4555579.

14. Singer KM, Roy SP. Osteochondrosis of the humeral capitellum. *Am J Sports Med.* 1984;12(5):351–360. https://doi.org/10.1177/036354658401200503. Available from: http://journals.sagepub.com/.

15. Jackson DW, Silvino N, Reiman P. Osteochondritis in the female gymnast's elbow. *Arthrosc J Arthrosc Relat Surg.* 1989;5(2):129–136. PMID:2736009.

16. Dexel J, Marschner K, Beck H, et al. Comparative study of elbow disorders in young high-performance gymnasts. *Int J Sports Med.* 2014;35(11):960–965. https://doi.org/10.1055/s-0034-1371835. Available from: http://www.thieme-connect.de/.

17. Eisenberg K, Wu M, Hart E, Williams K, Bae DS. Differences in clinical presentation of osteochondritis dissecans of the capitellum in males and females. *Orthop J Harvard Med Sch.* 2017;18(June 2017). Available from: http://www.orthojournalhms.org/18/article25_31.html.

18. Chen FS, Rokito AS, Jobe FW. Medial elbow problems in the overhead-throwing athlete. *J Am Acad Orthop Surg.* 2001:99–113.

19. Kajiyama S, Muroi S, Sugaya H, et al. Osteochondritis dissecans of the humeral capitellum in young athletes: comparison between baseball players and gymnasts. *Orthop J Sport Med.* 2017;5(3).

20. Morrey B. *Morrey's the Elbow and Its Disorders.* 2008.

21. Farana R, Strutzenberger G, Exell T, Skypala J, Wiltshire H, Irwin G. Gender differences in technique selection: elbow and wrist joint loading during round off in gymnastics. *ISBS Proc Arch.* 2018;36(1). Available from: https://commons.nmu.edu/.

22. Farana R, Strutzenberger G, Exell T, Skypala J, Wiltshire H, Irwin G. Sex differences in elbow and wrist joint loading during the cartwheel and round off with different hand positions performed by young gymnasts. *J Sports Sci.* 2019;37(13):1449–1456. https://doi.org/10.1080/02640414.2019.1565110. Available from: https://www.tandfonline.com/.

23. Hefti F, Beguiristain J, Krauspe R, et al. Osteochondritis dissecans: a multicenter study of the European pediatric orthopedic society. *J Pediatr Orthop B.* 1999;8(4).

24. Kessler JI, Jacobs JC, Cannamela PC, Shea KG, Weiss JM. Childhood obesity is associated with osteochondritis dissecans of the knee, ankle, and elbow in children and adolescents. *J Pediatr Orthop.* 2018;38(5):e296–e299. Available from: http://journals.lww.com/01241398-201805000-00018.

25. Jacobi M, Wahl P, Bouaicha S, Jakob RP, Gautier E. Association between mechanical axis of the leg and osteochondritis dissecans of the knee: radiographic study on 103 knees. *Am J Sports Med.* 2010;38(7):1425–1428. Available from: https://pubmed.ncbi.nlm.nih.gov/20351199/.

26. Lau BC, Pandya NK. Radiographic comparison of adolescent athletes with elbow osteochondritis dissecans to ulnar collateral ligament injuries and controls. *J Shoulder Elbow Surg.* 2017;26(4):589–595.

27. Schenck RC, Athanasiou KA, Constantinides G, Gomez E. A biomechanical analysis of articular cartilage of the human elbow and a potential relationship to osteochondritis dissecans. *Clin Orthop Relat Res.* 1994;(299): 305–312. Available from: https://pubmed.ncbi.nlm.nih.gov/8119034/.

28. Haraldsson S. On osteochondrosis deformas juvenilis capituli humeri including investigation of intra-osseous vasculature in distal humerus. *Acta Orthop Scand Suppl.* 1959;38.

29. Barrie HJ. Hypertrophy and laminar calcification of cartilage in loose bodies as probable evidence of an ossification abnormality. *J Pathol.* 1980;132(2):161–168. Available from: https://pubmed.ncbi.nlm.nih.gov/6775061/.

30. Barrie HJ. Hypothesis - a diagram of the form and origin of loose bodies in osteochondritis dissecans. *J Rheumatol.* 1984;11(4).

31. Matsuura T, Kashiwaguchi S, Iwase T, Takeda Y, Yasui N. Conservative treatment for osteochondrosis of the humeral capitellum. *Am J Sports Med.* 2008;36(5).

32. Mihara K, Tsutsui H, Nishinaka N, Yamaguchi K. Nonoperative treatment for osteochondritis dissecans of the capitellum. *Am J Sports Med.* 2009;37(2).

33. Takahara M, Mura N, Sasaki J, Harada M, Ogino T. Classification, treatment, and outcome of osteochondritis dissecans of the humeral capitellum. *J Bone Jt Surg.* 2007;89(6): 1205–1214. Available from: https://pubmed.ncbi.nlm.nih.gov/17545422/.

34. Kijowski R, De Smet AA. Radiography of the elbow for evaluation of patients with osteochondritis dissecans of the capitellum. *Skeletal Radiol.* 2005:266–271. https://doi.org/10.1007/s00256-005-0899-6. Available from: https://link.springer.com/.

35. Bowen RE, Otsuka NY, Yoon ST, Lang P. Osteochondral lesions of the capitellum in pediatric patients: role of magnetic resonance imaging. *J Pediatr Orthop.* 2001;21(3).

36. Pill SG, Ganley TJ, Milam A, Lou JE, Meyer JS, Flynn JM. Role of magnetic resonance imaging and clinical criteria in predicting successful nonoperative treatment of osteochondritis dissecans in children. *J Pediatr Orthop.* 2003;23(1).

37. Jans LBO, Ditchfield M, Anna G, Jaremko JL, Verstraete KL. MR imaging findings and MR criteria for instability in osteochondritis dissecans of the elbow in children. *Eur J Radiol.* 2012;81(6):1306–1310. Available from: https://pubmed.ncbi.nlm.nih.gov/21353415/.

38. Itsubo T, Murakami N, Uemura K, et al. Magnetic resonance imaging staging to evaluate the stability of capitellar osteochondritis dissecans lesions. *Am J Sports Med.* 2014; 42(8):1972–1977. Available from: https://pubmed.ncbi.nlm.nih.gov/24817006/.

39. Satake H, Takahara M, Harada M, Maruyama M. Preoperative imaging criteria for unstable osteochondritis dissecans of the capitellum elbow. *Clin Orthop Relat Res.* 2013;471(4):1137–1143. PMID: 22773394. Available from: https://pubmed.ncbi.nlm.nih.gov/22773394/.

40. Nguyen JC, Degnan AJ, Barrera CA, Hee TP, Ganley TJ, Kijowski R. Osteochondritis dissecans of the elbow in children: MRI findings of instability. *Am J Roentgenol.* 2019; 213(5):1145–1151. https://doi.org/10.2214/AJR.19.21855. Available from: https://www.ajronline.org/.

41. Niu EL, Tepolt FA, Bae DS, Lebrun DG, Kocher MS. Nonoperative management of stable pediatric osteochondritis dissecans of the capitellum: predictors of treatment success. *J Shoulder Elbow Surg.* 2018;27(11):2030–2037.

42. Bauer M, Jonsson K, Josefsson PO, Linden B. Osteochondritis dissecans of the elbow: a long-term follow-up study. *Clin Orthop Relat Res.* 1992;284.

43. Mitsunaga MM, Adishian DA, Bianco AJ. Osteochondritis dissecans of the capitellum. *J Trauma Inj Infect Crit Care.* 1982;22(1):53–55. Available from: http://journals.lww.com/00005373-198201000-00010.

44. Mcmanama GB, Micheli LJ, Berry MV, Sohn RS. The surgical treatment of osteochondritis of the capitellum. *Am J Sports Med.* 1985;13(1):11–21. https://doi.org/10.1177/036354658501300103. PMID: 3976976. Available from: http://journals.sagepub.com/.

45. Baumgarten TE, Andrews JR, Satterwhite YE. The arthroscopic classification and treatment of osteochondritis dissecans of the capitellum. *Am J Sports Med.* 1998;26(4).

46. Ruch DS, Cory JW, Poehling GG. The arthroscopic management of osteochondritis dissecans of the adolescent elbow. *Arthroscopy.* 1998;14(8).

47. Byrd JWT, Jones KS. Arthroscopic surgery for isolated capitellar osteochondritis dissecans in adolescent baseball players: minimum three-year follow-up. *Am J Sports Med.* 2002;30(4).

48. Brownlow HC, O'Connor-Read LM, Perko M. Arthroscopic treatment of osteochondritis dissecans of the capitellum. *Knee Surg Sport Traumatol Arthrosc.* 2006;14(2).

49. Rahusen FTG, Brinkman JM, Eygendaal D. Results of arthroscopic debridement for osteochondritis dissecans of the elbow. *Br J Sports Med.* 2006;40(12).

50. Shimada K, Tanaka H, Matsumoto T, et al. Cylindrical costal osteochondral autograft for reconstruction of large defects of the capitellum due to osteochondritis dissecans. *JBJS Essent Surg Tech.* 2012;2(2):e12. Available from: https://pubmed.ncbi.nlm.nih.gov/31321135/.

51. Lyons ML, Werner BC, Gluck JS, et al. Osteochondral autograft plug transfer for treatment of osteochondritis dissecans of the capitellum in adolescent athletes. *J Shoulder Elbow Surg.* 2015;24(7):1098–1105.

52. Nishinaka N, Tsutsui H, Yamaguchi K, Uehara T, Nagai S, Atsumi T. Costal osteochondral autograft for reconstruction of advanced-stage osteochondritis dissecans of the capitellum. *J Shoulder Elbow Surg.* 2014;23(12).

53. Funakoshi T, Momma D, Matsui Y, et al. Autologous osteochondral mosaicplasty for centrally and laterally located, advanced capitellar osteochondritis dissecans in teenage athletes: clinical outcomes, radiography, and magnetic resonance imaging findings. *Am J Sports Med.* 2018; 46(8):1943–1951.

54. Dunn JC, Kusnezov N, Orr J, Mitchell JS. Osteochondral defects of the upper extremity treated with particulated juvenile cartilage transfer. *Hand.* 2015;10(4).

55. Mirzayan R, Lim MJ. Fresh osteochondral allograft transplantation for osteochondritis dissecans of the capitellum in baseball players. *J Shoulder Elbow Surg.* 2016; 25(11).

56. Patzer T, Krauspe R, Hufeland M. Arthroscopic autologous chondrocyte transplantation for osteochondritis dissecans of the elbow. *Arthrosc Tech.* 2016;5(3):e633–e636.

57. Ueki M, Moriya K, Yoshizu T, Tsubokawa N, Kouda H, Endo N. Closed-wedge osteotomy of the distal humerus for treating osteochondritis dissecans of the capitellum in young patients. *Orthop J Sport Med.* 2019;7(10).

58. Westermann RW, Hancock KJ, Buckwalter JA, Kopp B, Glass N, Wolf BR. Return to sport after operative management of osteochondritis dissecans of the capitellum: a systematic review and meta-analysis. *Orthop J Sport Med.* 2016;4(6).

59. Matsuura T, Iwame T, Suzue N, et al. Long-term outcomes of arthroscopic debridement with or without drilling for osteochondritis dissecans of the capitellum in adolescent baseball players: a ≥10-Year follow-up study. *Arthrosc J Arthrosc Relat Surg.* 2020;36(5).

60. Allahabadi S, Bryant J, Mittal A, Pandya N. Outcomes of arthroscopic surgical treatment of osteochondral lesions of the elbow in pediatric and adolescent athletes. *Orthop J Sport Med.* 2020;8(11), 2325967120963054.

61. Nobuta S, Ogawa K, Sato K, Nakagawa T, Hatori M, Itoi E. Clinical outcome of fragment fixation for osteochondritis dissecans of the elbow. *Ups J Med Sci.* 2008;113(2).

62. Takeda H, Watarai K, Matsushita T, Saito T, Terashima Y. A surgical treatment for unstable osteochondritis dissecans lesions of the humeral capitellum in adolescent baseball players. *Am J Sports Med.* 2002;30(5):713–717.

63. Kuwahata Y, Inoue G. Osteochondritis dissecans of the elbow managed by Herbert screw fixation. *Orthopedics.* 1998;21(4).

64. Harada M, Ogino T, Takahara M, Ishigaki D, Kashiwa H, Kanauchi Y. Fragment fixation with a bone graft and dynamic staples for osteochondritis dissecans of the humeral capitellum. *J Shoulder Elbow Surg.* 2002;11(4).

65. Hennrikus WP, Miller PE, Micheli LJ, Waters PM, Bae DS. Internal fixation of unstable in situ osteochondritis dissecans lesions of the capitellum. *J Pediatr Orthop.* 2014; 35(5).

66. Uchida S, Utsunomiya H, Taketa T, et al. Arthroscopic fragment fixation using hydroxyapatite/poly-l-lactate acid thread pins for treating elbow osteochondritis dissecans. *Am J Sports Med.* 2015;43(5).

67. Sato K, Iwamoto T, Matsumura N, et al. Costal osteochondral autograft for advanced osteochondritis dissecans of the humeral capitellum in adolescent and young adult athletes clinical outcomes with a mean follow-up of 4.8 years. *J Bone Jt Surg Am.* 2018;100(11): 903–913.

68. Peterson L, Minas T, Brittberg M, Lindahl A. Treatment of osteochondritis dissecans of the knee with autologous chondrocyte transplantation: results at two to ten years. *J Bone Jt Surg Ser A*. 2003;85-A(Suppl 2):17–24.

69. Carey JL, Shea KG, Lindahl A, Vasiliadis HS, Lindahl C, Peterson L. Autologous chondrocyte implantation as treatment for unsalvageable osteochondritis dissecans: 10- to 25-year follow-up. *Am J Sports Med*. 2020;48(5): 1134–1140. PMID: 32181674.

70. Kiyoshige Y, Takagi M, Yuasa K, Hamasaki M. Closed-wedge osteotomy for osteochondritis dissecans of the capitellum: a 7- to 12-year follow-up. *Am J Sports Med*. 2000;28(4).

71. Maffulli N, Chan D, Aldridge MJ. Derangement of the articular surfaces of the elbow in young gymnasts. *J Pediatr Orthop*. 1992;12(3):344–350.

72. Jones KJ, Wiesel BB, Sankar WN, Ganley TJ. Arthroscopic management of osteochondritis dissecans of the capitellum: mid-term results in adolescent athletes. *J Pediatr Orthop*. 2010;30(1).

73. Yehyawi SE, Peck K, Bartkiw MJ, Hastings H. Five-year follow-up of adolescent gymnasts after surgical treatment of osteochondritis dissecans of the elbow. *J Hand Surg Am*. 2018;43(9).

CHAPTER 20

Epidemiology of Female Versus Male Athletic Injuries

HANNAH L. BRADSELL, BS • RACHEL M. FRANK, MD

INTRODUCTION

The world of sports has historically been dominated by males and much of our knowledge surrounding athletic injuries originates from our understanding of the male athlete. Data on injuries sustained by the female athlete is often underrepresented in sports medicine research, and as the number of female athletes participating in sports continues to grow, there is a significant need for an improved overall understanding of the female athlete and the associated injuries. Specifically, since 1972, the year Title IX was established, there has been a nearly 1000% increase in females playing high-school sports and a 600% increase in female participation in collegiate varsity sports.[1] Female athletes may be predisposed to specific risk factors that increase their chance of injury, such as differences in anatomy and biomechanics compared to males, and these risk factors can be easily overlooked when they are not fully understood. In order to counter these risks, acknowledgment of gender-based differences in injury presentation is necessary for proper injury assessment and treatment to allow for successful return to play and reduced risk of reinjury. A better understanding of injury patterns and an increase in prevention programs tailored specifically to the female athlete are important to ultimately provide the most effective care for this growing population.

With increasing representation of both males and females in a variety of sports, comparative studies focusing on gender differences in injury rates and mechanisms are also increasing. However, female athletes continue to be underrepresented in the development of solutions and interventions based on such studies. For example, FIFA 11+ is a well-established prevention program developed for soccer players to decrease the risk of anterior cruciate ligament (ACL) injuries. In a systematic review, a 30% reduction rate was reported for male soccer players and a 22% reduction was seen in females, but only three of the nine studies reviewed included female athletes.[2] Therefore there is a lack of data for females using this current prevention program, while females are two to eight times more likely to experience an ACL injury than males.[3] Additionally, a separate systematic review reported that current prevention programs for ACL injuries have reduced risk by 85% in males compared with only 52% in females.[4] Continuing to study the differences and applying them to the development of prevention programs and treatment methods specific to the female athlete is imperative in avoiding the physical, psychologic, and financial burdens that come with injuries. A greater understanding of the vast anatomic, physiologic, hormonal, and biomechanical gender differences is key to maintain successful female participation in athletics. This chapter will focus on the epidemiology of female athletic injuries, with the goal of providing clinicians evidence-based data to better understand just how common (or uncommon) certain injuries are, in order to be able to better guide patients, parents, and coaches.

EPIDEMIOLOGY BASICS

Numerous studies have reported the epidemiology of injuries in female athletes compared to male athletes. In more recent years, differences in the types of injury, mechanisms of injury, and potential biological and anatomic explanations for differences in rates have also been explored. In 2018, Lin et al.[3] performed a literature review of existing published data that discussed gender differences in epidemiology, risk factors, management, and outcomes among common sports injuries. Interestingly, there was a higher incidence in females in three main injury types: bone stress injuries, ACL injuries, and concussions. In 2019, Brant et al.[5] studied the rates of lower extremity injuries across gender-comparable sports at the high-school level

The Female Athlete. https://doi.org/10.1016/B978-0-323-75985-4.00011-8

over a period of 10 years. In all the eight sports studied, females had a higher rate of injury than males (9.14 vs. 7.30 injuries per 10,000 athlete exposures (AEs), respectively). Out of all the injuries reported, 56% of them were sustained by females. Additionally, females had a higher injury rate within each individual sport, the highest seen in soccer (15.87), and females sustained a greater number of injuries within each specific injury type in every sport studied, except track and field. Among the incidences, females also experienced a higher percentage of severe injuries, characterized by over 3 weeks of time away from participation or medical disqualification, in each sport except volleyball. This study also noted that among the incidences of injuries, magnetic resonance imaging evaluation was higher in females, relating to an increased medical cost for females who sustained injuries.[5]

In a separate study, Rechel et al.[6] reported the epidemiology of injuries at the high-school level that required surgery over a 5-year period and found an overall rate of 1.45 per 10,000 AEs and 6.3% of all high-school sport-related injuries nationally. Among gender-comparable sports, including soccer, basketball, and baseball/softball, females experienced a higher overall injury rate of 1.20 compared with males at 0.94 per 10,000 AEs ($P = .004$) and a significantly greater injury rate within soccer and basketball. Baseball and softball were the only gender-comparable sports where males had a higher rate of injury incidences, but it was not found to be significant. Of note, over half of soccer and basketball injuries were related to the knee and females made up a significantly greater proportion of those knee injuries in both sports (74.4% in soccer and 68.8% in basketball). Overall, 68.7% of injuries sustained by females were of the knee and 1.6% were of the shoulder when compared to males in whom 41.5% of injuries were o the knee and 11.1% were of the shoulder ($P < .001$). In addition, females experienced complete ligament sprains at a significantly higher rate than males (54.1% vs. 23.2%; $P < .001$), whereas males faced more fractures (30.0% vs. 17.5%; $P < .001$) and dislocations (9.1% vs. 1.1%; $P < .001$). Notably, 90.8% of complete ligament sprains occurred at the knee. Interestingly, of the 48% of injuries that required medical disqualification for the season, 45.3% were complete ligament sprains while 18.6% of injuries resulting in time loss of less than 1 week from participation were fractures. Furthermore, injuries resulting in medical disqualifications from sports activities for the season occurred in 55.6% of females compared to 45.0% of males.[6] In a separate study, Chan et al.[7] reported the epidemiology of

Achilles tendon injuries at the collegiate level. Although the injury rate was comparable between females and males, it is worth noting that females had greater time loss, higher rates of season-ending injuries, and higher operative rates, as well as poorer postoperative performance. Additionally, the recurrence rate among female athletes was almost twice as high compared to male athletes.[7]

In 2018, Baugh et al.[8] described the epidemiology of injuries specific to volleyball teams in the National Collegiate Athletic Association (NCAA) using data from 2013 to 2014 and 2014−15 seasons. Consistent with the previous epidemiologic studies mentioned, female athletes experienced injury at a significantly higher rate overall (7.07 per 10,000 AEs) compared with males (4.69) as well as a higher rate of time-loss injuries, indicated by greater than 24 h of participation restriction, compared with males (2.62 vs. 1.75). The lower extremities were found to be the most frequently injured location in both time-loss injuries and non-time-loss injuries, and females had a higher proportion of lower extremity injuries within both groups. Specific to time-loss injuries, ankle and knee injuries were the most frequent type sustained by female athletes, whereas concussions due to ball contact and hand and wrist sprains occurred most frequently in male athletes. It was noted that the higher injury rate seen in females could be attributed to the higher rates of injury during practices and in preseason compared with males.[8]

With respect to the mechanism of injury, each of the abovementioned studies that analyzed gender differences in this area reported that males were more likely to experience an injury after player-to-player contact, whereas females experienced primarily noncontact injuries.[5,6] In a similar sense, a higher rate of overuse-related injuries was found in females compared to greater ball contact-related injuries found in males.[8] Additionally, significantly higher rates of injury were sustained during competition compared to during practice among all athletes.[6,8] After providing possible explanations as to why this trend may exist (e.g., increased aggressiveness, exposure to high-risk activities and physical contact, and illegal activity), Rechel et al.[6] recommended developing new rules, strict officiating, and implementing drills in practice that teach high-risk skills to improve these rates. It is worth mentioning that this study also discussed areas to focus on when implementing prevention efforts for male-dominated sports, such as football and wrestling. However, prevention techniques for female athletes and even for gender-comparable sports were not described. For example, the authors provided explanations for understanding the mechanism of shoulder injuries and recommendations for potential solutions for prevention of these injuries, which occurred at a higher rate in male athletes, but at a lower overall rate compared with other injuries. No such suggestions for the prevention of knee injuries were mentioned, which made up the greatest proportion of total injuries requiring surgery and also had significantly higher rates in females. The authors merely suggested that efforts should be made and only cited other studies that have provided explanations as to why the gender differences may exist in complete ligament sprains of the knee.[6] On the contrary, Brant et al.[5] mentioned the importance of improving preventative care particularly for females, given their high risk of lower extremity sports injuries, in order to reduce rates of injury and the impact injuries can have on athletes. Similarly, Baugh et al.[8] discussed possible explanations and specific prevention methods that alluded to the gender differences found in the mechanisms of injury, type of injury, and the time during the season that the injury occurred. The authors also suggested that future research should address these differences.

CONCUSSION EPIDEMIOLOGY: GENDER-BASED DIFFERENCES

Studies on concussions have become increasingly popular, particularly in contact sports such as football and hockey, and mainly focus on male athletes involved in these sports. However, female athletes have been shown to have arguably higher rates of concussion incidences, especially in gender-comparable sports. Specifically, one literature review exploring gender differences in concussion incidence found that 9 out of the 10 studies reviewed had reports of higher concussion rates in females.[9] As an entire chapter is dedicated to understand concussions in the female athlete, this section will focus primarily on epidemiologic differences in concussions between males and females.

A study published in 2019 by Kerr et al.[10] described the epidemiology of sport-related concussions across 20 sports at the high-school level during the 2013–14 to 2017–18 school years. Overall, 9542 concussions were reported for an overall injury rate of 4.17 per 10,000 AEs, with football having the highest rate of 10.40. However, among gender-comparable sports (i.e., soccer, basketball, swimming, baseball/softball, cross-country, and track and field), females experienced higher concussion rates than males (3.35 vs. 1.51), as well as a larger proportion of recurrent concussions (9.3% vs. 6.4%). Interestingly, the rate of recurrent

concussions decreased over the course of the 5-year study period. This trend is most likely due to legislations implementing mandatory concussion protocols in youth and high-school athletics, which have been passed in all 50 American states and the District of Columbia beginning in 2009.[11,12]

Since the passing of these traumatic brain injury laws, studies have demonstrated an increase in concussion rates, possibly due to increased awareness and reporting, and a decrease in recurrent concussion rates, likely accredited to the improved management of removal from play and return-to-play requirements.[13] It is worth mentioning that studies consistently show higher rates of concussion incidences in females than males over time among gender-comparable sports, both before and an even greater increase after the passing of concussion policies ($P < .001$).[13] Similar results were found in a previous study looking at 20 sports among high-school players between 2008 and 2010.[14] Over the course of the study, 1936 concussions were reported for an overall rate of 2.5 per 10,000 AEs and accounted for 13.2% of the total injuries. Comparing all sports, football had the highest percentage of concussions (47.1%) and the highest rate (6.4). Within gender-comparable sports, females had a significantly higher concussion incidence rate than males (1.7 vs. 1.0), and in 18 out of the 20 sports studied, females experienced more recurrent concussions than males.[14]

O'Connor et al.[15] studied high-school concussion trends between 2011 and 2014 and reported a 56% higher incidence rate in females (1.56) than males (1.00) in gender-comparable sports. The researchers also found that although there was no gender difference in the number of symptoms, 44.4% of males reported symptom resolution within less than 7 days versus only 32.2% of females. The authors noted that a possible explanation for this trend could be based off of social norms and their influence on likeliness to report symptoms.[15] For example, male athletes may believe that they are expected to have a "tough attitude" about injury, whereas females may be less likely to be influenced by their peers' opinions on concussions.[16,17] At the collegiate level, Davis-Hayes et al.[18] studied sport-related concussions among the Columbia University varsity athletes in a 15-year retrospective cohort consisting of 68.5% males and 31.5% females. Despite the difference in representation, the prevalence of having at least one concussion was greater in female athletes than in male athletes (23.3% and 17.0%, respectively; $P = .01$). Notably, in contrast to the previously mentioned studies, no gender differences were found in the return-to-play duration, the number and types of symptoms, or the neurophysiologic test performance.[18] A study by Zuckerman et al.[19] reported that the relative risk of sustaining a concussion among female athletes at the collegiate level was 53% higher in basketball, 83% higher in soccer, and 265% higher in baseball/softball when compared with male athletes. Notably, this same study reported that the risk in women's lacrosse, a noncontact sport, was 64% higher than that in men's lacrosse, a contact sport, despite the rule changes implemented in women's lacrosse to reduce contact.[19] Generally speaking, reports consistently showed player-to-player contact as the most frequent mechanism of concussion injuries in male athletes, with incidence rates between 55% and 77% compared to 40%–53% in females. Player-to-playing surface contact or player-to-ball contact tend to be the most common cause of concussions in female athletes, with incidence rates reported between 34% and 45% compared to 18%–24% in males.[9,10,14,15]

Interestingly, a retrospective, self-report-based study in collegiate athletes observed association patterns between concussions and musculoskeletal injuries.[20] Overall, those who reported a history of concussion were more likely to also report a history of ankle sprains and knee injuries compared to those with no concussion history ($P = .004$). Females were found to have increased reports of concussions, ankle sprains, and knee injuries at rates of 29.5%, 48.9%, and 41.0%, respectively, compared with males with rates of 18.0%, 43.0%, and 23.0%, respectively. Specific to females, those who reported multiple concussions had significantly greater odds of also reporting ankle sprains and knee injuries compared to those without a concussion history (73.5% vs. 39.0%). However, this trend was not seen in females who reported a history of only one concussion and it was not found to be statistically significant in male athletes with a history of either one or multiple concussions. An important limitation of this study is that the type of relationship between concussions and musculoskeletal injuries was unclear with regard to which injury came first, as the study was conducted based on self-reported injury histories without a timeline, but the researchers did determine that a relationship existed in this population.[20]

Many researchers have attempted to provide reasonable explanations for gender-based differences observed in concussion rates, mechanisms, severity, and the associated number of symptoms. A range of potential factors that have been described include neck musculature and strength, cerebral blood flow and cerebrovascular organization, and differences in hormonal environments.[3,10] However, a physiologic basis for explaining the gender differences in the risk of sustaining a concussion is controversial because of the very limited evidence of supporting data and minimal understanding of the role these factors may play. Additional studies directly assessing a variety of factors and their relation to observed gender differences in concussion rates are necessary in order to ensure a proper approach toward prevention and treatment methods on an individual basis.

EPIDEMIOLOGY OF UPPER EXTREMITY INJURIES: GENDER-BASED DIFFERENCES
Shoulder Instability

While the topic of shoulder instability is described in detail in another chapter, it is important to highlight epidemiologic differences between males and females specific to this common shoulder pathology. Historical studies have typically reported anterior shoulder instability to be a male-dominated injury pattern, and most studies have few (or no) female patients, making it difficult to extrapolate findings to the female patient population. A study by Patzkowski et al.[21] analyzed shoulder instability in 36 collegiate female athletes who underwent surgical intervention. The authors noted that previous reports have shown higher instability rates in males, but they also had an underrepresentation of females in their respective studies. When comparing gender-comparable sports, the rates of shoulder instability were actually equal between males and females. Additionally, compared with previous studies that included both males and females, the authors of this study found a higher rate of labral tears and humeral avulsion of the glenohumeral ligament lesions in this female cohort. When compared with an equivalent population of male athletes from a separate study, females experienced greater injuries while participating in noncontact sports and had more combined (anterior and posterior) labral tears. The authors reported that females were two times more likely than males to experience shoulder instability after contact with an object or contact with the ground, whereas males were more frequently injured due to player-to-player collision.[21]

Researchers have attempted to identify potential underlying neuromuscular differences that may explain gender-based differences in the rates of shoulder instability seen in athletes. Often studied is the condition of general joint hypermobility, which has been suggested as a possible cause for increased incidences of joint instability, but the exact relationship is inconclusive. It is important to note that joint laxity, defined as the physiologic and asymptomatic motion of the glenohumeral joint that allows for normal range of motion, is not the same as joint instability, defined as symptomatic and abnormal motion of the glenohumeral joint that causes pain, subluxation, or dislocation of the shoulder.[22] Furthermore, hypermobility is considered when generalized joint laxity (four or more laxity test results are positive) is associated with musculoskeletal complaints, which appears to be more common in females.[22] One study found an association between general joint hypermobility, measured using the Beighton scale, and glenohumeral joint instability, reporting that patients with hypermobility (a Beighton scale score of 2 or more) were almost 2.5 times more likely to have a history of glenohumeral joint instability.[23] In this study, females were more likely to have general joint hypermobility and higher overall Beighton scale scores compared with males, but interestingly, patient gender was found to be unrelated to having a history of instability. Notably, Reuter and Fichthorn[24] reported that rates of general joint hypermobility were not significantly different between females (16.2%) and males (8.7%), but females did have a significantly higher rate of localized joint hypermobility than males. Additionally, fewer females had a Beighton scale score of 0 compared to males (22.6% vs. 44.2%). However, contrary to the findings by Cameron et al.[23] there was no increased risk for musculoskeletal injury in young female adults with general joint hypermobility. Johnson and Robinson[25] reviewed shoulder instability in patients with joint hyperlaxity and stated that male and female athletes were equally affected by acquired joint hyperlaxity.[25]

Other studies have reported that females undergoing surgery for shoulder instability have lower postoperative scores, greater functional deficits, and poorer outcomes compared with males.[26,27] The reason for this is unclear, and certainly, further research is needed to better delineate why female gender is a risk factor for worse outcomes.

LOWER EXTREMITY EPIDEMIOLOGY: GENDER-BASED DIFFERENCES

Ankle Injuries

Several studies have analyzed the epidemiology of ankle injuries in various sports and reported notable differences within multiple aspects of injury between female and male athletes. Hunt et al.[28] collected prospective data over a 2-year period to evaluate the epidemiology of foot and ankle injuries of NCAA

Division I athletes participating in 37 sports. Foot and ankle injuries accounted for 27% of all injuries, and women's gymnastics, women's cross-country, women's soccer, and men's cross-country were the four sports with the highest incidence rates. Overall, female athletes had a greater incidence of foot and ankle injuries than males (4.07 vs. 3.94 per 1000 AEs; $P < .05$) and sustained these injuries at a significantly higher rate (53% vs. 47%; $P < .05$). In addition, females experienced a significantly higher proportion of injuries resulting in at least 1 day of missed participation in comparison to males. Furthermore, the average number of days missed was 71.2 days for females and 43.8 days for males.[28]

Hosea et al.[29] explored gender-based differences in the epidemiology of ankle injuries in basketball players, including at both the collegiate and high-school levels. The authors found that females had a significantly greater risk than males of sustaining an ankle injury (a ratio of 1.25:1) both overall and specifically for Grade I ankle sprains, which accounted for 72% of the total ankle injuries documented ($P = .0001$). There was no significant difference in risk between males and females for Grade II and Grade III ankle sprains, fractures, or syndesmosis injuries. Additionally, as the level of competition increased from high school to college, the risk of suffering an ankle injury doubled for both genders.[29] Similar trends were observed in a separate study that investigated the effects of gender, level of competition, and sport on first-time ankle ligament trauma.[30] In this study, a total of 901 high-school and collegiate athletes (544 female and 347 male athletes) participating in basketball, soccer, lacrosse, and field hockey were included for analysis. Ankle ligament sprains due to an inversion injury occurred in 43 athletes (29 female and 14 male athletes), resulting in an incidence rate of 0.85 sprains per 1000 AEs. Overall, the risk of sustaining an ankle sprain was higher in females than in males, but it was not found to be statistically significant. Notably, female basketball players had a significantly greater risk than male basketball players.[30] Contrary to the study by Hosea et al.[29] the relative risk of suffering a first-time ankle injury was similar between high-school and collegiate athletes in this population.[30] On the other hand, it was noted by Beynnon et al.[30] that the complimentary data between these two studies suggests that there could be a gender bias for ankle ligament sprains that may depend on sport. Variations in anatomic alignment and neuromuscular control between males and females in combination with different demands in their respective sports could explain why this trend was observed. Additionally, differences in mechanisms of muscle recruitment that have been studied for ACL injuries have increased awareness that these same differences could also exist in ankle instability.[29]

Anterior Cruciate Ligament Injuries

Perhaps the most common acute injury that has been consistently reported to have a significantly higher incidence in females than males is ACL injuries. Over 50% of annual ACL injuries occur in high-school and collegiate athletes and females are two to eight times more likely than males to sustain an ACL injury.[3] In a systematic review, Montalvo et al.[31] reported rates of ACL injury risk across sports subclassified by the level of contact. In every category, females sustained ACL injuries at a higher rate than males. In contact sports, the total rate of injury was 1.51 per 10,000 AEs (females, 1.88; males, 0.87; $P < .0001$). For fixed-object high-impact rational landing activities (i.e., gymnastics, obstacle courses in military training and races, etc.), the overall injury rate was 2.62, with significantly higher rates in females than males (4.80 vs. 1.75, respectively, $P < .001$). In collision sports, limited-contact sports, and noncontact sports, females had higher ACL injury rates than males, but these results were not found to be statistically significant.[31]

A review of the difference between male and female ACL tears reported that the risk of ACL injury in collegiate soccer and basketball players was 4.4%–5% in females versus 1.7% in males.[32] The same review noted gender-based trends of surgical outcomes after ACL reconstruction and found that initial outcomes following surgery were poorer in females, but at 2 year after operation the results appeared to be equal.

Ryman Augustsson et al.[33] conducted a study in a youth athlete population to understand the role played by lower extremity muscle strength in traumatic knee injuries. In their study cohort, the authors found that 17% of females sustained an ACL injury compared to 2% of males ($P = .001$), and a significant majority of injured females were among the weak muscle strength group compared to the strong group. There was no difference observed in injury rates between the two weak and strong muscle strength groups within the male cohort. Within the weak muscle group, the rate of traumatic knee injury in females was significantly higher at 0.66 injuries per athlete compared with males who had a rate of 0.19 ($P < .0001$); within the strong muscle group, no gender difference was observed. With this data, the authors suggested that weaker lower extremity

muscle strength could be an important risk factor for ACL injuries in female athletes and that it should be included in screening for injury prevention training.[33] Additional anatomic and biomechanical risk factors that have been studied include gender differences in quadriceps angles, width of the intercondylar notch, ligament size, knee abduction during landing, and muscle activation patterns, among many others.[3,32,33]

OVERUSE INJURY EPIDEMIOLOGY: GENDER-BASED DIFFERENCES

Overuse injuries are incredibly common among all levels of female athletes. In a review describing stress fractures in female athletes, Abbott and colleagues[34] assessed risk factors and reported that overall, stress fractures account for up to 10% of orthopedic injuries and 20% of sports medicine injuries. Notably, up to 13% of stress fractures occur in females and between 80% and 95% are in the lower extremities. Several other studies have consistently reported higher rates of stress fracture injuries in females compared with males.[35–40]

In 2019, Valasek et al.[41] performed a retrospective chart review in pediatric patients to explore age and gender differences of overuse injuries. Males had higher proportions of apophysis, physis, and articular cartilage injuries particularly of the upper extremities, mainly attributable to overhead throwing in baseball, as this was the sport that resulted in the most injuries among males. On the other hand, females had higher rates of injuries to bones, injuries to tendons, and "other" problems, such as patellofemoral pain syndrome, medial tibial stress syndrome, and exertional compartment syndrome. Females additionally had greater lower extremity and pelvis overuse injuries, the majority of which were sustained during track and field and cross-country.[41]

Among some of the most common overuse injuries are stress injuries, including stress fractures and stress reactions, which are caused by cumulative and repetitive impact resulting in abnormal bone remodeling.[35,42] Rizzone et al.[35] researched the epidemiology of stress fractures in collegiate athletes over a 10-year period and reported an overall injury rate of 5.70 per 100,000 AEs and a total of 671 incidences of stress fractures during 11,778,145 AEs. Women's cross-country had the highest injury rate (28.59), followed by women's gymnastics (25.58) and women's outdoor track (22.26). Among gender-comparable sports, female athletes had a higher overall rate of stress fractures compared with male athletes (9.13 vs. 4.44), as well as higher rates within basketball, cross-country, soccer, indoor track, and outdoor track. Stress fractures sustained by female athletes occurred at the highest rate during preseason and more often in the foot and lower leg, while male athletes experienced greater stress fractures in the lower back, lumbar spine, and pelvis. Season-ending stress fractures and recurrent stress fractures did not differ between males and females, and they accounted for 20% and 22% of total stress fractures, respectively.[35] Additionally, the researchers observed higher rates of stress fracture incidence in collegiate athletes (5.70 per 100,000 AEs) compared to recent data on stress fracture incidence in high-school athletes (1.54 per 100,000 AEs).[35,36]

Frequently associated with stress fractures is the female athlete triad/RED-S (relative energy deficiency in sport), which consists of three components, namely, low energy availability with or without disordered eating, menstrual dysfunction, and low bone mineral density (BMD).[43] The presence of the components alone or in combination presents a significant health risk to physically active females, and having just one or two of the components can lead to a diagnosis of the female athlete triad.[44,45] Furthermore, as the number of female athlete triad-related risk factors an athlete has increases, the cumulative risk for bone stress injury also increases.[46] A study by Nose-Ogura et al.[43] assessed the risk of stress fractures due to the female athlete triad in elite female athletes and found that amenorrhea was present in 39.0% of female athletes, low energy availability was present in 14.0%, and low BMD was present in 22.7% of female athletes. A combined 19.4% of participants had a variation of two out of the three components of the female athlete triad and 5.3% had all three components.[43] The female athlete triad/RED-S and its impact on the female athlete is discussed in detail in a separate chapter. Overall, studies continue to show that all female athletes in general, not just endurance athletes, are at high risk for stress fracture development and various intrinsic and extrinsic risk factors are at play. Awareness of the epidemiology among female athletes and the knowledge of the risks and how these injuries present themselves can aid in an accurate, detailed diagnosis. Additionally, early screening for all contributing factors can facilitate quicker return to play while still allowing efficient bone healing. A multidisciplinary approach toward managing all potential causes of overuse injuries is necessary in creating effective individualized treatment strategies for the female athlete.[47] A compilation of recommendations for evidence-based care can be found in Table 20.1.

TABLE 20.1
Recommendations for Prevention and Care of Bone Stress Injury in Female Athletes.

PREVENTION

Prehabilitation at young age (i.e., physical therapy, gate training, etc.)

Early screening and management for female athlete triad components

Sufficient vitamin D intake during adolescence

Educate coaches, trainers, parents, and athletes on the epidemiology and recognizing the signs and symptoms

Monitor training load and utilize appropriate strength and conditioning regimens

TREATMENT

Use of a multidisciplinary approach for treatment of all contributing factors

Consideration of biological and anatomic variations

Activity modification

Non-weight-bearing to facilitate initial healing

Proper rest time and gradual return to play

Return to play once able to participate in activity pain free

SUMMARY

With the continuous growth of female participation in sports, it is critical to increase the knowledge and awareness of the epidemiology of female athletic injuries. Much of our current understanding of musculoskeletal injuries has originated from studying the male athlete, and further research is necessary to continue to establish important biological, anatomic, and biomechanical differences between males and females. A better understanding of gender-related differences and their direct relation to injury is important in ultimately developing more effective, individualized prevention programs and treatment methods.

REFERENCES

1. Ladd AL. The sports bra, the ACL, and title IX — the game in play. *Clin Orthop Relat Res.* 2014;472(6):1681−1684.
2. Al Attar WSA, et al. How effective are F-MARC injury prevention programs for soccer players? A systematic review and meta-analysis. *Sports Med.* 2016;46(2):205−217.
3. Lin CY, et al. Sex differences in common sports injuries. *PM R.* 2018;10(10):1073−1082.

4. Sadoghi P, Von Keudell A, Vavken P. Effectiveness of anterior cruciate ligament injury prevention training programs. *J Bone Joint Surg Am.* 2012;94(9):769–776.

5. Brant JA, et al. Rates and patterns of lower extremity sports injuries in all gender-comparable US high school sports. *Orthop J Sports Med.* 2019;7(10), 232596711987305.

6. Rechel JA, Collins CL, Comstock RD. Epidemiology of injuries requiring surgery among high school athletes in the United States, 2005 to 2010. *J Trauma.* 2011;71(4): 982–989.

7. Chan JJ, et al. Epidemiology of Achilles tendon injuries in collegiate level athletes in the United States. *Int Orthop.* 2020;44.

8. Baugh CM, et al. Descriptive epidemiology of injuries sustained in National Collegiate Athletic Association Men's and Women's Volleyball, 2013-2014 to 2014-2015. *Sport Health.* 2018;10(1):60–69.

9. Dick RW. Is there a gender difference in concussion incidence and outcomes? *Br J Sports Med.* 2009;43(Suppl_1): i46–i50.

10. Kerr ZY, et al. Concussion incidence and trends in 20 high school sports. *Pediatrics.* 2019;144(5):e20192180.

11. *Heads up on Concussion in Sports Policies*; January 13, 2020. Available from: https://www.cdc.gov/headsup/policy/index.html.

12. Green L. *Legal Perspectives, Recommendations on State Concussion Laws;* 2014. Available from: https://www.nfhs.org/articles/legal-perspectives-recommendations-on-state-concussion-laws/.

13. Yang J, et al. New and recurrent concussions in high-school athletes before and after traumatic brain injury laws, 2005-2016. *Am J Public Health.* 2017;107(12):1916–1922.

14. Marar M, et al. Epidemiology of concussions among United States high school athletes in 20 sports. *Am J Sports Med.* 2012;40(4):747–755.

15. O'Connor KL, et al. Epidemiology of sport-related concussions in high school athletes: national athletic treatment, injury and outcomes network (NATION), 2011-2012 through 2013-2014. *J Athl Train.* 2017; 52(3):175–185.

16. Bloodgood B, et al. Exploration of awareness, knowledge, and perceptions of traumatic brain injury among American youth athletes and their parents. *J Adolesc Health.* 2013;53(1):34–39.

17. Kroshus E, et al. *Social Norms Theory and Concussion Education.* Health Education Research; 2015:cyv047.

18. Davis-Hayes C, et al. Sex-specific outcomes and predictors of concussion recovery. *J Am Acad Orthop Surg.* 2017; 25(12):818–828.

19. Zuckerman SL, et al. Epidemiology of sports-related concussion in NCAA athletes from 2009-2010 to 2013-2014: incidence, recurrence, and mechanisms. *Am J Sports Med.* 2015;43(11):2654–2662.

20. Houston MN, et al. Sex and number of concussions influence the association between concussion and musculoskeletal injury history in collegiate athletes. *Brain Inj.* 2018;32(11):1353–1358.

21. Patzkowski JC, et al. Pathoanatomy of shoulder instability in collegiate female athletes. *Am J Sports Med.* 2019;47(8): 1909–1914.

22. Brown GA, Tan JL, Kirkley A. The lax shoulder in females. Issues, answers, but many more questions. *Clin Orthop Relat Res.* 2000;(372):110–122.

23. Cameron KL, et al. Association of generalized joint hypermobility with a history of glenohumeral joint instability. *J Athl Train.* 2010;45(3):253–258.

24. Reuter PR, Fichthorn KR. Prevalence of generalized joint hypermobility, musculoskeletal injuries, and chronic musculoskeletal pain among American university students. *PeerJ.* 2019;7:e7625.

25. Johnson SM, Robinson CM. Shoulder instability in patients with joint hyperlaxity. *J Bone Joint Surg Am.* 2010; 92(6):1545–1557.

26. Kaipel M, et al. Sex-related outcome differences after arthroscopic shoulder stabilization. *Orthopedics.* 2010; 33(3).

27. Largacha M, et al. Deficits in shoulder function and general health associated with sixteen common shoulder diagnoses: a study of 2674 patients. *J Shoulder Elbow Surg.* 2006; 15(1):30–39.

28. Hunt KJ, et al. Incidence and epidemiology of foot and ankle injuries in elite collegiate athletes. *Am J Sports Med.* 2017;45(2):426–433.

29. Hosea TM, Carey CC, Harrer MF. The gender issue: epidemiology of ankle injuries in athletes who participate in basketball. *Clin Orthop Relat Res.* 2000;(372):45–49.

30. Beynnon BD, et al. First-time inversion ankle ligament trauma. *Am J Sports Med.* 2005;33(10):1485–1491.

31. Montalvo AM, et al. Anterior cruciate ligament injury risk in sport: a systematic review and meta-analysis of injury incidence by sex and sport classification. *J Athl Train.* 2019;54(5):472–482.

32. Sutton KM, Bullock JM. Anterior cruciate ligament rupture: differences between males and females. *J Am Acad Orthop Surg.* 2013;21(1):41–50.

33. Ryman Augustsson S, Ageberg E. Weaker lower extremity muscle strength predicts traumatic knee injury in youth female but not male athletes. *BMJ Open Sport Exerc Med.* 2017;3(1):e000222.

34. Abbott A, et al. Part I: epidemiology and risk factors for stress fractures in female athletes. *Phys Sportsmed.* 2019: 1–8.

35. Rizzone KH, et al. The epidemiology of stress fractures in collegiate student-athletes, 2004-2005 through 2013-2014 academic years. *J Athl Train.* 2017;52(10):966–975.

36. Changstrom BG, et al. Epidemiology of stress fracture injuries among US high school athletes, 2005-2006 through 2012-2013. *Am J Sports Med.* 2015;43(1):26–33.

37. Chen Y-T, Tenforde AS, Fredericson M. Update on stress fractures in female athletes: epidemiology, treatment,

and prevention. *Curr Rev Musculoskelet Med.* 2013;6(2): 173–181.

38. Wright AA, et al. Risk factors associated with lower extremity stress fractures in runners: a systematic review with meta-analysis. *Br J Sports Med.* 2015;49(23):1517–1523.

39. Wentz L, et al. Females have a greater incidence of stress fractures than males in both military and athletic populations: a systemic review. *Mil Med.* 2011;176(4): 420–430.

40. Sonneville KR, et al. Vitamin D, calcium, and dairy intakes and stress fractures among female adolescents. *Arch Pediatr Adolesc Med.* 2012;166(7).

41. Valasek AE, et al. Age and sex differences in overuse injuries presenting to pediatric sports medicine clinics. *Clin Pediatr.* 2019;58(7):770–777.

42. Kiel J, Kaiser K. Stress reaction and fractures. In: *StatPearls.* Treasure Island (FL): StatPearls Publishing; 2020.

43. Nose-Ogura S, et al. Risk factors of stress fractures due to the female athlete triad: differences in teens and twenties. *Scand J Med Sci Sports.* 2019;29(10):1501–1510.

44. Nattiv A, et al. American College of Sports Medicine position stand. The female athlete triad. *Med Sci Sports Exerc.* 2007;39(10):1867–1882.

45. Matzkin E, Curry EJ, Whitlock K. Female athlete triad. *J Am Acad Orthop Surg.* 2015;23(7):424–432.

46. Barrack MT, et al. Higher incidence of bone stress injuries with increasing female athlete triad–related risk factors. *Am J Sports Med.* 2014;42(4):949–958.

47. Abbott A, et al. Part II: presentation, diagnosis, classification, treatment, and prevention of stress fractures in female athletes. *Phys Sportsmed.* 2019:1–8.

CHAPTER 21

Overuse Injuries in Females

ARIANNA L. GIANAKOS, DO • SCOTT BUZIN, DO • MARY K. MULCAHEY, MD

INTRODUCTION

Overuse injuries result from cumulative trauma or many repetitive minor insults, such that the body does not have adequate time to heal properly. These types of injuries typically occur in low-contact sports that require long training sessions and repetitive loading (e.g., running, jumping, rowing, and swimming) and can lead to loss of playing time, physiologic exhaustion, and pain.[1] Overuse injuries typically present with a gradual onset of pain, masking the true severity of the injury. Yang et al.[1] conducted a study evaluating acute and chronic injuries in professional athletes and reported that male athletes have higher rates of acute injuries than their female counterparts, but female athletes had higher rates of chronic overuse injuries. Previous studies have supported the findings that female athletes have an increased risk of overuse injuries than male athletes. Female rowers reported a significantly greater number of chest overuse injuries and female military recruits reported more stress fractures than male rowers and recruits, respectively.[2,3] Magnusson et al.[4] evaluated differences in the adaptability of tendons to loading between females and males and demonstrated that females have an attenuated tendon hypertrophy response to habitual training, a lower tendon collagen synthesis rate following acute exercise, further attenuation of collagen synthesis based on levels of estrogen, and lower mechanical strength in their tendons. Therefore female athletes may be at an increased risk for developing symptoms of tendonitis. The increase in female athletic involvement increases the risk for the development of overuse injuries. Therefore it is important to identify and properly manage these types of injuries in order to allow athletes to return to sport and prevent progression to more serious sequelae.

ACHILLES TENDON INJURIES

Achilles tendon pain is common among athletes and can be related to several conditions including tendinopathy, tendinosis, tendinitis, tenosynovitis, and rupture.

Maffulli et al.[5] described tendinopathy as a combination of tendon pain, swelling, and impaired performance, with peritendinitis and tendinosis found on histopathology. Acute tendonitis is defined by the presence of symptoms for less than 2 weeks, while symptoms lasting for more than 6 weeks are classified as chronic tendonitis. The Achilles tendon comprises the distal insertion of the gastrocnemius-soleus musculotendinous unit transmitting loads to the calcaneus in order to plantarflex the foot.[6] There is a relative zone of avascularity approximately 2−6 cm proximal to the tendon insertion, and therefore this area is at greatest risk for degeneration and rupture.[7]

Risk Factors

Achilles tendinopathy is most prevalent in athletes participating in middle- and long-distance running, tennis, volleyball, and soccer, with an incidence rate up to 9% of all top-level runners.[6,8] Biomechanical analyses have demonstrated that malalignment within the foot and ankle may predispose to Achilles tendon injuries. Kvist et al.[9] demonstrated that limited mobility of the ankle and subtalar joint may contribute to increased risk of injury. Muscle imbalance and decreased flexibility can lead to a loss of protection of the tendon during increased physical activity and load-bearing exercises.

Presentation/Examination Findings

Patients presenting with Achilles tendon injuries typically recall a change in activity levels that led to either an insidious or a gradual onset of discomfort over the Achilles tendon. The patient usually describes relief of symptoms with rest, but pain returns as soon as the patient resumes activity. Achilles tendon rupture often occurs acutely, with patients describing a "pop". On physical examination, there is usually a palpable defect over the area of ruptured tendon. Squeezing the calf in the prone position (i.e., Thompson test) does not elicit movement of the foot and can confirm diagnosis of rupture.[10]

The Female Athlete. https://doi.org/10.1016/B978-0-323-75985-4.00004-0

Imaging

Ultrasound is useful in providing information regarding changes of water content within the tendon as well as collagen integrity. Abnormal tendons usually demonstrate a larger tendon diameter with higher levels of water content and collagen discontinuity, and tendon sheath swelling.[10] Although ultrasound is useful, magnetic resonance imaging (MRI) remains the study of choice for diagnosing Achilles tendon injuries (Fig. 21.1).

Treatment

Initial management of Achilles tendinopathy includes activity modification, physical therapy, and antiinflammatory medications. Niesen-Vertommen et al.[11] reported

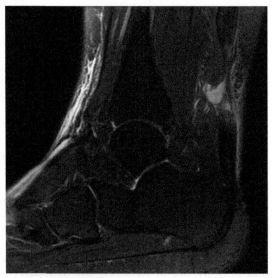

FIG. 21.1 Magnetic resonance image demonstrating Achilles tendon rupture.

that eccentric training was superior to concentric training in reducing pain in chronic Achilles tendinopathy. Deep friction massage accompanied by stretching is utilized to restore elasticity and reduce muscletendon strain.[12] It has been reported that 24%–45% of patients with Achilles tendon injuries fail conservative management, ultimately requiring surgical intervention.[6,13] Surgical treatments include open versus percutaneous Achilles tenotomy for tendinopathy and tendon repair for rupture (Fig. 21.2A–C). Testa et al.[14] evaluated 52 male and female elite middle- and long-distance runners with Achilles tendinopathy and reported good functional outcomes following percutaneous longitudinal tenotomies. Postoperatively, patients are often immobilized for 2 weeks and then transitioned to a CAM (controlled ankle motion) boot where they may begin ankle range of motion. Patients are often non-weight-bearing for as long as 6–8 weeks following repair.

PATELLAR TENDINOPATHY/TENDONITIS

Patellar tendinopathy, also referred to as "jumpers knee", is common in athletes involved in repetitive jumping, climbing, kicking, or running as a result of excessive pain over the patella tendon.[15] Repetitive motion of the extensor mechanism results in focal degeneration leading to fraying and microtearing of the tendon.[16,17]

Risk Factors

Patellar tendon injuries typically affect athletes involved in sports including basketball, volleyball, football, soccer, high/long jump, tennis, and running.[18] Torstensen et al.[19] demonstrated that elite athletes are more often

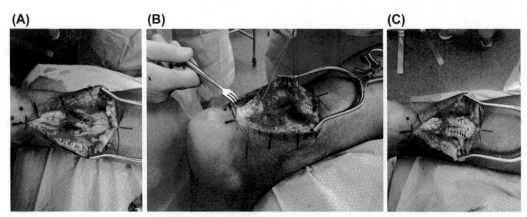

FIG. 21.2 **(A)** Acute Achilles tendon rupture. **(B)** Achilles tendon repair of proximal and distal ends utilizing the Krackow technique with FiberWire suture. **(C)** Repaired Achilles tendon.

affected than recreational athletes. Van der Worp et al.[20] conducted a meta-analysis reviewing risk factors for developing patellar tendinitis. The authors found that body mass index, waist-to-hip ratio, leg-length difference, arch height of foot, quadriceps/hamstring flexibility, quadriceps strength, and vertical jump all influence loading of the patellar tendon.[20] In addition, several factors related to training can contribute to the development of patellar tendinopathy/tendinitis, including quick acceleration, deceleration, stopping, and cutting actions.[21]

Presentation/Examination Findings

Athletes typically present with an insidious onset of pain that is related to the frequency and intensity of their training. Initially, pain presents as a dull ache on the anterior aspect of the knee just inferior to the patella. Patients often state that the pain is worse when walking or running upstairs and downstairs. The key finding is tenderness to palpation over the patellar tendon, which is usually worse in extension.

Imaging

Ultrasound and MRI are imaging modalities often utilized to confirm the diagnosis of patellar tendinopathy. Ultrasound can identify decreased echogenicity and irregularities within the tendinous envelope.[22] MRI can also demonstrate areas of higher signal intensity in the affected regions of the tendon.[22]

Treatment

Nonoperative intervention is the first line of treatment in patients with patellar tendinitis. Activity modification, antiinflammatory medication, and physical therapy are initially recommended. Rest is important in the early phases of recovery. Rehabilitation progresses from controlled exercises without load, to eccentric and concentric load, and finally to return to sports.[23] Other methods to reduce the load on the tendon include orthotics, braces, and straps. The Cho-Pat strap is commonly utilized to support the tibial attachment of the patellar tendon. Most athletes will be successfully treated with conservative measures alone.[23]

Patellar tendon surgery is typically reserved for patients who have failed at least 6 months of conservative therapy. Surgical interventions include drilling of the inferior pole of the patella, resection of the tibial attachment of the patellar tendon, repair of defects, tenotomy/tenoplasty, percutaneous needling, and excision of the inferior pole of the patella with repair.[22] Ferretti et al.[18] reported excellent results in 70% of male and female amateur and professional athletes with a mean age of 27 years treated with longitudinal splitting of the tendon and drilling of the inferior pole of the patella. Cucurulo et al. evaluated arthroscopic procedures in the treatment of patellar tendonitis in athletes, which involved controlled shaving of retrotendinous tissue and excision of damaged tendon. This study demonstrated good results in motivated athletes and reported equivalent outcomes in both open and arthroscopic techniques.[24]

ROTATOR CUFF TENDONITIS

Rotator cuff tendonitis is often used as a general term for athletes experiencing shoulder pain without a full-thickness rotator cuff tear or another identifiable cause for the pain. Rotator cuff tendonitis can often lead to tendinosis (i.e., degeneration of the tendon) and tear. The rotator cuff is composed of four muscles, namely, supraspinatus, infraspinatus, teres minor, and subscapularis, with all arising from the scapula. These four muscles combine to provide dynamic stability to the glenohumeral joint.

Risk Factors

Rotator cuff injuries are usually the result of overuse in athletes and rarely occur following a single traumatic event. Motions including overhead throwing, serving in tennis, and spiking the ball in volleyball increase the rotational forces on the shoulder during acceleration and deceleration phases and lead to an increased risk of injury.[25] Athletes with anterior glenohumeral instability have an increased risk of developing rotator cuff tendonitis, as there is increased stress across the rotator cuff with this condition. Impingement syndrome has been implicated as an underlying cause of multiple athletic shoulder injuries including rotator cuff tendonitis. External impingement occurs when the rotator cuff is compressed between the greater tuberosity and the acromion. Internal impingement occurs when the infraspinatus is compressed between the humeral head and the posterior superior glenoid rim with the arm in maximal external rotation as seen in overhead throwing athletes.[25–27]

Presentation/Examination Findings

The typical presentation of rotator cuff tendonitis is pain with overhead activity. Athletes typically note increased discomfort during maximal abduction and external rotation or during follow-through, when the rotator cuff is placed on maximal strain and tension.[26,28] Athletes initially describe discomfort during the painful activity that decreases with rest. Special tests can help isolate individual muscles of the rotator cuff. The empty can test and the drop arm test isolate the supraspinatus and may give positive results with rotator cuff tendonitis. The infraspinatus can be tested by external rotation, with the arm at the athlete's side. Patients with injuries affecting the teres minor may show external rotation weakness at 90 degrees of abduction with 90 degrees of external rotation (i.e., Hornblower's sign).[29] The lower subscapularis is tested using the belly press, while the upper aspect of the subscapularis is tested using the bear hug test. Other tests that may be beneficial in assessing an athlete with shoulder pain include Speed's test for biceps tendon pathology, O'Brien's test for labral pathology, and the apprehension test for glenohumeral instability.[29]

Imaging

Imaging studies for rotator cuff tendonitis should always begin with shoulder radiography including a Grashey view (true anteroposterior [AP] of the shoulder), scapular Y, and axillary lateral view. Superior migration of the humeral head may be found after rotator cuff tears; however, normal radiographs are common in athletes with rotator cuff tendonitis. Other modalities available include ultrasound to visualize the rotator cuff. It is less useful in cases of rotator cuff tendonitis; however, it can detect degeneration of the rotator cuff. MRI is the imaging modality of choice, as it provides much more detail of the soft tissue, rotator cuff tendons, and any fatty atrophy that occurs within the supraspinatus and other rotator cuff muscles.

Treatment

Initial treatment includes a short duration of rest (3–5 days) combined with nonsteroidal antiinflammatory drugs (NSAIDs).[30] A physical therapy program should be implemented focusing on stretching and strengthening of the shoulder girdle with emphasis on scapula stabilization and proper muscle activation during the athlete's specific sport. In addition, subacromial corticosteroid injections may be beneficial by reducing pain and inflammation.[30]

Surgical intervention is rarely utilized for rotator cuff tendonitis in the athletic population and is typically reserved for patients who have failed conservative management. Depending on the symptoms and imaging findings, surgical options include subacromial decompression, rotator cuff debridement, and rotator cuff repair (arthroscopic or mini-open technique). Surgical intervention is warranted in full-thickness tears of the rotator cuff, bursal sided tears >3 mm, and partial articular supraspinatus tendon avulsion lesions >7 mm or involving >50% of the tendon.[30] Athletes requiring surgical intervention have also shown good results. Reynolds et al.[31] evaluated 82 active male professional baseball pitchers who underwent arthroscopic debridement of a partial thickness rotator cuff tear and demonstrated that up to 76% were able to return to competitive pitching; however, only 50% returned to the same or higher level of competition. A systematic review by Klouche et al. evaluated return to sport in patients (all ages, participating in all sports at a variety of levels) with partial or full-thickness rotator cuff tears. This study demonstrated an overall return to sport of 84.7% following rotator cuff repair.[32] Of those athletes, 65% were able to return to their previous level of play and only 49% were able to return to their previous level of play in the professional and competitive athlete population.[32]

BICEPS TENDONITIS

Biceps tendonitis is an overuse injury often seen in overhead athletes due to the increased demands on the biceps tendon as it traverses through the narrow bicipital groove. Continued painful activity without rest can lead to tendinosis or degeneration of the biceps tendon. Biceps tendonitis typically occurs concomitantly with other shoulder injuries such as rotator cuff tendonitis/tears, subacromial impingement, superior labral tear from anterior to posterior (SLAP) tears, bursitis, and glenohumeral instability.[33,34]

Risk Factors

Overhead throwing athletes are at an increased risk of developing biceps tendonitis. Laudner and Sipes[25] reported a 12.1% incidence of biceps tendonitis in collegiate overhead throwing athletes. The authors demonstrated that biceps tendonitis was most commonly reported in swimming, baseball, softball, tennis, and volleyball. Oliver et al.[35] evaluated muscle activation patterns during windmill softball pitching and found the biceps brachii is most active during the acceleration phase of the pitch. Another possible risk factor for injury to the biceps tendon occurs with amateur athletes. Amateur throwing athletes have shown greater activity to the biceps during the acceleration and deceleration phases than their professional counterparts, whereas professional athletes demonstrate more efficient recruitment of rotator cuff muscles.[36]

Presentation/Examination Findings

Athletes with biceps tendonitis often complain of anterior shoulder pain; however, diagnosing biceps tendonitis versus other shoulder pathologies may be difficult, given the overlapping symptoms. Typically, biceps tendonitis occurs in conjunction with other pathologies within the shoulder; however, isolated pathology to the long head of the biceps tendon can occur in the younger and more athletic population.[34] Early signs of biceps tendonitis include pain after activity, with more severe presentations causing pain during activity and at rest. An audible snap or popping sensation in the anterior shoulder may signify subluxation of the biceps tendon. The two physical examination tests most commonly utilized in the diagnosis of biceps tendonitis are the Speed's test and Yergason's test. Speed's test is performed by resisted forward flexion of the shoulder to 90 degrees with the elbow fully extended and the forearm supinated. A positive test result is defined by pain within the bicipital groove.[37] Yergason's test is performed with the elbow at 90 degrees of flexion and the shoulder in neutral position. A positive test result is when pain is localized within the bicipital groove while undergoing resisted supination.[38]

Imaging

Initial imaging studies include standard shoulder radiography (i.e., Grashey, scapular Y, and axillary lateral views), which are typically normal. In addition, a magnetic resonance arthrogram may provide useful information regarding inflammation surrounding the biceps tendon. MRI provides information regarding soft tissue pathology surrounding the shoulder. However, it is poor at detecting biceps tendinopathy, having a concordance rate of only 37% with arthroscopy.[39]

Treatment

Initial treatment involves a period of rest combined with a multimodal approach including NSAIDs, activity modification, physical therapy, and corticosteroid injections. The sheath of the long head of the biceps is continuous with the glenohumeral synovium; therefore corticosteroid injections in the subacromial space (for patients also presenting with impingement syndrome) and glenohumeral joint can help decrease inflammation surrounding the biceps tendon within the bicipital groove.[40]

Surgical management is reserved for cases of biceps tendonitis who have failed nonoperative treatment as well as other more concerning issues with the long head of the biceps, such as partial tear of the biceps tendon (>25%), medial subluxation of the biceps tendon, subluxation in the setting of a subscapularis tendon tear, and SLAP tears.[33] In addition, visualizing an inflamed biceps tendon intraoperatively may prompt a decision to manage the biceps surgically. Management of pathology of the long head of the biceps tendon involves either tenotomy or tenodesis.[33] Both procedures may be performed either as open or arthroscopically depending on the experience and comfort level of the practicing surgeon. There is still no consensus as to which surgical option provides the best outcomes for the patient. In a systematic review and meta-analysis comparing biceps tenotomy and tenodesis, the authors found no difference between open or arthroscopic biceps tenodesis with regard to functional outcome.[41] They did note that patients who received a tenotomy were more likely to develop a Popeye deformity and cramping in the bicipital groove, which is consistent with previous literature.

There is limited research regarding outcomes of athletes undergoing surgical management of biceps tendonitis. This is likely because the majority of athletes improve following conservative management. Therefore activity modification, physical therapy, and antiinflammatory medication should be implemented as the first-line treatment for biceps tendonitis.

LATERAL EPICONDYLITIS

Lateral epicondylitis, also known as "tennis elbow", typically occurs in the fourth or fifth decades of life, but it can be found in patients ranging from 12 to 80 years old.[42] It is most commonly thought of as an overuse injury in relation to athletes and nonathletes playing tennis, although it can affect any athlete or worker whose occupation requires repetitive wrist extension activities.[43] About 50% of all tennis players will have lateral epicondylitis at least once in their career.[44] The greatest muscle activity during a ground stroke is found in the wrist extensors, more specifically the extensor carpi radialis brevis (ECRB), extensor carpi radialis longus, and the extensor digitorum communis.[45] Most notably, the ECRB demonstrates the greatest muscle activity and was most prominent during the acceleration and early follow-through phases. The repetitive stress on the ECRB leads to small tears in the tendon, resulting in an influx of fibroblasts with disorganization of parallel collagen and vascular hyperplasia.[42] Nirschl[46] described the microscopic appearance as "angiofibroblastic hyperplasia" and found the tendon to have varying amounts of grayish, homogenous, edematous, and friable tissue.

Risk Factors

Tennis players are at greatest risk for developing lateral epicondylitis.[42] The incidence and prevalence increase in patients over the age of 40 years, underscoring an overuse, degenerative process. Other risk factors include improper technique, poor equipment selection, and the type of tennis court being used. Studies have demonstrated that inexperienced players are more prone to have improper swinging mechanics and therefore greater mechanical stress at the elbow.[47,48] Grip size, racquet weight, racquet string tension, and the number of strings may also have an effect on how much force is transmitted through the hand and into the wrist extensors, thereby predisposing athletes to pain over the lateral epicondyle.

Presentation/Examination Findings

Lateral epicondylitis typically presents as lateral elbow pain that may or may not radiate down the forearm.[42] A history of repetitive activities that involve wrist extension is typical of these athletes. Patients often present with an insidious onset, reporting gradual worsening of symptoms. Other complaints include decreased grip strength, difficulty picking up objects, and increased pain with activities that involve wrist extension. On physical examination, patients will demonstrate tenderness to palpation over the ECRB tendon just distal and slightly anterior to lateral epicondyle. Reproducible pain will be noted with resisted wrist extension that is often increased with the elbow in full extension.[49] In addition, patients exhibit pain with resisted long finger extension as well as passive wrist flexion with the forearm in pronation.

Imaging

Initial imaging should include standard AP and lateral radiography of the elbow. The radiographs are typically normal in patients with lateral epicondylitis, but they can be helpful in ruling out other causes of lateral elbow pain. Ultrasound is a useful diagnostic tool for lateral epicondylitis. MRI can be used to evaluate for pathology associated with lateral epicondylitis, but it is not often necessary for the diagnosis (Fig. 21.3).[42]

Treatment

Nonoperative management is the first-line treatment for patients presenting with lateral epicondylitis, with the main goal being reduction of pain and other symptoms (e.g., weakness) and progression to improved strength and function.[42] Lateral epicondylitis is usually a self-limiting condition. Conservative treatment includes activity modification, rest, NSAIDs, cryotherapy, physical therapy, injections (corticosteroids, platelet-rich plasma, prolotherapy), extracorporeal shockwave therapy, bracing, iontophoresis, and laser therapy.[50] Current literature does not support the efficacy of one method over another. Surgical treatment is reserved for refractory cases in which the athlete continues to experience debilitating pain despite a well-organized and executed conservative management program for a minimum of 6–12 months. There are several surgical treatment options, but the most common is an extra-articular open procedure in which the pathologic tissue is excised and debrided, the defect is repaired, and the

(A)   **(B)**

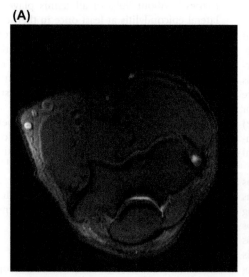 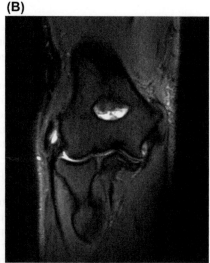

FIG. 21.3 **(A)** Axial and **(B)** coronal magnetic resonance images demonstrating increased signal around the common extensor tendon.

common extensor origin is then reattached to the lateral epicondyle.[42] In 1979, Nirschl and Pettrone[46] showed 85% of patients returning to full activities following surgical treatment of lateral epicondylitis. This was further supported by 93% of patients returning to sport following surgery at 10-year follow-up.[51] In a recent systematic review comparing open, percutaneous, and arthroscopic treatment of lateral epicondylitis, the authors found a greater proportion of patients were pain free in the open group than those in the arthroscopic group.[52] However, there was no difference among the three groups with regard to return to work, complication rate, or patient satisfaction.[52]

SPONDYLOLYSIS

Spondylosis is a stress reaction within the pars interarticularis of the lumbar spine, which connects the superior and inferior articular facets bilaterally.[53] If continued stress is placed on this anatomic structure, it has the potential to weaken leading to a fatigue fracture.[53] Spondylolysis is most commonly seen at L5 (85%), with L4 (15%) being the next most common location.[54] This condition can be either congenital or acquired. Rossi and Dragoni demonstrated an incidence of 13.9% in elite athletes who presented with low-back pain. Of those athletes who had spondylolysis, 47.5% of them developed a concomitant spondylolisthesis.[54] The lumbosacral articulation is exposed to the highest forces in the thoracolumbar spine.[55] The strength of the neural arch is suggested to increase up to the fourth or fifth decade of life, thus spondylolysis is typically seen in adolescent patients who experience repetitive stress to the lumbar spine (e.g., gymnasts, cheerleaders).[56,57]

Risk Factors

The risk of developing spondylolysis is often related to patient and/or environmental factors. Spondylolysis is common among adolescent athletes engaging in repetitive hyperextension of the lumbar spine (e.g., divers, gymnasts, dancers, football linemen, rowers, and soccer players). Although males are at increased risk for this condition, certain sports carry a higher risk for the female athlete. Female dancers and gymnasts specifically are at an increased risk of spondylolysis compared with their male counterparts.[58–60] In a study of 100 young female gymnasts engaged in high-level competition, the authors found 11% to be affected with a defect of the pars interarticularis, which was four times greater than their nonathletic female counterparts.[58] In a study by Goldstein,[60] 9% of pre-elite, 43% of elite, and 63%

of Olympic-level gymnasts had spine abnormalities including degenerative disk changes, spondylolysis, and spondylolisthesis as seen on MRI. Increased intensity and length of training correlated with an increase in these abnormalities seen. It has also been reported that the incidence of spondylolysis in dancers is two times more common in females.[59]

Presentation and Examination Findings

Low-back pain is a common complaint among the active pediatric and adolescent population. It is often the initial presenting symptom with vague pain and no specific inciting event. Patients with spondylolysis will usually have pain with activity that improves with rest; however, depending on the duration of symptoms, patients may have constant low-level pain. Patients often report participation in athletics requiring repetitive hyperextension of the lumbar spine. Radiation of pain into the buttock region may also be present. It is important to perform a thorough neurologic examination to rule out more severe causes of low-back pain. In addition, the patient should be evaluated for scoliosis. When assessing range of motion and movement of the lumbar spine, hyperextension may cause increased pain. Forward flexion can be limited, as patients with spondylolysis often have hamstring tightness. A single-leg hyperextension examination is used to help diagnose spondylolysis.[53]

Imaging

Athletes with a single inciting event or persistent back pain exacerbated by activity should be evaluated initially with AP, lateral, and lateral oblique lumbar spine radiography, which has been shown to be diagnostic in 86% of cases of spondylolysis (Fig. 21.4).[61] In refractory cases with negative radiographs, radionuclide bone scans and single-photon emission computed tomography (CT) can be used to pinpoint the location of the pars interarticularis defect.[62–64] CT scans are also particularly useful in diagnosing patients with spondylolysis, especially in athletes with back pain and normal radiographs.[65] MRI, on the other hand, can be very useful to rule out other potential spine pathologies that may be causing pain; however, MRI has a high false-positive result rate for the diagnosis of spondylolysis.[66] Given the lack of radiation in MRI, this study may be more desirable in the evaluation of adolescent female athletes.[56]

Treatment

Initial management consists of rest and activity modification including cessation of all sporting events for at

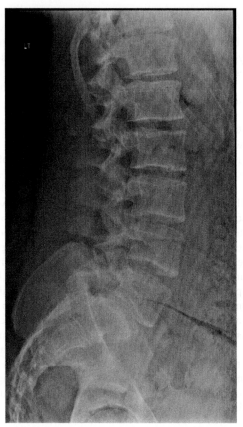

FIG. 21.4 Sagittal lumbar radiograph demonstrating L5 pars defect.

least 3 months or until pain free. Athletes should participate in a physical therapy program that includes stretching and strengthening in order to decrease the stress placed directly on the affected pars interarticularis. Core strengthening helps stabilize the lumbar spine and pelvis in dynamic activity, thus reducing stress placed on the lumbar spine. In addition, increasing the flexibility of tight muscles (e.g., hamstrings) is important in the rehabilitation process. Bracing and NSAIDs can also be used in the conservative management of spondylolysis. Previous studies have demonstrated that up to 87% of athletes returned to their sport at an average of 5.4 months after being treated nonoperatively with activity restriction and antilordotic lumbosacral bracing.[67] Athletes who are compliant with activity cessation for at least 3 months are 16 times more likely to have excellent results compared with those who do not comply with activity restrictions.[68]

Surgical intervention is not common for spondylolysis and used mostly in cases in whom conservative management has failed and patients have shown progression to spondylolisthesis or neurologic compromise.[53] Pars interarticularis repair using a pedicle screw is the least invasive of the options, but still requires a posterior midline approach.[69] Other options include adding posterior lumbar interbody fusion, which has shown promising results in patients with spinal stenosis.[70] A meta-analysis evaluating direct pars interarticularis repairs demonstrated that the use of pedicle screws resulted in the highest fusion and lowest complication rates compared to other interventions.[69] Surgical management has demonstrated a high level of success in getting athletes back on the field. A systematic review by Grazina et al. evaluated return to play after both conservative management and surgical treatment in athletes with spondylolysis. The review looked at 14 studies comprising 592 total subjects (59% male), aged 7—37 years, at varying levels of competition. The athletes participated in organized sports, with football, soccer, and baseball being the most common. The authors found that 81% and 89% of athletes returned to their preinjury level of competition after being treated surgically and conservatively, respectively. The time to return to sport was found to be 4.6 and 6.8 months in patients treated conservatively and surgically, respectively.[71]

ILIOTIBIAL BAND SYNDROME
Iliotibial band syndrome (ITBS) is an overuse injury in athletes who require repetitive knee flexion and extension. The iliotibial band (ITB) is a unique structure that originates from the connection between fascia from the tensor fascia latae and the gluteus maximus and medius. It extends distally along the lateral aspect of the thigh as a thickened band of fascia confluent with the fascia latae. The ITB continues over the lateral epicondyle of the femur, crosses the knee joint, and inserts into Gerdy's tubercle on the anterolateral aspect of the proximal tibia. As the ITB crosses the lateral aspect of the knee, it has both anterior attachments to the patella and femur and posterior attachments to the biceps femoris.[72] Orchard et al.[73] have suggested that an impingement zone exists at 20—30 degrees of knee flexion, where the distal fibers of the ITB compress and slide over the lateral femoral condyle.

The cause of ITBS remains controversial; however, the most widely accepted theory is that repetitive knee flexion and extension cause the ITB to continuously rub against the lateral femoral epicondyle, leading to inflammation and pain.[74] This is commonly seen in sports such as running and cycling. Fairclough et al.

proposed that the ITB is merely a thickened aspect of the fascia latae that is connected to the linea aspera through strong dense connective tissue and therefore is unable to slide over the lateral epicondyle. The perception of movement over the epicondyle is rather the change in tension in the anterior and posterior fibers of the ITB, and the pain may be due to compression and irritation of the tissue between the ITB and the lateral femur.[75]

Risk Factors

Anatomic factors, biomechanical factors, gender differences, and training errors have all been implicated in patients with ITBS. Anatomic factors that contribute to increased stress on the ITB include hip abductor weakness and increased internal rotation of the knee (tibial internal rotation or femoral external rotation).[76] Ferber et al.[77] demonstrated that athletes with ITBS exhibited greater peak rearfoot invertor moment, peak knee internal rotation angle, and peak hip adduction angle compared with athletes without ITBS. In addition, Frederickson et al.[78] noted increased hip abductor weakness in distance runners on the side affected by ITBS. It is common for runners to experience ITBS pain upon heel strike that increases when running downhill, as there is a higher degree of knee flexion at heel strike.[73] Training errors such as increased mileage without increased experience and cross-training with exercises that also encourage repetitive flexion and extension of the knee can also contribute to the development of ITBS.[79]

Presentation/Examination Findings

ITBS is a clinical diagnosis that relies heavily on the athlete's history and physical examination for accurate assessment of the disease process. Pain will often be localized over the lateral epicondyle approximately 3 cm proximal to the lateral joint line.[80] Radiating symptoms up the lateral thigh are sometimes present. Depending on how long the symptoms have been present, the athlete may describe mild symptoms after activity, symptoms during activity, or constant symptoms even while at rest.[80] It is imperative to rule out other causes of lateral knee pain before arriving at a diagnosis of ITBS. Standing lower extremity alignment should be initially evaluated in order to determine if there is increased varus/valgus alignment of the knee that could be putting stress on the lateral aspect of the knee.[80] It is also important to assess foot alignment and note any pronation and hindfoot eversion upon standing. Gait and biomechanics should be assessed to evaluate any muscle imbalances and altered mechanics that may be present and possibly causing

symptoms. There are two main provocative tests that are indicated when evaluating an athlete with ITBS: the Noble compression test and Ober's test. The Noble compression test is performed in the supine position with the knee bent to 90 degrees. Pressure is applied over the lateral epicondyle while the patient's knee is being extended. A positive test result is defined by increased pain at 30 degrees of knee flexion.[81] Ober's test is performed with the patient in the lateral decubitus position laying on the opposite site of the leg being tested. The hip is placed in line with the trunk and the knee is then flexed to 90 degrees. While holding the leg, the thigh is then allowed to adduct. A positive test result is defined by the inability of the leg to adduct, thus signifying a tight ITB.[82]

Imaging

Although ITBS is a clinical diagnosis and does not routinely require imaging, it can be useful to supplement the history and physical examination, especially if the examination does not elicit a clear diagnosis. Standard AP and lateral radiographs of the knee are warranted, but they are typically normal in cases of ITBS. These radiographs can however identify any bony pathology that may be causing the patient's pain (e.g., a prominent epicondyle, spur, and lateral compartment osteoarthritis). MRI, although not often indicated during initial evaluation, can be a useful diagnostic tool in cases refractory to conservative management by ruling out other potential causes of lateral knee pain.[80] Ekman et al.[83] found in their case series of seven patients that MRI can show thickening of the distal ITB as well as a fluid collection over the lateral epicondyle, deep to the ITB.

Treatment

ITBS is typically treated conservatively with rest, activity modification, equipment modifications, corticosteroid injections, physical therapy, and orthotics. Equipment modifications depend upon the specific sport being played, but examples include changing cleat position in baseball or softball players and altering the bicycle seat and handlebar positions in cycling.[84] Physical therapy can improve flexibility of the ITB, strengthen hip abduction and adduction, improve internal rotation of the knee, and correct overpronation of the foot.[80] In addition, foam rollers are often used in conjunction with physical therapy to help break up any soft tissue adhesions. NSAIDs and corticosteroid injections can help decrease inflammation and reduce painful symptoms. Surgery is only considered in athletes who have not improved after conservative management for at least 6 months. Several surgical options exist but most rely on open surgical excision of the posterior half of the ITB to eliminate any potential impingement. Additionally, in patients with a tight ITB, a z-lengthening can be used to help release stress on the distal ITB. Martens et al. demonstrated good results, low morbidity, and quick return to sport in their study of 23 athletes, mostly males, participating in football, running, and cycling affected with ITBS. They treated each athlete with a trial of physical therapy and proceeded with limited resection of a small triangular piece at the posterior aspect of the ITB directly over the lateral epicondyle when the patient's pain was refractory to conservative management. The mean time to reach previous level of activity was 7 weeks.[85] Another surgical option is arthroscopic resection of the lateral synovial recess. Michels et al. evaluated outcomes of arthroscopic debridement of the lateral synovial recess in 35 recreational or professional athletes (15 females, 21 males) with ITBS refractory to conservative treatment. Each athlete suffered from ITBS for an average of 18 months and participated in sports such as distance running, triathlons, cycling, rugby, soccer, swimming, and fencing. When assessing functional results, the authors found 80% excellent and 17.1% good results, with all athletes returning to their sports within 3 months after surgery.[86]

CONCLUSION

Overuse injuries are very common in female athletes. These injuries result from cumulative trauma or many repetitive minor insults and can lead to loss of playing time, physiologic exhaustion, and pain. Common injuries include Achilles tendonitis, patella tendonitis, biceps tendonitis, rotator cuff injury, lateral epicondylitis, spondylolysis, and ITBS. It is important to identify and properly manage these types of injuries in order to allow athletes to return to sport and prevent more serious sequelae.

REFERENCES

1. Yang J, Tibbetts AS, Covassin T, et al. Epidemiology of overuse and acute injuries among competitive collegiate athletes. *J Athl Train.* 2012;47(2):198–204.
2. Smoljanovic T, Bojanic I, Hannafin JA, et al. Traumatic and overuse injuries among international elite junior rowers. *Am J Sports Med.* 2009;37(6):1193–1199.
3. Gam A, Goldstein L, Karmon Y, et al. Comparison of stress fractures of male and female recruits during basic training in the Israeli anti-aircraft forces. *Mil Med.* 2005;170(8):710–712.
4. Magnusson SP, Hansen M, Langberg H, et al. The adaptability of tendon to loading differs in men and women. *Int J Exp Pathol.* 2007;88(4):237–240.
5. Maffulli N, Khan KM, Puddu G. Overuse tendon conditions: time to change a confusing terminology. *Arthroscopy.* 1998;14:840–843.
6. Paavola M, Kannus P, Jarvinen T, et al. Achilles tendinopathy. *J Bone Jt Surg.* 2002;84(11):2062–2076.
7. Carr AJ, Norris SH. The blood supply of the calcaneal tendon. *J Bone Jt Surg Br.* 1989;71(1):100–101.
8. Johansson C. Injuries in elite orienteers. *Am J Sports Med.* 1986;14:410–415.
9. Kvist M. Achilles tendon injuries in athletes. *Ann Chir Gynaecol.* 1990;80(2):188–201.
10. Cook JL, Khan KM, Purdam C. Achilles tendinopathy. *Man Ther.* 2002;7(3):121–130.
11. Niesen-Vertommen SL, Taunton JE, Clement DB, et al. The effect of eccentric versus concentric exercise in the management of Achilles tendonitis. *Clin J Sport Med.* 1992;2:109–113.
12. Maffulli N, Sharma P, Luscombe KL. Achilles tendinopathy: aetiology and management. *J R Soc Med.* 2004;97:472–476.
13. Maffulli N, Kader D. Tendinopathy of tendo Achillis. *J Bone Jt Surg Br.* 2002;84:1–8.
14. Testa V, Capasso G, Benazzo F, et al. Management of Achilles tendinopathy by ultrasound-guided percutaneous tenotomy. *Med Sci Sports Exerc.* 2002;34(4):573–580.
15. Lian O, Holen KJ, Engebretsen L, et al. Relationship between symptoms of jumper's knee and the ultrasound characteristics of the patellar tendon among high level male volleyball players. *Scand J Med Sci Sports.* 1996;6:291–296.
16. Hsu H, Siwiec RM. *Patellar tendon rupture.* Treasure Island (FL): StatPearls Publishing; January 2019. Available from: https://www.ncbi.nlm.nih.gov/books/NBK513275/.
17. Martens M, Wouters P, Burssens A, et al. Patellar tendinitis: pathology and results of treatment. *Acta Orthop Scand.* 1982;53(3):445–450.
18. Ferretti A, Conteduca F, Camerucci E, et al. Patellar tendinosis: a follow-up study of surgical treatment. *J Bone Jt Surg Am.* 2002;84(12):2179–2185.
19. Torstensen ET, Bray RC, Wiley JP. Patellar tendinitis: a review of current concepts and treatment. *Clin J Sport Med.* 1994;4:77–82.
20. Van de Worp H, dePoel HJ, Diercks RL, et al. Jumper's knee or lander's knee? A systematic review of the relation between jump biomechanics and patellar tendinopathy. *Int J Sports Med.* 2014;35(8):714–722.
21. Pezzullo DJ, Irrgang JJ, Whitney SL. Patellar tendinitis: jumper's knee. *J Sport Rehabil.* 1992;1(1):56–68.
22. Khan KM, Bonar F, Desmond PM, et al. Patellar tendinosis (jumper's knee): findings at histopathologic examination, US and MR imaging. *Radiology.* 1996;200:821–827.
23. Rutland M, O'connell D, Brismée JM, et al. Evidence-supported rehabilitation of patellar tendinopathy. *N Am J Sports Phys Ther.* 2010;5(3):166–178.

24. Cucurulo T, Louis ML, Thaunat M, et al. Surgical treatment of patellar tendinopathy in athletes a retrospective multicentric study. *Orthop Traumatol Surg Res.* 2009;95(8 Suppl 1):S78–S84.
25. Laudner K, Sipes R. The incidence of shoulder injury among collegiate overhead athletes. *J Intercoll Sport.* 2009;2(2):260–268.
26. Blevins FT. Rotator cuff pathology in athletes. *Sports Med.* 1997;24(3):205–220.
27. Page P. Shoulder muscle imbalance and subacromial impingement syndrome in overhead athletes. *Int J Sports Phys Ther.* 2011;6(1):51–58.
28. Tennent TD, Beach WR, Meyers JF. A review of the special tests associated with shoulder examination: part 1: the rotator cuff tests. *AJSM.* 2003;31(1):154–160.
29. Jain NB, Wilcox R, Katz JN, et al. Clinical examination of the rotator cuff. *HHS Public Access.* 2013;5(1).
30. Gomoll AH, Katz JN, Warner J, et al. Rotator cuff disorders. *Arthritis Rheum.* 2004;50(12):3751–3761.
31. Reynolds SB, Dugas JR, Cain EL, et al. Débridement of small partial-thickness rotator cuff tears in elite overhead throwers. *Clin Orthop Relat Res.* 2008;466(3):614–621.
32. Klouche S, Lefevre N, Herman S, et al. Return to sport after rotator cuff tear repair: a systematic review and meta-analysis. *Am J Sports Med.* 2016;44(7):1877–1887.
33. Nho SJ, Strauss EJ, Lenart BA, et al. Long head of the biceps tendinopathy: diagnosis and management. *J Am Acad Orthop Surg.* 2010;18(11):645–656.
34. Ahrens PM, Boileau P. The long head of biceps and associated tendinopathy. *J Bone Jt Surg Br.* 2007;89(8):1001–1009.
35. Oliver GD, Plummer HA, Keeley DW. Muscle activation patterns of the upper and lower extremity during the windmill softball pitch. *J Strength Cond Res.* 2011;25(6):1653–1658.
36. Gowan ID, Jobe FW, Tibone JE, et al. A comparative electromyographic analysis of the shoulder during pitching. *Am J Sports Med.* 1987;15(6):586–590.
37. Bennett WF. Specificity of the speed's test: arthroscopic technique for evaluating the biceps tendon at the level of the bicipital groove. *Arthroscopy.* 1998;14(8):789–796.
38. Yergason RM. Supination sign. *J Bone Joint Surg.* 1931;13(1):160.
39. Mohtadi NG, Vellet AD, Clark ML, et al. A prospective, double-blind comparison of magnetic resonance imaging and arthroscopy in the evaluation of patients presenting with shoulder pain. *J Shoulder Elbow Surg.* 2004;13(3):258–265.
40. Tallia AF, Cardone DA. Diagnostic and therapeutic injection of the shoulder region. *Am Fam Physician.* 2003;67(6):1271–1278.
41. Gurnani N, Van deurzen DF, Janmaat VT, et al. Tenotomy or tenodesis for pathology of the long head of the biceps Brachii: a systematic review and meta-analysis. *Knee Surg Sports Traumatol Arthrosc.* 2016;24(12):3765–3771.
42. Jobe FW, Ciccotti MG. Lateral and medial epicondylitis of the elbow. *J Am Acad Orthop Surg.* 1994;2(1):1–8.
43. Nirschl RP. Elbow tendinosis/tennis elbow. *Clin Sports Med.* 1992;11(4):851–870.
44. Allman FL. Tennis elbow, etiology, prevention and treatment. *Clin Orthop Relat Res.* 1975;111:308–316.
45. Morris M, Jobe FW, Perry J, et al. Electromyographic analysis of elbow function in tennis players. *Am J Sports Med.* 1989;17(2):241–247.
46. Nirschl RP, Pettrone FA. Tennis elbow: the surgical treatment of lateral epicondylitis. *J Bone Jt Surg Am.* 1979;61(6A):832–839.
47. Bernhang AM, Dehner W, Fogarty C. Tennis elbow: a biomechanical approach. *J Sports Med.* 1974;2(5):235–260.
48. Nirschl RP. Tennis elbow. *Prim Care.* 1977;4(2):367–382.
49. Tosti R, Jennings J, Sewards JM. Lateral epicondylitis of the elbow. *Am J Med.* 2013;126(4):357.e1–357.e6.
50. Sims SE, Miller K, Elfar JC, et al. Non-surgical treatment of lateral epicondylitis: a systematic review of randomized controlled trials. *Hand.* 2014;9(4):419–446.
51. Dunn JH, Kim JJ, Davis L, et al. Ten- to 14-year follow-up of the nirschl surgical technique for lateral epicondylitis. *Am J Sports Med.* 2008;36(2):261–266.
52. Riff AJ, Saltzman BM, Cvetanovich G, et al. Open vs percutaneous vs arthroscopic surgical treatment of lateral epicondylitis: an updated systematic review. *Am J Orthop.* 2018;47(6).
53. Standaert CJ, Herring SA, Halpern B, et al. Spondylolysis. *Phys Med Rehabil Clin.* 2000;11(4):785–803.
54. Rossi F, Dragoni S. The prevalence of spondylolysis and spondylolisthesis in symptomatic elite athletes: radiographic findings. *Radiography.* 2001;7(1):37–42.
55. Dietrich M, Kurowski P. The importance of mechanical factors in the etiology of spondylolysis. a model analysis of loads and stresses in human lumbar spine. *Spine.* 1985;10(6):532–542.
56. Standaert CJ, Herring SA. Spondylolysis: a critical review. *Br J Sports Med.* 2000;34(6):415–422.
57. Cyron BM, Hutton WC. The fatigue strength of the lumbar neural arch in spondylolysis. *J Bone Jt Surg Br.* 1978;60:234–238.
58. Jackson DW, Wiltse LL, Cirincoine RJ. Spondylolysis in the female gymnast. *Clin Orthop Relat Res.* 1976;117:68–73.
59. Hall H, Piccinin J. Dance. In: Watkins RG, ed. *The Spine in Sports.* St Louis: Mosby-Year Book; 1996:465–474.
60. Goldstein JD, Berger PE, Windler GE, et al. Spine injuries in gymnasts and swimmers. an epidemiologic investigation. *Am J Sports Med.* 1991;19(5):463–468.
61. Miller R, Beck NA, Sampson NR, et al. Imaging modalities for low back pain in children: a review of spondylolysis and undiagnosed mechanical back pain. *J Pediatr Orthop.* 2013;33(3):282–288.
62. Elliott S, Hutson MA, Wastie ML. Bone scintigraphy in the assessment of spondylolysis in patients attending a sports injury clinic. *Clin Radiol.* 1988;39(3):269–272.
63. Lowe J, Schachner E, Hirschberg E, et al. Significance of bone scintigraphy in symptomatic spondylolysis. *Spine.* 1984;9(6):653–655.

64. Bodner RJ, Heyman S, Drummond DS, et al. The use of single photon emission computed tomography (SPECT) in the diagnosis of low-back pain in young patients. *Spine*. 1988;13(10):1155–1160.

65. Congeni J, Mcculloch J, Swanson K. Lumbar spondylolysis. A study of natural progression in athletes. *Am J Sports Med*. 1997;25(2):248–253.

66. Harvey CJ, Richenberg JL, Saifuddin A, et al. The radiological investigation of lumbar spondylolysis. *Clin Radiol*. 1998;53(10):723–728.

67. Iwamoto J, Takeda T, Wakano K. Returning athletes with severe low back pain and spondylolysis to original sporting activities with conservative treatment. *Scand J Med Sci Sports*. 2004;14(6):346–351.

68. El rassi G, Takemitsu M, Glutting J, et al. Effect of sports modification on clinical outcome in children and adolescent athletes with symptomatic lumbar spondylolysis. *Am J Phys Med Rehabil*. 2013;92(12):1070–1074.

69. Mohammed N, Patra DP, Narayan V, et al. A comparison of the techniques of direct pars interarticularis repairs for spondylolysis and low-grade spondylolisthesis: a meta-analysis. *Neurosurg Focus*. 2018;44(1):E10.

70. Suk SI, Lee CK, Kim WJ, et al. Adding posterior lumbar interbody fusion to pedicle screw fixation and posterolateral fusion after decompression in spondylolytic spondylolisthesis. *Spine*. 1997;22(2):210–219.

71. Grazina R, Andrade R, Santos FL, et al. Return to play after conservative and surgical treatment in athletes with spondylolysis: a systematic review. *Phys Ther Sport*. 2019;37:34–43.

72. Terry GC, Hughston JC, Norwood LA. The anatomy of the iliopatellar band and iliotibial tract. *Am J Sports Med*. 1986;14(1):39–45.

73. Orchard JW, Fricker PA, Abud AT, et al. Biomechanics of iliotibial band friction syndrome in runners. *Am J Sports Med*. 1996;24(3):375–379.

74. Renne JW. The iliotibial band friction syndrome. *J Bone Jt Surg Am*. 1975;57(8):1110–1111.

75. Fairclough J, Hayashi K, Toumi H, et al. Is iliotibial band syndrome really a friction syndrome? *J Sci Med Sport*. 2007;10(2):74–76.

76. Noehren B, Davis I, Hamill J. ASB clinical biomechanics award winner 2006 prospective study of the biomechanical factors associated with iliotibial band syndrome. *Clin Biomech*. 2007;22(9):951–956.

77. Ferber R, Noehren B, Hamill J, et al. Competitive female runners with a history of iliotibial band syndrome demonstrate atypical hip and knee kinematics. *J Orthop Sports Phys Ther*. 2010;40(2):52–58.

78. Fredericson M, Cookingham CL, Chaudhari AM, et al. Hip abductor weakness in distance runners with iliotibial band syndrome. *Clin J Sport Med*. 2000;10(3):169–175.

79. Messier SP, Edwards DG, Martin DF, et al. Etiology of iliotibial band friction syndrome in distance runners. *Med Sci Sports Exerc*. 1995;27(7):951–960.

80. Strauss EJ, Kim S, Calcei JG, et al. Iliotibial band syndrome: evaluation and management. *JAAOS*. 2011;19(12):728–736.

81. Noble CA. Iliotibial band friction syndrome in runners. *Am J Sports Med*. 1980;8(4):232–234.

82. Ober FR. The role of the iliotibial band and fascia lata as a factor in the causation of low-back disabilities and sciatica. *J Bone Jt Surg*. 1936;18(1):105–110.

83. Ekman EF, Pope T, Martin DF, et al. Magnetic resonance imaging of iliotibial band syndrome. *Am J Sports Med*. 1994;22(6):851–854.

84. Wanich T, Hodgkins C, Columbier JA, et al. Cycling injuries of the lower extremity. *J Am Acad Orthop Surg*. 2007;15(12):748–756.

85. Martens M, Libbrecht P, Burssens A. Surgical treatment of the iliotibial band friction syndrome. *Am J Sports Med*. 1989;17(5):651–654.

86. Michels F, Jambou S, Allard M, et al. An arthroscopic technique to treat the iliotibial band syndrome. *Knee Surg Sports Traumatol Arthrosc*. 2009;17(3):233–236.

CHAPTER 22

Concussions in the Female Athlete

SHERRIE BALLANTINE-TALMADGE, DO, FACSM • HANNAH L. BRADSELL, BS

INTRODUCTION

Female athletes are more likely to sustain sport-related concussion than male athletes when playing equivalent sports.[1] Studies on middle-school to high-school females demonstrate that female athletes are at a higher risk of sustaining a concussion than their male counterparts.[2] A landmark study in 2017 by Schallmo et al.[3] was the first to report both gender differences and sport-specific differences in concussion. Despite significant educational efforts, athletes continue to underreport concussion symptoms. This chapter will discuss the evolving evidence surrounding gender differences in concussion, current trends, and future directions.

CLARIFYING TERMS

Since 2001, an international conference involving multidisciplinary experts has convened every 4 years to create an expert, consensus-based approach on how to review, discuss, and study concussion as it relates to sports.[4] Following each meeting, this group has produced a consensus paper with guidelines on the definitions, diagnosis, evaluation, and management of concussion.[5]

It is important to note the evolution of the term, "sport-related concussion (SRC)" versus "concussion." Concussion is a broad term applied to immediate and transient symptoms of traumatic brain injury (TBI).[6] Between the fourth and fifth International Conference on Concussion in Sport, SRC was more precisely described as, "a traumatic brain injury that is defined as a complex pathophysiological process affecting the brain, induced by biomechanical forces with several common features that help define its nature".[5,6] A consistent goal of the International Conference on Concussion in Sport is to streamline SRC definition, eliminating designation of severity ratings of concussion (i.e., mild vs. complex).[7]

This definition is incredibly important not only for the clinician but also for the patient to understand.

Important points from the Consensus Statement for the definition of SRC include the following:[5]
- SRC is an injury occurring as an induction of biomechanical forces.
- SRC can be caused by a direct blow to the head, face, neck, or elsewhere in the body (i.e., whiplash-type mechanism).
- SRC is a short-lived impairment of neurologic function, which resolves spontaneously. Special note should be taken, as both signs and symptoms can evolve over a period of minutes to hours.
- SRC results in many neuropathologic changes, but the more acute signs and symptoms manifest as a very functional change/disturbance versus a true structural change. This means that no abnormality is seen on a standard neuroimaging study, such as a magnetic resonance imaging or a computed tomographic scan.
- SRC may or may not involve loss of consciousness.
- SRC signs and symptoms will resolve over time with a "sequential course"; however, they can be prolonged in some cases.
- To clinically define a head injury as an SRC, the signs and symptoms need to be defined outside influences such as drug, alcohol, or medication use; other injuries; and/or other comorbidities.

The understanding of concussion is further complicated by it being largely a clinical diagnosis rather than a diagnosis based on an abnormal imaging study or a laboratory result.[6] Additionally, concussive symptoms, which help form the clinical diagnosis, are graded on a spectrum of severity from 1–6, rather than on black-and-white answers of yes or no.[7]

SPORT-SPECIFIC DIFFERENCES

In the popular press, concussion has long been portrayed largely through the eyes of male-dominated sports (e.g., football, boxing, combat sports, rugby, and ice hockey).[8] These sports may appear to have a

The Female Athlete. https://doi.org/10.1016/B978-0-323-75985-4.00018-0

higher risk of contact and collision, making it seem as though male athletes are more affected than females. However, when considering sports such as soccer, with similar rules for male and female athletes, some studies show an increased incidence of concussions in females compared with males.[9] In 2016, Covassin et al.[10] compiled injury surveillance data between the years 2004 and 2009 to evaluate gender-related differences in concussion rates and time loss from sport among National Collegiate Athletic Association (NCAA) athletes. This data yielded specifics about concussion rates among more traditional varsity sports such as soccer, basketball, ice hockey, lacrosse, softball, or baseball, showing increased risk for concussion in females. Using this NCAA Injury Surveillance Program, when specifically looking at gender-comparable sports, the authors found that females had an increased rate of concussion of 1.4 times higher overall than males. In addition, greater concussion rates were seen in women's baseball/softball, basketball, ice hockey, and soccer, as well as more time loss from sport due to concussion in female soccer and basketball players, as compared with males.[10]

Female athletes who play soccer seem to be at a particularly high risk of sustaining concussions. The United States has more registered female soccer players than all other countries combined, from youth athletes to professional teams.[11] Weber et al.[11] analyzed concussion injuries sustained by female collegiate soccer players in NCAA Division I athletics from the 2004 to 2017 seasons. Overall, the authors reported an average of 1.79 diagnosed concussions per year and an average annual incidence rate of 6.56% over the 14-year period.[11] In 2017, Schallmo et al.[3] evaluated high-school athletes to determine gender- and sport-specific trends in concussion injuries among them. Injury data was collected between 2005 and 2015, including all athletes participating in boys' football, boys' and girls' soccer, girls' volleyball, boys' and girls' basketball, boys' wrestling, boys' baseball, and girls' softball. This landmark study was the first to show that women's soccer has an even greater risk of concussion compared with all other sports.[1,3] This data highlights the need for not only expanding concussion protocols and prevention methods and improving the understanding of concussion in females but also evaluating concussions in female athletes in a more sport-specific manner.

Girls' lacrosse brings up many similar points and discrepancies between genders.[12] Lacrosse is a sport played by both genders, but there are some stark differences in terms of rules and protective equipment. In boys' lacrosse, full-contact body checking and stick checking is allowed. However, in girls' lacrosse, full-contact body checking is prohibited, but stick checking is permitted with restrictions. The "halo" or sphere rule applies in girls' lacrosse, dictating an imaginary sphere of 7 inches surrounding the athlete's head, which is not to be touched. In addition, the protective gear worn by male and female lacrosse players is different, with male athletes being required to wear hard-shell helmets with full face masks, mouth guards, shoulder/ arm pads, and padded gloves, whereas female athletes have to wear only mouth guards and protective eyewear. Owing to the play rules mentioned earlier, girls are prohibited from wearing the hard-shell, full-face-masked helmet. Despite these rules, greater concussions in female lacrosse players occur by contact with the stick or ball than by direct player contact.[12] This discrepancy raises the question of whether girls should be allowed to wear full hard-shell helmets, given the high risk of concussion that has been demonstrated in several studies.[12]

Many of our existing studies evaluating gender-related differences in concussion focus on more "traditional" varsity sports (e.g., soccer, basketball, lacrosse, and softball). However, there are several female-dominated sports (e.g., ballet and figure skating) that are not routinely studied but involve a high rate of concussion. These activities involve significant rotational components, which is a noteworthy aspect of investigation surrounding the mechanism of injury of concussion.[13] In 2015, Post and Blaine Hoshizaki[13] performed a review that studied mechanisms of concussion injury by investigating the relationship between rotational acceleration and brain tissue strains, which are said to be the root cause of concussion. The authors described that this relationship is important to take into account when determining ways to reduce the risk of concussion, but further research is warranted to clarify the role of all aspects of head kinematics, including linear components, in concussion mechanisms, prediction, and prevention.

UNIQUE FEATURES OF CONCUSSIONS IN FEMALE ATHLETES

Females tend to have a higher number of symptoms on the concussion grading scale at the time of initial presentation.[14-16] On concussion grading scales, symptom factors can be grouped into the following categories: (1) cognitive (difficulty concentrating, difficulty remembering, feeling mentally "foggy"), (2) emotional/affective (irritability, sadness, nervousness), (3) physical/somatic symptoms (headache, nausea, vomiting), and (4) sleep (trouble falling asleep, sleeping less than usual).[15] Several studies have shown that females report greater symptoms among all symptom categories compared with their male counterparts.[14,15] Clair and colleagues[14] observed symptom expression during concussion recovery in a pediatric population. The researchers found that in females, physical and cognitive symptoms presented more acutely (1- to 12-week time frame) following a concussion, as opposed to males. In later time periods (i.e., longer than 12 weeks after sustaining a concussion), males experienced higher physical and cognitive symptoms.[14] Concussive symptoms tend to take longer to resolve in female athletes.[16,17] Specifically, females have shown to take longer time to return to school without accommodations, to return to noncontact exercise, for full return to sport, to recovery on computerized neurocognitive function, and for full recovery of vision and vestibular dysfunction.[17]

Neuropsychologic testing demonstrates that female athletes struggle with more cognitive difficulties, worse emotional symptoms, and poorer visual memory than males following concussion.[15,16,18,19] Furthermore, significantly different outcomes in reaction time and concentration after concussion have been found when comparing the two genders.[19] In their review of the role of gender in assessing and managing SRC, Covassin and Elbin[19] mentioned that a proposed explanation for the variations in symptoms that exist is related to the differences in the nature of self-reporting symptoms between males and females. Previous studies have shown that female athletes are more concerned about their future health than males, while male athletes are pressured to show toughness and play through pain. These general findings of differences in sports environments can be translated to the setting of self-reporting concussion symptoms, where female athletes are more likely to report concussive symptoms, explaining in part the observed gender-based disparities in concussion symptoms.[19]

Vestibular/Ocular Motor Screening (VOMS), a patient-reported symptom provocation measure, was developed to better assess both vestibular and oculomotor dysfunction in patients following concussion.[20] This screening includes assessments in the following areas: (1) smooth pursuit, (2) horizontal and vertical saccades, (3) convergence, (4) horizontal vestibular ocular reflex, and (5) visual motion sensitivity.[20] Female athletes frequently demonstrate greater symptom provocation with vestibular and ocular testing. Specifically, utilizing VOMS, females were shown to often perform worse than their male counterparts.[16,17]

Females show delayed time to regain both vestibular and oculomotor deficits with smooth pursuits, saccades, gaze stability, near point of convergence, and balance.[17] Understanding this critical information is important when evaluating the concussed female athlete, as it directly relates to not only patient symptoms but also findings on physical examination, which will help guide the development of treatment plans.

The notable gender-based differences in vestibular and oculomotor dysfunction in combination with females typically presenting to specialty care for evaluation after SRC later than males are concerning.[17] This delay in obtaining proper care has been correlated to the prolonged recovery following concussion that is observed in females when compared to males.[17] As a result, with greater time and subsequent challenges to the reestablishment of proper eye tracking and vestibular function, female athletes will experience difficulties with reading, retaining information, and learning for a longer period. Overall, these effects produce physical symptoms manifested as fatigue, sleep irregularities, headache, and nausea. Therefore it is difficult to determine how much of the emotional symptoms of irritability, depressed mood, and anxiety are truly psychologic versus how much have their roots in oculomotor and vestibular dysfunction.

CONCUSSION IN FEMALES BEYOND THE ATHLETE

As we understand more about the differences between concussion in males and females, it is imperative to better understand the impact of concussion in females outside sports. Specifically, it is important to remember that concussions in females can happen outside the sporting arena. Females are more likely to be involved in domestic abuse situations, which can span across all races, ages, socioeconomic levels, education levels, and sports. According to the CDC's National Intimate Partner and Sexual Violence Survey (NISVS), about one in four females will experience sexual violence, physical violence, and/or stalking by an intimate partner in their lifetime.[21] This is in contrast to 1 in 10 males who will experience this type of violence. In addition, this violence can start as early as adolescence, with 11 million females and 5 million males reporting their first incidence of violence at an age less than 18 years.[21] Therefore injury can date back even before a college athlete presents to a student health or physician's office with symptoms. These violent episodes can not only directly result in concussion injuries but also contribute to other lasting mental health challenges, such as depression, anxiety, and posttraumatic stress disorder (PTSD).[22] Furthermore, traumatic events like abuse can increase the possibility of patients engaging in higher risk behaviors such as smoking, binge drinking, and higher risk sexual behavior.[21] These underlying issues, in addition to a concussion injury, make for an even more challenging situation. Therefore when working with female athletes who present with symptoms consistent with concussion, inquiring about the risk of abuse should not be overlooked.

The underresearched area of concussion caused by physical abuse carries significant weight when considering concussion in females. SRCs can certainly produce multiple concussions, but intimate partner abuse can result in far greater numbers of concussions/TBI over time.[23] It is not intuitive in the sporting context to think of the potential for athletes to have sustained a head injury from a physical abuse situation. This remains, however, an opportunity for healthcare providers surrounding these athletes to create treatment environments that support athlete disclosure related to potentially sensitive and emotional circumstances.

For future areas of continued study and the expansion of concussion assessment, establishing an informative link between SRC and intimate partner violence (IPV) could be very insightful. Determining their respective influences in both diagnosis and treatment could help further understand the gender differences in concussion. Smirl et al.[23] examined the degree of overlap between SRC and IPV symptoms pertaining to TBI in a population of female IPV survivors. Researchers compared the Brain Injury Severity Assessment (BISA) tool, an IPV-specific questionnaire, and the Sport Concussion Assessment Tool 5 (SCAT5), which is widely used for SRC evaluation.[24] Overall, it was found that in females who have experienced IPV, a greater number of TBIs were detected when using the BISA tool.[23] Traditionally, an SCAT-5 might not be included in the initial assessment of a female who has sustained IPV. The opposite is also true, where an athlete who has sustained a head injury may not be screened for potential IPV. Therefore the results from these authors indicate the potential for an enhanced ability to diagnose TBI by expanding screening tools used for athletes to include IPV-specific questionnaires, in addition to the SCAT-5 tool.[23] Furthermore, by including psychopathologic assessments for PTSD, depression, and anxiety, sports medicine teams may be able to gain a better understanding of the true incidence of TBI and assess the overall severity of these injuries.[22]

Although research such as this helps frontline staff to further identify TBI incidence and other challenges facing IPV survivors, the same should also be true for the sports medicine community.[23] This calls upon sport medicine physicians, athletic trainers, and other staff to understand the need to incorporate a more expansive view of the female athlete presenting with concussion-like symptoms. A female athlete who presents with symptoms of difficulty concentrating, fatigue, and "not feeling like themselves" very well may have concussion, but may also be a victim of abuse. As we learn more about the state of various forms of abuse that may be affecting athletes, it becomes clear that there is a stigma around reporting not only mental health issues but also abuse.[25] Even concussion itself continues to go underreported by female athletes in many sporting situations as a result of stigma.[26] Intertwining these stigmas with the additional aforementioned concerns, continued education surrounding the importance of all three of these issues (abuse, mental health, and concussion) is essential for the clinician to prioritize. Sports medicine providers need to create clinical environments that promote mindfulness of the possibility that female athletes can be at a greater risk for concussion from violence or abuse versus solely from SRC. In this environment, female athletes could also use the guise of potential diagnosis of concussion to get symptoms addressed from undisclosed abuse.

Yet another interesting facet of understanding concussions in female athletes involves the female military personnel population. Beginning in 2014, the fusion of two very similarly at-risk patient populations, collegiate student-athletes and military service academy students, formed the first large-scale prospective study on concussion and repetitive head injury.[27,28] The ongoing study, dubbed the Concussion Assessment, Research, and Education (CARE) Consortium, was launched and jointly funded by two organizations, the NCAA and the Department of Defense (DOD), and includes 30 campuses across the country. As both a clinical and neurobiological study, this incredible collection of data will be the first of its kind and will hopefully promote even more research based on its impending findings. Data and parameters will be measured with a sequence of tests at the immediate hours, days, and weeks from the head injury. Baseline testing was performed at the beginning of the study to ensure that new data following head injury has a standard of comparison. In addition, a secondary arm of the study will include following up patients long-term after they leave the college setting and for up to 4 years after they leave either their collegiate sport or their service academy career.[27]

Among the active population in a collegiate setting, both student-athletes and military personnel are not only alike in age but also highly motivated with similar reasons to potentially conceal their symptoms for fear of being taken out of activity. In both collegiate-level sports and military training, the risks and potential ramifications for the participant of sustaining a concussion can create difficulties with self-reporting, despite the extensive focus on education over the past decade.[29,30] Athletes have stated that they weigh the cost and benefits when considering reporting suspected concussive symptoms. Keeping in mind the health consequences of the potential concussion, they also worry about the impacts on their team if they are removed from play and receiving negative reactions from their teammates and coaches. These concerns are in addition to the potential cultural issues that surround various sports regarding performance pressures and expectations.[31] Although at present athletes receive significantly more education and have greater access to assistance than in the previous years, there are still substantial barriers to reporting concussion for fear of negative consequences.

A study by Rawlins et al.[32] analyzed the factors influencing concussion reporting in the United States Air Force Academy (USAFA) cadets. The researchers divided outcomes according to themes, which included perceived costs to physical fitness, military career aspirations, pilot qualifications, sports, reputation, academics, and lack of time. This study not only highlighted the complex nature and environment that these cadets must navigate but also illuminated a different barrier to reporting, with concern for future career ambitions. In finding a solution to these barriers, researchers suggested gearing more education toward helping cadets realize the importance of reporting concussions earlier, which in turn will get them back to military and sporting activity sooner. Intentional messaging around the themes identified to prevent reporting could also help minimize attempts at self-management of concussive symptoms.[32] Based on this study, continuing to debunk the stigma surrounding concussion disclosure would lower the fear of cadets' reputation being impacted and result in a greater inclination for this population to seek out necessary care.

Register-Mihalik and colleagues[33] looked at concussion education and reporting in first-year cadets, where 29% were also NCAA student-athletes and, notably, only 21.7% of the entire population studied were female. This study focused on using increasing concussion education as a tool to improve concussion disclosure among cadets. The authors found an association between being female and having lower odds of multiple concussion education exposures. In the same

study, however, a history of sport participation increased the likelihood of having received concussion education on multiple occasions through a variety of formats. More specifically, having played a contact sport in high school was tied to a greater likelihood of multiple education exposures, as did having a history of more than one concussion. Worth mentioning, however, females in this population were less likely to have a history of sustaining multiple concussions.[33] This particular study did not directly correlate more exposure to concussion education to increased knowledge, better attitudes, improved perceived norms, or higher intention to disclose concussion history. However, it did show that for those with a concussion history, exposure to multiple sources of concussion education had a nearly 40% increased prevalence of disclosing all concussions at the time of injury.[33] This was in contrast to those who had only one source of concussion educational exposure.[33] Furthermore, the female athlete/cadet may or may not have had the education exposure as those athletes who participate in contact sports, ultimately limiting her opportunity to receive proper, adequate concussion education, which should not be a deficiency in the female athletic or military experience. Moving forward, this information should motivate sports medicine departments and military programs involved at the collegiate level to ensure that all females continue to receive additional concussion education, as they may not have previously received it in high school. By correcting the disparity in the amount of concussion education exposure across all genders and sports, programs could improve concussion-related reporting and decision-making at the critical transition into collegiate athletics.[33]

THE FEMALE BODY AND CONCUSSION DIFFERENCES

The female brain is different than male brain in its composition and biochemistry, and the female physical body also has several variations. Research has shown that female and male brains differ in more than 100 ways involving structure, activity, chemistry, and blood flow.[34] Concussion affects all parts of the human body, including the brain and physical anatomy. Therefore taking a deeper dive into these gender-based differences is yet another important step in developing a better sense of concussion in females.

Understanding how female physiology may play a role in the concussion experience is one of the most underresearched topics facing the female athlete population. Female physiology provides constant fluctuations in daily hormonal status. Based on research performed on female athletes and anterior cruciate ligament injury risk, it is known that estrogen has effects on the musculoskeletal system with respect to muscle function and tendon and ligament strength. In addition, the female sex hormones, estrogen and progesterone, affect temperature regulation, central nervous system fatigue, substrate metabolism, and exercise performance.[35] Female athletes of all levels, from high school through Olympic and professional sport, note changes in their performance as well as the need for different nutrition, recovery, and injury prevention at various points in their monthly menstrual cycle.[36] How these all relate in the setting of concussion is still largely unknown. Growing numbers of case reports in the literature point to the potential of an altered neuroendocrine relationship in the postconcussion time frame.[37] In 2019, Di Battista et al.[38] evaluated correlations among levels of various neuroendocrine hormones, symptom burden based on the SCAT-5 questionnaire, and recovery time represented by time to physician medical clearance in a population of collegiate-level athletes participating in several different sports. Researchers clustered concussive symptoms into groups (somatic, cognitive, fatigue, and emotion) and observed their relationships to hormone levels, finding that lower levels of both dehydroepiandrosterone sulfate (DHEA-S) and progesterone were associated with an increased symptom burden and longer recovery times. Abnormally low cortisol levels were also reported to have similar effects. Interestingly, in cases of moderate to severe TBI, progesterone has been shown to have neuroprotective effects and other therapeutic benefits. However, owing to the complexities of TBI, there are varying conclusions about the true effect of progesterone, with contradictory results indicating that it likely still has mechanisms involved in injury pathophysiology.[38] Furthermore, at low levels of DHEA-S and progesterone in the setting of concussion, results showed greater mood symptoms corresponding to the presence of higher emotion-related symptom scores. This can be related to the general finding of improvements in mood and behavior seen with higher levels of both these hormones. The authors of this study also reported a positive correlation between prolactin hormone levels and recovery time, with higher levels of prolactin associated with more time to medical clearance and greater cognitive symptom reporting. The previously established relationship between elevated levels of prolactin following severe TBI was noted, as well as these results contradicted earlier studies, indicating the need for further research on the role of prolactin in concussion recovery.[38]

The aforementioned study did not control for menstrual cycle phase in the female athletes included, making it difficult to analyze the potential effect of menstrual phase at the time of concussion on the concussion experience and recovery. Few studies have addressed menstrual phase as a predictor of concussion outcomes in SRC; however, Wunderle and colleagues[39] studied this in 2014 among a population of females presenting to the emergency department with mild TBI. Researchers observed that females injured during the luteal phase of the menstrual cycle, indicated by increased progesterone concentration, experienced worse postconcussive symptoms and poorer quality of life at 1-month after injury compared with those injured during the follicular phase (low progesterone concentration). The authors posited that this occurs as a result of a sudden decrease in progesterone levels at the instance of injury, whereas preexisting low levels of progesterone seen during the follicular phase do not create the same sudden effect and, therefore, lead to better outcomes. This also in part explains gender-based differences in concussion symptoms, given that males have consistently low levels of progesterone and cannot experience the same abrupt fluctuation that is related to poorer outcomes in females. Interestingly, the same study found that females taking synthetic progestin as birth control reported greater quality-of-life outcomes, similar to females injured during the follicular phase, because of the consistency of high levels of progestin before and after injury.[39]

Understanding specific relationships between concentrations of female hormones and systemic inflammation may help clarify differences in concussion symptoms and severity between males and females. A study by Di Battista et al.[40] reported evidence of a significant association between levels of inflammatory biomarkers and symptom burden among all symptom clusters (somatic, cognitive, sleep, and emotion), showing differing results in female and male athletes. Future studies investigating the nature of gender-specific variations in symptom presentation and their potential relationships to female hormones are important for improving prognosis and management.

Evolving evidence surrounding gender-based musculoskeletal differences shows that these differences may also be important in how males and females experience concussion. Specifically, neck size, strength, and strength-to-head size ratios differ between the genders.[34,41] Decreased neck strength coupled with additional factors, such as greater peak angular acceleration and increased angular displacement, could all combine to give female athletes a "bobblehead" phenomenon.[41] Combining this information with considerations regarding sport type, mechanisms of injury, and sport demands brings us closer to understanding the role musculoskeletal deficits may have in female concussion. Soccer serves as an excellent example in understanding the pivotal role the head-and-neck anatomy have in concussion. The activity of heading in soccer has long come under fire as a large contributor to concussion. In soccer, both collisions and headers are well documented as sources of concussion that occur during both practice and competition/games.[11] Some studies have shown up to 40% of concussions occurring in practice and 40% of those caused by headers.[11] Addressing the relationship between this type of heading activity and concussion has shown growing support. There is value in not only changing how players are practicing with headers by incorporating more technique-focused repetitions but also placing limits on the number of repetitions in a given period. This would be a similar idea to following pitch counts in young baseball players, which ultimately limits harmful amounts of repetitions and ensures a proper rest and recovery period to avoid injury. Integrating neck strengthening and cervical proprioception into practice and training is yet another option to help combat this sport-specific risk of concussion in female athletes. Future studies geared toward establishing better tracking using impact monitors to evaluate frequency and strength of these contact episodes would help broaden our understanding of the cumulative effects of this type of activity. Thus combining knowledge of the differences in head/neck strength in females, cervical proprioception, and more precise data collection might help form more prospective, preventative strategies for female athletes.

Given the higher prevalence of concussion in females than males, observations regarding the actual play of different sports become important despite what popular press headlines read focusing on male-dominated sports. Drawing comparisons between female and male sports can be difficult, as not only can the sport itself but also the rules and protective equipment involved be different. However, interesting enough, when comparing sports that have somewhat similar rules and play, such as basketball and soccer, the gender-based differences in the mechanism of concussion injury are sustained. Across these types of sports, males tend to have a higher incidence of concussion from direct player contact, whereas females are more likely to have a concussion from contact with the ball or surface.[8,42] Relating position to concussion incidence is relevant in creating additional protection for these high-risk female athletes.

Better understanding of the specific scenarios where female athletes are at a greater risk of sustaining a concussion can help create additional education points for coaches, players, and referees. For example, concussions in soccer occur at higher rate during games than practice, and this information can help implement improved education to referees for better enforcement of rules as well as limit harmful contact between players.[11] These are just some of the tactics that could be useful in preventing concussions in a more sport-specific manner, and these concepts can be generalized and expanded across all sports.

As concussion is a clinical diagnosis, symptom reporting is a consistent measure across all concussion types by which conclusions can be drawn. When looking at the specifics of these concussive symptoms across studies, females fair worse in 85% of measured symptoms, consisting of poor memory, dizziness, fatigue, sensitivity to light and noise, impaired concentration, headache, anxiety, and depression.[8] Additionally, formal neurocognitive testing in females continues to show concerning data. Broshek et al.[43] evaluated gender differences in neurocognitive outcomes following concussion in both high-school and college athletes.[44] Compared with males, females showed significantly greater cognitive declines based on measures of simple and complex reaction times after concussion versus their preseason baseline levels.[44] Concussed female athletes have also shown significantly lower visual memory composite scores and perform worse up to 72 h after concussion compared with their male counterparts.[29] Furthermore, females continue to report more postconcussion symptoms and for longer periods compared with similar age-matched males, and they may exhibit longer neurocognitive impairments indicating potential long-term effects of SRC.[29] While the issue of "baseline testing" itself creates great debate among providers, these comparisons at a minimum highlight another area of research needed to understand why these differences exist in females.

MOVING TOWARD THE FUTURE

When considering ways for sports medicine teams, healthcare providers, military campuses, and schools to improve female athlete care, understanding and reviewing stigma and myths around the diagnosis of concussion continues to be crucial. Even outside the healthcare community, it is fair to say there is common knowledge that athletes knowingly play with concussion symptoms. A study of male and female high-school athletes demonstrated that over half of the athletes (60%) had played in practice or during a game with concussion symptoms.[45] This data is concerning as athletes continue to underreport concussions despite the tremendous efforts and advancements in concussion management, treatment, and education for both players and coaches over the past decade. Moving forward, creating educational forums specifically targeting the female audience has the potential to increase self-reporting and ultimately improve care for the female athlete. Evolving evidence shows that females also experience the stigma surrounding concussion, but studies indicate that females are more willing to report symptoms and have a greater intention to actually report compared with their male counterparts.[46] However, they may also have reduced access to concussion education, in comparison with males, prior to the collegiate experience.[45] This is a critical window for implementing interventions and addressing these gaps, as females possess the potential for increasing concussion knowledge and the capacity for direct reporting and continue to push the boundaries of participation in sports and military activities.

For future studies, it will be important to identify and correct the large test bias that often exists in the majority of concussion-related studies, which often lack female representation. Even in the case of postmortem brain studies, there is a significant male bias, as there are almost no female brains included in published research on chronic traumatic encephalopathy.[47] Research should be aimed at looking at how concussion studies are designed, conducted, and interpreted so that more accurate information can be gained in understanding the differences between concussion in males and females. Large-scale projects, such as the NCAA and DOD CARE Consortium, will likely provide vital information that will improve the lives of female athletes who sustain a concussion.

As we expand beyond sport-related concussion in females to include military personnel and victims of abuse, it will be essential to identify other associated diagnoses that may be present alongside concussions, such as depression, anxiety, and PTSD.[22] The intricate interweaving of these diagnoses and how they pertain specifically to females is crucial. Expanding education on these subject matters and enhancing screening for both concussion and other related conditions will be critical for improving the care of female patients. Furthermore, utilizing a multidisciplinary team of providers will deliver more thorough and well-rounded care to female athletes. Just as the female body is complex and multifaceted, so needs to be the team that

cares for and guides treatment of female athletes. The sports medicine provider may be at the heart of the concussion team, but additional access to psychologists, psychiatrists, sports nutritionists, physical therapists, massage therapists, optometrists, and speech therapists will provide female athletes with the highest level of care.

Now is the time for researchers and healthcare providers to band together to move the female athlete forward. As mental health is so pivotal to the overall health of athletes and patients, continuing to educate and help clinicians understand the closely intertwined relationship of psychologic pathology and concussion is key. Ensuring emotional symptoms are not mislabeled as anxiety and depression, but rather thoroughly investigated as potential concussive symptoms, will help identify and not overlook concussion in females. Bridging the gap between concussion in female and male athletes is the next step in understanding not only females in sports medicine but also concussion in a broader sense. By accomplishing this, clinicians will be an essential part of helping female athletes participate and stay in sport and ultimately build a foundation of positive self-image, confidence, and lifelong pursuit of physical activity.

REFERENCES

1. Cheng J, Ammerman B, Santiago K, et al. Sex-based differences in the incidence of sports-related concussion: systematic review and meta-analysis. *Sport Health.* 2019;11(6):486–491. https://doi.org/10.1177/1941738119877186.
2. Tsushima WT, Siu AM, Ahn HJ, Chang BL, Murata NM. Incidence and risk of concussions in youth athletes: comparisons of age, sex, concussion history, sport, and football position. *Arch Clin Neuropsychol.* 2019;34(1):60–69. https://doi.org/10.1093/arclin/acy019.
3. Schallmo MS, Weiner JA, Hsu WK. Sport and sex-specific reporting trends in the epidemiology of concussions sustained by high school athletes. *J Bone Jt Surg Am.* 2017;99(15):1314–1320. https://doi.org/10.2106/JBJS.16.01573.
4. Aubry M, Cantu R, Dvorak J, et al. Summary and agreement statement of the first international conference on concussion in sport, Vienna 2001. *Br J Sports Med.* 2002;36:6–7.
5. McCrory P, Meeuwisse W, Dvorak J, et al. Consensus statement on concussion in sport—the 5th international conference on concussion in sport held in Berlin, October 2016. *Br J Sports Med.* 2017;51:838–847.
6. McCrory P, Feddermann-Demont N, Dvořák J, et al. What is the definition of sports-related concussion: a systematic review. *Br J Sports Med.* 2017;51:877–887.
7. Eckner JT, Kutcher JS. Concussion symptom scales and sideline assessment tools: a critical literature update. *Curr*

Sports Med Rep. 2010;9(1):8−15. https://doi.org/10.1249/JSR.0b013e3181caa778.

8. Dick RW. Is there a gender difference in concussion incidence and outcomes? *Br J Sports Med.* 2009;43(1):i46−i50. https://doi.org/10.1136/bjsm.2009.058172.

9. Clay MB, Glover KL, Lowe DT. Epidemiology of concussion in sport: a literature review. *J Chiropr Med.* 2013;12(4):230−251. https://doi.org/10.1016/j.jcm.2012.11.005.

10. Covassin T, Moran R, Elbin RJ. Sex differences in reported concussion injury rates and time loss from participation: an update of the National Collegiate Athletic Association Injury Surveillance Program from 2004−2005 through 2008−2009. *J Athl Train.* 2016;51(3):189−194. https://doi.org/10.4085/1062-6050-51.3.05.

11. Weber AE, Trasolini NA, Bolia IK, et al. Epidemiologic assessment of concussions in an NCAA division I women's soccer team. *Orthop J Sport Med.* 2020;8(5). https://doi.org/10.1177/2325967120921746.

12. Comstock RD, Arakkal AT, Pierpoint LA, Fields SK. Are high school girls' lacrosse players at increased risk of concussion because they are not allowed to wear the same helmet boys' lacrosse players are required to wear? *Inj Epidemiol.* 2020;7(1):18. https://doi.org/10.1186/s40621-020-00242-5.

13. Post A, Blaine Hoshizaki T. Rotational acceleration, brain tissue strain, and the relationship to concussion. *J Biomech Eng.* 2015;137(3). https://doi.org/10.1115/1.4028983.

14. Clair R, Levin Allen S, Goodman A, McCloskey G. Gender differences in quality of life and symptom expression during recovery from concussion. *Appl Neuropsychol Child.* 2019:1−9. https://doi.org/10.1080/21622965.2018.1556102.

15. Kontos AP, Elbin RJ, Schatz P, et al. A revised factor structure for the post-concussion symptom scale: baseline and post-concussion factors. *Am J Sports Med.* 2012;40(10):2375−2384. https://doi.org/10.1177/0363546512455400.

16. Sufrinko AM, Mucha A, Covassin T, et al. Sex differences in vestibular/ocular and neurocognitive outcomes after sport-related concussion. *Clin J Sport Med.* 2017;27(2):133−138. https://doi.org/10.1097/JSM.0000000000000324.

17. Desai N, Wiebe DJ, Corwin DJ, Lockyer JE, Grady MF, Master CL. Factors affecting recovery trajectories in pediatric female concussion. *Clin J Sport Med.* 2019;29(5):361−367. https://doi.org/10.1097/JSM.0000000000000646.

18. Merritt VC, Padgett CR, Jak AJ. A systematic review of sex differences in concussion outcome: what do we know? *Clin Neuropsychol.* 2019;33(6):1016−1043. https://doi.org/10.1080/13854046.2018.1508616.

19. Covassin T, Elbin RJ. The female athlete: the role of gender in the assessment and management of sport-related concussion. *Clin Sports Med.* 2011;30(1):125. https://doi.org/10.1016/j.csm.2010.08.001.

20. Mucha A, Collins MW, Elbin RJ, et al. A brief vestibular/ocular motor screening (VOMS) assessment to evaluate concussions: preliminary findings. *Am J Sports Med.* 2014;42(10):2479−2486. https://doi.org/10.1177/0363546514543775.

21. cdc.gov/violenceprevention/intimatepartnerviolence/fastfact.html. April 2020.

22. Davis A. Violence-related mild traumatic brain injury in women: identifying a triad of postinjury disorders. *J Trauma Nurs.* 2014;21(6):300−308. https://doi.org/10.1097/JTN.0000000000000086.

23. Smirl JD, Jones KE, Copeland P, Khatra O, Taylor EH, Van Donkelaar P. Characterizing symptoms of traumatic brain injury in survivors of intimate partner violence. *Brain Inj.* 2019;33(12):1529−1538. https://doi.org/10.1080/02699052.2019.1658129.

24. Echemendia RJ, Meeuwisse W, McCrory P, et al. The sport concussion assessment tool 5th edition (SCAT5): background and rationale. *Br J Sports Med.* 2017;51(11):848−850. https://doi.org/10.1136/bjsports-2017-097506.

25. Reardon CL, Hainline B, Aron CM, et al. Mental health in elite athletes: International Olympic Committee consensus statement (2019). *Br J Sports Med.* 2019;53(11):667−699. https://doi.org/10.1136/bjsports-2019-100715.

26. McDonald T, Burghart MA, Nazir N. Underreporting of concussions and concussion-like symptoms in female high school athletes. *J Trauma Nurs.* 2016;23(5):241−246. https://doi.org/10.1097/JTN.0000000000000227.

27. Broglio SP, McCrea M, McAllister T, et al. A national study on the effects of concussion in collegiate athletes and US military service academy members: the NCAA-DoD concussion assessment, research and education (CARE) consortium structure and methods. *Sports Med.* 2017;47(7):1437−1451. https://doi.org/10.1007/s40279-017-0707-1.

28. http://www.ncaa.org/sport-science-institute/topics/ncaa-dod-care-consortium#:~:text=The%20NCAA%2DU.S.%20Department%20of,30%20campuses%20across%20the%20country. April 2020.

29. Weber ML, Suggs DW, Bierema L, Miller LS, Reifsteck F, Schmidt JD. Collegiate student-athlete sex, years of sport eligibility completed, and sport contact level influence on concussion reporting intentions and behaviours. *Brain Inj.* 2019;33(5):592−597. https://doi.org/10.1080/02699052.2019.1568573.

30. Register-Mihalik JK, Cameron KL, Kay MC, et al. Determinants of intention to disclose concussion symptoms in a population of U.S. military cadets. *J Sci Med Sport.* 2019;22(5):509−515. https://doi.org/10.1016/j.jsams.2018.11.003.

31. https://www.sciencedaily.com/releases/2019/05/190508142448.htm. May 2020.

32. Rawlins MLW, Johnson BR, Register-Mihalik JK, DeAngelis K, Schmidt JD, D'Lauro CJ. United States Air Force academy cadets' perceived costs of concussion disclosure. *Mil Med.* 2020;185(1−2):e269−e275. https://doi.org/10.1093/milmed/usz162.

33. Register-Mihalik JK, Kay MC, Kerr ZY, et al. Influence of concussion education exposure on concussion-related educational targets and self-reported concussion disclosure among first-year service academy cadets. *Mil Med.* 2020;185(3−4):e403−e409. https://doi.org/10.1093/milmed/usz414.

34. https://www.pinkconcussions.com/brain-injury. May 2020.

35. Emmonds S, Heyward O, Jones B. The challenge of applying and undertaking research in female sport. *Sport Med Open*. 2019;5(1):51. https://doi.org/10.1186/s40798-019-0224-x.

36. Constantini NW, Dubnov G, Lebrun CM. The menstrual cycle and sport performance. *Clin Sports Med*. 2005;24(2):e51—xiv. https://doi.org/10.1016/j.csm.2005.01.003.

37. Langelier DM, Kline GA, Debert CT. Neuroendocrine dysfunction in a young athlete with concussion: a case report. *Clin J Sport Med*. 2017;27(6):e78—e79. https://doi.org/10.1097/JSM.0000000000000408.

38. Di Battista AP, Rhind SG, Churchill N, et al. Peripheral blood neuroendocrine hormones are associated with clinical indices of sport-related concussion. *Sci Rep*. 2019;9(1). https://doi.org/10.1038/s41598-019-54923-3.

39. Wunderle K, Hoeger KM, Wasserman E, Bazarian JJ. Menstrual phase as predictor of outcome after mild traumatic brain injury in women. *J Head Trauma Rehabil*. 2014;29(5):E1—E8. https://doi.org/10.1097/HTR.0000000000000006.

40. Di Battista AP, Churchill N, Rhind SG, Richards D, Hutchison MG. The relationship between symptom burden and systemic inflammation differs between male and female athletes following concussion. *BMC Immunol*. 2020;21(1):11. https://doi.org/10.1186/s12865-020-0339-3.

41. Tierney RT, Sitler MR, Swanik CB, Swanik KA, Higgins M, Torg J. Gender differences in head-neck segment dynamic stabilization during head acceleration. *Med Sci Sports Exerc*. 2005;37(2):272—279. https://doi.org/10.1249/01.mss.0000152734.47516.aa.

42. Ling DI, Cheng J, Santiago K, et al. Women are at higher risk for concussions due to ball or equipment contact in soccer and lacrosse. *Clin Orthop Relat Res*. 2020;478(7):1469—1479. https://doi.org/10.1097/CORR.0000000000000995.

43. Broshek DK, Kaushik T, Freeman JR, Erlanger D, Webbe F, Barth JT. Sex differences in outcome following sports-related concussion. *J Neurosurg*. 2005;102(5):856—863. Retrieved Jun 30, 2020, from: https://thejns.org/view/journals/j-neurosurg/102/5/article-p856.xml.

44. Covassin T, Savage JL, Bretzin AC, Fox ME. Sex differences in sport-related concussion long-term outcomes. *Int J Psychophysiol*. 2018;132(Pt A):9—13. https://doi.org/10.1016/j.ijpsycho.2017.09.010.

45. https://www.pinkconcussions.com/brain-donation-faq. May 2020.

46. http://www.ncaa.org/sport-science-institute/concussion-educational-resources. May 2020.

47. https://www.cdc.gov/headsup/index.html. May 2020.

FURTHER READING

1. Sullivan L, Molcho M. Gender differences in concussion-related knowledge, attitudes and reporting-behaviours among high school student-athletes. *Int J Adolesc Med Health*. 2018. https://doi.org/10.1515/ijamh-2018-0031.

CHAPTER 23

Stress Fractures

KATHLEEN WEBER, MD, MS • JAMIE R. BIRKELO, PA-C • LUIS J. SOLIZ, MD

INTRODUCTION

Stress fractures are relatively common overuse injuries occurring in individuals participating in a variety of physical activities. They have been reported to account for up to 20% of all injuries seen in sports medicine clinics.[1] As an overuse injury, stress fractures occur by the accumulation of repetitive forces, which are lower than the force required to cause a fracture with a single load. Compression, tension, bending, torsion, or shear forces applied to the bone result in a deformation of the bone.[2] When the force exceeds the bone's elastic range, damage (e.g., microfracture) occurs.[3] Repeated stress of bone causes a disruption in the equilibrium between osteoclastic and osteoblastic activity. This results in an increased risk of microfractures to the bone as the repetitive mechanical loads result in a shift toward osteoclastic activity and thus overall bone resorption. Over time, osteoblasts are unable to keep up with bone remodeling demands and microfractures accumulate, which can lead to a disruption in the integrity of the bone and ultimately a fracture in the cortical bone.[4]

There are two types of stress fractures: fatigue and insufficiency fractures. An *insufficiency fracture* occurs when the bone quality is not able to withstand normal forces that are placed upon it. In these cases, compromised bone structure allows injury at otherwise normal physiologic strain levels. This can occur when a bone is weakened most commonly from osteoporosis, but it can also be attributed to various medications or other abnormal metabolic processes such as rheumatoid arthritis, fibromuscular dysplasia, Paget disease, osteogenesis imperfecta, osteomalacia, hyperparathyroidism, metastatic disease, or areas that have received radiotherapy.[5] In contrast, a *fatigue fracture* occurs as a result of repetitive forces on normal bone. In this situation, the subsequent frequency and/or intensity of the strain exceeds the bone's ability to adequately repair itself. When the bone fails to sufficiently keep up with the remodeling process required because of the excessive strain, microscopic fractures occur. If the frequency and/or intensity of loading of the bone is not diminished, the microfractures propagate and can result in a stress injury.

It is often a combination of several risk factors that lead to the development of a stress fracture. Risk factors are often described as either intrinsic or extrinsic (Table 23.1).[6] Muscle fatigue has been described as a possible risk factor for developing stress fractures.[7] During activity, muscles absorb, counteract, and redirect forces experienced by the bone. When the bone experiences a bending force, one side is subjected to a compressive force and the opposite side is subjected to a tensile force. An eccentric contraction of muscle on the tensile side serves to decrease the tensile force applied to the bone. As muscle becomes fatigue, this protective mechanism is weakened and as a result the bone is subjected to higher repetitive forces leading to bone fatigue. Muscle fatigue can result in the muscle's inability to decrease shear force seen in some individuals with poor gait mechanics. That section of bone is now subjected to higher levels of force resulting in increased microdamage.[8] Leg length discrepancies, pes planus, and pes cavus have been shown to play a role in increasing the risk of developing stress fractures.[5] Multiple studies have demonstrated that a decreased bone cross-sectional area increases the risk of developing stress fractures.[8,9] The importance of calcium and vitamin D in the role of bone health has been extensively described in the literature. Studies regarding the role of calcium and vitamin D in the prevention of stress fractures have shown mixed results.[10]

Females demonstrate an increased propensity of developing stress fractures compared with males.[11–13] Studies attribute this to hormonal, nutritional, biomechanical, and anatomic differences.[14,15] Females manifesting one or all of the components of the female athlete triad (or relative energy deficiency in sports) are at particularly high risk for developing stress

The Female Athlete. https://doi.org/10.1016/B978-0-323-75985-4.00014-3

TABLE 23.1
Risk Factors for Stress Fractures.

Intrinsic	Extrinsic
Decreased bone density	Muscle fatigue
Female gender	Poor footwear
Anatomic variants	Training surface
Medical conditions affecting metabolic/nutrition status	Impact sport/activity
Disruption of menstrual cycle	Low vitamin D levels
Bone cross-sectional area	Poor calcium intake
Previous history of stress fracture	Excessive or rapid change in activity level
	Smoking
	Poor biomechanics

fractures. The female athlete triad consists of low energy availability with or without concomitant eating disorder, menstrual disturbances, and altered bone mineral density.[16] The combination of decreased calorie intake and increased calorie expenditure from activity results in a low-energy or negative-energy state. This can result in estrogen deficiency and deficiency in other hormones that play a role in overall bone health.[17] Estrogen has the effect of protecting bone from resorption, and estrogen receptors have even been found on osteoblastlike cells.[18] When coupled with increased bone resorption from repetitive stresses, fracture risk further increases. Females experiencing oligomenorrhea or amenorrhea appear to have an increased risk of developing a stress fracture. Prepubescent females participating in high-intensity physical activity have been shown to be at increased risk of primary or secondary amenorrhea, stress, fractures, and nonhealing fractures.[19]

DIAGNOSIS

Diagnosis of stress fractures includes a thorough history including risk factor assessment, comprehensive physical examination, and imaging studies.[6] Important factors in the patient's health history include exercise regimen (e.g., change in type, intensity, and duration), dietary intake, history of prior stress fractures, past medical history, and menstrual cycle. Patients typically report an insidious onset of pain without an inciting event or trauma. They often describe symptoms with

activity that are relieved with rest.[6] Physical examination should involve the affected limb or body part, contralateral limb if applicable, as well as the joint above and below the involved body part. Palpation may reveal bony tenderness; however, owing to the depth of the overlying soft tissue, bony palpation may be difficult at certain anatomic locations. Tuning fork test, therapeutic ultrasound, percussion test, fulcrum test, and functional tests (e.g., hop test) may be performed to assist in the diagnosis.[1,3,20,21]

The clinical scenario, along with a thorough history and physical examination, should provide information to formulate and narrow the working differential. Additionally, appropriate diagnostic tests, when determined to be clinically necessary, assist in finalizing the diagnosis. The broad differential diagnoses to be considered when evaluating patients with a suspected stress fracture may include the following: bone contusion, surrounding soft tissue pathology (bursitis, tendinitis, muscle strain, ligament strain), infection, neoplasm, compartment syndrome, avascular necrosis (AVN), insufficiency fracture, contusion, nerve entrapment, vascular entrapment, arthritis, and sickle cell disease.[6]

IMAGING STUDIES

Imaging studies are readily used in the diagnosis of stress fractures. Plain radiography is typically the first study performed when evaluating for a suspected stress fracture.[22] In the early stages of the disease process, radiographs will often appear negative, thus resulting in an initial high false-negative result rate. Radiographic findings are highly dependent on the timing between onset of symptoms and obtaining the imaging study, as well as if the patient continued with the contributing activity.[23] In the early stages, radiographic findings vary depending on the type of bone and may include a lucency through the cortex without periosteal reaction or callus in long bones or a focal linear area of sclerosis perpendicular to the trabeculae in cancellous bone.[24] A periosteal thickening occurs as bone heals and ultimately, if previously seen, the fracture line disappears.[23] Obtaining serial radiographs over several weeks may not manifest characteristic evidence of fracture healing or new bony callus formation. Therefore when clinical suspicion remains despite negative radiographs, more advanced imaging techniques are required to confirm or rule out the diagnosis.

Nuclear medicine scintigraphy (bone scans) are highly sensitive and may aid in the early diagnosis of stress fractures.[22] A diagnostic bone scan will demonstrate radiotracer uptake in an area of bony remodeling, trabecular microfracture, periosteal reaction, or callus formation.[25] Nuclear scintigraphy is sensitive to early bony remodeling changes and can detect stress fractures or reactions within 72 h after the initial injury.[26] Although bone scans are very sensitive for bone turnover and remodeling, they are not always specific for stress fractures. Any condition producing increased bone turnover, such as osteogenic tumors, infection, trauma, or inflammation, will result in increased radiotracer uptake.[27] Conversely, a negative bone scan allows for the exclusion of a stress fracture. A bone scan involves radiation exposure approximately 44 times that of a standard chest radiography, which should be considered when choosing an imaging study.[28]

Magnetic resonance imaging (MRI) can detect early bone marrow changes and bone remodeling related to stress reaction and fractures. MRI also offers more intricate detail of surrounding soft tissue, which could potentially be the source of the patient's pain. Use of water-sensitive pulse sequence (e.g., fat suppression) allows for the detection of endosteal bone marrow edema, which is one of the earliest changes seen in stress fractures.[29] When compared to nuclear scintigraphy, MRI allows for a more precise location of fractures, allows for a comprehensive evaluation of the surrounding structures including soft tissue, and does not have radiation exposure. Given that MRI is sensitive for bone marrow edema, MRI findings must be correlated with the patient's clinical presentation, as bone marrow edema may be detected on asymptomatic patients/athletes and it may persist after diagnosis and treatment of stress fractures, even as cortical healing continues.[30]

Computed tomographic (CT) imaging is not as commonly used to diagnose stress fractures and is used primarily when the patient is unable to undergo an MRI or to further delineate a fracture line.[22] CT does not have the ability to show bone marrow edema and lacks the precision to determine the acute or chronic nature of the lesion.[30] Diagnostic musculoskeletal ultrasound is another emerging diagnostic tool in the evaluation of stress fractures. Cortical buckling and hypoechogenic callous formation have been seen in superficial bones such as the distal tibia and metatarsals.[27] The usefulness of ultrasound remains limited and has not been recommended as a stand-alone diagnostic tool.[20]

MANAGEMENT

Education and prevention are the cornerstones for management and prevention of stress fractures. Proper identification and education of patients at risk of developing stress fractures can assist in the prompt diagnosis of stress fractures once they occur, thus typically resulting in improved outcomes as well as avoidance of complications and recurrence.[11]

Fortunately, nonoperative management often yields excellent outcomes.[11,31] Initially, the goal of treatment should be aimed at pain control, which can typically be achieved through medication, cryotherapy, elevation, and most importantly rest from the aggravating activity. In addition to activity modification, rest involves off-loading the involved bone/extremity. Medications often include acetaminophen, nonsteroidal antiinflammatory drugs (NSAIDs), and rarely narcotics. There is some controversy regarding the risk of delayed healing or developing a nonunion with the use of NSAIDs[32-34]; therefore the treating physician should take into account the current evidence when considering the use of NSAIDs. Additionally, use of medication may decrease the patient's symptoms, thus prompting the patient to increase the use of the involved body part prior to sufficient healing.

Stress fractures typically heal over a period of 4–8 weeks, depending on the severity, the location, and the age of the patient; however, in some cases, healing may take up to 12 weeks.[6,11] Some stress fractures require strict non-weight-bearing (NWB) status or immobilization with a cast, splint, or controlled ankle motion (CAM) boot, whereas others may require only restriction of activity. Although typically not indicated, except in the case of nonunions, low-intensity pulsed ultrasound could be considered as a tool to increase bone healing; however, the literature has been mixed with its use in treating stress fractures.[35,36] Planned follow-up including repeat clinical examinations and, when deemed necessary by the treating physician, repeat imaging studies may be important to ensure appropriate healing of the stress fracture.

Patients may benefit from a structured multidisciplinary program guided and overseen by their treating physician as the stress fracture heals and activity is reinitiated. This medical team typically includes the treating physician, a physical therapist, and/or a certified athletic trainer. During the initiation of increased activity, careful attention should be paid to the patient's symptoms as they progress to higher levels of activity. In the setting of pain, the patient should not be allowed to progress to the next phase, as the presence of pain indicates that additional time is required for adequate healing. Provided the athlete is pain free, conditioning exercises that do not stress the involved bone are permitted. During the rehabilitation stage, biomechanical errors or other predisposing factors leading to the development of the stress fracture should be identified and corrected in order to effectively manage and prevent the recurrence of stress fractures. Some physicians prescribe over-the-counter or custom orthotics to improve biomechanics and provide shock absorption, which may play a role in the prevention of stress fractures.[10] A review of the individual's prior training regimen, along with functional testing and a gait analysis, may guide the rehabilitation and return-to-play program. Once the stress fracture is healed and the functional deficits are addressed, an emphasis should be placed on gradual return to full activity. Female athletes diagnosed with one or more stress fractures should be screened for the female athlete triad. The screening should be part of the history taking and should include a menstrual history, dietary assessment, and, when appropriate, consideration of obtaining bone density testing.[17,19] Treatment of the female athlete triad requires a multidisciplinary approach.

Although most stress fractures can be treated nonoperatively, surgical intervention may be required in the setting of high-risk stress fractures or stress fractures that have failed conservative management. High-risk stress fractures are more likely to progress to complete fracture, result in delayed union or nonunion, and/or are on the tensile side of the natural biomechanical axis (Table 23.2).[6,10,22]

SPECIFIC STRESS FRACTURES

Femoral Stress Fractures

Stress fractures of the femur are the fourth most common type of stress fracture.[31] Military recruits, dancers, distance runners, jumpers, female athletes, and older

TABLE 23.2
High-Risk Stress Fractures.
Tension-side femoral neck
Patella
Anterior tibia
Medial malleolus
Talus
Tarsal navicular
Jones fracture (proximal fifth metatarsal)
Talar neck
Base of the second metatarsal
Great toe sesamoid

athletes are at higher risk of developing a femoral stress fracture.[30,37] Determining the true incidence of femoral stress fractures is difficult, and these fractures are thought to be underdiagnosed. It is estimated that up to 75% of femoral stress fractures are missed or misdiagnosed on initial evaluation.[38] Patients often present with vague, nonspecific complaints. A high index of suspicion combined with a thorough history, comprehensive physical examination, and obtaining the appropriate imaging studies can confirm the diagnosis. Arriving at a prompt diagnosis may result in improved patient outcomes with a decreased risk of complications.[11]

Femoral stress fractures are often classified based on their anatomic location. Although they can occur at any location along the femur, they are most commonly seen at the femoral neck.[30] Stress fractures involving the femoral neck are of particular importance, given the risk of serious complication including fracture displacement. With regard to the femur, the mechanical axis falls medial to the majority of the femur, thus the compression side is the medial aspect of the femoral neck and the lateral side is considered the tensile side.[30] Compression-sided femoral neck stress fractures (Fig. 23.1) are typically treated nonoperatively with a period of rest, which initially includes a limited weight-bearing status followed by a gradual progression of activity.[11] If the patient fails conservative measures, he/she may require referral for surgical consultation. Although there have been some studies demonstrating successful conservative management of tension-sided femoral neck stress fractures with extensive periods of protected weight-bearing,[39] early surgical intervention continues to be favored due to the risk of displacement.[11] A displaced femoral neck stress fracture is at risk of progression to nonunion or osteonecrosis of the femoral head and is therefore considered a surgical emergency.[40]

Stress fractures of the subtrochanteric region and shaft are less common and occur most often along the medial or posteromedial cortex. When diagnosed early, they can be managed nonoperatively.[41] In cases of displacement or continued pain despite conservative measures, operative fixation is indicated.[30] The long-term use of bisphosphonates has been identified as a risk factor for developing an atypical subtrochanteric femur fractures. The risk and benefits of these medications in the treatment of osteoporosis should be weighed before initiating treatment.[13] Stress fractures of the femoral shaft (Fig. 23.2) have been described more frequently in military recruits and athletes and often involve the posteromedial aspect of the proximal

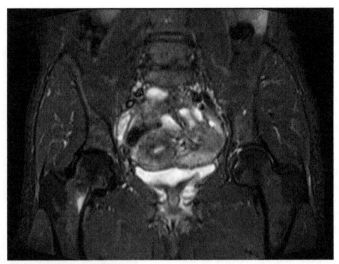

FIG. 23.1 **Femoral compression-side stress injury.** Magnetic resonance T2 coronal image showing edema along the medial aspect of the right femoral neck compression-side stress reaction without discrete fracture line.

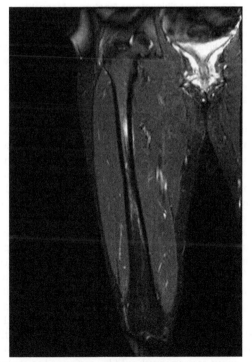

FIG. 23.2 **Femoral shaft.** Magnetic resonance T2 coronal image showing edema midshaft consistent with stress injury.

third of the femur.[42–44] Distal femur stress fractures are even more rare; however, this should remain in the physician's differential diagnoses when the patient presents with a concerning history and physical examination finding.

The patient's history often involves an insidious onset of gradually worsening leg, thigh, or hip pain that may worsen with activity. Athletes with femoral neck stress fractures may report symptoms as early as 2 weeks after increasing exercise intensity and typically report pain in the groin.[45] Patients with femoral shaft stress fractures often report activity-related pain in the thigh or ipsilateral knee[46] but typically lack tenderness or swelling.[43] Pain may limit athletes from participation in athletic activities and sometimes may be associated with night pain.

The general location of the pain may guide physical examination, although the clinical presentation can be variable. Typically, muscle tone and bulk are normal. Due to the overlying soft tissue, the point of maximal tenderness may be difficult to elicit with proximal femur and femoral shaft stress fractures, although some distal femoral stress fractures may demonstrate tenderness to palpation. Pain at the end range of passive hip motion or straight leg raise as well as a positive log roll test result may be present in patients with femoral neck stress fractures.[30] A positive hop test result has been strongly associated with femoral stress fracture.[47] The fulcrum test has proven to be beneficial in the diagnosis of femoral shaft stress fractures.[42] Both the hop and fulcrum tests should be performed with caution so as to not complete a fracture.

When a femoral stress fracture is clinically suspected based on history and physical examination, imaging begins with plain radiography. In the early stages of the disease process, radiographs are often negative, and in fact, radiographic evidence of femoral stress fracture is present in only 10% of cases within the first week.[48] New periosteal bone formation may be noted approximately 10 days after the injury begins, with peak formation at 6 weeks.[23,49] When suspicion of a femoral stress fracture remains despite negative serial radiographs, additional imaging becomes necessary. MRI is often the test of choice, although CT or nuclear scintigraphy may be considered. MRI provides a more precise location of the fracture and allows evaluation of the surrounding tissue pathology. It should be noted that MRI may show persistent bone marrow edema at the site of the femoral stress fracture for up to 6 months after injury.[50]

In summary, the mainstays of conservative care consist of rest and activity modification.[44] Displaced or high-risk fractures typically require surgical intervention. Depending on the location and severity of the femoral stress fracture, the degree of rest and unloading varies from weight-bearing as tolerated to strict NWB.[26,37] The healing process primarily occurs over a period of 6–8 weeks but may take up to 12 weeks.[28,42]

Tibial Stress Fractures

Stress fractures occur most commonly at the tibia, accounting for 25.9%–49.1% of all stress fractures.[51] Developing as a result of recurrent high load-bearing activities, tibial stress fractures have an incidence as high as 10%–20% in distance runners.[52] Stress fractures of the tibia are typically transverse. Longitudinal fractures, although more rare, are at an increased risk of delayed union or nonunion.[53,54] The majority of tibial stress fractures (Fig. 23.3) occur at the diaphysis and are often broken up into two groups based on location and risk classification.[55,56] The majority of tibial stress fractures occur posteromedially and are considered low risk, while stress fractures located anteriorly are classified as high risk.[57] With regard to the tibia, the tension side is anterior and the compression side is posterior.[58] Runners are at an increased risk of developing posterior tibial stress fractures, while the anterior tibial stress fractures are seen more frequently in athletes who participate in jumping/landing activities.[59] Smaller tibial cross-sectional dimensions have been associated with an increased risk of developing a tibial stress fracture.[60] Although treatment for both begins with a trial of

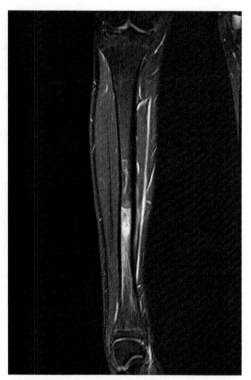

FIG. 23.3 Right tibial stress fracture. Magnetic resonance coronal short tau inversion recovery image showing diffuse endosteal and periosteal marrow edema in the lower tibia extends proximally to mid-one-third diaphysis. Posterior tibial cortex is discretely disrupted with elevated cortical ridges suggesting cortical fracture. Mild intermuscular edema noted between tibialis anterior and tibialis posterior.

nonoperative management, the clinical course and outcomes for anterior and posterior tibial stress fractures vary significantly. Posterior tibial stress fractures demonstrate significantly shorter return-to-sport times compared with anterior tibial stress fractures, which may ultimately require surgical intervention and can be career threatening.[56,58]

Patients typically present with an insidious onset of pain, which initially occurs only during the inciting activity, but may progress to daily weight-bearing activity.[60] Pertinent physical examination findings include focal tenderness over the involved bony area. Swelling may be noted and percussion away from the fracture site may elicit pain. Special tests including the hop test and fulcrum test may be performed, but they should be conducted with caution.[61] A lower limb alignment assessment should be performed to evaluate for possible contributing factors, including mechanical overload.[61–63]

Early recognition of tibial stress fractures is important to minimize the patient's recovery time as well as avoid potentially devastating complications. When there is clinical suspicion for a tibial stress fracture, radiographs should be ordered. Although early in the process they demonstrate a low sensitivity of 10%, they may confirm the diagnosis.[1,27] Although often of limited utility, radiographs may demonstrate the "dreaded black line" indicating the presence of a high-risk anterior cortex tibial stress fracture.[62] It may take 3 weeks for periosteal reaction and cortical irregularities to be visualized under radiography, and thus additional imaging is recommended when clinical suspicion remains high despite negative radiographs.[57,64] MRI is considered the imaging modality of choice given its high sensitivity (86%–100%) and specificity (100%).[51,55] MRI also has the benefit of evaluating the surrounding soft tissue, which can assist in confirming other diagnoses such as medial tibial stress syndrome if no stress fracture is identified. Bone scans are also capable of identifying tibial stress fractures early; however, they lack the specificity of MRI.[61] CT scans may be useful, but are not as sensitive as MRI.[57]

Conservative management (e.g., rest, pneumatic bracing) of posterior tibial stress fractures demonstrates excellent outcomes with return rates of 100%.[56] Multiple studies have shown evidence of significant clinical benefit including earlier return to participation with the use of low-intensity pulsed ultrasound.[36,65] These fractures typically heal in 4–8 weeks.[61] Aerobic fitness, especially low- or no-impact activities (e.g., cycling or swimming), should be encouraged during the treatment.

Management of low-grade anterior cortex tibial stress fractures typically resolve without surgery with a period of relative rest, immobilization, and modified weight-bearing.[60] However, higher grade stress fractures may require early surgical intervention.[52] Treatment recommendations should be based on the fracture site, grade, and level of sport participation.[10] Return to activity is only considered when complete healing of the fracture has been confirmed to avoid progression to a complete fracture.[52,66] Anterior tibial cortex stress fractures are associated with lower rates of return to activity. Of those who are able to return to full participation, the mean time of return to activity varies in the literature from 5 to 7 months.[37,54] Once the patient no longer demonstrates tenderness to palpation, experiences no pain with normal ambulation, has normalized joint range of motion, and has addressed strength deficits, the patient may initiate a guided return to running program. The sports medicine physician should monitor for any recurrence of pain as the athlete gradually increases to preinjury activity levels.

Foot and Ankle Stress Fractures

Stress fractures in the foot and ankle can be categorized as either low-risk or high-risk stress fractures (Table 23.3).[67] High-risk fractures are typically located on the tension side of the bone, develop in locations with limited vascularity, have a tendency to have delayed union or nonunion, and may require surgical intervention.[52]

As with other stress fractures, foot and ankle stress fractures are associated with repetitive submaximal load that over time result in the stress injury. If not diagnosed early and the inciting activity continues, the stress injury can result in a complete fracture. Foot type, training errors, and poor footwear may predispose the athlete to a higher risk for developing these stress injuries. This section will focus on the tibial stress fracture, navicular stress fracture (NSF), and metatarsal stress fracture, but the reader should be aware that no foot or ankle bone is spared from a stress injury.

Common symptoms of foot and ankle stress fractures are similar to those of other stress fractures in that they typically develop gradually. The clinical history is of a gradual pain that first occurs with weight-bearing activity, improves with rest, and worsens during normal activities if the inciting activity is not modified or discontinued. In the foot, unlike some other sites of stress injury, swelling or bruising may be visible.

Plain radiographs may not demonstrate the stress fracture, and these injuries often go unidentified on plain radiographs for several weeks or may never be identified by plain radiographs.[31,68] If plain

TABLE 23.3
Most Common Low-Risk and High-Risk Foot and Ankle Stress Fractures.

Low-Risk	High-Risk
Postero-medial tibia	Anterior tibial cortex
Calcaneus	Medial malleolus
Second metatarsal	Talus
Third metatarsal	Navicular
	Base of the second metatarsal
	Jones Fracture (Proximal fifth metatarsal)
	Tibial sesamoid

radiographs are negative in a clinical scenario suspicious for a stress injury, treatment should be initiated (i.e., activity modification, modified weight-bearing, and/or immobilization) with either follow-up plain radiographs or further imaging with MRI or technetium bone scan to confirm the diagnosis.[69,70]

Navicular Stress Fractures

NSFs are high-risk stress fractures involving the foot and ankle.[67] If poorly managed or treated, these fractures can lead to detrimental consequences for the injured athlete, including persistent pain, functional deficits, and AVN. Up to 20% of all sports medicine clinic visits are for foot and ankle stress fractures.[67] In particular, NSFs represent up to 14%−35% of all foot and ankle stress fractures, with the majority occurring in elite track-and-field athletes.[71−73] Almost three-quarters of all stress fractures diagnosed in elite track-and-field athletes are navicular.[74]

The anatomy of the navicular bone is complex with a tenuous blood supply.[74] The structure of the overall foot is defined by a rigid lateral column and a flexible medial column, with the navicular bone being the cornerstone of the medial column prone to mechanical impingement from the talar head and cuneiform.[67,75] Furthermore, most of the motion of the hindfoot occurs at the talonavicular joint.[74] This puts significant medial stress at the navicular bone, which ultimately affects the central one-third.[72] The tibialis posterior tendon inserts into the navicular medial tuberosity and can also be a source of pain.[75] The navicular bone has a watershed blood supply.[67,72] The medial side of the navicular bone receives its blood flow from the tibialis posterior artery, while the dorsalis pedis artery supplies its lateral half. There is a zone of central avascularity, which is prone to poor healing.

Individuals with NSFs typically present with midfoot pain that worsens with activity.[67,74] Most patients' symptoms tend to be vague in nature, with chronicity spanning at least 6 months to the point where severe pain is no longer relieved with rest.[67,72,75] Pain is characteristically described as achy that radiates to the medial arch.[75] It is usually worse with running and jumping, with bilateral symptoms being rare. On examination, there is usually focal tenderness and swelling over the "N" spot or dorsal navicular prominence.[67,74,75] Pain is often increased with the hop test as well as standing on toes in the equinus position.[74,75]

Potential risk factors for NSF development include altered gait mechanics with decreased forefoot use, long second metatarsal, metatarsal adduction, equinus contracture, and pes planovalgus deformity.[72,74,75] It

is also theorized that the severity of pes planus correlates with the amount of stress placed at the central dorsal location of the navicular bone during axial loading.[72] Initial workup for a suspected NSF involves obtaining three-view weight-bearing radiographs to help rule out other pathologies, as NSFs tend to be difficult to visualize on plain films.[67,72,74] If there remains clinical concern for an NSF, an MRI (Figs. 23.4 and 23.5) can be ordered to look for a stress fracture or an occult injury.[67,74] Some authors have advocated the use of a triple-phase bone scan as the next diagnostic test of choice after radiography partly due to its lower cost.[75] This scan shows positive results early and localized lesions well, but it is a nonspecific test.

Once a stress fracture is confirmed, a CT scan (Fig. 23.6) is recommended to help characterize the anatomic details of the stress fracture and guide treatment, as MRI tends to provide inferior visualization of disrupted trabecular bone compared with CT.[67,74−77] NSFs on CT scan are defined by the Saxena Classification as followed: Type 1, only a dorsal cortical break; Type 2, cortical break with extension into the navicular body; and Type 3, involvement of any two cortices.[67,77]

Although there appears to be good support in the literature for both nonoperative and operative management of NSFs, it is generally accepted that the gold standard of care for nondisplaced, noncomminuted fractures is NWB cast immobilization for 6 weeks.[72,74−76] Indications for operative management

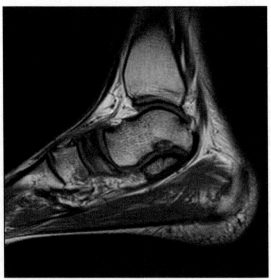

FIG. 23.4 **Magnetic resonance T1 image showing navicular stress fracture.** Low T1 signal present in navicular bone consistent with a fracture.

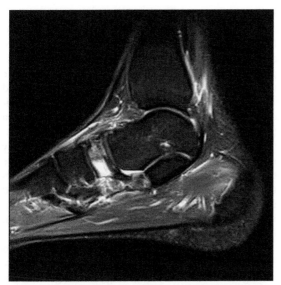

FIG. 23.5 Magnetic resonance T2 image showing navicular stress fracture. Extensive bone marrow edema present within the navicular bone. Incidental minimal fluid in retrocalcaneal bursa and posterior subtalar joint.

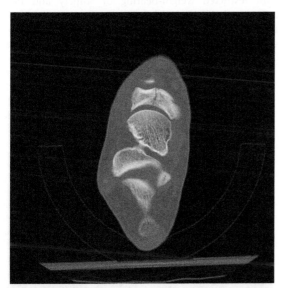

FIG. 23.6 Computed tomography (CT) of navicular stress fracture. CT axial hindfoot revealing minimally displaced fracture of the right navicular bone.

of NSFs with open reduction internal fixation (ORIF) include any displacement, comminution, and delayed union/nonunion fractures.[72,75] Postoperative care includes splinting for 2 weeks followed by NWB casting for an additional 4 weeks.[72] Reported complications

of operative care include deep venous thrombosis, AVN, nonunion, infection, secondary osteoarthrosis, and secondary surgery for hardware retrieval.[78] For cases of failed ORIF or AVN, autologous bone grafting from the cuneiforms is typically performed.[72]

It is generally not recommended to monitor progress with serial CT scans, as CT scans tend to lag behind clinical symptoms and improvement with no obvious correlation.[71,76] However, CT scanning to assess osseous healing for operatively treated NSFs is not uncommon.[72] Another alternative to monitor recovery from NSFs is therapeutic ultrasound.[79] One prospective clinical case series determined that in elite track-and-field athletes, therapeutic ultrasound correlated well with visual analog scores and grade of fracture demonstrated on MRI. The authors concluded that ultrasound was a safe and reproducible method of monitoring resolution of these fractures. However, at this time, ultrasound has not been recommended as a stand-alone diagnostic tool.[20]

One systematic review that included eight studies of NSFs determined that return-to-sport time was 16 weeks for the surgically treated group as opposed to 22 weeks in the conservatively treated group.[58] Saxena et al., in a prospective study of elite athletes, reported that the return-to-activity time between nonoperatively managed Type 1 NSFs and operatively managed Type 2 and Type 3 NSFs was comparable among all groups at approximately 4 months duration.[77] However, some literature suggests that at least for elite athletes, return-to-activity duration tends to be longer, approaching 6−12 months in length.[72] Regardless of whether nonoperative or operative management is pursued, any period of limited weight-bearing during the treatment process brings with it the risk of complications including delayed healing and nonunion.[76]

The functional rehabilitation protocol after a successfully treated NSF typically lasts 6 weeks,[75] but it should be individualized to the athlete's needs incorporating strengthening, restoration of range of motion, and progressive aerobic activity. During the first 2 weeks, swimming and water running are permitted. In weeks 3−4, jogging on grass for 5 min on alternate days is permitted. By weeks 5−6, individuals are able to run at 50% of their maximum speed with walking on alternate days. Finally, by weeks 6 and beyond, there is a gradual return to full training activity.

First Through Fourth Metatarsal Stress Fractures

First metatarsal stress fractures are uncommon,[67,80] and when diagnosed, they typically occur at the proximal metaphyseal/diaphyseal junction. Increased medial stress on the foot is thought to be a factor in their development.[81] Metatarsal stress fractures of digits 2 through 4 are commonly seen in runners and ballet dancers,[51,82,83] but they can be seen in other sports[84,85] that require forefoot loading.[86] These fractures are also known as "march fractures," as they occur frequently in military recruits.[67] The second through fourth metatarsals are cross-sectionally weaker,[87] likely contributing to stress injuries that are common to these metatarsals. While the second through fourth metatarsal stress fractures primarily involve the diaphysis, stress fractures at the base of the second metatarsal (Fig. 23.7) are known to occur in ballet dancers, but are also seen in nondancers.[67,88,89] The high stress loads placed on the forefoot during ballet dance movements, such as *en pointe*, likely contribute to the second metatarsal base stress fractures seen in these dancers.[90,91]

In general, metatarsal shaft stress fractures heal well with conservative treatment, in contrast to the high rate of nonunion seen in the base of the second metatarsal stress fractures. Chuckpaiwong et al.[89] reported that 12 base of the second metatarsal stress fractures were treated nonoperatively and found that 50% developed nonunions and 5% underwent subsequent surgery.

Fifth Metatarsal Stress Fractures

A widely accepted classification by Lawrence and Botte[92] divides fifth metatarsal fractures into three zones. Zone 1 is the tuberosity, the most proximal portion of the fifth metatarsal; zone 2 is the metaphyseal-diaphyseal junction (Jones fracture); and zone 3 is the proximal diaphyseal. Stress fractures typically occur in the proximal to mid-diaphyseal area (Fig. 23.8), but all three zones are subject to stress injury. The proximal diaphysis has a poor blood supply increasing the risk of delayed union or nonunion, while the rich network of arteries that supply metaphysis fracture allow for them to heal well.[93] Management should include NWB immobilization in a cast. Close follow-up is advised, as these stress fractures may require surgical intervention.

Most foot and ankle stress fractures are considered low risk and tend to heal well.[67] These injuries can be managed conservatively with weight-bearing immobilization and activity modification, typically healing in 4–8 weeks. However, some higher risk stress fractures, such as navicular or the fifth metatarsal, are at high risk for nonunion. They are typically immobilized with restricted weight-bearing or surgery and take longer to heal. High-risk stress fractures require close follow-up and should be managed by individuals with expertise in treating these injuries. Returning to

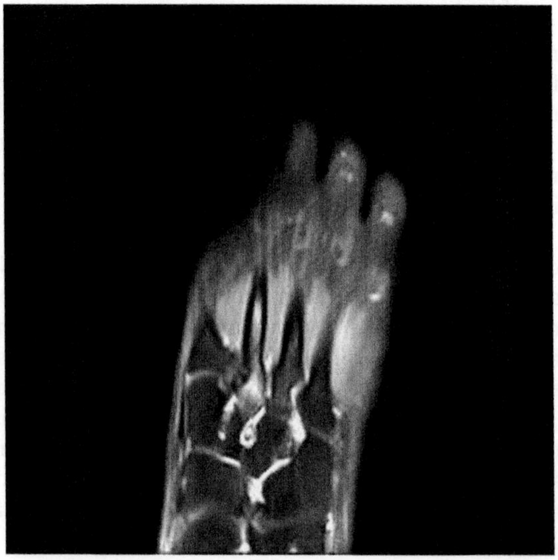

FIG. 23.7 **Base of the second metatarsal stress injury.** Magnetic resonance imaging: increased T2 and amorphous low T1 signal (not pictured) throughout the proximal aspect of the second metatarsal with extension to the mid-diaphysis with no focal linear low T1 (not pictured) areas of signal to suggest a fracture.

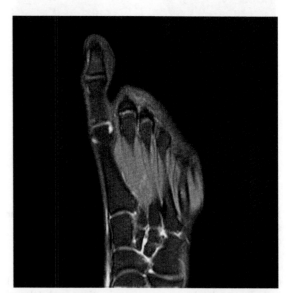

FIG.   23.8 **Fifth   metatarsal   diaphysis.** Magnetic resonance imaging T2 hyperintensity noted in the left fifth metatarsal diaphysis without a corresponding T1 signal abnormality (not pictured) consistent with stress reaction.

activities too rapidly can delay healing, increase the risk of completing the fracture, or result in a nonunion.

Stress Fractures of the Spine and Sacrum

Stress fractures of the axial spine most commonly involve defects within the pars interarticularis, secondary to chronic low-grade trauma or repetitive loading.[94] The term for this is known as spondylolysis. Sometimes this results in instability of the posterior elements of the spine, which can lead to isthmic spondylolisthesis in which one vertebral body slips forward to the vertebral body below it. Specifically, the prevalence of spondylolysis within the general population is 6%–8%, with a disproportionately higher incidence in athletic populations who require repetitive hyperextension of the spine within their sport.[94,95]

One prospective study calculated an overall prevalence of spondylolysis as high as 40% in athletic patients younger than 19 years presenting with persistent low-back pain for greater than 2 weeks.[96] Within the high-school population, it was calculated that 1.54 stress fractures occur for every 100,000 athlete-exposures.[97] About 63% of all these stress fractures occurred in girls and 37% in boys, and 15% of the stress fractures involved the lumbar spine or pelvis area. Although rare, new-onset spondylolysis can also be seen in high-level adult athletes.[98] Spondylolysis most commonly involves the L5 vertebra, but it can occur at any level, including the thoracic spine.[99,100] Almost three-quarters of individuals with spondylolysis will develop spondylolisthesis.[99] Bilateral pars interarticularis defects occur in approximately 80% of cases.

Spondylolysis is typically an asymptomatic presentation found incidentally on radiography.[99] Individuals who are symptomatic usually present with localized and insidious low-back pain that radiates to the buttocks.[94,99] Athletes typically report a history of activity that involves repeated extension or rotation of the lumbar spine that makes their pain worse. Pertinent examination findings can include hamstring tightness, prominent loss of lumbar lordosis, presence of functional scoliosis, and a palpable step-off. One systematic review reported that the one-legged hyperextension test had low-to-moderate sensitivity (50%–73%) and low specificity (17%–73%).[94]

Imaging modalities for workup of spondylolysis include radiography, planar scintigraphy, single-photon emission computed tomography (SPECT), CT, and MRI.[99] Plain radiography of the lumbar spine is generally ordered initially and should include standing anteroposterior and a lateral view to assess for the degree of vertebral body slippage.[94,101] Radiographic signs of spondylolysis include lateral deviation of the spinous process and unilateral pedicle sclerosis.[102] MRI is generally recommended if initial radiographs are negative and is the initial imaging modality of choice with select patient populations, including juveniles and pregnant women, given ionizing radiation is not used.[101] SPECT is a more sensitive test than planar scintigraphy in detecting lesions, and a normal planar scintigraphy cannot rule out a stress fracture until SPECT is performed.[103] Furthermore, SPECT has been found to be useful in both adolescent and young adult populations. Combined SPECT/CT is useful in detecting both the metabolic activity and the structural components of spondylolysis.[102] The MRI sequence short tau inversion recovery has been helpful in distinguishing painful from painless pars fractures.[104]

Nonoperative management with bracing and physical therapy is considered the gold standard of care in treating symptomatic spondylolysis.[95,99] Some physicians do not use bracing, but rather treat with rest and activity modification and avoidance of extension activities.[105] If bracing is not incorporated from the onset of treatment then the lack of symptom improvement by 2–4 weeks, evidence of fracture, or lack of patient compliance with restrictions would indicate the need to incorporate bracing.[106,107] One retrospective case series estimated a 95% success rate with nonoperative care (including custom-fitted thoracolumbar orthosis, activity cessation for 3 months, and a physical therapy program) in juveniles and adolescents with symptomatic isthmic spondylolysis that was confirmed by either SPECT or CT.[108] Furthermore, all individuals in the study were able to return to their preinjury level of activity, with no individual requiring any surgical intervention. A retrospective review of 63 pediatric patients with symptomatic lumbar spondylolysis (LS) also reported excellent outcomes with conservative treatment.[109] They found a bony healing rate of 100% in very early stage LS, with an average treatment period of only 2.5 months. In early stage LS, the bony healing rate fell slightly down to 94%, with an average treatment length of 2.6 months. For progressive stage LS, the bony healing rate was 80%, with an average treatment length of 3.6 months. Surprisingly, the recurrence rate of LS was 26.1%, but fortunately, all the pediatric patients with recurrence achieved bony healing.

Operative management with pars repair and fusion is indicated for failed conservative care for more than 6 months, persistent back pain, pars nonunion at 9–12 months, and any neurologic impairment. Return to play after surgery is typically 6–12 months, with prohibition of contact sports thereafter. In children with a history of spondylolysis, it is generally recommended that 25-hydroxyvitamin D levels be checked routinely and treated if levels are not sufficient.[110] Previous studies have demonstrated either deficient or insufficient levels within this vulnerable population.

In addition to stress fracture of the pars interarticularis, stress fractures of the spine can involve the pedicles[111] and, more commonly, the sacrum.[95,112-117] Sacral stress fractures most commonly occur in high-level running sports and female athletes, as well as during pregnancy.[95,112-114] Individuals often present with low-back and pelvic pain, as well as gait disturbances.[112] Risk factors include abnormal menstrual history, dietary deficiencies, and low bone mineral density.[113] MRI has 100% sensitivity in detecting these sacral stress fractures and is the imaging modality of choice.[102] Treatment typically involves limited weight-bearing with progressive mobilization with physical therapy.[95] Most female athletes are able to return to sport within 2 months.

CONCLUSION

Stress fractures are a common overuse injury among female athletes. Early recognition, diagnosis, and management are important, as a delay in the diagnosis can be associated with prolonged pain, disability, and delayed healing and may result in a nonunion requiring surgery.

REFERENCES

1. Fredericson M, Jennings F, Beaulieu C, Matheson GO. Stress fractures in athletes. *Top Magn Reson Imag.* 2006;17(5):309–325.
2. Romani WA, Gieck JH, Perrin DH, Saliba EN, Kahler DM. Mechanisms and management of stress fractures in physically active persons. *J Athl Train.* 2002;37(3):306–314.
3. Matcuk Jr GR, Mahanty SR, Skalski MR, Patel DB, White EA, Gottsegen CJ. Stress fractures: pathophysiology, clinical presentation, imaging features, and treatment options. *Emerg Radiol.* 2016;23(4):365–375.
4. Frost HM. Some ABC's of skeletal pathophysiology. 5. Microdamage physiology. *Calcif Tissue Int.* 1991;49(4):229–231.
5. Tsao R, Weber K. Stress fractures of the hip and pelvis. In: Nho SJ, Leunig M, Larson CM, Bedi A, Kelly BT, eds. *Hip Arthroscopy and Hip Joint Preservation Surgery.* New York, NY: Springer New York; 2015:1015–1025.
6. Denay KL. Stress fractures. *Curr Sports Med Rep.* 2017;16(1):7–8.
7. Markey KL. Stress fractures. *Clin Sports Med.* 1987;6(2):405–425.
8. Yoshikawa T, Mori S, Santiesteban AJ, et al. The effects of muscle fatigue on bone strain. *J Exp Biol.* 1994;188:217–233.
9. Beck TJ, Ruff CB, Mourtada FA, et al. Dual-energy X-ray absorptiometry derived structural geometry for stress fracture prediction in male U.S. Marine Corps recruits. *J Bone Miner Res.* 1996;11(5):645–653.
10. Chen YT, Tenforde AS, Fredericson M. Update on stress fractures in female athletes: epidemiology, treatment, and prevention. *Curr Rev Musculoskelet Med.* 2013;6(2):173–181.
11. Nelson BJ, Arciero RA. Stress fractures in the female athlete. *Sports Med Arthrosc Rev.* 2002;10(1):83–90.
12. Wentz L, Liu PY, Haymes E, Ilich JZ. Females have a greater incidence of stress fractures than males in both military and athletic populations: a systemic review. *Mil Med.* 2011;176(4):420–430.
13. Jones BH, Bovee MW, Harris 3rd JM, Cowan DN. Intrinsic risk factors for exercise-related injuries among male and female army trainees. *Am J Sports Med.* 1993;21(5):705–710.
14. Milgrom C, Finestone A, Levi Y, et al. Do high impact exercises produce higher tibial strains than running? *Br J Sports Med.* 2000;34(3):195–199.
15. Royer M, Thomas T, Cesini J, Legrand E. Stress fractures in 2011: practical approach. *Jt Bone Spine.* 2012;79(Suppl 2):S86–S90.
16. Nazem TG, Ackerman KE. The female athlete triad. *Sport Health.* 2012;4(4):302–311.
17. Nattiv A, Loucks AB, Manore MM, Sanborn CF, Sundgot-Borgen J, Warren MP. American College of Sports Medicine position stand. The female athlete triad. *Med Sci Sports Exerc.* 2007;39(10):1867–1882.
18. Eriksen EF, Colvard DS, Berg NJ, et al. Evidence of estrogen receptors in normal human osteoblast-like cells. *Science.* 1988;241(4861):84–86.
19. Braam LA, Knapen MH, Geusens P, Brouns F, Vermeer C. Factors affecting bone loss in female endurance athletes: a two-year follow-up study. *Am J Sports Med.* 2003;31(6):889–895.
20. Schneiders AG, Sullivan SJ, Hendrick PA, et al. The ability of clinical tests to diagnose stress fractures: a systematic review and meta-analysis. *J Orthop Sports Phys Ther.* 2012;42(9):760–771.
21. Fatima ST, Jeilani A, Mazhar ud D, et al. Validation of tuning fork test in stress fractures and its comparison with radionuclide bone scan. *J Ayub Med Coll Abbottabad.* 2012;24(3–4):180–182.
22. Astur DC, Zanatta F, Arliani GG, Moraes ER, Pochini Ade C, Ejnisman B. Stress fractures: definition, diagnosis and treatment. *Rev Bras Ortop.* 2016;51(1):3–10.
23. Daffner RH, Pavlov H. Stress fractures: current concepts. *Am J Roentgenol.* 1992;159(2):245–252.
24. Savoca CJ. Stress fractures. A classification of the earliest radiographic signs. *Radiology.* 1971;100(3):519–524.
25. Nussbaum AR, Treves ST, Micheli L. Bone stress lesions in ballet dancers: scintigraphic assessment. *Am J Roentgenol.* 1988;150(4):851–855.
26. Deutsch AL, Coel MN, Mink JH. Imaging of stress injuries to bone. Radiography, scintigraphy, and MR imaging. *Clin Sports Med.* 1997;16(2):275–290.

27. Sofka CM. Imaging of stress fractures. *Clin Sports Med.* 2006;25(1):53–62 (viii).

28. DeFranco MJ, Recht M, Schils J, Parker RD. Stress fractures of the femur in athletes. *Clin Sports Med.* 2006;25(1): 89–103 (ix).

29. Kiuru MJ, Niva M, Reponen A, Pihlajamaki HK. Bone stress injuries in asymptomatic elite recruits: a clinical and magnetic resonance imaging study. *Am J Sports Med.* 2005;33(2):272–276.

30. Haro M, Bruene J, Weber K, Bach B. Stress fractures of the femur. In: *Stress Fractures in Athletes: Diagnosis and Management.* 2015:111–124.

31. Matheson GO, Clement DB, McKenzie DC, Taunton JE, Lloyd-Smith DR, MacIntyre JG. Stress fractures in athletes. A study of 320 cases. *Am J Sports Med.* 1987; 15(1):46–58.

32. Dimmen S, Nordsletten L, Engebretsen L, Steen H, Madsen JE. Negative effect of parecoxib on bone mineral during fracture healing in rats. *Acta Orthop.* 2008;79(3): 438–444.

33. Dodwell ER, Latorre JG, Parisini E, et al. NSAID exposure and risk of nonunion: a meta-analysis of case-control and cohort studies. *Calcif Tissue Int.* 2010;87(3):193–202.

34. Ziltener JL, Leal S, Fournier PE. Non-steroidal anti-inflammatory drugs for athletes: an update. *Ann Phys Rehabil Med.* 2010;53(4):278–282.

35. Rue JP, Armstrong 3rd DW, Frassica FJ, Deafenbaugh M, Wilckens JH. The effect of pulsed ultrasound in the treatment of tibial stress fractures. *Orthopedics.* 2004;27(11): 1192–1195.

36. Uchiyama Y, Nakamura Y, Mochida J, Tamaki T. Effect of low-intensity pulsed ultrasound treatment for delayed and non-union stress fractures of the anterior mid-tibia in five athletes. *Tokai J Exp Clin Med.* 2007;32(4): 121–125.

37. Arendt E, Agel J, Heikes C, Griffiths H. Stress injuries to bone in college athletes: a retrospective review of experience at a single institution. *Am J Sports Med.* 2003;31(6): 959–968.

38. Provencher MT, Baldwin AJ, Gorman JD, Gould MT, Shin AY. Atypical tensile-sided femoral neck stress fractures: the value of magnetic resonance imaging. *Am J Sports Med.* 2004;32(6):1528–1534.

39. Aro H, Dahlstrom S. Conservative management of distraction-type stress fractures of the femoral neck. *J Bone Jt Surg Br.* 1986;68(1):65–67.

40. Swiontkowski MF, Winquist RA, Hansen Jr ST. Fractures of the femoral neck in patients between the ages of twelve and forty-nine years. *J Bone Jt Surg Am.* 1984;66(6): 837–846.

41. Ivkovic A, Bojanic I, Pecina M. Stress fractures of the femoral shaft in athletes: a new treatment algorithm. *Br J Sports Med.* 2006;40(6):518–520. discussion 520.

42. Johnson AW, Weiss Jr CB, Wheeler DL. Stress fractures of the femoral shaft in athletes—more common than expected. A new clinical test. *Am J Sports Med.* 1994;22(2): 248–256.

43. Kang L, Belcher D, Hulstyn MJ. Stress fractures of the femoral shaft in women's college lacrosse: a report of seven cases and a review of the literature. *Br J Sports Med.* 2005;39(12):902–906.

44. Hershman EB, Lombardo J, Bergfeld JA. Femoral shaft stress fractures in athletes. *Clin Sports Med.* 1990;9(1): 111–119.

45. Fullerton Jr LR, Snowdy HA. Femoral neck stress fractures. *Am J Sports Med.* 1988;16(4):365–377.

46. Provost RA, Morris JM. Fatigue fracture of the femoral shaft. *J Bone Jt Surg Am.* 1969;51(3):487–498.

47. Monteleone Jr GP. Stress fractures in the athlete. *Orthop Clin N Am.* 1995;26(3):423–432.

48. Shin AY, Morin WD, Gorman JD, Jones SB, Lapinsky AS. The superiority of magnetic resonance imaging in differentiating the cause of hip pain in endurance athletes. *Am J Sports Med.* 1996;24(2):168–176.

49. Knapp TP, Garrett Jr WE. Stress fractures: general concepts. *Clin Sports Med.* 1997;16(2):339–356.

50. Slocum KA, Gorman JD, Puckett ML, Jones SB. Resolution of abnormal MR signal intensity in patients with stress fractures of the femoral neck. *Am J Roentgenol.* 1997;168(5):1295–1299.

51. Behrens SB, Deren ME, Matson A, Fadale PD, Monchik KO. Stress fractures of the pelvis and legs in athletes: a review. *Sport Health.* 2013;5(2):165–174.

52. Boden BP, Osbahr DC. High-risk stress fractures: evaluation and treatment. *J Am Acad Orthop Surg.* 2000;8(6): 344–353.

53. Clayer M, Krishnan J, Lee WK, Tamblyn P. Longitudinal stress fracture of the tibia: two cases. *Clin Radiol.* 1992; 46(6):401–404.

54. Schraml FV, Riego De Dios RL, Flemming DJ. Exercise-related longitudinal tibial stress fracture in a young person. *Ann Nucl Med.* 2006;20(6):441–444.

55. Bennell KL, Brukner PD. Epidemiology and site specificity of stress fractures. *Clin Sports Med.* 1997;16(2): 179–196.

56. Robertson GA, Wood AM. Return to sports after stress fractures of the tibial diaphysis: a systematic review. *Br Med Bull.* 2015;114(1):95–111.

57. McCormick F, Nwachukwu BU, Provencher MT. Stress fractures in runners. *Clin Sports Med.* 2012;31(2):291–306.

58. Mallee WH, Weel H, van Dijk CN, van Tulder MW, Kerkhoffs GM, Lin CW. Surgical versus conservative treatment for high-risk stress fractures of the lower leg (anterior tibial cortex, navicular and fifth metatarsal base): a systematic review. *Br J Sports Med.* 2015;49(6):370–376.

59. Orava S, Hulkko A. Stress fracture of the mid-tibial shaft. *Acta Orthop Scand.* 1984;55(1):35–37.

60. Kahanov L, Eberman LE, Games KE, Wasik M. Diagnosis, treatment, and rehabilitation of stress fractures in the lower extremity in runners. *Open Access J Sports Med.* 2015;6:87–95.

61. Feldman JJ, Bowman EN, Phillips BB, Weinlein JC. Tibial stress fractures in athletes. *Orthop Clin N Am.* 2016;47(4): 733–741.

62. Maitra RS, Johnson DL. Stress fractures. Clinical history and physical examination. *Clin Sports Med.* 1997;16(2): 259–274.

63. Brockwell J, Yeung Y, Griffith JF. Stress fractures of the foot and ankle. *Sports Med Arthrosc Rev.* 2009;17(3): 149–159.

64. Spitz DJ, Newberg AH. Imaging of stress fractures in the athlete. *Radiol Clin N Am.* 2002;40(2):313–331.

65. Brand Jr JC, Brindle T, Nyland J, Caborn DN, Johnson DL. Does pulsed low intensity ultrasound allow early return to normal activities when treating stress fractures? A review of one tarsal navicular and eight tibial stress fractures. *Iowa Orthop J.* 1999;19:26–30.

66. Kaeding CC, Najarian RG. Stress fractures: classification and management. *Phys Sportsmed.* 2010;38(3):45–54.

67. Mandell JC, Khurana B, Smith SE. Stress fractures of the foot and ankle, part 2: site-specific etiology, imaging, and treatment, and differential diagnosis. *Skeletal Radiol.* 2017;46(9):1165–1186.

68. Greaney RB, Gerber FH, Laughlin RL, et al. Distribution and natural history of stress fractures in U.S. Marine recruits. *Radiology.* 1983;146(2):339–346.

69. Kola S, Granville M, Jacobson RE. The association of iliac and sacral insufficiency fractures and implications for treatment: the role of bone scans in three different cases. *Cureus.* 2019;11(1):e3861.

70. Schilcher J, Bernhardsson M, Aspenberg P. Chronic anterior tibial stress fractures in athletes: no crack but intense remodeling. *Scand J Med Sci Sports.* 2019;29(10): 1521–1528.

71. Burne SG, Mahoney CM, Forster BB, Koehle MS, Taunton JE, Khan KM. Tarsal navicular stress injury: long-term outcome and clinicoradiological correlation using both computed tomography and magnetic resonance imaging. *Am J Sports Med.* 2005;33(12): 1875–1881.

72. Gross CE, Nunley JA. Navicular stress fractures. *Foot Ankle Int.* 2015;36(9):1117–1122.

73. Torg JS, Moyer J, Gaughan JP, Boden BP. Management of tarsal navicular stress fractures: conservative versus surgical treatment: a meta-analysis. *Am J Sports Med.* 2010; 38(5):1048–1053.

74. Sangeorzan BJR UE, Beuchel MW. Fractures and dislocations of the tarsal navicular. *J Am Acad Orthop Surg.* 2016;24(6).

75. Coris EEL JA. Tarsal navicular stress fractures. *Am Fam Physician.* 2003;67(1).

76. Robinson M, Fulcher M. Delayed healing of a navicular stress fracture, following limited weight-bearing activity. *BMJ Case Rep.* 2014;2014.

77. Saxena A, Fullem B. Navicular stress fractures a prospective study on athletes. *Foot Ankle Int.* 2006;27(11).

78. Coulibaly MO, Jones CB, Sietsema DL, Schildhauer TA. Results and complications of operative and non-operative navicular fracture treatment. *Injury.* 2015; 46(8):1669–1677.

79. Malliaropoulos NA D, Konstantinidis G, Papalada A, Tsifountoudis I, Petras K, Maffulli N. Therapeutic ultrasound in navicular stress injuries in elite track and field athletes. *Clin J Sport Med.* 2017;27(3).

80. Meurman KO. Less common stress fractures in the foot. *Br J Radiol.* 1981;54(637):1–7.

81. Crotty JG, Berlin SJ, Donick II . Stress fracture of the first metatarsal after Keller bunionectomy. *J Foot Surg.* 1989; 28(6):516–520.

82. Mayer SW, Joyner PW, Almekinders LC, Parekh SG. Stress fractures of the foot and ankle in athletes. *Sport Health.* 2014;6(6):481–491.

83. Boden BP, Osbahr DC, Jimenez C. Low-risk stress fractures. *Am J Sports Med.* 2001;29(1):100–111.

84. Iwamoto J, Takeda T. Stress fractures in athletes: review of 196 cases. *J Orthop Sci.* 2003;8(3):273–278.

85. Childers Jr RL, Meyers DH, Turner PR. Lesser metatarsal stress fractures: a study of 37 cases. *Clin Podiatr Med Surg.* 1990;7(4):633–644.

86. Weinfeld SB, Haddad SL, Myerson MS. Metatarsal stress fractures. *Clin Sports Med.* 1997;16(2):319–338.

87. Griffin NL, Richmond BG. Cross-sectional geometry of the human forefoot. *Bone.* 2005;37(2):253–260.

88. Albisetti W, Perugia D, De Bartolomeo O, Tagliabue L, Camerucci E, Calori GM. Stress fractures of the base of the metatarsal bones in young trainee ballet dancers. *Int Orthop.* 2010;34(1):51–55.

89. Chuckpaiwong B, Cook C, Nunley JA. Stress fractures of the second metatarsal base occur in nondancers. *Clin Orthop Relat Res.* 2007;461:197–202.

90. Khan K, Brown J, Way S, et al. Overuse injuries in classical ballet. *Sports Med.* 1995;19(5):341–357.

91. Harrington T, Crichton KJ, Anderson IF. Overuse ballet injury of the base of the second metatarsal. A diagnostic problem. *Am J Sports Med.* 1993;21(4):591–598.

92. Lawrence SJ, Botte MJ. Jones' fractures and related fractures of the proximal fifth metatarsal. *Foot Ankle.* 1993; 14(6):358–365.

93. Smith JW, Arnoczky SP, Hersh A. The intraosseous blood supply of the fifth metatarsal: implications for proximal fracture healing. *Foot Ankle.* 1992;13(3):143–152.

94. Alqarni AM, Schneiders AG, Cook CE, Hendrick PA. Clinical tests to diagnose lumbar spondylolysis and spondylolisthesis: a systematic review. *Phys Ther Sport.* 2015; 16(3):268–275.

95. Bono CM. Low back pain in athletes. *J Bone Jt Surg.* 2004; 86(2).

96. Nitta A, Sakai T, Goda Y, et al. Prevalence of symptomatic lumbar spondylolysis in pediatric patients. *Orthopedics.* 2016;39(3):e434–437.

97. Changstrom BG, Brou L, Khodaee M, Braund C, Comstock RD. Epidemiology of stress fracture injuries among US high school athletes, 2005–2006 through 2012–2013. *Am J Sports Med.* 2015;43(1):26–33.

98. Tezuka FS F, Sakai T, Dezawa A. Etiology adult spine stress fracture. *Clin Spine Surg.* 2017;30(3):E233–E238.

99. Bouras T, Korovessis P. Management of spondylolysis and low-grade spondylolisthesis in fine athletes. A comprehensive review. *Eur J Orthop Surg Traumatol.* 2015;25(Suppl 1):S167–S175.

100. Jha SCS T, Hangai M, Toyota A, Fukuta S, Nagamachi A, Siryo K. Stress fracture of the thoracic spine in an elite rhythmic gymnast a case report. *J Med Invest.* 2016;63.

101. Bencardino JT, Stone TJ, Roberts CC, et al. ACR appropriateness criteria((R)) stress (fatigue/insufficiency) fracture, including sacrum, excluding other vertebrae. *J Am Coll Radiol.* 2017;14(5S):S293–S306.

102. Murthy NS. Imaging of stress fractures of the spine. *Radiol Clin N Am.* 2012;50(4):799–821.

103. Garces GLG-M,I, Rasines JL, Stantonja F. Early diagnosis of stress fracture of the lumbar spine in athletes. *Int Orthop.* 1999;23:213–215.

104. Yamashita K, Sakai T, Takata Y, et al. Utility of STIR-MRI in detecting the pain generator in asymmetric bilateral pars fracture: a report of 5 cases. *Neurol Med -Chir.* 2018;58(2):91–95.

105. Omidi-Kashani F, Ebrahimzadeh MH, Salari S. Lumbar spondylolysis and spondylolytic spondylolisthesis: who should be have surgery? An algorithmic approach. *Asian Spine J.* 2014;8(6):856–863.

106. Congeni J, McCulloch J, Swanson K. Lumbar spondylolysis. A study of natural progression in athletes. *Am J Sports Med.* 1997;25(2):248–253.

107. Jackson DW, Wiltse LL, Dingeman RD, Hayes M. Stress reactions involving the pars interarticularis in young athletes. *Am J Sports Med.* 1981;9(5):304–312.

108. Kurd MFP D, Norton R, Picetti G, Friel B, Vacarro AR. Nonoperative treatment of symptomatic spondylolysis. *J Spinal Disord Tech.* 2007;20(8).

109. Sakai T, Tezuka F, Yamashita K, et al. Conservative treatment for bony healing in pediatric lumbar spondylolysis. *Spine.* 2017;42(12):E716–E720.

110. McClellan III JW, V BA, White MA, Stamm S, Ryschon KL. Should 25-hydroxyvitamin D and bone density using DXA be tested in adolescents with lumbar stress fractures of the pars interarticularis? *J Spinal Disord Tech.* 2012; 25(8).

111. Amari R, Sakai T, Katoh S, et al. Fresh stress fractures of lumbar pedicles in an adolescent male ballet dancer: case report and literature review. *Arch Orthop Trauma Surg.* 2008;129(3):397–401.

112. Hilal N, Nassar AH. Postpartum sacral stress fracture: a case report. *BMC Pregnancy Childbirth.* 2016;16:96.

113. Johnson AWW CB, Stento K, Wheeler DL. An atypical cause of low back pain in the female athlete. *Am J Sports Med.* 2001;29(4).

114. Perdomo AD, Tome-Bermejo F, Pinera AR, Alvarez L. Misdiagnosis of sacral stress fracture: an underestimated cause of low back pain in pregnancy? *Am J Case Rep.* 2015;16:60–64.

115. Skaggs DL, Avramis I, Myung K, Weiss J. Sacral facet fractures in elite athletes. *Spine.* 2012;37(8):E514–E517.

116. Slipman CW, Gilchrist RV, Isaac Z, Lenrow DA, Chou LH. Sacral stress fracture in a female field hockey player. *Am J Phys Med Rehabil.* 2003;82(11):893–896.

117. Takahashi Y, Kobayashi T, Miyakoshi N, et al. Sacral stress fracture in an amateur rugby player: a case report. *J Med Case Rep.* 2016;10(1):327.

CHAPTER 24

Chronic Exertional Compartment Syndrome

HANNAH L. BRADSELL, BS • KATHERINE C. BRANCHE, MD •
RACHEL M. FRANK, MD

INTRODUCTION

Chronic exertional compartment syndrome (CECS) most commonly affects the young, military, and athletic populations and can be debilitating for active individuals. Typical symptoms include pain, paresthesias, muscle weakness, and discomfort described as squeezing or cramping that occur during exercise and intensify as exertion continues, but disappears when activity stops. Although the specific source of pain in CECS is not entirely understood, the condition is caused by a rise in intracompartmental pressure within an osteofascial space likely related to increased blood flow to muscles during exercise. CECS primarily affects the lower limb, but it can also occur in the thigh, hand, and forearm compartments. Originally thought to be a diagnosis of exclusion, CECS is now thought to be underdiagnosed, and thus increased understanding and awareness of this condition are critical. The symptoms can often be nonspecific, and the broad differential for lower leg pain can interfere with diagnostic clarity.[1-4]

Owing to the difficulty and delay in diagnosis, the true epidemiology of lower leg CECS in the general population remains unclear.[2] However, incidence rates among athletes and military members have been provided by individual studies, giving an idea of the prevalence of CECS within at-risk populations. In a large population of active military members, Waterman et al.[7] reported an overall incidence rate of 0.49 cases per 1000 person-years. In a different cohort of recreational runners and military members, patients presenting with lower leg pain were evaluated[5] and CECS was diagnosed in 27%–33% of all cases of lower leg pain. Davis et al.[6] confirmed CECS diagnosis in 153 of 226 patients (67.7%; 250 of 393 legs) who presented with the appropriate symptoms and were suspected to have CECS. Among the group with confirmed CECS, 92.2%

were active athletes.[6,7] Worth noting, and discussed by de Bruijn et al.[8] who analyzed CECS in a large, mixed population, CECS is not completely limited to the athletic patient population and can also be found in less active individuals and diabetics.

ANATOMY

Compartments are fascia-surrounded groupings of muscles, blood vessels, and nerves categorized by specific anatomic areas in the extremities. The fascia is relatively inelastic, keeping these structures in place and inhibiting stretching and expansion of the compartment space. The lower leg is divided into four compartments: anterior, lateral, superficial posterior, and deep posterior. The anterior compartment consists of the tibialis anterior, extensor hallucis longus, extensor digitorum longus, and peroneus tertius muscles, as well as the deep peroneal nerve and anterior tibial artery and vein. The main functions of the muscles in this compartment are dorsiflexion of the foot and ankle and extension of the toes, as well as inversion and weak eversion of the foot. The lateral compartment includes the peroneus longus and peroneus brevis muscles and the superficial peroneal nerve. These muscles primarily function in eversion of the foot and ankle and secondarily in plantar flexion of the ankle. The superficial posterior compartment comprises the gastrocnemius, soleus, and plantaris muscles and the sural nerve. Finally, the deep posterior compartment consists of the tibialis posterior, popliteus, flexor hallucis longus, and flexor digitorum longus muscles, as well as the posterior tibial artery, peroneal artery, and tibial nerve. The musculature of the combined posterior compartments function in plantar flexion and inversion of the foot.[9-12]

PATHOPHYSIOLOGY AND RISK FACTORS

There are several proposed mechanisms leading to the development of CECS. The exact cause is not well understood. In normal functioning of the muscles of the lower leg, intracompartmental pressures increase and muscles enlarge with exertion and return to baseline within a few minutes of rest. Related to the pathophysiology of CECS is the capability of muscles to expand up to 20% in volume and weight during exercise, along with a rise in intracompartmental pressures against the surrounding inelastic fascia secondary to an increase in blood flow and edema.[12,13] Muscular hypertrophy that occurs over time in chronic exercise, particularly the involvement of repetitive activities, as well as fascial thickening, can lead to a reduction in the reserve volume available within the compartment.[13] Moreover, compartment noncompliance found in individuals with CECS can cause an abnormal elevation in tissue pressure during normal muscle enlargement throughout exercise, leading to lower functioning and tolerance that typically returns to normal when activity stops and muscles return to resting size.[12,13] In some cases, although this is not necessarily a defining feature of CECS, patients can have elevated intracompartmental pressures that are sustained at rest.[14] Long-standing, persistent abnormal pressures lead to the development of pain and may result in neurovascular compromise, paresthesias, and/or muscle weakness.[12,15,16] An additional proposed contribution to the noncompliant compartments of the lower leg includes stiffer and thicker fascia, specifically reported of the anterior compartment, found in patients with CECS compared to unaffected patients.[15] Furthermore, eccentric activities/moments may be a contributing factor, as patients with CECS have been shown to be more susceptible to pain with eccentric muscle contractions, which is indicated by studies reporting increases in compartment noncompliance as a result of eccentric exercise over time.[15,16] As summarized by Schubert,[15] additional intrinsic and extrinsic factors may contribute to the development of CECS. Potential intrinsic factors include leg length discrepancy and malalignment, while extrinsic factors may consist of decreased strength, endurance, or flexibility; improper biomechanics; and insufficient training volume, intensity, or frequency.[15,17] Braver[18] has also suggested genetic predisposition as a contributing factor in some individuals.

It was originally proposed that CECS-related pain may be the result of ischemia caused by microvascular compromise related to the elevated intramuscular and intracompartmental pressures that follow a significant volume increase in a relatively tight space.[2,13,15,16]

However, this implication as a cause of pain is ambiguous and not universally accepted among researchers. It may be more likely that pain results from receptor stimulation through increased pressure.[13,16] A more widespread theory is related to abnormal muscle perfusion and alterations in gradients caused by pressure imbalances.[2,15,16] Strenuous exercise can lead to microtrauma of muscular tissue and thus inflammation of the muscle and capillary bed.[15] This can ultimately increase the pressure of the interstitial space through increased fluid flow from the capillaries into this space, subsequently producing the symptoms of CECS.[15] This fluid shift can also be a result of impaired functioning of muscle tissue perfusion and deoxygenation that occurs as a result of intracompartmental pressure increase.[2] As described by Brennan and Kane,[16] when peripheral muscles are relaxed, they undergo perfusion and the arterial/venous gradient increases as a result. For the perfusion gradient to occur, it must be able to overcome normal resting intramuscular pressure and therefore be ≥30 mm Hg.[16] In the case of CECS where pressures are greater than normal, this perfusion gradient is lost or reduced to the point of inadequacy for tissue viability.[19] This results in reduced blood flow and subsequent pain that will only subside when these overriding pressures decline and the gradient returns to normal.[16,19] Previous studies have presented the results of imaging patients with CECS that demonstrate lack of perfusion in affected muscles after exercise, supporting this concept.[20] Moreover, Fraipont and Adamson[21] discussed the observation of greater deoxygenation of the muscle during exercise and delayed reoxygenation after exercise in patients with CECS compared to unaffected patients.

In 2013, Davis et al.[6] performed a large-scale retrospective study over a 12-year period to examine the characteristics of patients who develop CECS. In the population studied, 60.1% (92 of 153) were females, with an overall average age of 24 years (range, 13–69 years) and an average body mass index of 25 (range, 18–38). A majority of patients (63.4%) presented with bilateral CECS, and the number of compartments affected within a single extremity ranged from one to all four compartments. The anterior compartment was most frequently affected, followed by the lateral compartment, deep posterior compartment, and finally the superficial posterior compartment. Of the 153 patients, 141 (92.2%) had symptoms present with activity only, while 12 patients reported symptom onset in daily activity alone. The patients who reported exercise-induced symptoms were predominantly competitive athletes (63.1%), whereas others participated only in recreational sports (36.9%). Among the competitive athletes, 64.1% (57 of 89) were involved in team sports, 28.1% (25 of 89) participated in individual sports, and 7 athletes reported activity in both. Among the competitive and team sports, patients who participated in soccer and competitive running (track or cross-country) had the highest proportion of affected athletes, followed by lacrosse and field hockey. Interestingly, each of these sports had noticeably more females diagnosed with CECS than males. In a review by Campano et al.[22] a total of 1596 patients with diagnosed CECS were analyzed for demographics and characteristics across 24 publications. The authors found males to be predominately affected (70%). In addition, the authors found that 54% of the population consisted of military service members and that 29% were athletes (9% collegiate level and 8% professional level). This particular review reported bilateral CECS in 79% of patients, but reported the same findings of the most commonly affected compartments.[22] Characteristic and risk factor studies have also been applied to the military population owing to the high incidence rates of CECS among active service members. Within this population, factors such as gender, age, race, military rank, and branch of service have all been associated with incidence rates.[7] Understanding patterns in the characteristics of patients who develop CECS can provide useful insight on the diagnosis and treatment for both healthcare providers and patients. Likewise, determining specific risk factors can influence patient and provider decision-making and improve our understanding of the underlying causes leading to the development of CECS. Known risk factors include the use of creatine supplementation and anabolic steroids, which result in increased muscle volume and potential cause for abnormally high intracompartmental pressures.[2,16,23] As previously mentioned, eccentric exercise and irregular biomechanics during running, such as rear-foot landing or overprotonation, can also increase the risk of experiencing CECS.[2,16] Finally, in addition to the aforementioned commonalities such as age and type of sport, the associated risk factors that have been suggested include overuse, history of trauma, and diabetes.[24]

SIGNS AND SYMPTOMS

CECS is often misdiagnosed in the athletic population because it can present with a variety of symptoms. Generally, CECS causes exercise-induced pain in the lower leg that is localized to the affected compartment or compartments.[3,25] Typically, the pain is described as a dull, aching, cramping, or burning pain with a feeling of tightness or bursting in the lower leg. The pain begins within 15–20 min of the start of exercise and increases in intensity until the participant is forced to stop. There is typically no history of trauma or direct injury associated with the condition, and most often, there is a gradual onset of symptoms that arise after a long and intense period of exercise, unrelated to impact or weight-bearing. Occasionally, although transient, patients may experience accompanying motor weakness or neurologic symptoms, including numbness and tingling along the distribution of the nerve(s) within the affected compartment(s). Patients with CECS frequently report that the pain completely resolves shortly after discontinuing the aggravating activity.[2,3,25] The condition often occurs bilaterally, with numerous studies reporting bilateral pain in 60% –90% of cases.[8,26,27] In 2018, de Bruijn and colleagues[8] analyzed the primary factors in predicting CECS of the lower leg. The authors found that within their large, heterogeneous population, gender, age, clinical history, bilateral symptoms, and painful or tensed compartment were associated with predicting CECS. According to the study, males and younger patients were more prone to develop CECS, in whom the median age at diagnosis was 25 years and the prevalence reduced as age increased. The researchers noted that their results confirmed previously reported findings.

Having a high level of suspicion based on patient history is critical for making a proper diagnosis, as physical examination of CECS can often be unremarkable because of the absence of symptoms when not engaging in exercise.[2,3] Therefore it has been recommended that if CECS is suspected, physical examination should be performed before exercise and immediately after exercise.[2,25] Findings after exercise often include pain on palpation of the affected muscles, pain during passive stretching of the muscle, and firmness of the compartments involved.[2] Fascial defects may also be palpated in some instances.[2,3] Pronation and pes planus are often present in patients with CECS; therefore a gait analysis can be helpful as part of the overall evaluation.[2,25] Preexercise physical findings are usually normal; however, in severe and prolonged cases of CECS, atrophy of the affected compartment may be observed.[3]

In the lower leg, any of the four compartments can be affected by CECS and differentiating symptoms may assist when determining which compartment or compartments are involved. The most commonly affected are the anterior and lateral compartments, followed by the deep and superficial posterior compartments.[2] When the anterior compartment is affected, patients often complain of dorsal foot numbness and weakness with dorsiflexion of the toes and ankle. With involvement of the lateral compartment of the lower leg, patients experience dorsal foot numbness and eversion weakness. Involvement of the superficial posterior compartment results in lateral ankle or foot numbness, distal calf numbness, and posterior leg cramping. Patients with CECS of the deep posterior compartment develop weakness of plantar flexion, plantar foot numbness, and posterior leg cramping.[2,3,10,28,29]

DIFFERENTIAL DIAGNOSES AND DIAGNOSTIC TESTING

A variety of conditions are important to consider in both avoiding misdiagnosis and ensuring certainty in pursuing the official diagnosis of CECS, as diagnostic testing for this condition can be invasive. A summary of diagnoses to consider in patients presenting with symptoms similar to CECS is provided in Table 24.1.[1–3,30] Common diagnostic tests that can assist in narrowing down the differential diagnosis include magnetic resonance imaging (MRI), electromyography, radiography, and bone scintigraphy.[30]

Once CECS is suspected, objective diagnostic testing can be performed to confirm the diagnosis. Diagnostic testing for CECS includes the assessment of intramuscular compartment pressure (IMP) in the lower limb; however, this should only performed when clinical diagnosis is highly suspected due to the invasiveness of the technique. The most frequently utilized system for IMP testing is the Stryker catheter, a handheld needle device with a pressure scale that is placed into the compartment.[2] In 1990, Pedowitz et al.[20] established the diagnostic criteria of CECS based on IMP values,

which are still commonly used by most clinicians. The criteria for diagnosis include one or more of the following: preexercise pressure, ≥ 15 mm Hg; 1-min postexercise pressure, ≥ 30 mm Hg; or 5-min postexercise pressure, ≥ 20 mm Hg. Before the development of these criteria, Puranen and Alavaikko[31] proposed a during-exercise IMP value of ≥ 50 mm Hg in 1981 that may also be used as a reference for diagnosis.

Notably, several recent studies have questioned the accuracy of these existing measurements and proposed improved techniques. In 2011, Roberts and Franklyn-Miller[32] performed a review to determine the validity of the diagnostic criteria, specifically in the anterior compartment. The authors found that much of the current criteria overlapped with the range found in healthy patients. Additionally, some of the studies included in the review reported average pressures that would typically suggest CECS but found that those patients did not report symptoms. The researchers also mentioned that at the suggested time points for testing, IMP values can vary as a result of other factors aside from CECS. Based on the potential for misleading results, the authors recommended the use of the average upper confidence limits at each point noted as having more sensitivity than using the maximum upper confidence limits. These values are as follows: 14 mm Hg before exercise or 18 mm Hg at relaxation, 54 mm Hg during exercise, 36 mm Hg at 1 min after exercise, and 23 mm Hg at 5 min after -exercise. In 2015, Roscoe, along with Roberts and Hulse,[14] suggested a new diagnostic criteria with improved value by recording IMP measurements of the anterior compartment continuously during exercise and comparing the values to a control group. The recordings were taken by an indwelling electronic catheter system and were collected throughout the following phases: (1) resting supine for 2 min, (2) standing in a relaxed resting state for 30 s, (3) exercising on a treadmill following a three-phase protocol to the end or until the point of maximal pain, and (4) resting supine for 5 min after exercise recovery (5-s averages taken at 1 and 5 min). The authors found no significant difference between the patient and control groups for preexercise supine pressures, but the patient group had significantly higher IMP values at all other time points. Based on these findings, the authors demonstrated relatively poor validity of the widely accepted Pedowitz criteria[20] and suggested the use of continuous dynamic IMP measurements, as measurements taken during exercise had greater diagnostic value and were well-tolerated and safe.[14] More specifically, phase 2 of the exercise phase, which was walking on a treadmill at a set pace of 6.5 km/h for 5 min at a 5%

TABLE 24.1
Differential Diagnoses to Consider When Evaluating Chronic Exertional Compartment Syndrome of the Lower Leg.

Stress fracture
Medial tibial stress syndrome ("shin splints")
Tendon pathologies
Deep vein thrombosis
Fascial defects
Nerve entrapment syndromes
Popliteal artery entrapment syndrome
Claudication (peripheral artery disease)

incline while carrying a 15-kg backpack, provided the greatest diagnostic accuracy (sensitivity = 63%, specificity = 95%). A cutoff of 105 mm Hg during this phase proved to be of greater value in diagnosing CECS than the cutoffs of 30 mm Hg 1 min after exercise and 20 mm Hg 5 min after -exercise set by Pedowitz. Although these results added significant value over existing techniques, further research is necessary to establish a full protocol to confirm certainty or to determine if measuring phase 2 alone or the maximal tolerable pain is sufficient for diagnosis.[14]

Lindorsson et al.[33] investigated differences in IMP between compartments of the lower leg to determine if altered diagnostic criteria was indicated. Measurements were taken at 1 min after exercise in the affected compartments of patients with CECS and compared to the IMP values of the corresponding compartments taken from patients presenting with exertional lower leg pain, but without CECS. This study demonstrated significantly lower IMP values in the lateral and both posterior compartments compared with the IMP values in the anterior compartments, leading the authors to suggest lowering the 1-min postexercise cutoff value for diagnosing CECS.[33]

Gill and colleagues[3] have discussed other methods of diagnosing CECS that have also been proposed by other studies, such as MRI, near-infrared spectroscopy, and thallium-201 SPECT (single photon emission computed tomography) scanning to evaluate for muscle ischemia. The MRI of an affected individual appears normal at rest but shows a T2-weighted signal in the affected compartment or compartments after exercise.[3] MRI may also be useful in detecting muscle atrophy, fatty infiltration of muscles, and fascial thickening.[3] Ultrasound can also be used,[32] but IMP measurements remain the more efficient and accurate method to confirm diagnosis of CECS.

TREATMENT AND OUTCOMES

In many cases, CECS with minor symptoms is treated nonoperatively, although surgery is considered the "gold standard" and recent evidence suggests that it results in higher rates of satisfaction and return to activity.[34] In a 2019 review of current management strategies of CECS, Buerba et al.[30] noted that conservative management begins with discontinuing all activities that cause symptoms, but this can be unsuccessful because patients, especially professional athletes, are reluctant to give up sport or activity. Gait retraining, massage, arch supports and shoe modifications, traditional physical therapy, and botulinum injections are among the

other attempted methods of nonoperative treatment.[30,34] Gait retraining, in the form of running modifications, was reported to be effective by Helmhout et al.[35] in 2015 using a 6-week training program that was aimed at adopting a forefoot strike technique (landing on the ball of the foot). Similarly in 2016, Helmhout and colleagues[36] reported improvements of CECS in a small cohort of military service members through modifications in marching technique. In their review, Rajasekaran and Hall[37] also described multiple studies indicating gait changes to be effective and reported that a 5-week massage treatment and home-stretching program significantly reduced pain in patients with CECS. These authors also discussed that using a negative sole (heel rocker) decreased anterior compartment pressure by reducing abnormal loads on the muscles, specifically the tibialis anterior.[37] Arch support inserts have also been studied as a method of altering biomechanical loads on the lower leg.[30]

Notably, in a 2016 case report of a triathlete diagnosed with bilateral CECS in the anterior and posterior compartments of the lower leg, Collins and Gilden[38] treated the patient with physical therapy targeting myofascial restrictions, neuromuscular function, and motor control deficits. After 23 visits over three and a half months, the patient was able to return to training pain free with a significantly improved functional score and minimal postexercise tightness. IMP measurements of the left leg had returned to normal 4 months after completing physical therapy. In addition, the patient was able to complete an Olympic triathlon with no pain at 6 months following intervention and remained pain free at a 3-year follow-up.[38] Lastly, a preliminary study performed in 2013 by Isner-Horobeti et al.[39] and more recently in separate case studies of a runner[40] and military service member,[41] reported the efficacy of botulinum injections as a potential long-term and low-risk, nonsurgical treatment.

The surgical management of CECS consists of opening the surrounding fascia of the affected compartment by a fasciotomy, which can be performed through various techniques.[34] Some of these variations include traditional open fasciotomy, minimal incision(s) fasciotomy, and minimally invasive endoscopic techniques.[30,34] The surgical techniques of a traditional open fasciotomy have been described in detail,[21,42,43] originally portrayed by Rorabeck et al.[42] in 1988, and generally consist of making one or two appropriately located larger incisions for the release of the affected compartment or compartments. As CECS often presents bilaterally, bilateral simultaneous fasciotomies have also reported to be successful with low complication rates and early return to activity.[27] In single minimal incision fasciotomy, a smaller incision between 2.5 and 4 cm in length is used to release the affected compartment.[26,44] High satisfaction and return to activity rates have been reported by both Maffulli et al.[44] in 2016 and Drexler et al.[26] in 2017, with few cases of complications and recurrence. Maffulli and colleagues[44] reported significant improvements in self-reported outcomes from preoperative baseline to the last follow-up at an average of 36 months after operation. In addition, prior to surgery, a majority of patients were unable to participate in any activity and some were only able play at a lower level than their preinjury level of play.[44] After a single minimal incision fasciotomy was performed, 17 of the 18 participants were able to return to the same or greater level of activity. The average time of return to training and return to competitive sport was 8 and 13 weeks, respectively.[44] Of the 27 minimal incision fasciotomies performed, no recurrence of symptoms occurred, but a few complications were reported in 6 patients, although most were not severe and were resolved.[44] Drexler et al.[26] performed a larger retrospective study including 95 legs of 53 patients, reporting a 75.5% satisfaction rate and long-term improvements in activity and quality of life, with minimal complications and only 8 cases of recurrence.[26] Endoscopy-assisted fasciotomy is a less invasive technique described to be safe and to have relatively positive outcomes. This is a particularly favorable surgical method for younger patients.[30,45] Depending on the affected compartment or compartments, a 3-cm incision is made over the appropriate area and dissection is carried through the skin and subcutaneous tissue to the fascia.[30] An arthroscope allows direct visualization for an additional incision and use of meniscal knives to identify and release the compartment fascia.[30] Several studies have reported the efficacy of this procedure,[46–48] with an 80% return-to-sports rate in a pediatric population. However, 19% of the legs treated in this population had recurrent CECS that required reoperation.[46] Interestingly, the same study[46] found a correlation between presentation and surgery, where each additional month between the time points decreased the odds of recurrence by 12%. Based on studies of adult populations,[47,48] a majority of outcomes were good or excellent with minimal complications. In a study by Wittstein and colleagues,[48] endoscopic fasciotomy was performed for the treatment of 14 legs in 9 patients. No recurrences of symptoms were reported in the seven patients who were followed up at 3.75 years after operation, and eight of the patients were able to return to the preinjury level of

activity, including collegiate and recreational levels of sport.[48] No neurovascular injuries occurred in this population, but postoperative hematomas were observed and resolved in two patients.[48] Lohrer and Nauck[47] also reported positive outcomes in a separate study, but they recommended an endoscopy-assisted compartment release be performed for CECS of the anterior and lateral compartments because of the lower rates of complications compared with the deep posterior compartment release, which led to the risk of hemorrhage.

In 2016, Campano et al.[22] performed a systematic review of studies reporting clinical outcomes of surgical management of CECS with an average follow-up of 48.8 months. Of the entire population included between 24 studies, 96% eventually underwent surgical treatment, including 86% undergoing compartment-specific open fasciotomy, 12% undergoing fasciotomy with partial fasciectomy, and less than 2% undergoing endoscopic fasciotomy.[22] Overall, the authors found a cumulative success rate of 66%, with a 6% risk of reoperation and a 13% risk of perioperative complications (i.e., postoperative neurologic dysfunction, infection, hematomas, etc.), and 84% patient satisfaction of surgical outcomes.[22] Ding et al.[49] performed a review comparing functional outcomes and symptom resolution of surgical intervention to nonoperative techniques in managing CECS, and while the literature was not able to determine the superiority of one approach over another, the authors noted fasciotomy to be safe and effective, with satisfaction rates as high as 94%.[49] Based on their findings, the authors determined that fasciotomy appears to be a safe and promising long-term option when surgical management is warranted. In a separate 2020 review, Vogels et al.[34] analyzed outcome parameters following treatment, comparing surgical and conservative interventions. Overall, a few studies discussing conservative treatments, including gait retraining and botulinum injection, reported decreased IMP measurements and led to a 47% rate of satisfaction and 50% rate of return to physical activity.[34] On the other hand, multiple studies providing surgical intervention outcomes also reported a significant reduction in postoperative IMP measurements compared with preoperative measurements, with an overall satisfaction rate of 85% and an average rate of return to activity of 80%.[34] Worth noting, however, the average rate of returning to previous level of play was 69% and 65% for return to full activity.[34] Overall, Vogels and colleagues[34] concluded that although additional research is needed because of the low evidence and limited number of studies, surgical treatment resulted in higher rates of satisfaction and return to activity compared with conservative methods. Thein et al.[50] further supported this in their 2019 study, finding that among the patients studied with CECS of the anterior compartment, 25% (3 of 12) of the conservative group returned to prediagnosis activity level compared with 77.4% (24 of 31) of the surgical group that underwent traditional open fasciotomy. Finally, in 2020, Salzler et al.[51] reported surgical outcomes in a population of runners for the treatment of CECS via fasciotomy. Overall, of the 32 runners included in the study, significant improvements in pain were observed in a majority of the patients, with 78.1% reporting satisfaction with their procedure and 84% were able to return to sports.[51] However, 19% developed recurrent symptoms leading to a revision surgery and 28% of patients did not return to running sports (16% due to recurrent pain with running) and of the 56% that did return, the average weekly running distance decreased postoperatively.[51]

CONCLUSIONS

CECS is a well-recognized condition that greatly impacts the active population. Continued research for a better understanding of cause of pain, related symptoms, and the risk factors involved in the development of CECS can improve care and treatment of the condition. Furthermore, additional studies are necessary to resolve the discrepancies pertaining to a standard method of diagnosis. Lastly, special attention should be placed on the management of CECS, keeping in mind that reducing activity level and attempting nonoperative treatment should be considered before considering surgical intervention.

REFERENCES

1. Chandwani D, Varacallo M. Exertional compartment syndrome. In: *StatPearls*. Treasure Island (FL): StatPearls Publishing Copyright © 2020, StatPearls Publishing LLC.; 2020.
2. Tucker AK. Chronic exertional compartment syndrome of the leg. *Curr Rev Musculoskelet Med*. 2010;3:32−37.
3. Gill CS, Halstead ME, Matava MJ. Chronic exertional compartment syndrome of the leg in athletes: evaluation and management. *Phys Sportsmed*. 2010;38:126−132.
4. Joubert SV, Duarte MA. Chronic exertional compartment syndrome in a healthy young man. *J Chiropr Med*. 2016; 15:139−144.
5. Breen DT, Foster J, Falvey E, Franklyn-Miller A. Gait re-training to alleviate the symptoms of anterior exertional lower leg pain: a case series. *Int J Sports Phys Ther*. 2015;10: 85−94.
6. Davis DE, Raikin S, Garras DN, Vitanzo P, Labrador H, Espandar R. Characteristics of patients with chronic exertional compartment syndrome. *Foot Ankle Int*. 2013; 34:1349−1354.
7. Waterman BR, Liu J, Newcomb R, Schoenfeld AJ, Orr JD, Belmont PJ. Risk factors for chronic exertional compartment syndrome in a physically active military population. *Am J Sports Med*. 2013;41:2545−2549.
8. de Bruijn J, van Zantvoort A, van Klaveren D, et al. Factors predicting lower leg chronic exertional compartment syndrome in a large population. *Int J Sports Med*. 2018;39: 58−66.
9. Khan IA, Mahabadi N, D'Abarno A, Varacallo M. Anatomy, bony pelvis and lower limb, leg lateral compartment. In: *StatPearls*. Treasure Island (FL): StatPearls Publishing Copyright © 2020, StatPearls Publishing LLC.; 2020.
10. Lezak B, Summers S. Anatomy, bony pelvis and lower limb, leg anterior compartment. In: *StatPearls*. Treasure Island (FL): StatPearls Publishing Copyright © 2020, StatPearls Publishing LLC.; 2020.
11. Mostafa E, Graefe S, Varacallo M. Anatomy, bony pelvis and lower limb, leg posterior compartment. In: *StatPearls*. Treasure Island (FL): StatPearls Publishing Copyright © 2020, StatPearls Publishing LLC.; 2020.
12. Liu B, Barrazueta G, Ruchelsman DE. Chronic exertional compartment syndrome in athletes. *J Hand Surg Am*. 2017;42:917−923.
13. Bong MR, Polatsch DB, Jazrawi LM, Rokito AS. Chronic exertional compartment syndrome: diagnosis and management. *Bull Hosp Jt Dis*. 2005;62:77−84.
14. Roscoe D, Roberts AJ, Hulse D. Intramuscular compartment pressure measurement in chronic exertional compartment syndrome. *Am J Sports Med*. 2015;43: 392−398.
15. Schubert AG. Exertional compartment syndrome: review of the literature and proposed rehabilitation guidelines following surgical release. *Int J Sports Phys Ther*. 2011;6: 126−141.
16. Brennan FH, Kane SF. Diagnosis, treatment options, and rehabilitation of chronic lower leg exertional compartment syndrome. *Curr Sports Med Rep*. 2003;2:247−250.
17. Roberts A, Roscoe D, Hulse D, Bennett AN, Dixon S. Biomechanical differences between cases with suspected chronic exertional compartment syndrome and asymptomatic controls during running. *Gait Posture*. 2017;58:374−379.
18. Braver RT. Chronic exertional compartment syndrome. *Clin Podiatr Med Surg*. 2016;33:219−233.
19. Frank RM, Hearty T, Chiampas GT, Kodros SA. Acute bilateral exertional lateral leg compartment syndrome with delayed presentation: a case report. *JBJS Case Connect*. 2012;2:e81.
20. Pedowitz RA, Hargens AR, Mubarak SJ, Gershuni DH. Modified criteria for the objective diagnosis of chronic compartment syndrome of the leg. *Am J Sports Med*. 1990;18:35−40.
21. Fraipont MJ, Adamson GJ. Chronic exertional compartment syndrome. *J Am Acad Orthop Surg*. 2003;11: 268−276.
22. Campano D, Robaina JA, Kusnezov N, Dunn JC, Waterman BR. Surgical management for chronic exertional

compartment syndrome of the leg: a systematic review of the literature. *Arthroscopy.* 2016;32:1478–1486.

23. Dunn JC, Waterman BR. Chronic exertional compartment syndrome of the leg in the military. *Clin Sports Med.* 2014; 33:693–705.

24. Rynkiewicz KM, Fry LA, Distefano LJ. Demographic characteristics among patients with chronic exertional compartment syndrome of the lower leg. *J Sport Rehabil.* 2020:1–4.

25. Chatterjee R. Diagnosis of chronic exertional compartment syndrome in primary care. *Br J Gen Pract.* 2015;65: e560–e562.

26. Drexler M, Rutenberg TF, Rozen N, et al. Single minimal incision fasciotomy for the treatment of chronic exertional compartment syndrome: outcomes and complications. *Arch Orthop Trauma Surg.* 2017;137:73–79.

27. Raikin SM, Rapuri VR, Vitanzo P. Bilateral simultaneous fasciotomy for chronic exertional compartment syndrome. *Foot Ankle Int.* 2005;26:1007–1011.

28. Murdock CJ, Mudreac A, Agyeman K. Anatomy, abdomen and pelvis, rectus femoris muscle. In: *StatPearls.* Treasure Island (FL): StatPearls Publishing Copyright © 2020, StatPearls Publishing LLC.; 2020.

29. Cantrell AJ, Imonugo O, Varacallo M. Anatomy, bony pelvis and lower limb, leg bones. In: *StatPearls.* Treasure Island (FL): StatPearls Publishing Copyright © 2020, StatPearls Publishing LLC.; 2020.

30. Buerba RA, Fretes NF, Devana SK, Beck JJ. Chronic exertional compartment syndrome: current management strategies. *Open Access J Sports Med.* 2019;10:71–79.

31. Puranen J, Alavaikko A. Intracompartmental pressure increase on exertion in patients with chronic compartment syndrome in the leg. *J Bone Joint Surg Am.* 1981;63: 1304–1309.

32. Roberts A, Franklyn-Miller A. The validity of the diagnostic criteria used in chronic exertional compartment syndrome: a systematic review. *Scand J Med Sci Sports.* 2011;22: 585–595.

33. Lindorsson S, Zhang Q, Brisby H, Rennerfelt K. Significantly lower intramuscular pressure in the posterior and lateral compartments compared with the anterior compartment suggests alterations of the diagnostic criteria for chronic exertional compartment syndrome in the lower leg. *Knee Surg Sports Traumatol Arthrosc.* 2021;29:1332–1339.

34. Vogels S, Ritchie ED, Dongen TTCF, Scheltinga MRM, Zimmermann WO, Hoencamp R. Systematic review of outcome parameters following treatment of chronic exertional compartment syndrome in the lower leg. *Scand J Med Sci Sports.* 2020;30.

35. Helmhout PH, Diebal AR, Van Der Kaaden L, Harts CC, Beutler A, Zimmermann WO. The effectiveness of a 6-week intervention program aimed at modifying running style in patients with chronic exertional compartment syndrome. *Orthop J Sports Med.* 2015;3, 232596711557569.

36. Helmhout PH, Diebal-Lee MA, Poelsma LR, Harts CC, Zimmermann LW. Modifying marching technique in military service members with chronic exertional compartment syndrome: a case series. *Int J Sports Phys Ther.* 2016; 11:1106–1124.

37. Rajasekaran S, Hall MM. Nonoperative management of chronic exertional compartment syndrome. *Curr Sports Med Rep.* 2016;15:191–198.

38. Collins CK, Gilden B. A non-operative approach to the management of chronic exertional compartment syndrome in a triathlete: a case report. *Int J Sports Phys Ther.* 2016;11:1160–1176.

39. Isner-Horobeti ME, Dufour SP, Blaes C, Lecocq J. Intramuscular pressure before and after botulinum toxin in chronic exertional compartment syndrome of the leg: a preliminary study. *Am J Sports Med.* 2013;41:2558–2566.

40. Baria MR, Sellon JL. Botulinum toxin for chronic exertional compartment syndrome. *Clin J Sport Med.* 2016; 26:e111–e113.

41. Hutto WM, Schroeder PB, Leggit JC. Botulinum toxin as a novel treatment for chronic exertional compartment syndrome in the U.S. Military. *Mil Med.* 2019;184: e458–e461.

42. Rorabeck CH, Fowler PJ, Nott L. The results of fasciotomy in the management of chronic exertional compartment syndrome. *Am J Sports Med.* 1988;16:224–227.

43. Scully WF, Benavides JM. Surgical tips for performing open fasciotomies for chronic exertional compartment syndrome of the leg. *Foot Ankle Int.* 2019;40:859–865.

44. Maffulli N, Loppini M, Spiezia F, D'Addona A, Maffulli GD. Single minimal incision fasciotomy for chronic exertional compartment syndrome of the lower leg. *J Orthop Surg Res.* 2016;11.

45. Knight JR, Daniels M, Robertson W. Endoscopic compartment release for chronic exertional compartment syndrome. *Arthrosc Tech.* 2013;2:e187–190.

46. Beck JJ, Tepolt FA, Miller PE, Micheli LJ, Kocher MS. Surgical treatment of chronic exertional compartment syndrome in pediatric patients. *Am J Sports Med.* 2016;44: 2644–2650.

47. Lohrer H, Nauck T. Endoscopically assisted release for exertional compartment syndromes of the lower leg. *Arch Orthop Trauma Surg.* 2007;127:827–834.

48. Wittstein J, Moorman 3rd CT, Levin LS. Endoscopic compartment release for chronic exertional compartment syndrome: surgical technique and results. *Am J Sports Med.* 2010;38:1661–1666.

49. Ding A, Machin M, Onida S, Davies AH. A systematic review of fasciotomy in chronic exertional compartment syndrome. *J Vasc Surg.* 2020;72.

50. Thein R, Tilbor I, Rom E, et al. Return to sports after chronic anterior exertional compartment syndrome of the leg: conservative treatment versus surgery. *J Orthop Surg.* 2019;27, 230949901983565.

51. Salzler M, Maguire K, Heyworth BE, Nasreddine AY, Micheli LJ, Kocher MS. Outcomes of surgically treated chronic exertional compartment syndrome in runners. *Sports Health.* 2020;12:304–309.

CHAPTER 25

The Female Athlete Triad/Relative Energy Deficiency in Sports

KAREN M. SUTTON, MD • SARAH M. CHENEY, BS • ELIZABETH A. FIERRO, DO • ELLEN K. CASEY, MD

INTRODUCTION

The female athlete triad (triad) is a medical condition often observed in physically active girls and women. The three interrelated components of the triad are energy availability (EA), menstrual status, and bone health. These components each present along a physiologic spectrum: EA ranges from optimal to low EA to eating disorder (ED), menstrual function ranges from eumenorrhea to oligomenorrhea to amenorrhea, and bone health ranges from normal to low bone mineral density (BMD) to osteoporosis.[1,2]

Optimum health in the female athlete is indicated by optimal EA, eumenorrhea, and optimal bone health, whereas at the other end of the spectrum, the most severe presentation of the triad is characterized by low EA with or without disordered eating/eating disorder (DE/ED), functional hypothalamic amenorrhea (FHA), and osteoporosis. An athlete's condition moves along each spectrum at different rates depending on her diet and exercise behaviors. The relationships among these three components are illustrated in Fig. 25.1.[3]

Relative energy deficiency in sports (RED-S) is a broader, more comprehensive term used more recently in the literature defining a syndrome that occurs in both female and male athletes (Fig. 25.2). Low EA may lead to altered reproductive hormones (including menstrual dysfunction in the female) and/or low BMD, as well as abnormalities in other systems (e.g., metabolic, cardiovascular, gastrointestinal, immunologic), that may have both health and performance consequences.[4,5] For the purposes of this chapter, we will focus on the specific causes and consequences of the triad on the female athlete.

In the 2017 Consensus Statement, Female Athlete Issues for the Team Physician, it was noted that it is essential for the team physician to recognize that the components of the triad are interrelated and emphasized the comprehensiveness of evaluating female athletes who may fall into this category.[1] Team physicians should coordinate a multidisciplinary healthcare team to address the medical, nutritional, psychologic, and sports-participation-related issues and develop a return-to-play protocol.

LOW ENERGY AVAILABILITY IN THE FEMALE ATHLETE

What is Low Energy Availability?

EA has been defined as the dietary energy intake (measured in kilocalories) minus the energy cost of exercise (measured in kilocalories) relative to fat-free mass (FFM, measured in kilograms).[6] For an athlete, this value is the amount of energy remaining for physiologic processes and activities of daily living after accounting for exercise training. Failure to balance energy intake and exercise energy expenditure will result in a negative energy balance.[5]

This energy deficiency, known as low EA, occurs when an athlete has insufficient energy to support normal physiologic functions. Low EA is defined as <30 kcal/kg FFM per day and negative implications begin to arise below this value.[6] Low EA predisposes athletes to possible physical injury, systemic pathology, psychologic stress, and poor athletic performance. Optimal EA is >45 kcal/kg FFM per day.[1,6,7] Low EA occurs with a reduction in energy intake and/or an increased exercise load. Consequences of various levels of EA are delineated in Table 25.1.

Female athletes are particularly susceptible to inadequate EA due to lack of nutritional education, higher prevalence of DE/ED, and prioritizing leanness more often in women's sports, even those with male equivalents (gymnastics, figure skating, ballet, beach volleyball). Genetics and age may alter an individual's

The Female Athlete. https://doi.org/10.1016/B978-0-323-75985-4.00030-1

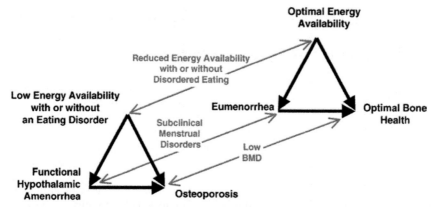

FIG. 25.1 Female athlete triad. The spectrums of energy availability, menstrual function, and bone mineral density (BMD) along which female athletes are distributed (*narrow arrows*). An athlete's condition moves along each spectrum at a different rate, in one direction or the other, according to her diet and exercise habits. Energy availability, defined as dietary energy intake minus exercise energy expenditure, affects BMD both directly via metabolic hormones and indirectly via effects on menstrual function and thereby estrogen levels (*thick arrows*).

initial condition and sensitivity to low EA, and therefore a high index of suspicion is necessary when evaluating female athletes. Importantly, it has been demonstrated that low EA, not the stress of exercise, will have negative implications on many hormonal, metabolic, and functional mechanisms.[6,9,10]

Low EA is prevalent across a variety of sports, not only those that encourage leanness.[11] A study of female high-school varsity athletes participating in a range of sports found that 36% presented with low EA, with 6% at <30 kcal/kg lean body mass (LBM).[14] A study of female Division 1 soccer players over the course of a season revealed mean EA was lowest midseason,

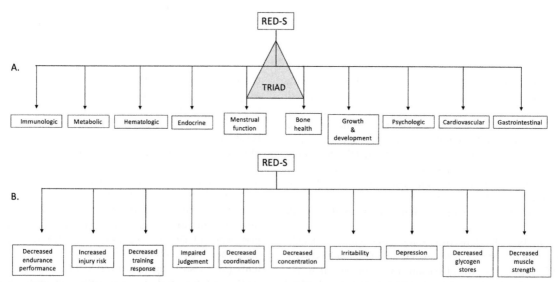

FIG. 25.2 **(A)** Health consequences of relative energy deficiency in sports (RED-S) showing an expanded concept of the female athlete triad. **(B)** Potential performance (aerobic and anaerobic) consequences of RED-S.

TABLE 25.1	
Loucks' Proposed Energy Availability Ranges for Different Athletic Functions.	
Energy Availability Range	**Effect on Body Mass/Composition**
>45 kcal/kg FFM/day (>188 kJ/kg FFM/day)	Gain of body mass, muscle hypertrophy, carbohydrate loading
~45 kcal/kg FFM/day (188 kJ/kg FFM/day)	Maintenance of body size and mass; focus on skill development
30–45 kcal/kg FFM/day (125–188 kJ/kg FFM/day)	Loss of body mass or fat

FFM, fat-free mass.
Adapted from Loucks[8].

with 33.3% of athletes demonstrating low EA at <30 kcal/kg LBM.[11] Young female athletes, especially those participating in aesthetic or weight-restrictive sports, are often at risk.

Low Energy Availability and Disordered Eating

There are three main mechanisms by which athletes commonly reduce EA. First, by intentionally modifying body size and composition for performance. These methods, which include skipping meals, fasting, using diet pills, using laxatives, or self-induced vomiting, may be used for sport-specific short-term weight loss or may illustrate a long-term pattern of behavior. The tactics may be short-term diets or long-term patterns of behavior.[4] Although these restrictive eating behaviors are considered DE, they do not involve any psychopathologic underpinnings.

In contrast, compulsively acting in a psychopathologic pattern of DE[15] may indicate a clinical ED. EDs are classified by the *Diagnostic and Statistical Manual of Mental Disorders* (Fifth Edition) (*DSM-5*) as psychiatric disorders often including a distortion of body image and often resulting in significant nutritional and medical complications. These include anorexia nervosa, bulimia nervosa, binge ED, or other specified EDs.[16] *Anorexia athletica* refers to a DE pattern often observed in the female athlete who has an intense fear of gaining weight, despite being underweight. She reduces energy intake and body mass despite high physical performance.[17,18] *Anorexia athletica* has some, but not all, of the criteria of EDs, so it is considered a DE or a subclinical ED.[17]

Third and finally, low EA may occur inadvertently, due to lack of knowledge about appropriate nutrition and the lack of biological drive to match energy intake to activity-induced energy expenditure.[19] While DE very commonly underpins cases of low EA,[5,15] an athlete may in fact unknowingly fail to attain her energy requirements after a sudden increase in exercise commitment, because of time restraint, or due to lack of nutritional knowledge.[18,20] The athlete may lack the appetite necessary to ensure proper dietary energy intake to compensate for the energy expenditure of intense exercise.[21]

Athletes participating in sports involving aesthetics, endurance, and weight classifications (i.e., gymnastics, ballet, figure skating, lightweight rowing, running) are at a particularly high risk for DE/ED and therefore low EA (Table 25.2).[22] In these high-risk sports, a greater percentage of female athletes demonstrated clinical EDs compared with athletes in other sports and nonathletic controls.[25] The prevalence of EDs is also higher in female athletes of all sports as compared with their male counterparts.[24] The risk factors associated with DE behavior that may put any individual, athlete or not, at risk include psychologic factors such as low self-esteem, perfectionism, and body image dissatisfaction and sociocultural factors such as peer pressure, media influence, family influence, or bullying. History of physical or sexual abuse may also be a contributing factor. Additionally, athlete- or sport-specific risk factors for DE may include frequent weight regulation, external pressure, lack of nutritional knowledge and energy requirements, traveling, lack of time, overtraining, injuries, and coaching behavior.[26]

DE, clinical EDs, anorexia athletica, and inadvertent low energy intake will all affect the EA of an athlete. Understanding the cause of an individual athlete's low EA will allow the sports medicine team to generate a more effective treatment plan.

Physiologic Consequences of Low Energy Availability

Nearly every system of the human body may be affected by low EA. The nutritional deficiencies and electrolyte

TABLE 25.2
High-Risk Stress Fractures: Characteristics and Initial Treatment.

Site	Stress Fractures (%)	Common Sports	Initial Treatment
Femoral neck	<5%	Running, endurance athletes	Compression-side: NWB × 4–6 week Tension-side: surgical referral Displaced: urgent surgical referral
Patella	<1%	Running, basketball, gymnastics	Low grade[a]: activity restriction, WB as tolerated High grade[a]: NWB, knee extension brace immobilization × 4–6 week Displaced: surgical referral
Anterior tibia	0.8%–7%	Basketball, gymnastics	NWB × 6–8 week[b] Surgical referral if poor healing at 3–6 months
Medial malleolus	0.6%–4.1%	Running, track and field, basketball, gymnastics	NWB and cast immobilization × 4–8 week[b] Displaced: Surgical referral
Talus	–	Running, pole vaulting, basketball, gymnastics	NWB × 6 week with or without cast immobilization
Navicular	14%–25%	Track and field, football, basketball	Type 1: NWB and cast immobilization ≥6 week[b] Type 2 or 3: surgical referral
Proximal fifth metatarsal	<1%	Soccer, basketball, football	Low grade[a]: NWB and immobilization × 6 week High grade (types 1–3)[a]: surgical referral
Sesamoid	–	Dance, gymnastics, racquet sports, basketball, soccer, volleyball, running, sprinting	NWB and immobilization × 6 week; orthotics Surgical referral if poor healing at 3–6 months

NWB, non-weight-bearing; *WB*, weight-bearing.
[a] Low grade, stress reaction; high grade, fracture line.
[b] Early surgical intervention considered; may allow quicker return to play but further research is needed.

imbalances have implications on reproductive function,[27] bone health,[31] immune function, gastrointestinal problems (e.g., dental, gingival, bleeding, ulceration, bloating, constipation), cardiovascular abnormalities (e.g., arrhythmias, heart block, endothelial dysfunction),[32] renal dysfunction (e.g., urinary incontinence),[33] and psychiatric concerns (e.g., depression, anxiety, suicide).[34] Comorbid EDs pose even greater health risks: EDs have one of the highest mortality rates of any mental health condition[16,35] most often caused by suicide or cardiac arrhythmia.[36,37]

Athletic performance may suffer before the severe consequences of low EA are manifested. The loss of fat and LBM, electrolyte imbalances, and dehydration contribute to poor sport performance and increased risk of musculoskeletal injury.[38,39] The effects of low EA on the menstrual cycle and BMD are a specific concern in the female athlete.

Treatment of Low Energy Availability

The primary goal of treatment for any component of the triad is to increase EA. This may be accomplished by modifying the athlete's diet and exercise regimen to reduce energy expenditure and/or maximize energy intake. In order to remain at or above an EA level of 30 kcal/kg FFM per day, nutritional intake must be optimized. This is best accomplished by an interdisciplinary team including a sports medicine physician, dietitian, or nutritionist and possibly a mental health professional. Additionally, it is imperative to ensure the athlete has social support throughout the process, including coaches, athletic trainers, and family members.

Recovery of energy status may result in restimulation of anabolic hormones and bone formation, as well as reversal of energy conservation adaptations. This may be achieved in days or weeks.[2] Fig. 25.3 depicts the various short-term and long-term consequences that may result from low EA. For many athletes with DE behavior, providing healthy nutritional information and monitoring behavior is sufficient. With cases of clinical EDs, however, psychotherapy may be necessary.

Primary prevention and early identification should be the highest priority of sports medicine teams. Screening for risk factors of DE behaviors may be performed at preparticipation physical examinations. Several nutritional assessments have been developed and validated for screening of EDs specifically for female athletes.[40] Additionally, the Female Athlete Triad Consensus Panel Cumulative Risk Assessment tool provides an objective method of determining an athlete's risk using risk stratification and evidence-based risk factors.[41] Beyond early screening, promoting healthy body image, providing nutritional information, dispelling misconceptions about body weight and composition relating to athletic performance, and discussing healthy weight control are important primary interventions that we can use with our athletes.

MENSTRUAL DYSFUNCTION IN THE FEMALE ATHLETE

The Menstrual Cycle

The menstrual cycle is a complex, coordinated sequence of events that involves the hypothalamus, anterior pituitary, ovary, and endometrium. The menstrual cycle can be easily disrupted by a variety of environmental factors including stress, extreme exercise, EDs, and obesity.[42] It is important to understand the hormones underlying the normal menstrual cycle before studying menstrual dysfunction.

The hypothalamus secretes the gonadotropin-releasing hormone (GnRH), which stimulates the anterior pituitary to secrete follicle-stimulating hormone (FSH) and luteinizing hormone (LH). The levels and timing of secretion of each gonadotropin is correlated by GnRH, feedback from sex steroid hormones, and other autocrine and paracrine factors.[42] The relationship among these hormones is depicted in Fig. 25.4.

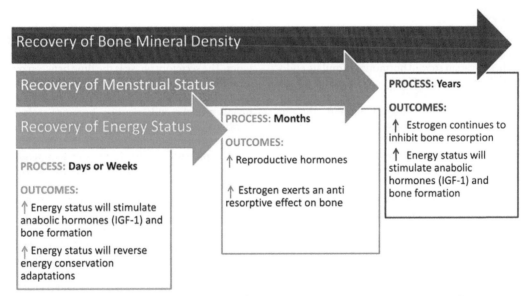

FIG. 25.3 Treatment of the triad. The recovery of the three components of the triad occurs at different rates with appropriate treatment. Recovery of energy status is observed typically after days or weeks of increased energy intake and/or decreased energy expenditure. Recovery of menstrual status is observed typically after months of increased energy intake and/or decreased energy expenditure, which improves energy status. Recovery of bone mineral density may not be observed until years after recovery of energy status and until menstrual status has been achieved. *IGF-1*, insulinlike growth factor 1.

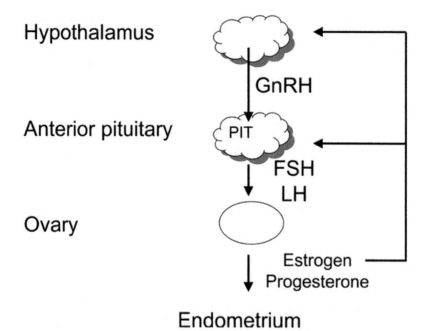

Endometrium

FIG. 25.4 General overview of the important factors in the menstrual cycle. Regulation of the menstrual cycle begins with influences at the level of the hypothalamus. The hypothalamus stimulates the anterior pituitary that stimulates the ovaries. One of the end organs for the ovarian sex hormones is the endometrium. The menstrual cycle is regulated by feedback and cross talk between these different components. *FSH*, follicle-stimulating hormone; *GnRH*, follicle-stimulating hormone; *LH*, luteinizing hormone; *PIT*, pituitary.

The gonadotropins FSH and LH stimulate the ovary to produce the steroid hormones, estrogen and progesterone. These ovarian steroid hormones stimulate endometrial proliferation and affect many other end organs. The feedback of estrogen and progesterone occurs primarily at the level of the anterior pituitary, through the release of GnRH. Folliculogenesis, ovulation, luteinization, and endometrium growth and shedding during the menstrual cycle depend on the factors produced from this hypothalamus-anterior pituitary-ovarian axis.[43]

The menstrual cycle is most commonly broken up into the follicular and luteal phases as characterized by changes within the ovary. The endometrium cycles through the proliferative and secretory phases that correspond to the follicular and luteal phases in the ovary, respectively. The first day of the menstrual cycle is defined as the first day of menstrual bleeding. During this menstrual phase, the endometrium is sloughed because of low levels of estrogen. The proliferative phase is described as the time between menses and ovulation and is characterized by rising levels of estrogen, while progesterone levels remain low. As estrogen levels rise, the endometrial lining thickens with proliferation of stroma, glands, and elongation of the spiral arteries. The secretory phase is the time between ovulation and the next menses. After ovulation, progesterone levels rise, leading to the secretion of glycogen and mucus and the endometrium becomes receptive to a fertilized embryo. In the late secretory phase, in the absence of pregnancy and with the fall in both estrogen and progesterone levels, the spiral arteries vasoconstrict and the endometrium involutes, resulting in menses.[43]

The average length of a menstrual cycle is approximately 28 days,[44] with substantially large 95% confidence intervals (CIs) ranging from 23 to 32 days.[45] Along with interwoman cycle variability, there is also intrawoman cycle variability. Cycle-to-cycle variability has been found to be >7 and <14 days in 42%—46% of females aged 18—44 years.[46,47] Creinin et al.[47] found that 1 in 5 females had cycle-to-cycle variability of 14 days or more. Owing to the large inter- and intra-woman variability in cycle length, it cannot be assumed that all females have 28-day cycles or that any one female will always have consistent cycle lengths.[44] Of note, most changes in cycle length occur in the 1–3 years leading up to menopause,[48] and this is unlikely to begin before the age of 44 years.[49]

In addition to total cycle length variability, there has been found to be follicular and luteal length variability.[44] Most menstrual cycle disturbances have been presumed to be reflective of changes in the follicular phase length; however, luteal phase length variability must also be considered. It is therefore important to have a greater understanding of the cycle phase dynamics when evaluating athletes with deviations from the 28-day cycle. In a study of 165 premenopausal females, electronic fertility monitors characterized 1060 menstrual cycles and demonstrated the average follicular and luteal phase lengths to be 16.5 ± 3.4 days and 12.4 ± 2.0 days, respectively; however, the 95%CI for each phase was 9–23 days and 8–17 days, respectively.[46] Another study used daily urine samples to determine cycle phase characteristics based on the timing of LH peak and reported mean follicular and luteal phase lengths of 14.7 ± 2.4 days and 13.2 ± 2.0 days, and 95%CI for each phase of 10–20 days and 9–17 days, respectively.[45] In addition, when daily urine samples were collected from one female for eight consecutive menstrual cycles, total cycle length varied from 25 to 29 days and follicular and luteal lengths ranged from 10 to 17 days and 11–17 days, respectively.[45] Interestingly, four of the eight cycles had a total length of 27 days, yet the follicular and luteal lengths ranged from 10 to 15 days and 12–17 days, respectively, indicating that even when multiple cycles from the same individual are equal in total length, both follicular and luteal phase lengths can vary.[45]

Types of Menstrual Dysfunction

Menstrual dysfunction is the physiologic consequence of hypoestrogenism, which ranges from amenorrhea to subclinical conditions such as luteal phase defects and anovulation.[20] These conditions lie on a spectrum based on estrogen levels, as shown in Fig. 25.5, with amenorrhea resulting from the most extreme deficiency in estrogen and subclinical conditions resulting from less severe deficits in estrogen.

Primary amenorrhea is the delay of menarche beyond age 15 years in the presence of normal secondary sexual development.[50] Secondary amenorrhea occurs after menarche and is defined as the absence of menstrual cycles lasting more than 3 months.[50] In athletes, amenorrhea is most commonly hypothalamic in origin with low and chronically suppressed levels of circulating gonadotrophins, estrogen and progesterone, and with unaltered responsiveness of the pituitary gland and ovaries.[51]

In females with luteal phase defects, the ovarian system functions to ovulate but is unable to support implantation, which is highly dependent upon progesterone during the luteal phase. The presentation of luteal phase defects that occurs in athletes is also referred to as luteal phase insufficiency to describe the poor quality of the endometrium secondary to low progesterone levels.[20]

Oligomenorrhea is defined as irregular and inconsistent menstrual cycles lasting from 36 to 90 days in length. Owing to the inconsistent nature of this abnormality, no definitive data exists on the prevalence of this menstrual abnormality in athletes, except to note that cycles of irregular length are often reported in female athletes.[52] Oligomenorrheic cycles may be ovulatory

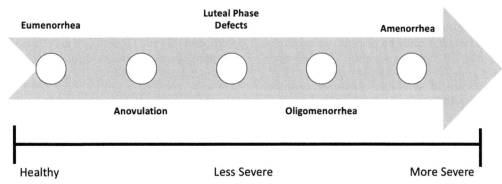

FIG. 25.5 Menstrual disturbances in the female athlete lie along a continuum ranging from eumenorrhea to amenorrhea. Eumenorrhea is considered optimal menstrual health, where regular ovulatory menstrual cycles occur. Amenorrhea is considered the most severe menstrual disturbance, which is characterized by the absence of menses for at least 3 months.

or anovulatory, as the defining event is the sloughing of the endometrial lining, which occurs in response to increasing estrogen levels that are independent of ovulation.[20]

Anovulation is defined as the absence of ovulation in the setting of low levels of LH and FSH, associated with reduced estrogen levels.[20] As cycle length can vary in anovulatory cycles, anovulation can be associated with oligomenorrhea. This type of menstrual dysfunction is generally not noticed by the athlete until she is trying to conceive.

Amenorrhea in athletes can occur for other reasons besides the triad. Polycystic ovarian syndrome (PCOS) is associated with menstrual dysfunction and androgen excess. PCOS is characterized by menstrual disturbances ranging from dysfunctional uterine bleeding to oligomenorrhea and amenorrhea, hyperandrogenism, and infertility.[53] To be classified as having PCOS, an individual must have two out of three of the following features[1]: oligo- and/or anovulation,[2] clinical and/or biochemical signs of hyperandrogenism (hirsutism, acne, androgenic alopecia),[3] and ultrasound evidence of polycystic ovaries.[54] Serum androgen levels usually range from upper normal to twofold higher than normal in females with PCOS.[53]

Prevalence of Menstrual Dysfunction in Female Athletes

Clinical manifestations of menstrual dysfunction have been shown to range from 1% to 61% in exercising females and are documented at much higher rates than that in nonathletic, premenopausal females.[13] Specifically, the more severe presentations of menstrual disturbances in athletes, such as oligomenorrhea and amenorrhea, have been reported to range from 6% to 43% in runners and 1% to 31% in both high-school and collegiate athletes from a variety of different sports.[13] There is evidence suggesting that half of exercising females experience subclinical menstrual dysfunction, including luteal phase defect and anovulation, and that self-reporting menstrual history alone does not provide the appropriate information to indicate the presence of subclinical menstrual dysfunction.[55] Because the method of self-report can only identify those components of menstrual dysfunction readily apparent to females as an absence of menses for greater than 3 months, or irregularities in menstrual cycle length, investigators reporting on the prevalence of menstrual dysfunction using self-report methods are likely to have underestimated the percentage of females with menstrual dysfunction.[13]

Menstrual dysfunction affects many athletes, particularly those participating in leanness sports such as distance running, cycling, swimming, lightweight rowing, wrestling, gymnastics, and figure skating.[56] Participants in these sports tend to reach menarche later than other athletes and nonathletes.[57] One study assessed the menstrual patterns of 38 adolescent female ballet dancers and 77 age-matched controls and found that 42% of dancers versus 14% of controls had oligomenorrhea.[58] Of 82 elite rhythmic gymnasts, 55% of postmenarcheal participants had a history of menstrual dysfunction, with 20% having amenorrhea.[59] Among runners, menstrual dysfunction has been reported in 26%–43%.[60] Of 21 elite lightweight rowers, 91% reported a history of oligomenorrhea.[63]

How Low Energy Availability Leads to Menstrual Dysfunction

The cause of menstrual disturbances in female athletes has been linked to inadequate EA.[20] When the body has low EA, energy is conserved for the most vital physiologic processes and away from processes such as fat accumulation, growth, and reproduction. Female athletes are particularly susceptible to inadequate EA, as menstruation and pregnancy are energetically expensive.

Previous authors have demonstrated that in regularly menstruating, sedentary females, aged 18–30 years, short-term manipulation of EA, in a tightly controlled setting, affects LH pulsatility. When EA decreased below 30 kcal/kg FFM per day, the LH pulse amplitude increased and frequency decreased.[6] Ovarian function relies on LH pulsatility. Therefore 30 kcal/kg FFM per day is crucial for normal functioning of the hypothalamic-pituitary-gonadal axis.

Reproductive suppression in times of low EA is a form of FHA, which manifests as persistent anovulation with no identifiable organic cause. Aberrant GnRH pulsatility at the hypothalamus leads to abnormal pituitary secretion of FSH and LH, resulting in decreased estrogen and progesterone levels, inadequate folliculogenesis, and anovulation. Alterations in gonadotropin secretions have been attributed to alterations in secretion of kisspeptin, cortisol, insulin, insulinlike growth factor 1 (IGF-1), and appetite-regulating hormones, such as leptin, ghrelin, and peptide YY.[64] Athletes with FHA typically have lower EA than eumenorrheic athletes and nonathletic controls, although a specific EA threshold cannot necessarily predict the menstrual status of all females.[65] In a prospective study of typically sedentary, eumenorrheic females aged 18–30 years, manipulations of EA by diet and exercise led to EA as low as 58% of baseline. The probability of developing menstrual dysfunction was greater than 50% as absolute EA dropped below 30 kcal/kg FFM per day. There was a dose-response relationship between relative energy deficit (percentage decrease in EA from baseline) and frequency of menstrual disturbances (luteal phase defects, anovulation, and oligomenorrhea), but the severity of menstrual disturbances did not correlate with the magnitude of energy deficiency.[27,66]

Treatment Strategies for Menstrual Dysfunction Often Target Low Energy Availability

In order to treat menstrual dysfunction in the female athlete, low EA must be addressed. Treatment typically begins with increasing nutritional intake to ensure the athlete has adequate EA. Restoration of menses can take several months, and the athlete should be counseled as such. In a retrospective study of 373 female collegiate athletes, 18% of athletes with oligo-amenorrhea resumed menses with nonpharmacologic treatment, with a mean time of menstrual restoration of 15.6 months. Weight gain and increased body mass index (BMI) were the primary differentiating factors between athletes who did or did not resume menses.[67] Another study found that a 9-month nutritional intervention in adolescent and young adult dancers and athletes led to improved nutritional intake and LH concentration after 3 months in athletes and 9 months in dancers.[68] Of the 52 dancers and athletes with menstrual dysfunction, 10 resumed regular menstruation after intervention, and these individuals had on average a greater percentage of body fat mass than those whose menses did not resume.[68] Weight gain can lead to restoration of normal menses, along with improvements in BMD and endothelial function.[69,70]

As discussed in the previous section on low EA, the treatment plan for low EA with ED may include psychotherapy. Cognitive behavior therapy (CBT) may help females with EDs and those without EDs—CBT focuses on identifying and restructuring irrational thoughts to change maladaptive behaviors. A study of 16 females with FHA without ED showed that after 20 weeks, 7 of 8 females who received CBT recovered ovarian function, compared with 2 of 8 females who received no CBT.[71]

Prescribing combined oral contraceptive pills for the purpose of resuming menstrual function and improving BMD is not recommended. These formulations result in a cyclic withdrawal bleed by modifying endogenous hormone concentrations, without addressing the FHA.

As the cyclical bleeding mimics a physiologic menses, the underlying low EA is masked. The Endocrine Society's systematic review evaluated the effects of oral contraceptive pills on BMD in females with FHA and showed the absence of any clear benefits on bone parameters. This is likely due to additional neuroendocrine disruptions, with reductions in IGF-1 concentrations, a potent bone anabolic hormone.[64]

There is evidence suggesting that transdermal 17β-estradiol and cyclic oral micronized progesterone can be used as an adjunct treatment to improve bone density outcomes in athletes with FHA. Significant increases in BMD at the spine and femoral neck were seen over the course of a year in young adult athletes with oligo-amenorrhea who received 100 μg transdermal 17β-estradiol and cyclic oral micronized progesterone (200 mg per day, for 12 days per month).[64,72]

LOW BONE MINERAL DENSITY
Epidemiology

Athletes are at risk for impaired BMD with the female athlete triad. Risk factors for low BMD include dietary restraint, low BMI, reduced lean tissue, late menarche, menstrual dysfunction, and prior stress reaction/stress fracture.[62] Gibbs et al.[73] showed that of these risk factors, low BMI and late menarche were the strongest for low BMD. Furthermore, Tenforde et al.[74] found that each triad risk factor was individually associated with low BMD, and in multivariate analysis, only low BMI and oligomenorrhea/amenorrhea were associated with low BMD ($P < .05$). There may be an association with multiple triad risk factors and increased risk for low BMD, suggesting a dose-response relationship.[73]

As with low EA, sport type may also contribute to increased risk of low BMD: athletes in sports that emphasize leanness may have impaired bone density, likely due to behaviors that contribute to energy deficiency.[75] Tenforde et al.[74] studied 239 female athletes participating in 16 collegiate sports and evaluated dual energy X-ray absorptiometry (DXA) scans to measure BMD z-scores of the lumbar spine and total body. Athletes with the lowest average BMD z-scores included those who participated in synchronized swimming, swimming/diving, crew/rowing, and cross-country. Highest BMD were seen in athletes playing gymnastics, volleyball, basketball, and softball. The sports most commonly associated with low BMD can be seen in Table 25.3. The authors concluded that athletes who participated in high-impact and multidirectional sports have approximately five times the BMD of athletes who participated in low-impact sports.[74]

TABLE 25.3
LS BMD z-Score, TB BMD z-Score, and BMC z-Score and Percentage of Athletes With Low BMD (z-Score < −1.0 for LS and/or TB BMD) in 239 Athletes.

Sport	No. of Athletes	LS BMD z-Score, Mean (SD)	TB z-Score, Mean (SD)	BMC z-Score, Mean (SD)	% Low BMD
Swimming/diving[a]	21	0.34 (0.92)	−0.06 (0.81)	0.78 (0.87)	24
Sailing	3	−0.20 (1.22)	0.13 (1.39)	0.20 (1.14)	33
Synchronized swimming[a]	11	−0.34 (1.28)	0.21 (1.19)	0.29 (1.29)	45
Crew/rowing[a]	30	0.27 (0.89)	0.62 (0.72)	1.24 (1.14)	0
Cross-country[b]	47	0.29 (1.46)	0.91 (1.06)	1.15 (1.21)	19
Water polo	16	0.86 (0.93)	1.04 (0.88)	1.84 (0.97)	0
Tennis	7	1.44 (1.35)	1.08 (0.64)	1.18 (0.98)	0
Fencing	5	0.84 (0.66)	1.10 (0.58)	0.98 (0.53)	0
Lacrosse	16	1.09 (0.95)	1.21 (0.78)	1.44 (1.04)	0
Field hockey	21	0.76 (1.13)	1.22 (0.95)	1.15 (1.01)	5
Track and field	4	0.68 (1.34)	1.33 (1.01)	1.43 (0.67)	0
Soccer	5	0.68 (1.42)	1.43 (0.45)	1.95 (0.51)	20
Gymnastics[a]	16	1.96 (1.13)	1.37 (1.33)	1.10 (0.90)	0
Softball[b]	19	1.68 (1.04)	1.78 (0.94)	1.96 (1.00)	0
Volleyball[b]	9	1.90 (1.39)	1.74 (1.06)	2.56 (1.20)	11
Basketball[b]	9	1.73 (1.42)	1.99 (0.86)	3.01 (0.96)	0

Table organized by lowest to highest average TB BMD z-scores.
BMD, bone mineral density; LS, lumbar spine; SD, standard deviation; TB, total body.
[a] LS and TB BMD significantly different than the rest of the sample.
[b] Only spine BMD significantly different than the rest of the sample.

It has also been reported that prior participation in multidirectional loading sports, such as soccer and basketball, during adolescence reduces the risk of stress fracture by half in older track-and-field athletes, except in females with current menstrual irregularities (Fig. 25.6).[76]

Physiology/Pathophysiology

Peak bone mass occurs around 19 years in females. Estrogen increases uptake of calcium into the blood and deposition into the bone, with progesterone being a beneficial accessory. Testosterone has anabolic effects on bone, stimulating osteoclasts and increasing bone formation and calcium absorption. The bones of athletes with chronic amenorrhea benefit less from the osteogenic effects of exercise. Low BMD was initially attributed to hypoestrogenism of menstrual dysfunction, but low EA is now proven to be an independent factor of poor bone health at all levels of energy deficiency due to decreased IGF-1 and bone formation

marker levels.[77] Bone loss in these athletes may be irreversible.[78]

Evaluation and Treatment

BMD is assessed using DXA. Low BMD is defined as a BMD z-score of ≤−2.0, adjusted for age, gender, and body size, as necessary.[2] Importantly, z-scores < −1.0 are classified as "lower than expected" and are also worthy of additional workup.[79] All female athletes considered to be either high risk or moderate risk for triad risk factors are indicated for DXA scans.[2,79] The criteria for classifying these athletes can be seen in Table 25.4. The frequency of DXA testing will depend on the athlete's initial BMD and ongoing clinical status (e.g., where there is ongoing bone loss). Adult women aged 20 years or older are screened at weight-bearing sites (posteroanterior spine, total hip, and femoral neck). If for any reason weight-bearing sites cannot be assessed, the radius may be screened as an alternative. Children and adolescent women aged <20 years will

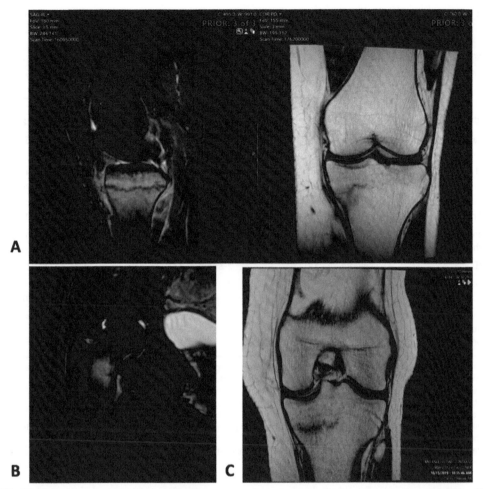

FIG. 25.6 A series of noncontrast magnetic resonance images demonstrating common stress fractures. **(A)** Left knee image showing a nondisplaced stress fracture of the medial tibial plateau. Patient is a 44 year-old female who presented with worsening medial sided knee pain 2 weeks after running a 50-mile endurance race. **(B)** Right hip image showing a femoral neck stress fracture. Demonstrates progression of the basicervical stress fracture with persistent fracture line extended further along the anterior cortex and more edema in the underlying bone. Patient is a 24 year-old female presenting with worsening hip pain, no acute injury. She has a history of previous eating disorder and osteopenia. **(C)** Left knee image showing a nondisplaced stress fracture of the medial tibial plateau. Patient is a 47-year-old healthy female presenting with mild medial sided pain after resuming exercising including light jogging.

be screened for posteroanterior lumbar spine bone mineral content and areal BMD and/or whole body less head if possible. In this population, adjustments for growth or maturational delay may be necessary.[2]

It is important to screen athletes in higher risk sports, such as cross-country, swimming/diving, synchronized swimming, and crew/rowing. These athletes and other female athletes with low BMI and/or current oligomenorrhea/amenorrhea would benefit from a thorough assessment of nutrition to ensure adequate EA, calcium,

vitamin D, and other nutritional needs to optimize skeletal health. Early data also suggest instituting cross-training activities with high skeletal impacts to stimulate improvement in bone strength in at-risk athletes.[74]

CONCLUSION

The components of the female athlete triad (EA, menstrual status, and bone health) are part of a highly interconnected system. In this chapter, we reviewed the

TABLE 25.4

Triad: Cumulative Risk Assessment. The Cumulative Risk Assessment Provides an Objective Method of Determining an Athlete's Risk Using Risk Stratification and Evidence-Based Risk Factors for the Triad. This Assessment is Then Used to Determine an Athlete's Clearance for Sport Participation.

Risk Factors	MAGNITUDE OF RISK		
	Low Risk = 0 Point Each	Moderate Risk = 1 Point Each	High Risk = 2 Points Each
Low EA with or without DE/ED	No dietary restriction	Some dietary restriction[e]; current/past history of DE	Meets *DSM-5* criteria for ED[a]
Low BMI	BMI, >18.5 or ≥90% EW[b] or weight stable	BMI, 17.5 < 18.5 **or** <90% EW **or** 5 to <10% weight loss/month	BMI, ≤17.5 **or** <85% EW **or** ≥ 10% weight loss/month
Delayed menarche	Menarche, <15 years	Menarche, 15–<16 years	Menarche, >16 years
Oligomenorrhea and/or amenorrhea	>9 Menses in 12 months[a]	6–9 Menses in 12 months[a]	<6 Menses in 12 months[a]
Low BMD	z-score, ≥−1.0	z-score, −1.0[c] <−2.0	z-score, ≤−2.0
Stress reaction/fracture	None	1	≥ 2; ≥1 High risk or of trabecular bone sites[d]
Cumulative risk (total each column and then add for total score)	_____ points +	_____ points +	_____ points = _____ total score

BMD, bone mineral density; *BMI*, body mass index; *DE/ED*, disordered eating/disordered eating; *DSM-5, Diagnostic and Statistical Manual of Mental Disorders* (Fifth Edition); *EA*, energy availability; *EW*, expected weight.

[a] Currently experiencing or has a history.[3,29]
[b] ≥90% EW; absolute BMI cutoffs should be not used for adolescents.
[c] Weight-bearing sport.
[d] High-risk skeletal sites associated with low BMD and delay in return to play in athletes with one or more components of the triad include stress reaction/fracture of trabecular sites (femoral neck, sacrum, and pelvis).
[e] Some dietary restriction as evidenced by self-report or low/inadequate energy intake on diet logs.

common risk factors associated with low EA, menstrual dysfunction, and low BMD and the influence of each element on another. The type of sport has been associated with each component of the triad and therefore likely has a significant impact on risk in a female athlete. Sports that focus on leanness are associated with low EA and menstrual dysfunction, while high-impact, multidirectional sports may protect against low BMD. The female athlete triad is often denied, not recognized, and underreported. Multidisciplinary teams of sports medicine professionals must be aware of the interrelated and varied components of the triad. Recognizing, diagnosing, and treating or referring female athletes with any one component of the triad is critical. While the triad has the potential to become a vicious cycle, preventative measures such as nutritional education can create a system of optimal energy, eumenorrhea, and optimal skeletal health.

REFERENCES

1. Herring SA, Bergfeld JA, Boyajian-O'Neil LA, et al. Female athlete issues for the team physician: a consensus statement—2017 update. *Med Sci Sports Exerc.* 2018; 50(5):1113−1122.
2. Joy E, De Souza MJ, Nattiv A, et al. 2014 female athlete triad coalition consensus statement on treatment and return to play of the female athlete triad. *Curr Sports Med Rep.* 2014;13(4):219−232.
3. Nattiv A, Loucks AB, Manore MM, Sanborn CF, Sundgot-Borgen J, Warren MP. American College of Sports Medicine position stand. The female athlete triad. *Med Sci Sports Exerc.* 2007;39(10):1867−1882.
4. Mountjoy M, Sundgot-Borgen J, Buke L, et al. The IOC consensus statement: beyond the female athlete triad – relative energy deficiency in sport (RED-S). *Br J Sports Med.* 2014;48:491−497.
5. Mountjoy M, Sundgot-Borgen JK, Burke LM, et al. IOC Consensus statement on relative energy deficiency in sport

(RED-S): 2018 update. *Br J Sports Med.* 2018;52(11): 687−697.

6. Loucks AB, Thuma JR. Luteinizing hormone pulsatility is disrupted at a threshold of energy availability in regularly menstruating women. *J Clin Endocrinol Metab.* 2003;88: 297−311.

7. Thomas DT, Erdman KA, Burke LM. Position of the academy of nutrition and dietetics, dietitians of Canada, and the American college of sports medicine: nutrition and athletic performance. *J Acad Nutr Diet.* 2016;116(3): 501−528.

8. Loucks AB. *Energy balance and energy availability.* In: *The Encyclopaedia of Sports Medicine: An IOC Medical Commission Publication.* Lausanne, Switzerland: International Olympic Committee; 2013;19:72−87.

9. Loucks AB, Verdun M, Heath EM. Low energy availability, not stress of exercise, alters LH pulsatility in exercising women. *J Appl Physiol (1985).* 1998;84(1):37−46.

10. Hilton LK, Loucks AB. Low energy availability, not exercise stress, suppresses the diurnal rhythm of leptin in healthy young women. *Am J Physiol Endocrinol Metab.* 2000; 278(1):E43−E49.

11. Reed JL, De Souza MJ, Williams NI. Changes in energy availability across the season in Division I female soccer players. *J Sports Sci.* 2013;31(3):314−324.

12. Koehler K, Achtzehn S, Braun H, Mester J, Schaenzer W. Comparison of self-reported energy availability and metabolic hormones to assess adequacy of dietary energy intake in young elite athletes. *Appl Physiol Nutr Metab.* 2013; 38(7):725−733.

13. Gibbs JC, Williams NI, De Souza MJ. Prevalence of individual and combined components of the female athlete triad. *Med Sci Sports Exerc.* 2013;45(5):985−996.

14. Hoch AZ, Pajewski NM, Moraski L, et al. Prevalence of the female athlete triad in high school athletes and sedentary students. *Clin J Sport Med.* 2009;19(5):421−428.

15. Herring SA, Kibler WB, Putukian M, et al. Psychological issues related to illness and injury in athletes and the team physician: a consensus statement-2016 Update. *Med Sci Sports Exerc.* 2017;49(5):1043−1054.

16. American Psychiatric Association. *Diagnostic and Statistical Manual of Mental Disorders.* 5th ed. Arlington, VA: American Psychiatric Association; 2013.

17. Sudi K, Ottl K, Payerl D, Baumgartl P, Tauschmann K, Müller W. Anorexia athletica. *Nutrition.* 2004;20(7−8): 657−661.

18. Nazem TG, Ackerman KE. The female athlete triad. *Sports Health.* 2012;4(4):302−311.

19. Loucks AB. Low energy availability in the marathon and other endurance sports. *Sports Med.* 2007;37(4−5):348−352.

20. De Souza MJ, Williams NI. Physiological aspects and clinical sequelae of energy deficiency and hypoestrogenism in exercising women. *Hum Reprod Update.* 2004;10(5): 433−448.

21. Blundell JE, King NA. Effects of exercise on appetite control: loose coupling between energy expenditure and energy intake. *Int J Obes Relat Metab Disord.* 1998;22(Suppl. 2):S22−S29.

22. Loucks AB. Energy balance and body composition in sports and exercise. *J Sports Sci.* 2004;22(1):1−14.

23. Costello LE. Eating disorders in athletes. In: Madden C, Putukian M, McCarty E, Young C, eds. *Netter's Sports Medicine.* 2nd ed. Philadelphia, PA: Elsevier; 2017:191−196 (in press).

24. Sundgot-Borgen J, Torstveit MK. Prevalence of eating disorders in elite athletes is higher than in the general population. *Clin J Sport Med.* 2004;14(1):25−32.

25. Torstveit MK, Rosenvinge JH, Sundgot-Borgen J. Prevalence of eating disorders and the predictive power of risk models in female elite athletes: a controlled study. *Scand J Med Sci Sports.* 2008;18(1):108−118.

26. Sundgot-Borgen J, Meyer NL, Lohman TG, et al. How to minimise the health risks to athletes who compete in weight-sensitive sports review and position statement on behalf of the Ad Hoc Research Working Group on Body Composition, Health and Performance, under the auspices of the IOC Medical Commission. *Br J Sports Med.* 2013;47(16):1012−1022.

27. Williams NI, Leidy HJ, Hill BR, Lieberman JL, Legro RS, De Souza MJ. Magnitude of daily energy deficit predicts frequency but not severity of menstrual disturbances associated with exercise and caloric restriction. *Am J Physiol Endocrinol Metab.* 2015;308(1):E29−E39. https://doi.org/10.1152/ajpendo.00386.2013.

28. Vanheest JL, Rodgers CD, Mahoney CE, De Souza MJ. Ovarian suppression impairs sport performance in junior elite female swimmers. *Med Sci Sports Exerc.* 2014;46(1): 156−166.

29. Muia EN, Wright HH, Onywera VO, Kuria EN. Adolescent elite Kenyan runners are at risk for energy deficiency, menstrual dysfunction and disordered eating. *J Sports Sci.* 2016; 34(7):598−606.

30. Lagowska K, Kapczuk K, Friebe Z, Bajerska J. Effects of dietary intervention in young female athletes with menstrual disorders. *J Int Soc Sports Nutr.* 2014;11(21). https://doi.org/10.1186/1550-2783-11-21.

31. Ihle R, Loucks AB. Dose-response relationships between energy availability and bone turnover in young exercising women. *J Bone Miner Res.* 2004;19(8):1231−1240.

32. Hoch AZ, Papanek P, Szabo A, Widlandsky ME, Schimke JE, Gutterman DD. Association between the female athlete triad and endothelial dysfunction in dancers. *Clin J Sport Med.* 2011;21(2):119−125.

33. Whitney KE, Holtzman B, Parziale A, Ackerman KE. Urinary incontinence. *Orthop J Sports Med.* 2019;7(3) (suppl 1).

34. Logue D, Madigan S, Delahunt E, Heinen M, McDonnell SJ, Corish CA. Low energy availability in athletes: a review of prevalence, dietary patterns, physiological health, and sports performance. *Sports Med.* 2018;48(1): 73−96.

35. Marquez S. Eating disorders in sports: risk factors, health consequences, treatment and prevention. *Nutr Hosp.* 2008;23(3):183−190.

36. Arcelus J, Mitchell AJ, Wales J, Nielsen S. Mortality rates in patients with anorexia nervosa and other eating disorders.

A meta-analysis of 36 studies. *Arch Gen Psychiatry*. 2011; 68(7):724–731.

37. Crow SJ, Peterson CB, Swanson SA, et al. Increased mortality in bulimia nervosa and other eating disorders. *Am J Psychiatry*. 2009;166(12):1342–1346.

38. El Ghoch M, Soave F, Calugi S, Dalle Grave R. Eating disorders, physical fitness and sport performance: a systematic review. *Nutrients*. 2013;5(12):5140–5160.

39. Thein-Nissenbaum JM, Rauh MJ, Carr KE, Loud KJ, McGuine TA. Associations between disordered eating, menstrual dysfunction, and musculoskeletal injury among high school athletes. *J Orthop Sports Phys Ther*. 2011;41: 60–69.

40. Knapp J, Aerni G, Anderson J. Eating disorders in female athletes: use of screening tools. *J Curr Sports Med Rep*. 2014;13(4):214–218.

41. Barrack MT, Gibbs JC, De Souza MJ, et al. Higher incidence of bone stress injuries with increasing female athlete triad-related risk factors: a prospective multisite study of exercising girls and women. *Am J Sports Med*. 2014;442(4): 949–958.

42. Hawkins SM, Matzuk MM. Menstrual cycle: basic biology. *Ann NY Acad Sci*. 2008;1135(1):10–18. https://doi.org/ 10.1196/annals.1429.018.

43. Speroff L, Fritz MA. *Clinical Gynecologic Endocrinology and Infertility*. Lippincott Williams & Wilkins; 2005.

44. Vescovi J. The menstrual cycle and anterior cruciate ligament injury risk. *Sports Med*. 2011;41(2):91–101.

45. Cole LA, Ladner DG, Byrn FW. The normal variabilities of the menstrual cycle. *Fertil Steril*. 2009;91(2):522–527. https://doi.org/10.1016/j.fertnstert.2007.11.073.

46. Fehring RJ, Schneider M, Raviele K. Variability in the phases of the menstrual cycle. *J Obstet Gynecol Neonatal Nurs*. 2006;35(3):376–384.

47. Creinin MD, Keverline S, Meyn LA. How regular is regular? An analysis of menstrual cycle regularity. *Contraception*. 2004;70(4):289–292.

48. Ferrell RJ, Simon JA, Pincus SM, et al. The length of perimenopausal menstrual cycles increases later and to a greater degree than previously reported. *Fertil Steril*. 2006;86(3):619–624.

49. O'Connor KA, Holman DJ, Wood JW. Menstrual cycle variability and the perimenopause. *Am J Hum Biol*. 2001; 13(4):465–478.

50. American Society of Reproductive Medicine Practice Committee. Current evaluation of amenorrhea. *Fertil Steril*. 2008;90(5 Suppl):S219–S225. https://doi.org/10.1016/ j.fertnstert.2008.08.038.

51. Veldhuis JD, Evans WS, Demers LM, Thorner MO, Wakat D, Rogol AD. Altered neuroendocrine regulation of gonadotropin secretion in women distance runners. *J Clin Endocrinol Metab*. 1985;61(3):557–563.

52. Loucks AB, Horvath SM. Athletic amenorrhea: a review. *Med Sci Sports Exerc*. 1985;17(1):56–72.

53. Legro RS. Polycystic ovary syndrome: the new millennium. *Mol Cell Endocrinol*. 2001;184(1–2):87–93.

54. Rotterdam ESHRE/ASRM-Sponsored PCOS Consesus Workshop Group. Revised 2003 consensus on diagnostic criteria and long-term health risks related to polycystic ovary syndrome. *Fertil Steril*. 2004;81(1):19–25.

55. De Souza MJ, Toombs RJ, Scheid JL, O'Donnell E, West SL, Williams NI. High prevalence of subtle and severe menstrual disturbances in exercising women: confirmation using daily hormone measures. *Hum Reprod*. 2010;25(2): 491–503. https://doi.org/10.1093/humrep/dep411.

56. Ackerman K, Misra M. Amenorrhea in adolescent female athletes. *Lancet Child Adolesc Health*. 2018;2(9):677–688.

57. Beunen G, Malina RM. Growth and biological maturation: relevance to athletic performance. In: Hebestreit H, Bar-Or O, eds. *The Young Athlete*. Blackwell Publishing. International Olympic Committee; 2008:3–17.

58. Castelo-Branco C, Reina F, Montivero AD, Colodrón M, Vanrell JA. Influence of high-intensity training and of dietetic and anthropometric factors on menstrual cycle disorders in ballet dancers. *Gynecol Endocrinol*. 2006;22(1):31–35.

59. Maïmoun L, Coste O, Georgopoulos NA, et al. Despite a high prevalence of menstrual disorders, bone health is improved at a weight-bearing bone site in world-class female rhythmic gymnasts. *J Clin Endocrinol Metab*. 2013; 98(12):4961–4969. https://doi.org/10.1210/jc.2013-2794.

60. Barrack MT, Rauh MJ, Nichols JF. Prevalence of and traits associated with BMD among female adolescent runners. *Med Sci Sports Exerc*. 2008;40(12):2015–2021. https:// doi.org/10.1249/MSS.0b013e3181822ea0.

61. Austin TM, Reinking MF, Hayes AM. Menstrual function in female high school cross-country athletes. *Int J Adolesc Med Health*. 2009;21(4):555–565.

62. Tenforde AS, Fredericson M, Sayres LC, Cutti P, Sainani KL. Identifying sex-specific risk factors for low bone mineral density in adolescent runners. *Am J Sports Med*. 2015; 43(6):1494–1504. https://doi.org/10.1177/0363546515 572142.

63. Dimitriou L, Weiler R, Lloyd-Smith R, et al. Bone mineral density, rib pain and other features of the female athlete triad in elite lightweight rowers. *BMJ Open*. 2014; 4(2):e004369. https://doi.org/10.1136/bmjopen-2013-004369.

64. Gordon CM, Ackerman KE, Berga SL, et al. Functional hypothalamic amenorrhea: an endocrine society clinical practice guideline. *J Clin Endocrinol Metab*. 2017;102(5): 1413–1439. https://doi.org/10.1210/jc.2017-00131.

65. Elliott-Sale KJ, Tenforde AS, Parziale AL, Holtzman B, Ackerman KE. Endocrine effects of relative energy deficiency in sport. *Int J Sport Nutr Exerc Metab*. 2018;28(4): 335–349. https://doi.org/10.1123/ijsnem.2018-0127.

66. Lieberman JL, DE Souza MJ, Wagstaff DA, Williams NI. Menstrual disruption with exercise is not linked to an energy availability threshold. *Med Sci Sports Exerc*. 2018; 50(3):551–561. https://doi.org/10.1249/MSS.000000 0000001451.

67. Arends JC, Cheung MY, Barrack MT, Nattiv A. Restoration of menses with nonpharmacological therapy in college athletes with menstrual disturbances: a 5-year retrospective study. *Int J Sport Nutr Exerc Metab*. 2012;22(2): 98–108.

68. Lagowska K, Kapczuk K, Jeszka J. Nine-month nutritional intervention improves restoration of menses in young female athletes and ballet dancers. *J Int Soc Sports Nutr.* 2014; 11(1):52. https://doi.org/10.1186/s12970-014-0052-9.

69. Misra M, Prabhakaran R, Miller KK, et al. Weight gain and restoration of menses as predictors of bone mineral density change in adolescent girls with anorexia nervosa-1. *J Clin Endocrinol Metab.* 2008;93(4):1231–1237.

70. Hoch AZ, Jurva JW, Staton MA, et al. Athletic amenorrhea and endothelial dysfunction. *WMJ.* 2007;106(6):301–306.

71. Berga SL, Marcus MD, Loucks TL, Hlastala S, Ringham R, Krohn MA. Recovery of ovarian activity in women with functional hypothalamic amenorrhea who were treated with cognitive behavioral therapy. *Fertil Steril.* 2003; 80(4):976–981.

72. Ackerman K. Transdermal 17-β estradiol has a beneficial effect on bone parameters assessed using HRpQCT compared to oral ethinyl estradiol-progesterone combination pills in oligo-amenorrheic athletes: a randomized control trial. *Am Soc Bone Mineral Res.* 2017:1119, 2017 Annual Meeting; Denver, CO, USA. Sept 8-11.

73. Gibbs JC, Nattiv A, Barrack MT, et al. Low bone density risk is higher in exercising women with multiple triad risk factors. *Med Sci Sports Exerc.* 2014;46(1):167–176.

74. Tenforde AS, Carlson JL, Sainani KL, et al. Sport and triad risk factors influence bone mineral density in collegiate athletes. *Med Sci Sports Exerc.* 2018;50(12):2536–2543.

75. Barrack MT, Van Loan MD, Rauh MJ, Nichols JF. Body mass, training, menses, and bone in adolescent runners: a 3-yr follow-up. *Med Sci Sports Exerc.* 2011;43(6): 959–966.

76. Fredericson M, Ngo J, Cobb K. Effects of ball sports on future risk of stress fracture in runners. *Clin J Sports Med.* 2005;15(3):136–141.

77. Lambrinoudaki I, Papadimitriou D. Pathophysiology of bone loss in the female athlete. *Ann N Y Acad Sci.* 2010; 1205:45–50.

78. Keen AD, Drinkwater BL. Irreversible bone loss in former amenorrheic athletes. *Osteoporos Int.* 1997;(7):311–315.

79. Nichols DL, Sanborn CF, Essery EV. Bone density and young athletic women. *Sports Med.* 2007;27:1001–1014.

FURTHER READING

1. Holtzman B, Ackerman KE. Measurement, determinants, and implications of energy intake in athletes. *Nutrients.* 2019;11(665):1–13.

CHAPTER 26

Exercise Considerations Before, During, and After Pregnancy

STEPHANIE CHU, DO • SARAH WEINSTEIN, DO • KELSEY ANDREWS, BS

INTRODUCTION

Over the past decade, there has been an increased interest in the topic of physical activity during pregnancy. This is likely due to the increasing number of studies that have shown what benefits exercise can have during this unique time in a woman's life. Physicians and patients often express uncertainty regarding physical activity during pregnancy out of concern for the safety of both the mother and fetus. Previous studies have shown that physical activity is not associated with critical outcomes such as miscarriage, neonatal death, preterm birth, or birth defects.[1] The dramatic rise in obesity, hypertension, and diabetes over the past few decades is well-documented in the literature. Subsequently there has been a similar increase in pregnancy complications such as gestational diabetes, gestational hypertension, and preeclamspsia.[1] For this reason, there is an emphasis on using physical activity to help decrease the risk of these complications and optimize maternal-fetal health during pregnancy.[1]

Pregnancy no longer needs to be thought of as a time to cease all activity, and it is important to counsel patients that there can be more complications by not exercising. Exercise throughout all three trimesters of pregnancy is safe, does not lead to an increase in major complications, and improves overall pregnancy outcomes.[5] While the benefits almost always outweigh the risks for the general pregnant population, it is important to be aware of contraindications and to know when to refrain from certain activities. The goal of this chapter is to discuss the specific considerations and recommendations for exercise during pregnancy and the peripartum period based on the most updated guidelines, explain how the physiologic changes throughout pregnancy may impact the ability to perform physical activity, and describe appropriate precautions to take before engaging in physical activity.

PATHOPHYSIOLOGY

Pregnancy has a profound effect on multiple body systems, and the subsequent physiologic adaptations can be a large factor in determining the level of participation in physical activity for a pregnant woman. In the section, we will discuss the relevant adaptations and physiologic changes during pregnancy.

Anatomic/Musculoskeletal Considerations

There are various anatomic changes that occur throughout pregnancy that may affect a woman's ability to participate in certain activities or sports, of which the most obvious and noticeable is gestational weight gain. For a female with a normal prepregnancy body mass index (BMI) ($18.5-24.9 \text{ kg/m}^2$), the optimal weight gain is between 25 and 35 pounds, with an average of 1 pound per week in the second and third trimesters.[7] Increased mass may transfer significant force across the larger weight-bearing joints such as the knees and hips.[4] Over time, this may cause discomfort and limit the ability to participate in activities or sports requiring full load bearing, such as running.

Throughout pregnancy, both the expanding uterus and enlarging breasts will displace the center of gravity. Increased lumbar lordosis and subsequent anterior pelvic rotation on the femur occur in pregnancy, changing a woman's center of gravity.[3] This is important for activities that require optimal balance such as cycling on a nonstationary bike or walking on uneven ground.[1]

Finally, ligamentous laxity increases throughout pregnancy, secondary to the effects of increased levels of estrogen and relaxin, which can predispose a female to joint instability and the theoretic risk of increased strains and sprains.[3,4,6]

Hemodynamic Adaptations

Significant hemodynamic changes occur during pregnancy, including increased cardiac output, increased resting heart rate, increased stroke volume, and decreased systemic vascular resistance.[3,4] Cardiac output may increase by as much as 50% in the third trimester.[3,9] These changes are to supply sufficient blood to the placenta and the growing fetus.[3,8] During exercise, there can be up to a 50% decrease in splanchnic blood flow and subsequently blood flow to the uterus, as blood is redirected to the exercising muscles.[13] This raises the hypothetical risk of fetal hypoxemia during exercise, which has been the subject of multiple reports. However, flow velocity profiles in the fetal aorta and umbilical circulation in various studies resulted in contradictory and inconclusive results.[4,14,15] At this time, the general consensus is that an increase in fetal heart rate between 10 and 30 beats per minute (bpm) over baseline during maternal exercise does not have a negative sequela on the fetus and that overall fetal injuries are unlikely during a normal uncomplicated pregnancy.[4]

An important consideration is the effect of supine positioning on the fetus, both at rest and during exercise. Primarily after the first trimester, compression of the inferior vena cava by the enlarged uterus reduces cardiac output.[3,4] A similar phenomenon has been seen with motionless standing for prolonged periods, which leads to decreased venous return and a subsequent increased risk of hypotension.[10–12] For this reason, it is best to assume a right or left lateral side lying position and avoid motionless standing as pregnancy progresses, especially if one is experiencing hypotensive episodes. Equally important is avoiding supine exercises such as bench press or sit-ups.

Respiratory Adaptations

Along with the cardiovascular adaptations during pregnancy, significant respiratory changes occur. As the uterus enlarges, the diaphragm displaces superiorly, which ultimately causes a profound increase in tidal volume and subsequently minute ventilation, decreasing arterial carbon dioxide.[3,4,16] All these adaptations protect the fetus from an acidic environment, which may significantly affect the function of various organ systems, such as the cardiovascular and central nervous systems, ultimately lowering APGAR (appearance, pulse, grimace, activity, and respiration) scores.

The pressure of the enlarged uterus on the diaphragm causes a decrease in oxygen availability and thereby increased work of breathing and feelings of respiratory discomfort late in pregnancy.[3,4] In response to increased oxygen requirements of the fetus, there are mild increases in tidal volume and oxygen consumption in pregnant women. To meet the greater oxygen demand during physical activity, pregnant women will have an increase in respiratory frequency and oxygen consumption with just mild exercise.[3,4,13,16] Studies have demonstrated that during pregnancy, the subjective effort to perform aerobic exercise is increased and maximum voluntary exercise performance is decreased.[3,4,13]

Thermoregulatory Adaptations

Metabolic rate increases throughout pregnancy subsequently increasing heat production.[4,13] In the first trimester, core temperatures above 39°C (103°F) should be avoided because of an increased risk of neural tube defects.[3,4,13] In the second and third trimesters, thermoregulatory control improves, during which fetal temperature is maintained approximately 1°C above maternal core temperature, due to fetoplacental metabolism.[3,4,13] Core temperature does not increase significantly with steady-state moderate exercise, which is approximately 60%–70% Vo_2max.[3,4] It is critical that heat dissipation remains greater than heat production to protect the fetus and ensure adequate uterine blood flow. For this reason, exercising in hot, humid environments or engaging in strenuous and high-intensity activities should be avoided.[3]

BENEFITS OF EXERCISE IN PREGNANCY

Exercise during pregnancy has been shown to have immense cardiac, metabolic, and mental health benefits. According to the 2019 Canadian guidelines for physical activity in pregnancy, there is a strong recommendation for all females without contraindications to be physically active throughout pregnancy.[1] Contraindications will be discussed in another section of this chapter. Contrary to certain myths that have prevailed over the years, recent research has shown that there is no association between physical activity and increased risk of miscarriage, preterm birth/rupture of membranes, low birth weight, congenital defects, neonatal death, hypoglycemia, or birth complications.[1,30] Some of the many maternal benefits of physical activity during pregnancy include reduced risk of gestational diabetes, gestational hypertension, preeclampsia, and excessive gestational weight gain.[1] There has also been shown to be a reduced risk of cesarean and assisted vaginal delivery.[1,27] Another very important benefit of exercise during pregnancy is the reduction of prenatal depressive symptoms, as well as reduction of stress and anxiety and feelings of overall improved quality of life.[1,28,29]

GENERAL RECOMMENDATIONS

Similar to the general population, females without contraindications to exercise should aim for 150 min of moderate intensity exercise per week, accumulated over a minimum average of 3 days per week.[1,17] It is best however to be active daily, if possible. Unfortunately, less than 15% of pregnant women achieve the goal of 150 min of moderate intensity activity per week.[1] Intensity can best be assessed via the "talk test." Moderate-intensity exercise raises the heart rate enough that an individual is still able to carry on a conversation but would not be able to sing a song.[1,21] Examples of moderate-intensity exercises include resistance training, brisk walking, stationary cycling, and water aerobics.[1] Heart rate ranges have also been established by the American College of Sports Medicine and the Canadian Guidelines to help better define moderate-intensity activity, based on age, fitness level, and BMI (Table 26.1).[17,34,38]

There remains a paucity of information related to the effects of more vigorous activity levels during pregnancy, which is challenging for medical professionals caring for elite athletes and high-intensity recreational athletes. A study revealed vigorous intensity exercise during the third trimester in uncomplicated pregnancies did not result in increased poor birth outcomes.[18] Studies are still limited on vigorous intensity activity in the first and second trimesters and primarily consist of media reporting on high-profile athletes.[18] It is of utmost importance for any female who wishes to exercise, especially at a high intensity, to have a conversation with a trained medical professional to individualize her exercise program during pregnancy.

EXERCISE PRESCRIPTION

With any exercise prescription and fitness counseling, the main factors that should be discussed are frequency, intensity, time, and type of exercise. The same concepts apply to pregnant women as with the general population; however, the provider must be aware of the contraindications of exercise during pregnancy. In this section, the focus will be on the different types of exercise that can be done safely in pregnancy. In general, a combination of aerobic and resistance exercises has shown greater benefit than just aerobic exercise alone and adding yoga and/or stretching may provide added benefits.[1]

FIRST STEPS AND HOW TO START EXERCISING DURING PREGNANCY

Given all the benefits of exercise during pregnancy are previously discussed, it is important to know appropriate resources and how to safely engage in an exercise program during pregnancy for females who may be naïve to routine physical activity. A resource for both clinicians and pregnant women is *PARmed-X for Pregnancy*, also known as the Physical Activity Readiness Medical Examination (available through the Canadian Society for Exercise Physiology's (CESP) website at www.csep.ca/forms.asp). PARmed-X for Pregnancy was established by CESP and has since been adopted by other institutions to help medical professionals provide individualized counseling to their patients on exercise during pregnancy.[1,34] Further research is still needed on the effects of high-intensity activity during pregnancy, but it can be said with confidence that unless there are contraindications, all pregnant women should be engaging in moderate-intensity physical activity most days of the week.[4,17,33]

Aerobic Exercises

Aerobic exercises that are advisable in pregnancy include those that focus on the larger muscle groups and those in which intensity is easily modified based on the goal heart rate or the talk test, as mentioned in the section General Recommendations. Brisk walking, jogging, swimming, cycling, rowing, dancing, and cross-country skiing are all examples of aerobic activities that one can partake in while pregnant.[4] Again,

TABLE 26.1
Heart Rate Ranges Defining Moderate-Intensity Activity, Based on Age, Fitness Level, and BMI.

HEART RATE RANGES FOR PREGNANT WOMEN		
Maternal Age (Years)	**Fitness Level or BMI**	**Heart Rate Range (beats/min)**
Less than 20	—	140–155
20–29	Low	129–144
	Active	135–150
	Fit	145–160
	BMI >25 kg/m²	102–124
30–39	Low	128–144
	Active	130–145
	Fit	140–156
	BMI > 25 kg/m²	101–120
>40	*No written guidelines due to insufficient information*	

Target heart rate ranges were derived from peak exercise tests in medically prescreened low-risk pregnant females (established by the American College of Sports Medicine and the Canadian Guidelines). *BMI*, body mass index.

this must be catered to each patient and pregnancy based on individual risk factors, previous experience, and preferences.

Strength Training

Overall, there is much less evidence with regard to strength training, especially heavy lifting, during pregnancy. Based on findings from recent studies, lower weights and higher repetitions did not have negative impacts on pregnancy outcomes.[4,19,22,23] Although evidence is lacking regarding heavier weight strength training or Olympic lifts, it is advisable to refrain from any lifts that require a Valsalva maneuver. The Valsalva maneuver increases intra-abdominal pressure and in turn hypothetically reduces blood flow and oxygen supply to the fetus, in addition to the potential of damaging pelvic floor muscles.[2,4,20] Pelvic floor muscle training, if done correctly, has been shown to treat and prevent urinary incontinence both during pregnancy and after delivery. Females should aim to perform these exercises at least three times per day on most days of the week for the greatest benefit.[2,31] It may be prudent to avoid heavy lifts or physical strain during the 6−9 days after estimated ovulation; limited evidence has shown a slightly increased risk of miscarriage during this time of implantation.[26] If done in the appropriate manner, weight lifting during pregnancy can have beneficial effects on the mother without negatively impacting the health of the baby.

Flexibility

Recent studies have shown that prenatal yoga is a promising treatment for maternal depression, providing beneficial effects on maternal comfort during labor, as well as reduced stress, reduced anxiety, and overall improved quality of life.[24,25] Increased ligamentous laxity during pregnancy causes pelvic instability and misalignment of the spine, which can result in pain and discomfort. Maintaining flexibility during pregnancy enables a female to adapt effectively, efficiently, and safely to pregnancy-associated changes in alignment, joints, tendons, and ligaments. Stretching during pregnancy should focus on maintaining a normal range of motion required for activity, stretching the muscle belly rather than at the tendon or ligament, and performing stretches in a slow and controlled manner for maximum effectiveness.[4]

CONTRAINDICATIONS TO EXERCISE DURING PREGNANCY

Although the benefits of exercise during pregnancy far outweigh the risks, this primarily applies to uncomplicated pregnancies. It is essential to be aware of both relative and absolute contraindications, as well as warning signs for when to stop exercising. For this reason, there is a need to emphasize individualized exercise programs for each patient and have a discussion regarding risks and benefits. Table 26.2 has been adopted by the 2019 Canadian guidelines for exercise in pregnancy and outlines the absolute and relative contraindications. Table 26.3 demonstrates the warning signs to terminate exercise during pregnancy, as detailed by the American College of Obstetricians and Gynecologists (ACOG).

HIGH-RISK SPORTS TO AVOID

It is advised to avoid contact sports with an increased risk of blunt abdominal trauma during pregnancy; this includes but is not limited to boxing, soccer, basketball, ice hockey, wrestling, and football.[4] Additionally, sports with an increased risk of falls such as skiing (downhill and water), horseback riding, gymnastics, and ice skating should be avoided because of changes in the center of gravity as pregnancy progresses.[1,13] Scuba diving should be avoided throughout pregnancy, as this places the fetus at an increased risk of decompression sickness and gas embolism.[1,32]

ALTITUDE TRAINING

Exercising at altitudes less than 2500 m (8200 feet) has not been shown to have any adverse effects on the fetus in an otherwise uncomplicated pregnancy.[1,4,32] Exercising at altitudes over 2500 m carries a hypothetical risk of hypoxia and decreased uteroplacental perfusion, especially in those who are not acclimatized or who have high-risk pregnancies.[2,32] Uncomplicated pregnant women who are not acclimatized should limit exercise to altitudes less than 2000 m (6500 feet).[2]

EXERCISE CONSIDERATIONS DURING THE POSTPARTUM PERIOD AND RETURN TO SPORT

Similar to exercise prescriptions during pregnancy, returning to sport during the postpartum period must be individualized and the exact time to return is influenced by several factors. It is important for patients to be aware that regardless of prior activity level, resumption of activity after pregnancy should be gradual and should progress along a continuum. Return to sport can begin as soon as it is medically and physically safe, which is variable, and often depends on the type of delivery (cesarean section, instrumental delivery, or

TABLE 26.2
Contraindications to Exercise During Pregnancy.

Absolute Contraindications	Relative Contraindications
• Ruptured membranes, premature labor	• Recurrent pregnancy loss
• Unexplained persistent vaginal bleeding	• History of spontaneous preterm birth
• Placenta previa after 28 weeks gestational age	• Gestational hypertension
• Preeclampsia	• Symptomatic anemia
• Incompetent cervix	• Malnutrition
• Intrauterine growth restriction	• Eating disorder
• High-order multiple pregnancy (i.e., triplets)	• Twin pregnancy after 28th week
• Uncontrolled type I diabetes, uncontrolled hypertension, or uncontrolled thyroid disease	• Mild/moderate cardiovascular or respiratory disease
• Other serious cardiovascular, respiratory, or systemic disorders	• Other significant medical conditions

TABLE 26.3
Warning Signs to Discontinue Exercise in Pregnancy.

- Vaginal bleeding
- Regular painful contractions
- Amniotic fluid leakage
- Dyspnea before exertion
- Dizziness
- Headaches
- Chest pain
- Muscle weakness affecting balance
- Calf pain or swelling

vaginal delivery), extent of damage to the pelvic floor muscles, or any type of incision that may have been made.[4]

Low-impact endurance training such as brisk walking or cross-country skiing can begin soon after birth, as this does not place excessive pressure on the healing pelvic floor muscles.[2] Higher impact endurance training as well as strength training should be resumed in a step-by-step manner, initially focusing on regaining pelvic floor muscle strength.[2] Following strengthening of the pelvic floor, emphasis should be on core strengthening, specifically the abdomen and back.[2] If a female exercised at a moderate- to high-intensity level during pregnancy, she can expect her Vo_2max to return to pre-pregnancy levels, or possibly even increase.[2]

BREASTFEEDING

Breastfeeding and return to exercise are also important topics. The World Health Organization recommends breastfeeding for at least the first 6 months of pregnancy due to the numerous benefits for both mother and infant.[35] For mothers who want to engage in moderate-to high-intensity activity post partum, it is best to nurse just prior to exercise.[2,4] This will allow for increased comfort from decreased engorgement, as well as decreased risk of acidity in breast milk, as lactic acid builds with prolonged exercise.[4] While some mothers may be concerned about reduced production of breast milk with increased activity, some studies show performing high-volume aerobic exercises during breastfeeding resulted in both slightly greater quality and quantity of breast milk.[36,37]

CONCLUSIONS

Pregnancy is a critical time in a woman's life and is characterized by numerous physiologic and anatomic changes. Physical activity is highly beneficial during pregnancy and is recommended for all patients with uncomplicated pregnancies. Engaging in physical activity has shown a variety of benefits for the mother and the fetus, including reduced risk of gestational hypertension, gestational diabetes, and preeclampsia, as well as a reduction in prenatal depressive symptoms, all without increasing adverse effects. Exercise programs should be tailored to each pregnancy based on patient-specific risk factors and should include a combination of aerobic and resistance training for maximum benefit. It is important as healthcare providers and medical professionals to reassure our pregnant patients that not only will exercise improve overall health but also it has been shown to improve pregnancy outcomes.

REFERENCES

1. Mottola MF, Davenport MH, Ruchat S-M, et al. 2019 Canadian guideline for physical activity throughout pregnancy. *Br J Sports Med*. 2018;52:1339–1346.
2. Bo K, Artal R, Barakat R, et al. Exercise and pregnancy in recreational and elite athletes: 2016/2017 evidence summary from the IOC expert group meeting, Lausanne. Part 5. Recommendations for health professionals and active women. *Br J Sports Med*. 2018;52:1080–1085.
3. Bo K, Artal R, Barakat R, et al. Exercise and pregnancy in recreational and elite athletes: 2016/2017 evidence summary from the IOC expert group meeting, Lausanne. Part 1 - exercise in women planning pregnancy and those who are pregnant. *Br J Sports Med*. 2018;50:571–589.
4. Artal R, O'Toole M. Guidelines of the American College of Obstetricians and Gynecologists for exercise during pregnancy and the postpartum period. *Br J Sports Med*. 2003;37:6–12.
5. Davies G, Artal R. It's time to treat exercise in pregnancy as therapy. *Br J Sports Med*. 2019;53:81.
6. Dumas GA, Reid JG. Laxity of knee cruciate ligaments during pregnancy. *J Orthop Sports Phys Ther*. 1997;26:2–6.
7. ACOG Committee opinion no. 548: weight gain during pregnancy. *Obstet Gynecol*. 2013;121:210–212.
8. Morris EA, Hale SA, Badger GJ, et al. Pregnancy induces persistent changes in vascular compliance in primiparous women. *Am J Obstet Gynecol*. 2015;212, 633. E1–6.
9. Pivarnik J. Cardiovascular responses to aerobic exercise during pregnancy and postpartum. *Semin Perinatol*. 1996;20:242–249.
10. Ibrahim S, Jarefors E, Nel DG, et al. Effect of maternal position and uterine activity on periodic maternal heart rate changes before elective cesarean section at term. *Acta Obstet Gynecol Scand*. 2015;94:1359–1366.
11. Avery ND, Stocking KD, Tranmer JE, et al. Fetal responses to maternal strength conditioning exercises in late gestation. *Can J Appl Physiol*. 1999;24:362–376.
12. Jeffreys RM, Stepanchak W, Lopez B, et al. Uterine blood flow during supine rest and exercise after 28 weeks of gestation. *Br J Obstet Gynaecol*. 2006;113:1239–1247.
13. Wang TW, Apgar BS. Exercise during pregnancy. *Am Fam Physician*. 1998;57:1846–1852.
14. Collings CMS, Curet LB, Mullin JP. Maternal and fetal responses to a maternal aerobic exercise program. *Am J Obstet Gynecol*. 1983;145:702–707.
15. Carpenter MW, Sady SP, Hoegsberg B, et al. Fetal heart rate response to maternal exertion. *J Am Med Assoc*. 1988;259:3006–3009.
16. LoMauro A, Aliverti A. Respiratory physiology of pregnancy: Physiology masterclass. *Breathe*. 2015;11:297–301.
17. American College of Sports Medicine. In: Riebe D, Ehrman JK, Liguori G, Magal M, eds. *American College of Sports Medicine's Guidelines for Exercise Testing and Prescription*. 10th ed. Philadelphia: Wolters Kluwer; 2018.
18. Beetham KS, Giles C, Noetel M, Clifton V, Jones JC, Naughton G. The effects of vigorous intensity exercise in the third trimester of pregnancy: a systematic review and meta-analysis. *BMC Pregnancy Childbirth*. 2019;19:281.
19. Hall DC, Kaufmann DA. Effects of aerobic and strength conditioning on pregnancy outcomes. *Am J Obstet Gynecol*. 1987;157:1199–1203.
20. Johnson J. Exercise in pregnancy. *Sport Med Today*; 2016. https://www.sportsmedtoday.com/exercise-in-pregnancy-va-126.htm.
21. Nascimento S, Surita F, Cecatti J. Physical exercise during pregnancy: a systematic review. *Curr Opin Obstet Gynecol*. 2012;24:387–394.
22. Barakat R, Lucia A, Ruiz JR. Resistance exercise training during pregnancy and newborn's birth size: a randomised controlled trial. *Int J Obes*. 2009;33:1048–1057.
23. Zavorsky G, Loongo L. Adding strength training, exercise intensity, and caloric expenditure to exercise guidelines in pregnancy. *Obstet Gynecol*. 2011;117:1399–1402.
24. Babbar S, Agatha C, Parks-Savage S. Yoga during pregnancy: a review. *Am J Perinatol*. 2012;29:459–464.
25. Ng QX, Venkatanarayanan N, Loke W, et al. A meta-analysis of the effectiveness of yoga-based interventions for maternal depression during pregnancy. *Compl Ther Clin Pract*. 2019;34:8–12.
26. Bo K, Artal R, Barakat R, et al. Exercise and pregnancy in recreational and elite athletes: 2016 evidence summary from the IOC expert group meeting, Lausanne. Part 2 - the effect of exercise on the fetus, labour and birth. *Br J Sports Med*. 2016;50:1297–1305.
27. Tinloy J, Chuang CH, Zhu J, et al. Exercise during pregnancy and risk of late preterm birth, cesarean delivery, and hospitalizations. *Wom Health Issues*. 2014;24:e99–104.
28. Davenport MH, McCurdy AP, Mottola MF, et al. Impact of prenatal exercise on both prenatal and postnatal anxiety and depressive symptoms: a systematic review and meta-analysis. *Br J Sports Med*. 2018;52:1376–1385.
29. Kolomanska D, Zarawski M, Mazur-Bialy A. Physical activity and depressive disorders in pregnant women—a systematic review. *Medicina*. 2019;55:212.
30. Barakat R, Pelaez M, Menotejo R, et al. Exercise during pregnancy does not cause preterm delivery: a randomized, controlled trial. *J Phys Activ Health*. 2014;11:1012–1017.
31. Boyle R, Hay-Smith EJ, Code JD, et al. Pelvic floor muscle training for prevention and treatment of urinary and faecal incontinence in antenatal and postnatal women. *Cochrane Database Syst Rev*. 2012;10:CD007471.
32. Artal R, Fortunato V, Welton A, et al. A comparison of cardiopulmonary adaptations to exercise in pregnancy at sea level and altitude. *Am J Obstet Gynecol*. 1995;172:1170–1180.
33. Bo K, Artal R, Barakat R, et al. Exercise and pregnancy in recreational and elite athletes: 2016/2017 evidence

summary from the IOC expert group meeting, Lausanne. Part 4. Recommendations for future research. *Br J Sports Med.* 2018;51:1724–1726.

34. *PARmed-X for Pregnancy: Canadian Society for Exercise Physiology.* 2013.

35. World Health Organization (WHO). *Recommendations on Exclusive Breast Feeding.* 2017.

36. Bo K, Artal R, Barakat R, et al. Exercise and pregnancy in recreational and elite athletes: 2016/17 evidence summary from the IOC expert group meeting, Lausanne. Part 3 - exercise in the postpartum period. *Br J Sports Med.* 2017;51: 1516–1525.

37. Lovelady CA, Lonnerdal B, Dewey KG. Lactation performance of exercising women. *Am J Clin Nutr.* 1990;52: 103–109.

38. Mottola MF, Davenport MH, Brun CR, et al. VO2 peak prediction and exercise prescription for pregnant women. *Med Sci Sports Exerc.* 2006;38:1389–1395.

FURTHER READING

1. Barakat R, Pelaez M, Montejo R, et al. Exercise during pregnancy improves maternal health perception: a randomized controlled trial. *Am J Obstet Gynecol.* 2011;204: 402.e1–402.e7.

2. Campolong K, Jenkins S, Clark MM, et al. The association of exercise during pregnancy with trimester-specific and postpartum quality of life and depressive symptoms in a cohort of healthy pregnant women. *Arch Womens Ment Health.* 2018;21:215–224.

3. Mottola M. Chapter 12: Performance in the pregnant woman: maternal and fetal considerations. In: Taylor N, Groeller H, eds. *Physiological Bases of Human Performance During Work and Exercise.* USA: Elsevier; 2008:225–237.

4. Jean D, Moore LG. Travel to high altitude during pregnancy: frequently asked questions and recommendations for clinicians. *High Alt Med Biol.* 2012;13:73–81.

Index

Note: Page numbers followed by "f" indicate figures and "t" indicate tables.

Printed and bound by CPI Group (UK) Ltd, Croydon, CR0 4YY

03/10/2024

01040300-0007